Communication Skills for the Health Care Professional

Context, Concepts, Practice, and Evidence

THIRD EDITION

Gwen van Servellen , PhD, RN, FAAN
Professor Emeritus
School of Nursing
University of California, Los Angeles

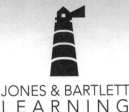

JONES & BARTLETT
LEARNING

World Headquarters
Jones & Bartlett Learning
5 Wall Street
Burlington, MA 01803
978-443-5000
info@jblearning.com
www.jblearning.com

Jones & Bartlett Learning books and products are available through most bookstores and online booksellers. To contact Jones & Bartlett Learning directly, call 800-832-0034, fax 978-443-8000, or visit our website, www.jblearning.com.

Production Credits

VP, Product Management: David D. Cella
Director of Product Management: Michael Brown
Product Manager: Sophie Fleck Teague
Product Specialist: Danielle Bessette
Production Manager: Carolyn Rogers Pershouse
Vendor Manager: Juna Abrams
Senior Marketing Manager: Susanne Walker
Manufacturing and Inventory Control Supervisor: Amy Bacus
Composition: codeMantra U.S. LLC
Project Management: codeMantra U.S. LLC

Cover Design: Scott Moden
Text Design: Kristin E. Parker
Director of Rights & Media: Joanna Gallant
Rights & Media Specialist: Merideth Tumasz
Media Development Editor: Shannon Sheehan
Cover Image (Title Page, Part Opener, Chapter Opener):
  © Excellent backgrounds/Shutterstock
Printing and Binding: McNaughton & Gunn
Cover Printing: McNaughton & Gunn

Library of Congress Cataloging-in-Publication Data
Names: Van Servellen, Gwen Marram, author.
Title: Communication skills for the health care professional : context, concepts, practice,
   and evidence / Gwen van Servellen, PhD, RN, FAAN, Professor Emeritus.
Description: Third edition. | Burlington, MA: Jones & Bartlett Learning, 2018. |
   Includes bibliographical references and index.
Identifiers: LCCN 2018013611 | ISBN 9781284141429 (paperback)
Subjects: LCSH: Allied health personnel and patient. | Interpersonal communication. |
Communication in medicine. | BISAC: HEALTH & FITNESS / Health Care Issues.
Classification: LCC R727.3 .V36 2018 | DDC 610.73/7069—dc23
   LC record available at https://lccn.loc.gov/2018013611

6048

Printed in the United States of America
22 21 20 19 18   10 9 8 7 6 5 4 3 2 1

To Health Providers and the Patients and Families They Serve

As health care professionals and providers, we have a duty and commitment to enhance and restore health care quality, and this goal is achieved in the context of an ever increasingly complex health care delivery system. The goal is achieved not just by a single health professional but multiple health providers who interact with patients and families throughout a continuum of care from health promotion and disease prevention to end-of-life care. They include physicians and surgeons, nurses, nurse practitioners, dentists, pharmacists, pharmacy technicians, dietitians, occupational therapists, respiratory therapists and physical therapists, exercise physiologists, radiation therapists, medical and clinical diagnostic technologists, and emergency medical technicians. This list does not exhaust the range and number of health providers that interact directly with patients and their families. Many interact with each other in integrative service teams. They advise and apply principles of health promotion and deliver direct patient care with the ultimate goal of meeting the needs of individuals, communities, and populations. The opportunities to make a contribution are multiple and varied.

Communication knowledge and skills make this possible. This text is dedicated to enhancing students' knowledge and skills in using effective health care communications. Students are guided by professors and seasoned health care professionals in understanding the significance of effective communications and their application in *real-time* patient–provider interactions. This revision of the text adds an important advantage: its expansion to cover important content and skills needed by graduate students in the health professions. In particular, the new Part VIII of the text includes four new chapters that focus on evidence of the impact of interventions or programs altering health care communications. Skills and knowledge of using this evidence from research and evaluation studies to evaluate changes in communication strategies are discussed in depth in these new chapters.

Finally, the content in the text promotes the message that to provide health care effectively we need to look through the special lens of patient–family–provider interactions. These interactions mirror the impact of patient health status and health literacy, provider knowledge, patient and family cultural and religious beliefs, and the systems of care that either support or diminish the therapeutic effects of communications.

As miraculous as our ability to communicate is, not all patients and families can speak to be heard, listen to know, understand to respond appropriately and in a timely manner, or even remember what we write or say. In fact, the patient might tell us the same about health care professionals. The reasons are many but it is always important to assume little and consistently assess the communication that has occurred in the interactions between patients, providers, and families. Let it be our goal to not miss one or more critical components that will result in compromised health care. And most of all let us never give up on the power of effective communications.

Contents

What's New in the Third Edition?

This important revision of the text provides an improved and updated version of the context, concepts, practice, and evidence supporting our knowledge and skill in communicating effectively with patients and their families. The text is an excellent addition to a course on interviewing and therapeutic management of health provider and patient alliances. While the text has been used effectively in college pre-licensure programs, this revision makes the content also applicable to some graduate-level courses.

This edition introduces another important topic: the *context* for health care communications in an evolving health care system. Context means the history of the evolution of health care delivery system as well as recent changes in health care delivery that impact our understanding of health care communications. We are continually reminded that communication is affected by both micro- and macrolevel factors. At the microlevel are the specific interviewing skills needed to assess and motivate patients who represent a wide range of groups and cultures. At the macrolevel are social, economic, and political events as well as technological advances that serve as facilitators or barriers to health care communications and sometimes both. The latter is the focus of the new Part I addressing the overall context of health care communications.

Two new chapters in new Part I examine the context for health care communications: advances in health information technology and problems in access to and availability of health care. These topics are introduced and their impact on patient–provider and provider–provider communications is explored. In recent decades, advancements in health information technology (HIT) have opened the possibility for more-informed patient consumers. At the same time, the problem in access and availability of health care services reminds us that health communications in real-time are both the outcome of and pathway to advancing quality health care.

The revision of the text maintains the value that health care communications are vital to quality care and patient safety. The Third Edition retains the same general structure but adds two new divisions: Part I: "The Context for Health Care Communications in an Evolving Health Care System" and Part VIII: "Evidence Supports the Importance of Effective Communication." The two new chapters in Part I are foundational and the four new chapters in Part VIII present more advanced discussions of how communication strategies and programs might enhance or restore patient safety and quality care.

All other chapters addressing essential concepts and practice remain but have been updated. They contain revised chapters that address basic principles of communication and practice skills. The content of the chapters in Part III addressing specific therapeutic communications competencies (confirmation, empathy, and compassionate caring; communications contributing to trust; the use of questions; uses of silence and pauses; the impact and limitations of self-disclosure; the place of advisement; the use of reflections and interpretations; and the judicious use of confrontation, orders, and commands) has been updated. The important concept and role of compassionate caring in responding empathetically to patients and their families has been added to the chapter on confirmation and empathy. In Parts IV through VII the original content has been retained and updated. The emphasis on effective communications between patient and provider and across provider groups and work teams is pervasive throughout all chapters. The intent is to strengthen students' ability to understand the importance of communication skills and the link between health care communications and quality care.

In summary, new chapters have been added and original chapters have been updated. For both new and updated chapters, relevant objectives, key terms, and references are provided. Definitions of key terms are provided both in the introduction of each chapter as well as in an updated glossary at the end of the text. Chapter citations and references are updated, and where possible, web-links have been provided to ease access to valuable bibliography detail. Numerous tables and figures are provided throughout the chapters and help to alert students to key important content in the text. Photographs depicting the themes discussed in each chapter have been added to bring attention to certain ideas and points. Additional inserts encourage students to apply what they are reading to specific patient cases and selected research studies. These valuable inserts are one of the following types: **RED FLAG BOXES, DIALOGUE BOXES, CITED STUDY BOXES,** and what is **EVIDENCE FOR/MORE TO KNOW BOXES** that summarize research and evaluation studies.

The placement of these illustrative inserts depends upon the focus of the chapter. For example, **RED FLAG BOXES** serving as patient care alerts are separated from the text and bring attention to the need to consider wisely the contribution of health information technology advances in health care (Part I, Chapter 2). **DIALOGUE BOXES** are particularly useful in Part III (Chapters 7–14) because they give concrete examples of dialog using the various therapeutic response modes discussed in this section of the text. **CITED STUDY BOXES** summarize a selected research study to illustrate the importance of topics discussed and are found in Part I (Chapter 2) and Part VIII (Chapters 26–29). **MUST READ BOXES** bring attention to important summaries of the literature and are found in Part III (Chapter 6) and Part VIII (Chapters 26–29). Finally, **EVIDENCE FOR/MORE TO KNOW BOXES** that summarize selected research and evaluation studies are found in Part VIII (Chapters 26–29).

The following is a detailed listing summarizing the changes and additions in this revision:

Part I, "The Context for Health Care Communications in an Evolving Health Care System" is new and has a total of three instead of four chapters. Chapter 1, entitled "Evolution of Health Care Delivery and Implications, for Health Providers Communications," describes both the evolution of health care and more recent events that shape health care delivery and communications today and in the future. The Agency for Healthcare Research and Quality report *National Healthcare Disparities Report—2008* and the Institute of Medicine's report *Crossing the Quality Chasm: A New Health System for the 21st Century* are discussed. Chapter 2, entitled "Technological Advances Have Changed the Way Health Professionals and Patients Communicate," explores how recent innovations in health care information technology (HIT) have significantly altered patient–provider and provider–provider communications. There are several national agendas identified and the Office of the National Coordinator for Health Information Technology's *Federal Health Information Strategic Plan—2011-2015* is cited. Chapter 3, entitled

"Problems in Access to and Availability of Health Care Intimately Linked to Patient–Provider Communication," addresses the issues of access to and availability of health care services and implications for provider–patient communications. **CITED STUDY BOXES** are included in the Part I chapters.

Chapters in Parts II through VII remain but have been revised and updated substantially. The concept of compassionate caring is added to the discussion of empathy and confirmation in Part III, Chapter 7, entitled "The Pervasive Role of Empathy, Confirmation, and Compassionate Caring." In selected chapters, **CITED STUDY** and **MUST READ BOXES** are included.

Finally, a new section, Part VIII entitled "Evidence Supports the Importance of Effective Communications" with four new chapters has been added. This section is particularly responsive to both advanced baccalaureate and graduate curricula programs that incorporate critical thinking skills applied to reviews of research studies. These chapters include (all prefaced with evidence of effective communications making a difference): Chapter 26, entitled "Bringing Health Provider Communication to the Patient, Not Patient to Provider;" Chapter 27, entitled "Communications to Promote Behavior Change;" Chapter 28, entitled "Collaborative Care to Promote Treatment Adherence and Effective Mental Health Care;" and Chapter 29, entitled "Communications for Advance Care Planning." **CITED STUDY, MUST READ,** and **EVIDENCE FOR/MORE TO KNOW BOXES** are included in these chapters.

▶ Key Features

In-depth discussions of the context, concepts, practice, and evidence for effective communication approaches are provided and organized into logically presented sections. These sections are Parts I and II, the importance and value of effective patient–provider communications and basic principles of communications; Part III, discussions of therapeutic communication skills, one technique at a time (e.g., empathy, confirmation, and compassion; trust; questioning; use of silence; reflection; and interpretation), and skills needed to ensure therapeutic communications under challenging patient circumstances (e.g., patients in crisis, coping with chronic illness, and with limited literacy skills); Part IV, communication patterns within and across providers and families; Part V, within and across health care providers; Part VI, ethics and health care communications; Part VII, transforming health care through system changes and behavior change; and Part VIII, the text concluding with evidence supporting the importance of effective communications using selected research and evaluation reports.

Key features of the text include learning objectives for each chapter, questions to address with respect to communication as a science, examples of dialogue from interactions between providers and patients, illustrations of the actual use of specific skills, explanations of the principles underlying the use of various skill-sets, easy-to-read and understanding summaries, notations about regulatory issues and standards of practice as appropriate, lists of resources pertinent to the subject of the chapter, and a complete glossary of key terms to assist students in understanding chapter concepts. As previously noted in this revision of the text, there are additional aids to enhance learning and understanding of the content. These include **RED FLAG, DIALOGUE, CITED STUDY, MUST READ,** and **EVIDENCE FOR/MORE TO KNOW BOXES.**

Acknowledgments

As is the case for most extensive writing efforts, many people are to be thanked for their assistance along the way. Their names are not acknowledged on the cover but their input was essential. Special thanks to faculty and students in the several universities and colleges I have taught who offered their helpful advice and enthusiasm about what needs to be covered and how. Insights from instructing undergraduate students in the health sciences at a variety of universities as well as graduate students in the Schools of Nursing and Public Health and Department of Psychology contributed to the development of the text. Clearly, it was these individuals and the keen insight of Mike Brown, Director of Product Management, Jones & Bartlett Learning, who persistently saw and understood the value of educating health professionals about the concepts and skills needed to communicate effectively in health care settings. Those who granted permission to reprint excerpts of their work are appreciated. In some cases, the classic early work of those cited is invaluable to our in-depth understanding of communication processes. The professors and instructors reviewing selected chapter content as it appeared in drafts was very important and helped clarify students' needs for information and how best to present the material. I would like to extend my appreciation to Danielle Bessette, Product Specialist for Public Health and Health Administration, for her ongoing support and assistance throughout the production process, and to those in the editing department of Jones & Bartlett Learning for their extensive efforts in preparing chapter tables and illustrations and reviewing and recommending changes, including a tweaking here and a tweaking there.

Preface

This text presents the context, concepts, practice, and evidence for the use of communication skills in both patient–family–provider and provider–provider encounters. While health care communication skills and knowledge are the subject of many health professional educational programs, these skills and knowledge might not receive the attention they deserve. If taught, they might be introduced in a course on assessment or diagnostic interviewing. True, interviewing for the purpose of making an assessment or diagnosis of patients' health care problems is critical in health care. However, this skill does not speak to the many times when talking to patients (and their families) is not a diagnostic interview but *purposeful conversation*.

Conversations are usually thought of as informal exchanges between two or more people, and the development of conversational skills is an important part of our personal and social development. It is familiar and comfortable. The ability to switch from conversation to diagnostic questions and back to conversation when talking with patients and their families can distinguish seasoned health care professionals. It is also a message to patients and their families that *we are human too*, and prepared to respect the human aspects of their experience and their cultural differences. Also, starting with conversation may ease the transition to diagnostic interviewing.

There is still another category important in what we do that can be termed *purposeful conversation*. Purposeful conversation includes the deliberate use of messages to achieve an important outcome relevant to the health and well-being of patients and their families. Purposeful conversation can be health care communication that is effective rather than non-effective or neutral; that is, therapeutic rather than nontherapeutic. Students' grasp of these important but sometimes subtle distinctions is important in their understanding of their roles and should be a focus of educational programs.

It cannot be stressed enough that it is critical that health professionals be able to communicate with a variety of patients from different age groups, cultures, ethnicities, economic strata, and with different levels of education and health literacy. Sometimes *conversation* is a critical skill in initially engaging patients and families in health care decision-making. The basics and advanced use of communications should be integral in health professional educational programs. But even if students have mastered the art of conversation and effective communications, this does not mean they will be able to use these skills and knowledge in all cases. Among other barriers, the most frequently mentioned barrier is the current unwieldy health care delivery system. Even when adequately primed to function, providers often face the reality that there is not enough time to use these skills and not enough venues to practice them. This is an important barrier, and very bothersome since providers recognize they cannot afford *not* to use these skills and knowledge.

There is ample evidence that health professionals do not communicate as well as they should. Noted scholars and professional organizations emphasize that communication skills are critical to providing patient-centered care. The Institute of Medicine (IOM) report on health professions and training (IOM, 2003) sent a strong message that health professionals lack adequate training and education to provide high-quality patient-centered care. The report reached out to educators and licensing organizations to strengthen health professional training requirements to include patient-centered communication skills. The deficit in communication skill training is important across the board but particularly in the care of persons with serious illness (Clayton et al., 2012; Curtis et al., 2013; Hoffman, Ferri, Sison, Roter, Schapira, & Baile, 2004). High-quality patient-centered care models emphasize health care communications which are based upon core communication competencies. These core competencies, including active listening, empathy, the use of open-ended questions, and reflection are the focus of a significant portion of this text, namely eight chapters, and are picked up again in other chapters throughout the book.

Good communication skills can help in numerous and important ways. They facilitate the accurate identification of patients' problems, engage patients and patients' families in shared decision-making, support patients and families in adjusting to the psychosocial stress of their illness, and produce patients who are more likely to adhere to the advice and follow the treatment regimen prescribed by their health care professional. Patient satisfaction is greater but so is that of their health professionals themselves. There is some evidence that work stress can be lower in those professionals practicing strong communication skills. Still, the majority of practitioners do not feel confident in their communication skills or perhaps had no formal training at all. If their skills were improved, it follows that the quality of care would improve and the costs of this care could be reduced.

These statements require further elaboration. Effective communications are at the core of quality patient care. Patients and families require the help and support of health professionals. Every contact with a patient or potential patient and their family requires courteous, considerate, respectful, and helpful communication. When patients and their families feel respected and get the responses they need and want, they feel good about their encounter with health care providers, and their need for positive interaction is satisfied. When they feel good about their experience, they are more willing to cooperate and are more likely to repeat their contacts with us. If their experience is negative, however, they are likely to avoid and limit further contact. Depending on what is required to complete their care, patients' avoidance may have very serious consequences. It may cause them to avoid getting needed help or it may cause them to ignore the health care instructions they have been given.

Negative communication experiences can cause anger and resentment toward providers and the health care system as a whole. If patients and their families come to a health care facility, for example, and get routed to several providers without getting the help they need and seek, they are likely to feel resentful. Depending upon future interactions, this resentment can build. One negative experience can require many additional positive interactions before the effects are completely erased.

It is possible that some negative interactions are never forgotten, and triggers in subsequent interactions can bring them to the surface causing stress in both patients and their families and health professionals. This can happen even if the current health professionals had nothing, or very little, to do with the initial interaction. The value of a positive provider–patient and provider–patient–family relationship where good communication skills are practiced cannot be underestimated. In addition to being the doorway to quality care, the provider–patient–family relationship nurtured by effective patient-centered communications is regarded to be the most essential component of the health care delivery system as a whole.

Communication skills are best taught using a variety of teaching modalities, examples, and evidence behind the importance of communication in patient–provider encounters. Just reading about communication is not sufficient. Therapeutic response modes and communication knowledge and skills cannot be learned from textbooks alone. The critical test of providers' competency is how they put these principles and skills into practice with patients. Because of this, interactive classroom and laboratory experiences in which students test out and practice therapeutic responsiveness are critical in their professional role development. Practice and feedback can significantly affect students' abilities and feelings of self-efficacy in their communications with patients and their families. Despite the importance of communication, health provider communication skills training is often conducted using singular methods, such as lectures, that have not been shown to result in behavior change.

Experiential learning such as with role playing exercises can be very helpful because they encourage students to practice communications before they use them in real-time interactions with patients and families. Role playing opportunities are also helpful because students, as well as faculty, observing the role-playing activity provide feedback about what they saw and what they think happened. Those playing the roles of provider and patient can offer insight about what they experienced and how communications can be improved. In the Instructor's Manual for this text, group experiential and role-playing exercises are included. Role playing where students demonstrate and evaluate their skills is enormously helpful in aiding learners to examine their expertise and where they need improvement. These exercises should be conducted in a supportive, nonthreatening manner to maximize students' comfort in demonstrating how they would implement effective communication principles and practices.

Role playing exercises need to be augmented with supervised practice with patients and patients' families. What is practiced in role playing exercises may not be completely transformable to clinical practice. Practice experience with actual patient situations, such as in clinical rotations initially supervised by faculty and/or clinical preceptors, is critical. Because of this, even when in-class role playing exercises are a part of the curricula, faculty observation and feedback about the student's use of effective communication principles and concepts in the clinical setting can reinforce strengths and guide areas needing improvement. It is very possible that when students receive content about effective communications and read about the topic but do not demonstrate these skills in actual patient and family encounters, they lack the necessary supervision and follow-up they need.

Student evaluations of courses aimed at teaching communication skills are usually very positive, indicating that students recognize that their knowledge of communication skills and interviewing are improved with this course work. They generally like the content and see the applicability to a variety of settings and roles. Communications are so linked to quality patient care that any undergraduate or graduate health care professional training program that denies students formalized instruction and supervision in communication skills and principles not only produce an incompletely trained provider but those who are not adequately armed to provide quality care and protect patient safety.

The purpose of this textbook is to both inform and enhance the reader's effective communication knowledge and skills, including aspects of context, concepts, practice, and evidence. Becoming proficient in communicating with a variety of patients and their families in varying health care settings and circumstances is a requirement of all health care professionals. However, effective communicative behavior with other health professionals is also mandated in this era of increased inter-professional collaboration. The literature (e.g., research reports, a review of the literature, consensus recommendations, affirmed experience, or any case studies and patient self-reports) is replete with examples of how improved provider-provider communication can or did make a difference. A special section in this revision of the book is dedicated to examining the evidence that reports how changes in the organization of care delivery can impact patient–provider and provider–provider communications and consequently improved patient care.

In summary, professors, instructors, and other teaching staff who use this text will find the material detailed and informative. The text is intended to be applicable to upper-division undergraduate students as well as first-level graduate students and practicing health professionals. Most universities with health professional schools have an undergraduate core curriculum in which communication content and experiential learning is a requirement. Therefore, the text is extremely useful to students who are entering the health professions but who have not yet encountered many patient–provider contacts. The text is designed to be useful cross-disciplinarily, and examples using these providers are used generously in the discussion. The importance of effective communication skills in all health care professions is undeniably important.

References and Resources

Clayton, J. M., Adler, J. L., O' Callaghan, A., Martin, P., Hynson, J., Bulow, P. N., ... Back, A. L. (2012). Intensive communication skills teaching for specialist training in palliative medicine: Development and evaluation of an experiental workshop. *Journal of Palliative Medicine, 15*(5), 585–591. doi:10.1089/jpm.2011.0292

Curtis, J. R., Back, A. L., Ford, D. W., Downey, L., Shannon, S. E., Doorenbos, A. Z., ... Engelberg, R. A. (2013). Effect of communication skills training for residents and nurse practitioners on quality of communication with patients with serious illness: A randomized trial. *Journal of American Medical Association, 310*(21), 2271–2281. doi:10.1001/jama.2013.282081

Hoffman, M., Ferri, J., Sison, C., Roter, D., Schapira, L., & Baile, W. (2004). Teaching communication skills: An AACE survey of oncology training programs. *Journal of Cancer Education, 19*(4), 220–224. doi:10.1207/s15430154jce1904_8

Institute of Medicine. (2003). *Health professions education: A bridge to quality.* Washington, DC: National Academies Press. Retrieved from https://www.ncbi.nlm.nih.gov/books/NBK221528/

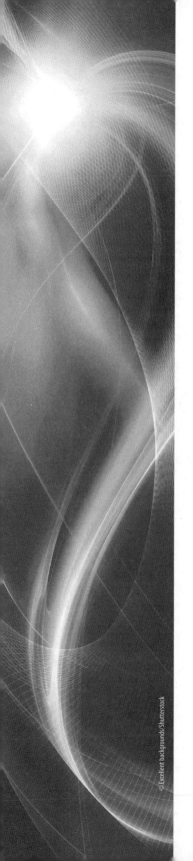

PART I

The Context for Health Care Communications in an Evolving Health Care System

Part I of this text introduces contemporary topics that have significant importance in the delivery of health care and the context for effective health professional–patient communications. Chapter 1, *Evolution of Health Care Delivery and Implications for Health Providers,* addresses the historical roots shaping the delivery of care and more recent approaches to shape health care and health care delivery system in the United States. This chapter is important because it lays the foundation for discussing, more specifically, current advances and issues impacting both quality care and patient–provider and provider–provider communications. The topics introduced cover the range of health services required, from health-promotion and disease prevention to end-of-life care. The argument is made that health care must accommodate self-care, community-based programs, and interprofessional coordination of health care service delivery.

Models of care are discussed, especially those that significantly impact health care communications. Arguments presented from patients, their families, and health professionals themselves illustrate what needs to be changed. These targets for change include not only system-level changes but also provider skills and knowledge that have a direct impact on their relationships with patients and patients' families and their ability to engage in the process of shared decision-making.

Chapter 2, *Technological Advances Have Changed the Way Health Professionals and Patients Communicate,* addresses the role of technological advances in health care in greater depth. Technological innovations in health care almost always alter, at least to some degree, the ways health professionals communicate with patients and their families and with each other. These advances also play an important role in patients' access to health care, data gathering and assessment, care delivery, and evaluation of the efficacy of treatment. One example of this phenomenon is the widespread use of health information technologies (HITs) (e.g., health and medical care websites). These websites are responsive to patients and families who are seeking answers to "What's wrong with me?" and "What should I do?" These websites are only one facet of HIT reshaping and impacting patient care. Others include patient health records, electronic health records, patient portals, telemedicine, m-Health, sensory technology, and self-service health kiosks. Each of these advanced health information technologies is discussed in depth in Chapter 2. Additionally, particular attention is given to how these innovations impact health provider communication with patients, patients' responses to health providers, and shared data across health professionals and health care institutions.

The major ideas and goals of health information technology at the national level are discussed providing background information about why there is support for these innovations and perspectives on the needs to guide their development and monitor their impact. Because HIT can have potential drawbacks, the structure and design of these technologies need to be monitored closely. The discussions in Chapter 2 address these issues and the role of HIT particularly as they impact patient safety and quality care by altering the way providers and patients communicate with one another. These advances play a role in patients' access to health care, data gathering and assessment, care delivery, and evaluation of the efficacy of treatment.

Chapter 3, *Problems in Access to and Availability of Health Care Intimately Linked to Patient–Provider Communications,* takes up issues initially raised in Chapter 1, but discusses these issues in more depth. Problems in access to health care, health, and patient well-being are raised, and the differences in related concepts—availability, affordability, accessibility, and acceptability of health care services—are clarified. Foundations for health care reform, its history and current agenda, are reviewed. Patterns of disparities in health and health care are discussed in depth, and the importance of patients' and families' abilities to navigate the complex health care system is stressed. New roles, such as the patient navigator, are presented, and the benefits and liabilities associated with assisting patients and families to navigate the health care system while at the same time adding a new layer of provider contact are raised. Finally, whether access to available care can ensure effective communications between patients and providers is explored.

In this section of the text, Part I, there are study aids that add depth and richness to each chapter discussion. They include **RED FLAG** boxes alerting the reader to examples of faulty communications that might compromise health care. For example, in Chapter 2, there is a **RED FLAG** box highlighting the problem of patients self-diagnosing a health care problem based on Web-based information without checking out assumptions with a health care professional. Another addition is the **Cited Study** box that presents a research or evaluation study highlighting a concept covered in the chapter. For example, in Chapter 3, a community-based breast health navigation program study is cited, summarized, and discussed. These additions are included not only to illustrate the topic but also to build interest in the content and in the importance of effective health care communications.

CHAPTER 1

Evolution of Health Care Delivery and Implications for Health Providers Communications

CHAPTER OBJECTIVES

- Discuss the evolution of the health care system in the United States over the last 300 years.
- Identify key elements shaping the trend in health care services delivery over time.
- Describe and discuss the current crisis in health care delivery from the perspective of quality care and cost of and access to health care.
- Discuss how the problems of affordability, accessibility, and accountability shape the need for health care reform.
- Using examples from the list of comments and voices of patients and their families provided, identify needed changes in health care communications. Discuss how these examples may reflect health care delivery system-level problems.

KEY TERMS

- Accessibility of health care
- Accountability in health care
- Affordability
- Case management
- Community-based programs
- Health care delivery system
- Health care quality
- Health maintenance organizations (HMOs)
- Health promotion
- Interprofessional collaboration
- Managed care
- Preferred provider organizations (PPOs)
- Self-care

▸ Introduction

Powerful new tools emerging from advanced technology and organizational change continue to revolutionize our current **health care delivery system**, and these changes are felt in our methods of communicating with patients. **Managed care** is the primary mode of organizing health care and continues to be in the form of integrated delivery systems. These approaches impact communications within and across the health care delivery system.

Managing Health Care While Incorporating New Technologies

Health care communications are expected to be, on the one hand, more focused and, on the other hand, less direct as episodes of care are managed on the outskirts of the provider–patient–family relationships. Ironically, care may be more comprehensive than ever before, and patients may be more informed and engaged in decision-making about their care. The compelling push for managing patients' illness, but also wellness, over time is distinctively different. Today, the trajectory of care is disease prevention and **health promotion**, illness treatment, restorative interventions, and end-of-life care. As some providers explain: "From the womb to the tomb." The need to actively engage patients and their families in health-promoting behaviors emphasizes a holistic approach. Providers' needs for communication skills to engage, persuade, and facilitate change remain critical.

Emerging in this biotechnological revolution are two primary issues: how will care be delivered and what will be required of providers in these new delivery systems? The first issue deals with health care delivery systems; the second deals with the prevailing mode of interaction between provider and client. Just what shapes health care and health care delivery systems and how these factors play a role in the evolution of health care in the United States is addressed in this chapter. A paradigm for viewing health care from a health promotion model is presented. Implications for provider–patient and provider–provider relationships and communications are discussed. The role of communications in the provision of care is examined, and needs for commitment, caring, and partnership are highlighted in selected examples of patient and family dialogue with health care providers.

In this section of the text, the history of the American health care system is briefly summarized. The current crisis in health care delivery is discussed in detail, enumerating the many important reasons for continued health care reform. It is important to understand potential threats to patient–provider communications as system barriers to adequate health care. The prerequisites for therapeutic alliances today include reassurances that problems at the system level will not impair interactions between patient and provider and providers with providers.

The voices of patients and their families depict the priorities for change and are presented here. Patients' and families' complaints, comments, and associated observations of their needs launch the text. What follows is specific communication skills, strategies, and programs known to improve communications and strengthen the provider–patient–family and provider–provider partnerships.

Health Care Delivery in the United States—1600s to 2025

The evolution of health care and changes in the health care delivery system over the last 500 years is significant. If we were to trace the evolution of health care in the United States from its inception in the early 1600s to today's system of health care delivery, our first conclusion might be it is not possible to draw comparisons because there are far too many differences to show clear trends over time. The health care system in the early colonial days (1620) was very different from the system we have today. Still, factors impacting health care in the 1600s are also those influencing health care today, as the following discussion demonstrates.

Factors Influencing Health Care Delivery Systems

Factors influencing the design of health care systems 500 years ago are in fact much the same as they are today. Those who study trends in health care delivery systems usually identify at least four elements that have stimulated change over time: (1) societal influences, (2) public health programs, (3) existing health problems, and (4) levels of technology. Factors underlying changes in hospital care systems are similar with some significant differences. Systems of care in hospitals have been influenced by (1) advances in medical science, (2) the development of specialized technology, (3) the development of professional training, (4) the growth of health insurance, and (5) the role of government.

Elements important in shaping health care delivery 500 years ago can be studied for their role in shaping health care today. If we took a trip back in time during the colonial period (roughly 1620–1781), we would identify several important factors. Society in the colonial period revolved around small agricultural communities. Trade was important, and several port towns (Boston, New York, and Charleston) were the chief points of entry for intercontinental trade. There were distinct health problems that reflected this social structure—epidemics were of concern and these port towns were havens for communicable diseases (e.g., yellow fever).

Physicians and nurses were few, but they participated in initiating quarantine standards. The clergy played a significant role in caring for the ill, and visiting patients and their families at home. Voluntary boards of concerned citizens were also involved in public health concerns, but governmental involvement was negligible. Medical technology was insufficient to control health problems. However, ordinances were passed to control problems of sanitation, waste disposal, and public markets in the port towns to curb the spread of infectious disease.

In the 500 years that have ensued, vast changes in society and in health care make the problems and issues just cited vastly outdated. Important social events such as the Civil War, and later, World War I and World War II, the Vietnam War, and the Gulf War with prolonged involvement in the Middle East have greatly influenced the evolution of our health care delivery system.

From the close of World War II through 1965, the delivery of health care shifted dramatically from curbing infectious disease to care of the infirmed and injured patient population in hospitals. Urban areas became more prominent fixtures and rural areas shifted to large farms. Housing improved and immunizations continued to improve our ability to fend off disease—this time, polio. With acute problems and infectious diseases more under control, chronic diseases raised concern.

Diseases such as arthritis, heart failure, asthma, and diabetes drew our attention. Hospitals dominated the health care delivery system; however, community programs were staffed to help patients and their families cope with chronic illness. New agencies for health care and promotion included public health department programs and visiting nurses' associations. In 1950, the U.S. government made its first significant contribution to health care, investing $3.6 billion for all health purposes and $83 million in medical research

(Reed & Hanft, 1966). This sum in 1950 would calculate to be $746,802,372 (with an annual inflation rate of 3.53%) today.

The Vietnam War, extending from 1964 through 1973, influenced not only our social–political structure but also the structure of our health care system. Prevention of chronic diseases was still important, but the realization that these diseases would not be eradicated without significant changes in the health habits of the population prevailed. Health promotion programs to control smoking, diet, and substance abuse were stressed. By 1985, there were a total of 6,872 hospitals; the majority (5,784) of them were designated short-term acute-care hospitals. The federal government administered a mere 343 hospitals, while state and local governments administered only about 1,600 of the hospitals. While acute-care hospitals dominated, long-term care and nursing home facilities also existed, but in much smaller numbers. Home health agencies continued to deliver care to chronically and terminally ill patients in the home.

Changes occurring from 1984 to date reflect tremendous shifts in health care. Public health problems continued to include environmental threats (e.g., pollution), but health problems once defined as disease and injury shifted to include societal problems. What then were considered society's problems—teen pregnancy, drug abuse, mental illness, and domestic violence—were now being classified as significant threats to the nation's health. Along with the continued focus on health maintenance and quality of life for those with chronic illnesses and disabilities, the support for healthy living became increasingly important to the effective management of health problems.

A change in the country's commitment to medical technology and research was also on the horizon. Funding for medical research increased dramatically from the expenditure of $73 million in 1950 to billions of dollars today. The National Institutes of Health (NIH)

budget for medical research rose to an annual $30.1 billion in 2017 (NIH, 2017).

Our Current Health Care Delivery System: In Crisis or Major Problems?

Arising out of mid-century 1900s was the realization that a focus on treatment of acute illnesses and injuries was insufficient. Early on, the role of the health care system was to protect us from infectious diseases and then treat acute illnesses in the confines of the inpatient hospital setting. We woke to a significant problem not fully anticipated. Our focus on acute illnesses and their treatment underestimated the growing problems of managing health and illness on an ambulatory basis (outside the walls of inpatient hospitals and centers). We faced the potential travesty of building a vast and costly acute-care delivery system while neglecting the need to strengthen health promotion at the population and community level.

Significant shifts toward a focus on health promotion and disease prevention occurred requiring the adoption of health promotion models. While we disagree about the role of social issues (violence, homelessness, drug abuse, and teen pregnancy) and individual health behaviors (diet and exercise), there is general consensus that these problems impact our ability to remain healthy. Additionally, these problems both affect and reflect the state of our nation's health and significantly impact the ability of families and communities to stay healthy.

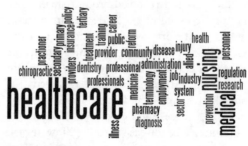

© Tang Yan Song/Shutterstock.

Health care reform was one of the major issues in the 1990 Conference of Governors, in the 1992 presidential campaign, later with the enactment of our national health care reform bill in 2011 (Affordable Care Act (ACA)), and most recently in Congressional efforts to address the problems of previous health care reform legislation. Legislators continue to study and search for solutions to needed reform, but the search for needed change occurs at different levels. One level is the need for change in health care costs and coverage; another level is the need for change in equal access to quality care.

Much has been reported in both public announcements and scholarly reports to describe the health care delivery crisis in the United States. Some describe the situation as a system facing major problems but not at the level of a crisis. Is the system facing a crisis or just major problems? Is it a question of quality of care received or the cost and coverage of this health care? The answer is that it is both. The question needs to be examined in detail because there are multiple sources of opinions and reports, and the quality of health care received and patient satisfaction with care are two different things. Also, views of **health care quality** are different from views of health care costs and coverage.

Recent Gallup polls report that Americans tend to view the quality of health care they personally receive and believe is available nationally as quite positive. However, they rate health care costs and coverage much lower. Their high opinions of the quality of care received are in contrast with their lower ratings of health care cost and coverage. Findings from this Gallup poll reinforce the idea that Americans' issues may not be so much with the actual medical treatment they receive but more about how that treatment is paid for.

There is also evidence that the public places priority in coverage to minimize health care disparities between the rich and the poor. The majority of those surveyed on Health Care Priorities for 2017 agreed that future directions should guarantee a certain level of health coverage and financial help for seniors and lower-income Americans even if it meant spending more federal dollars (Kirzinger, Wu, & Brodie, 2017). These findings support reports that even after the enactment of the ACA, more than 8 in 10 voters believed that the rich get better care than the poor.

At the same time, professionally led pushes for changes in health care responded to documented health care deficits and health care delivery system problems which created health disparities among at-risk populations in the United States. While health care reform has taken center stage in arguments about accessibility and **affordability**, concerns about the delivery of quality care have occupied our public health service system and the Institute of Medicine (IOM) over several years.

In a series of reports by the IOM (2000, 2001, 2003, 2004, 2007, and 2009), major problems in delivering care that was safe and of high quality as well as recommendations were addressed. In a recent report in the *New England Journal of Medicine* (Blendon, Benson, & Casey, 2016), the gap in care between the rich and poor was documented. Further, this problem, likely a crisis, was acknowledged in voter polls during the 2016 presidential election. Even after the enactment of ACA, more than 8 in 10 voters (82%) believed that the rich get better care than the poor (Blendon, Benson, & Casey, 2016, p. 6).

Three basic concepts relevant to the organization of health care emerged in new directions for health care reform. These were regarded as deficiencies in the current health care system and included (1) affordability, (2) accessibility, and (3) accountability. We will refer to them as the 3 As. The concepts of affordability and accessibility are discussed in greater depth in Chapter 3; but for discussion purposes these concepts, along with accountability for health care outcomes, are briefly mentioned here since they are key elements pushing the efforts to reform health care.

Affordability

Affordability of health care refers to individual, family, or community capacity to purchase needed health care in a timely manner. A primary aim of national health care reform has been to make health care affordable to everyone. Affordability of health care services from a broader context refers to the relative costs of delivering care as a portion of the nation's gross national product (GNP). To understand the problem of affordability of health care in the United States, it is important to examine more broadly how the costs of health care have escalated and are expected to soar in decades to come.

In 1940, just prior to WWII, the nation spent $4 billion on health care. By 1950, these costs had tripled. In the Centers for Medicare and Medicaid Services report for 2015 (CMS, 2017), the nation spent $3.2 trillion, or $9,990 per person, in 2015 for health care. CMS projected expenditures for 2016–2025 are expected to grow at an annual rate of 5.6% and 4.7% on a *per capita* basis.

Although the largest percentage of health spending comes from investments by the federal government (28.7% of the total expenditures), actual and projected expenditures also take into account the contributions of individual households, private businesses, and state and local governments. Reports such as these remind us that health care is expensive and health care costs keep rising. But, the problem is far more complicated. Despite a significant investment in health care, the inaccessibility of care for some is alarming. It has become clearer that even with the advent of managed care systems to streamline health care, the nation's health care expenditures are high and headed higher without the promise of reaching all those in need for these services, a problem of lack of access to care.

Accessibility

Access to health care is sometimes used to refer to how easily the patient can physically reach the health provider's location. In actuality, the notion of access is more general and not just a measure of geographic accessibility. It refers to the timely use of health care services to achieve quality care. Economists describing the problem of **accessibility of health care** estimate that millions of people go uninsured despite the fact that the United States spends more of the GDP on health care than any other country in the world. The IOM's report describing the plight of the uninsured (2009) explains that uninsured people are more likely to receive too little medical care and receive it too late, resulting in their getting sicker and dying sooner.

How can this be? Despite the fact that the American health care system is one of the most technically advanced in the world and that so much is spent on health care, a substantial proportion of the population is locked out of the system. The problem is described as one of both the uninsured and underinsured. This, however, is not the only basis for the problem of access. Surely the lack of health care services in rural areas, and even in some urban areas, contributes to the problem of accessibility, and therefore, health care disparities.

Accountability

The third and less frequently discussed issue in health care delivery is the problem of accountability. It is shocking to realize that despite the extremely large amounts of money expended for health care, we need to know more about its outcomes. Is it effective? Is it even safe? Is it efficient? (It has already been accused of being too costly!) There is now a continued effort to identify outcomes and to examine where problems exist. An example of this is the emphasis on assessing medication errors in health care (within and outside the hospital setting), their source, their costs, and how they may have been prevented.

In summary, the problems of affordability, accessibility, and **accountability in health care** have generated a platform for health care reform in which all aspects are attended

---

EXHIBIT 1-1 Rallying Points to Enhance Affordability, Accessibility, and Accountability

1. Universal
2. Continuous
3. Affordable for all individuals and families
4. Sustainable and provide consumers with choices
5. Enhance health and well-being by promoting access to high-quality care that is effective, efficient, safe, timely, patient-centered, and equitable

---

to simultaneously (**EXHIBIT 1-1**). Guidelines for resolving the problems of affordability, accessibility, and accountability have been captured in the following rallying points.

A Paradigm for Ensuring Better Health to Larger Numbers

Those who attempt to predict or influence the shape of health care reform usually recognize that any change that does occur must address all three elements—affordability, accessibility, and accountability—and address them simultaneously. Most importantly, we are now not only faced with health care problems of affordability, accessibility, and accountability, as we have known them for years, but we are also faced with major problems in our system of health care delivery. The challenge of reducing health care disparities (ensuring better health to larger numbers of people) and delivering that care equitably raises several complex issues: What is health? How is it established and maintained? How is this objective met with the largest numbers of Americans?

Health Care Reform and the Need for Health Promotion Models

Former notions of public health and individual entitlement tended to de-emphasize the dynamics of several factors that affect the health status of most persons. A social ecological orientation to health considers the interaction of numerous social, political,

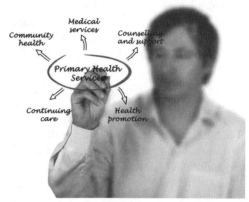

© Arka38/Shutterstock.

and environmental as well as physical and emotional conditions that affect individuals' quality of life. At the risk of being too abstract, a paradigm that ensures better health to larger numbers of people includes all of these factors and affects and is affected by public policy.

A basic assumption behind such a paradigm is that health is a multifaceted phenomenon encompassing emotional well-being, physical health, and social integration. It is a model that recognizes the interplay among individuals, families, and groups that are set within particular socioculturally defined fields. It is a model that views health and illness on a continuum and estimates years of health based on projections of life span.

A critical departure in the adaptation of a health-promotion model is the adherence to concepts that are foreign to more traditional medical model approaches (e.g., the traditional medical model stresses patho-physiology). Specific disease processes, characteristic of both illness and injury, are judged in relation to body systems and specific clinical evidence, such as lab tests and blood pressure measurement. Medical interventions (e.g., medications to lower blood cholesterol) aim to reduce death due to coronary heart disease.

Biological models are used to justify this choice of treatment, and the model argues that there is a benefit to this treatment because it reduces deaths from coronary heart disease. In contrast, a quality-of-life health-promotion model gives significantly more weight to a variety of factors, including treatment benefits, estimates of the relative value of treatment versus no treatment, and side-effects that occur in relation to the treatment chosen. Decisions about treatment become quite specific with clarification of what intervention is essential, very important, or only valuable to certain groups of individuals.

The Promotion of Self-Care and Community-Based Programs

The demand for inpatient care relative to outpatient treatment and management has decreased. Acute care that predominated decades ago is no longer the model for the American health system. Health care policy makers have come to realize that community-based systems, whether founded on a public health model or medical group practice (or some combination of the two), are the foundation for an effective new system of care. This model stresses health promotion and active participation on the part of patients, families, and communities who are no longer passive recipients of health care. As definitions of health care have expanded to include health promotion, there has been an increase in **community-based programs**. These programs are located in a wide variety of community organizations including schools and community and neighborhood centers promoting general health and well-being.

An outcome associated with newer health-promotion models is the achievement of high levels of **self-care** potential. Self-care refers to the actions performed by patients themselves (or their significant others) directed at alleviating the effects of illness and its treatment. These actions emphasize the important role of patients or consumers in protecting and promoting their health and well-being. Because patients' and their families' views of their health and well-being are critical, understanding "where the patient is coming from" is paramount in encounters with them. The many sociocultural interpretations that patients and families make in understanding health needs and problems, as well as their personal goals relative to these health problems, provide valuable information needed to form effective therapeutic alliances.

One of the variables repeatedly cited in providing quality care through health promotion is the character of the patient–family–provider relationship, particularly communications. Features of these relationships found to be associated with positive patient behaviors included (1) the friendly and accepting attitude of the provider, (2) patients' perceptions that the health professional has spent time with them, (3) their feelings that they had control in the interaction and input in decisions about their treatment or therapy, (4) their satisfaction with the care they received, (5) a treatment program that was actually tailored to them as individuals, (6) situations in which they felt that information was willingly shared with them, (7) absence of formal disagreements, and (8) provider–patient relationship continuity. Although the largest proportion of these data focused specifically on patient–physician encounters, the conclusions have validity for encounters between other health providers and patients.

In summary, it is clear from current trends that not only will the patient and family be instrumental in deciding the impact of health care reform, but also whole communities will shape the manner in which health care will be rendered. Proportionately, less care will occur in acute-care hospitals, while more care will occur in brief urgent-care centers or community centers. An increasingly significant proportion of the care of the very ill will occur outside the hospital. Providers are currently and will continue to be asked to assist in this transition as well as deliver care in settings distant from their health care work setting.

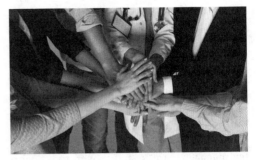

© Sheff/Shutterstock.

Managed Care and Interprofessional Collaboration

A health-promotion model of care has direct implications for the collaborative relationships and communications between health providers, and within integrative service teams. Endorsing a focus on health and recognizing the value of patients' quality of life leaves us open to health in a broader context, not just the absence of disease. This perspective encourages recognition of the importance of multiple health and human service providers, including professionals, paraprofessionals, and community service workers.

The overall goal—maintaining the patient's optimal level of health and increasing the patient's years of freedom from disease and disability—frees us to think out of the box, not only of formal approaches to cure and care administered by physicians, nurses, dentists, pharmacists, and many other providers, but also of contributions of a multitude of alternative health care approaches.

This health-promotion perspective emphasizes both the advantages and the appropriateness of multilevel interventions. Many of these interventions are complementary. Reducing stress, for example, can occur through medical management and medication; it can also be reduced through relaxation and massage programs organized and led by paraprofessionals. Other approaches are synergistic, building on one another to produce desired results.

What concept of interprofessional teamwork is appropriate? If we are to operate within integrative service teams, what does this mean for leadership within the team? Under the old disease-oriented approach, providers were relegated to positions of importance with respect to their role in ridding individuals of disease. Physicians, under this model, were at the top of the hierarchy for several reasons. They had the authority to cure disease. Under this model, because disease is paramount in directing health care providers, physicians automatically assumed the primary leadership role.

Managed care is the prevailing system of health care delivery today and is likely to be in the future with some movement toward integrated delivery systems. It is a system through which health care services are coordinated and delivered, putting resources to best use in optimizing patient care. This system integrates the payment and delivery of health care and services to consumers in an effort to deliver the highest quality services at the lowest possible cost. It is regarded as a potential solution to containing health care costs, while at the same time, ensuring equitable care to all Americans. According to many providers, managed care of the ill requires, at the very minimum, multidisciplinary teams consisting of physicians, nurses, home-care providers, and ambulatory-care practitioners. Under managed care, the aim is to provide a range of services in such a way that these services and their costs will be scrutinized and controlled. Three basic managed care programs exist at present:

health maintenance organizations (HMOs), **preferred provider organizations (PPOs),** and fee-for-service plans.

HMOs and PPOs have been criticized for their drawbacks. Despite the fact that they were designed to provide preventive health care services and to improve the continuity of quality of care, the results reveal problems. Healthier individuals are favored by managed care systems over those who are at high-risk, those who require high-cost procedures, and those who are chronically ill and need long-term care. Managed care has also been criticized for overlooking quality of care in order to meet the basic aim of cost containment.

Managed Care Versus Case Management

Managed care is a system of managing and financing health care delivery to ensure that services are needed, are efficiently provided, and are appropriately priced. Through a variety of means, including preadmission certification, concurrent review of necessity of services, and financial incentives, managed care attempts to contain costs, ensure optimal patient outcomes, and maximize the efficient use of service utilization.

As previously indicated, managed care is one system of delivery that is proposed to correct the problems of inefficient and costly health care delivery. Managed care has rapidly changed traditional approaches to health care. Current and future developments in managed care suggest that it has fulfilled its promise in supporting quality care but also cost-containment concerns remain.

Frequently associated with the concept of managed care is the term **case management**. Although managed care and case management are sometimes used interchangeably, they refer to distinctly different phenomena. Managed care is the way care is structured for reimbursement. Case management, however, is a technique used to monitor and coordinate treatment, usually for specific diagnoses. Traditionally a utilization review process, case management means that care is closely monitored and coordinated, particularly with regard to high-cost service-intense diagnoses. Case management includes activities of assessment, treatment planning, referral, and follow-up to ensure that comprehensive and continuous services are provided. Case management oversees reimbursement for care in that it ensures that the coordinated payment and reimbursement of services is properly executed.

The emergence of managed care is congruent with case management because both aim to ensure quality and control costs. Managed care systems have been widely endorsed as necessary options in health care reform. The goals of these organizations—to ensure maximum value from available resources—are congruent with the basic philosophy of health care professionals. This philosophy holds in high esteem a focus on the total needs of an individual, not just on the disease process and on maintaining health to minimize the need of future expensive health care intervention.

Underlying Problems and Issues with Managed Care and Case Management

Health care reform is not new and different; reform can be traced back in time to the health initiatives of President John F. Kennedy's New Frontier and President Lyndon B. Johnson's Great Society. Because health care reform spans several decades, we can safely conclude that reform in the United States is a continuous process.

Managed care, though, has come under criticism. Primarily, this criticism is leveled at the premise that accessibility, affordability, and accountability can be present simultaneously. Some providers claim that addressing any one of those three elements will inevitably compromise another; for example, promising accessibility may change the affordability of care. Otherwise, choices need to be made, and these choices may preclude the possibility of simultaneous significant improvement in all areas.

In part, concerns about case management surfaced because of the rapid proliferation of case management systems. The current managed care industry is criticized because it is felt that case managers were needed before adequate planning for their preparation could occur. Essentially, the professionals managing care may not have the expertise to execute their roles. No real data, however, are available to adequately judge the quality of care under case management. While data about patients' responses to case management are limited, patients and their families are said to value the system because it eases the burden in managing their own care.

Shifts in Care Delivery

In keeping with the need for health care reform and the methods used to secure affordability, accessibility, and accountability, certain predictable trends are shaping health care. These trends have implications for provider encounters with patients and their families.

To Community Ambulatory Care

Diminishing hospital use and vast expansion of ambulatory care has occurred. Health promotion and disease prevention—high-priority aims in health care reform—are achieved largely in community ambulatory care settings.

To Disease Management

These predicted shifts in the focus of care clearly indicate that the majority of services will continue to occur in the community ambulatory care settings. This does not, however, mean that disease is no longer a concern. A newer term, *disease management*, describes a community approach to treating chronic conditions. Diseases such as cancer, cardiovascular disease, diabetes, stroke, chronic obstructive pulmonary diseases, mental illness, HIV, and other chronic, potentially debilitating conditions are examples. The care processes of disease management also include prevention and health promotion. Early identification of disease; assessment of problems secondary to disease; and development, implementation, and evaluation of a plan of care are encompassed in this approach to disease management.

Disease management consists of taking a primary health problem such as cancer, cardiovascular disease, or diabetes (conditions known to be chronic) and applying regular interventions to achieve high-quality care outcomes consistently. Early identification is critical to patients who can benefit from early detection. The unique needs of the patient and family are understood to be the essential part of assessing the problem as well as in developing appropriate plans of care. Care is individualized and patient–family-centered reflecting data obtained in interactions with patients and also their families.

In plan development, the protocol for care is based on evidence-based practice and promotes health rather than simply treating disease. This care recognizes that patients require attention to other health needs and illnesses that can coexist with their primary illness. For example, depression can co-occur with cardiovascular diseases and diabetes and can make the plan of care more complicated than a simple strategy to manage the primary illness. The plan is put into action using health-promotion strategies, and the plan of care is evaluated regularly, but also is not confined to measures of treatment. Rather, evaluation also includes measures of patients' reported quality of life and sustained health and well-being over time.

To Extensive Interprofessional Collaboration and Consultation

Interprofessional collaborations and consultations are requirements under managed care and case management. To develop and implement successful managed care approaches, support from key participants—administrators, physicians, nurses, and many other professional and paraprofessional health care providers—is required. The ability to work with other individuals and within a team on a continuous basis is essential to the success of case management. Case management within and outside hospitals requires consultation with employees who have no responsibilities for direct patient care (e.g., finance personnel and administrators, as well as a wide range of providers [e.g., dietitians, physicians, social workers, physical therapists, and nurses]) to obtain relevant information about potential problems.

The idea is to communicate and collaborate with many in order to design and execute health care strategies. This is central to successful managed care. Case managers are health professionals or other key health providers who take a leadership role in managing care. These professionals communicate with provider groups to identify problems, plan strategies, execute these strategies, and evaluate outcomes of the efforts of the integrated service team. Within case management, therapeutic relationships with patients and families are very important. Case managers rely on these relationships to achieve mutually acceptable outcomes. Consultation with patients and families and the development of collaborative relationships with patients and families are as important as those are between health providers within the integrated health care team.

Skills and Knowledge of Providers in a Managed Care Environment

Generic to All Providers

The skills and knowledge that are necessary for providers who work in managed care environments are defined, in part, by the expected outcomes of managed care and case management approaches.

Managed care includes a commitment to reduce cost, make services accessible, and control and monitor quality. Managed care is expected to (1) positively reduce or limit the cost of service, (2) improve provider consultation and communication, (3) engage other key providers in participating in care planning, and (4) improve continuous quality improvement through the design of critical-care pathways (**EXHIBIT 1-2**). Additionally, patients should be positively

---

EXHIBIT 1-2 Service Components of Case Management Models

Although there are a variety of case management models, common to all are the following service components:

- Client identification and outreach
- Individual client assessment and diagnosis
- Service planning and resource identification
- Linking clients to needed services
- Actual service implementation and coordination
- Monitoring service delivery activities
- Patient advocacy to reduce problems of access to care
- Evaluation of services and measurement of expected outcomes

affected in that their care is coordinated for them and that there is a reduction in unpredictable outcomes. Thus, patients and families should be more knowledgeable and better prepared to understand and participate collaboratively in the planning and evaluation of their care.

To accomplish these goals, providers need to function as both multidisciplinary and multiservice integrators. Integrators operate at the hub of the wheel as they bring together and coordinate broad-based services.

Functions Specific to the Role of Case Manager

Case managers perform the primary functions of case management. Case managers in managed care organizations steer, guide, and track patients through a variety of care activities, thus enhancing continuity of care. A major instrument in this tracking process is critical-pathway analysis directing the patient's plan of care. Critical pathways and critical-path tools are based on the critical path method (CPM).

Patient care plans identify a "critical pathway" of key events (activities and interventions) that must occur if the desired patient outcomes are to be achieved within a specified time period. The case manager oversees these pathways and facilitates interventions to ensure that patients progress appropriately and satisfactorily. The coordination and collaborative consultation that occurs requires skillful assessment, negotiation, and collaboration with the client or patient and health care professionals involved in care. Patient and family assessment, planning, facilitation and advocacy, patient and family education, resource and risk management, benefits interpretation, and provider liaison are all aspects of this role.

The Role of Communication in the Delivery of Health Care

Explaining the importance of communication skills and knowledge to providers is somewhat like discussing the need for eyes in order to see. Most providers would not argue about the relevance or importance of these skills and knowledge. The issue is rather what communication skills and knowledge are needed and how they are acquired. Additionally, in this era of evidence-based practice, providers can no longer be satisfied with knowing how to do it. They must understand why and what evidence there is to support these selected approaches.

In this text, dimensions of the phenomena of human communication and, more specifically, health care communication are explored in depth. Essentially, every provider needs a foundation in the basic "anatomy and physiology" of communication. Providers need to know the variables that affect reception, processing, and expression of messages. They need to understand the relationship of communication to quality care outcomes. They also need to understand the multicultural context in which communication occurs.

Providers deliver health care services, all of which—disease prevention, health promotion, health screening, and health education—require foundations in therapeutic communications. Therapeutic response modes are needed not just to successfully assess individuals and families but also to manage care and to increase patient awareness and capacity for health management and self-care. Specialized knowledge and skill are needed to relate effectively in these capacities when crisis or prolonged chronic illness are the target of health care management.

Further, to participate fully in interprofessional managed health care teams that are collaborating with other providers and patients and their families, knowledge of the dynamics of group and family communication patterns is required. Communicating effectively with all relevant constituencies—patients, providers, and regulatory agencies—calls for effective negotiation skills. The ethical precepts of communicating in managed care, particularly with regard to patients' rights to informed choice and informed consent, must serve to critically guide practice in these emerging models that now dominate health care delivery in the United States. Finally, advanced issues (e.g., communication and models of behavior change, communication and the use of health information technology, and communications as a function of systems of care) further extend the coverage of the topic of how the provider will use and alter factors that enhance communications.

▶ Summary

In summary, significant changes have occurred in the U.S. health care delivery system over the past 300 years. These changes are the product of many factors, including the advancement of medical technology, the evolving social structure, and threats to health and equitable health care delivery that have plagued us over time. With a seemingly unwavering belief in our system of health care, the American dream was beginning to be realized as one of absence of disease and remarkable chances of recovery from extraordinary debilitating conditions.

The fulfillment of this dream was abruptly met with awareness of significant health disparities—not all Americans were beneficiaries or benefited equally. Fulfilling the promise of affordable, accessible care that was monitored and held accountable for positive outcomes became the core premise behind restructuring the health care delivery system.

Affordability, accessibility, and accountability are major recurrent system barriers to the delivery of effective health care services. They are not isolated problems; they affect providers' encounters with patients and their families and provider-to-provider communications. Patients' reactions to providers reflect their fears and concerns that basic health care is costly, may not always prove adequate, and is frequently administered by an unresponsive system. These fears and concerns are translated into communication difficulties where patients mistrust providers' intentions and the system as a whole.

While public opinion polls report faith in the health care available to them personally and on a national level, other data substantiate significant problems with equitable distribution of high-quality patient care. Patients' and families' attitudes of mistrust and fear of neglect, if they do exist, are not without basis in reality. While they may be deemed to be without much substance or even unimportant in the broader context of care delivery and curing disease, they are important.

Today there is substantial evidence that effective patient–provider relationships and communications are associated with a number of important health care outcomes. These include greater patient satisfaction, improved comprehension and retention of health information, improved adherence to treatment regimens, and even reductions in rehospitalization rates. In summary, effective communications have been shown to result in better care and better outcomes of this care. Thus, it becomes even more imperative that providers be guided by sound principles of interpersonal communication.

Reforming health care and health care delivery systems will continue to be a topic of interest and debate. But, key principles are likely to remain in place. These include goals for health promotion where patients and families practice certain self-care behaviors never before expected of them. Further, additional reform will occur outside the hospital, in neighborhoods, and in community settings. It will require new concepts of collaboration within and across integrative health care teams of physicians, nurses, therapists, and a broad range of professional and paraprofessional health care providers. Finally, it will require a growing sensitivity and awareness of patient-family-provider encounters that work and do not work. Certainly, the trust, confidence, and security that providers evoke in their encounters—an element of professional practice always held in high esteem—will play a critical role in the reform that takes place at the system level.

The capacity for providers to compensate for system deficits through enhanced communication skills is clear. To this end, the parameters of good interpersonal communications are the "handbook" for all health professionals. Provider–patient–family and provider–provider communications are both a determinant and a by-product of successful health care delivery. Patients and their families do value providers and often comment on what they appreciate; these include acts of provider compassion, caring, and kindness (**EXHIBIT 1-3**).

Just as patients and their families comment on the qualities they appreciate and look for, they also comment about what upsets and worries them. In **EXHIBIT 1-4**, there are several statements that describe patient- and family-perceived difficulties in making themselves understood and constitute potentially important communication deficits. With each statement, a possible unexpressed concern or request gives possible clues about what might be the root cause of the problems they mention. Take the opportunity to discuss the root cause of these problems and examine the

EXHIBIT 1-3 Positive Statements of Patients and Families About Health Care Services Received

The following are some specific examples of positive statements from patients and their family members:

"We were very pleased with the professional demeanor of the doctor and staff. Lots of compassion too! The information we received was very helpful."

"No matter what your circumstances, they treat you with respect and dignity."

"They treated us like family and have been instrumental in providing him (my spouse) with the most advanced and comprehensive medical treatment available. This is not drive-thru medicine as is found in other medical institutions which we have visited."

"I have never felt better when she (my mother) comes here because I always feel that they not only want my mother to get better, but that they actually care about not only her, but everyone else like if they were family."

"He was kind, positive, friendly, and exuded expertise and professionalism."

EXHIBIT 1-4 Patients' Descriptions of Difficulties in Communicating With Providers and the Underlying Meanings

"Having to tell my story over again and again." Please save me the energy and humiliation.

"Not having doctors get together on their opinions—each one telling me something different." If my doctors are not together on what they think, how can I trust what they say or do at all?

"The RNs, doctors, and physical therapists communicate poorly (to one another)… and they do not follow-up on the information they give." Do they think I don't notice this and worry, or worse yet, do they even care?

[What is difficult is] "wanting to speak to someone who really cares (and not having anyone)." I'm lonely and isolated, somebody recognize that I need someone to show they really care about me.

"I get frustrated, irritated when nurses are not able to respond because they are overwhelmed." What is their work if it isn't to care for me?

"When nurses say, 'I'll be back in 5 minutes' and don't come back at all or it takes a long time." How can I trust what they say to me? What else should I not trust?

(continues)

EXHIBIT 1-4 Patients' Descriptions of Difficulties in Communicating With Providers and the Underlying Meanings
(continued)

"Having them lie to me (e.g., about not having blankets)." Why would they do that? What can I really believe?

"The staff didn't involve my family (in discharge planning)." My family needs support and counseling—I'm afraid they won't get it.

"I rarely ask for a nurse unless I really need one—nurses don't come when you call them—I ask the nurse for minor things and don't get them." Will I always know when I need a nurse? What happens when I really need one but I'm not able to ask for one?

"I don't know what is expected of me—I don't want to be a bother." If I ask them what is expected, will I bother them too much?

"Night nurses don't answer call lights." Sometimes I wonder if there really is someone out there behind that door.

"I'm beginning to feel like an inmate—not a patient…staff are more concerned about hospital procedures than patient needs." I feel locked up and punished by the way they treat me.

"People are non-entities—I feel like a prisoner, alone in my room." Non-entities are not entitled to anything.

"People come into your room without permission. They come in and don't identify themselves. I feel like a guinea pig." How can I tell if they should be here or not? What are they going to do to me?

"Some staff are more professional than others. Some bring their problems to work. Their attitudes are reflected in their work…causes you to wonder if they really care about you. You feel dependent and worry if they really care. You feel helpless." If they can be both professional and unprofessional, how can I make sure I get the professional one?

"When I ask one member of the medical team a question, he always answers, 'You'll have to ask Dr. D.'—don't get information when I want it." Does he know the answer; is he withholding it when he really knows? It would be nice to have the information; I'm not sure when I'm going to see the doctor.

"(Staff) is not present to support my wife with the stress she is experiencing due to my illness." I don't think they realize how she must feel.

"Medical students who don't know what they are doing—come in at 2:00 AM to take my blood, drop equipment, say 'my resident/teacher will probably tell me to go back and try it again.'" Are medical students given the right education to do things right?

"(I worry about) morale and high turnover. I don't want to worry about my care, but some staff work two or three shifts in a row." How can they be up to speed when they work too much? Am I going to suffer because of this?

"Lack of communication between doctors, hospital, and volunteers. More competition than cooperation." Too many staff are involved in my care. I worry that they might not be communicating… that orders from one doctor might conflict with orders from another.

"It is very bothersome when I have to fill a doctor in on the aspects of my care." What would happen if I leave out something important or wasn't able to monitor my own care?

"Not always understanding answers to my questions, I ask a question and get a *nonanswer* for an answer. I am supposed to be satisfied with that!" Do they think they are really helping by treating me this way?

"When you push the call light and the nurse doesn't come—a volunteer comes instead. This happened with my roommate: My roommate yelled all night for the nurse."
What does it take to get a nurse?

"I've tried to get a vegetarian diet. I'm still getting a regular diet despite 5 days of asking for a change, talking to the dietitian, etc." I can't get through to the dietitian no matter what.

"They don't think about how it must feel to be a patient." They are insensitive to my needs.

"I'm afraid my doctor is not telling me the truth (cancer diagnosis)." I can't trust what he says.

"The nurse got mad when I told her I couldn't take my pill with water." Why is she mad at me? Doesn't this ever happen with other patients?

"There is really only one staff who takes the time to talk to me." I must make sure I get *that* nurse again.

"Not having answers about why I'm sick." Do they know and are just not telling me?

"Too many different staff; hard to form a relationship with one—causes you to hesitate to open up and confide (in them)." There is no one person that really knows me and knows how to take care of me.

"Doctors not knowing what's wrong with me—not taking my symptoms (diarrhea) seriously." My communications don't count. I don't count.

"I go for my annual checkup and my doctor keeps talking about his special projects...finally I had to say to him: 'what about *me* doc?" Maybe I don't have any major problems, but still I want my doctor to ask me about my health and any concerns I have even though he might not think I have a problem.

"I had some legitimate questions but the nurse practitioner got defensive...was demeaning, she raised her voice and called me: 'Dear,''Sweetheart,''Honey'...that just made me more frustrated, and I thought it was very inappropriate. She didn't speak English very well. I just wanted concrete answers and she contradicted herself." When I ask questions, I think I deserve an answer; how could they assign me someone who couldn't even understand me or answer my questions? The nurse needs help, but I am not here to help her; I am here to get help.

"I told my doctor that I had a problem with my sinuses. She said she didn't think it was a sinus infection. I saw my dentist and he ordered an antibiotic for a tooth infection. Believe it or not, this antibiotic took care of my sinus infection. I think my doctor didn't do enough to diagnose my problem; thanks to my dentist for seeing the problem and taking care of it. Now when I see my doctor and I have a problem, if she says she doesn't see a problem I ask how she knows." Health professionals need to thoroughly evaluate and assess a health problem; did she not believe me?

extent to which problems in accessibility and accountability cause or contribute to these common complaints.

These examples of patient (and family) complaints or comments about their care providers give important clues about potential deficits in communications during provider–patient–family face-to-face encounters, or in some cases, lack of encounters. This list of patient statements reveals specific kinds of communication problems that may threaten quality patient care, trust, and a willingness to see the same provider again. The list also raises the question of how current health care delivery problems affect or exacerbate patient- (and family-) perceived problems with the health care and treatment they receive.

One category emerging from this list of complaints and comments was the feeling of not being cared about. This was revealed in comments about providers not listening, being too preoccupied with personal issues, or institutional policies that may limit the time to engage in meaningful patient-centered dialogue. Lack of caring was also mentioned in patients' descriptions of their family members not getting the support they needed. Another category emerging from this list is providers' communicating disrespect either by expressing anger, speaking in a demeaning manner, or entering the patient's room unannounced (not identifying who they were or waking them up from a sound sleep to perform tests). Disjointed communications and communication contradictions that are not corrected is still another category.

Disjointed communications were expressed in patients' descriptions of provider–provider communications that lacked adequate follow-up of their requests. Poor follow-up, lack of care continuity, and poor coordination was implicated in complaints (e.g. never seeing the same staff, providers not doing what they said they would do, and observations of poor health-provider team-coordinated care).

These comments are, unfortunately, not uncommon. Health professionals are aware of these kinds of patient and family complaints and observations. Knowing that these types of concerns do frequently occur, health providers have an opportunity to avoid them and their potential consequences. So, why do these complaints and comments arise repeatedly? There are several factors that might be responsible. First, health providers may lack adequate training in patient-centered care and effective health care communications. Second, providers may have been initially prepared but also have found it difficult to use these skills in each encounter, especially when feeling tired and overwhelmed.

Patients and families also have something to do with these encounters. There are patients that act inappropriately or too harshly criticize. Finally, there are system factors that contribute to these problem encounters. Poor alignment of staff-to-patient needs and characteristics, lack of qualified staff, provider pressure to take on too many tasks simultaneously, and ineffective supervision and leadership are factors that can lead to poor communication encounters or exacerbate already existing tense encounters.

The value of this text is the breadth and depth of discussion about not only what effective communication is and what communication skills work, but also what leads to failed communications. Most importantly, the text discusses the potential consequences of poor communications on the quality of care as well as the consequences of therapeutic communications on improving quality care and patent and family satisfaction with care. In the following chapters, the context, concepts, practice, and evidence for understanding the importance of effective and ineffective communications continues.

Discussion

1. Compare and contrast the differences between today's health care delivery system and that of over 300 years ago in the United States.
2. Identify two or more threats to quality care today.
3. Identify two or more threats to access to care for minority communities in the United States.
4. Analyze the importance of health care affordability, accessibility, and accountability in shaping the legislation for health care reform.
5. Using examples from the list of comments and voices of patients and their families provided, identify needed changes in health care communications.

References

Blendon, R. J., Benson, J. M., & Casey, L. S. (2016, October 27). Health care in the 2016 election—A view through voters' polarized lenses. *The New England Journal of Medicine, 375*(e37). doi:10.1056/NEJMsr1606159

Centers for Medicare and Medicaid Services. (2017). *National health expenditure data, NHE Fact Sheet.* Retrieved from CMS.gov

Institute of Medicine Reports. (2000). *To err is human: Building a safer health system.* Washington, DC: The National Academies Press. doi:https://doi.org/10.17226/9728

Institute of Medicine Reports. (2001). *Crossing the quality chasm: A new health system for the 21st century.* Washington, DC: The National Academies Press. doi:https://doi.org/10.17226/10027

Institute of Medicine Reports. (2003). *Priority areas for national action: Transforming health care quality.* Washington, DC: The National Academies Press. doi:https://doi.org/10.17226/10593

Institute of Medicine Reports. (2004). *Patient safety: Achieving a new standard for care.* Washington, DC: The National Academies Press. doi:https://doi.org/10.17226/10863

Institute of Medicine Reports. (2007). *Preventing medication errors.* Washington, DC: The National Academies Press. doi:https://doi.org/10.17226/11623

Institute of Medicine Reports. (2009). *America's uninsured crisis: Consequences for health and health care.* Washington, DC: The National Academies Press. doi:https://doi.org/10.17226/12511

Kirzinger, A., Wu, B., & Brodie, M. (2017, January 6). *Kaiser health tracking poll: Health care priorities for 2017.* Retrieved from KFF.org

National Institutes of Health. (2017). *National Institutes of Health: Turning discovery into health.* U.S. Department of Health & Human Services. Retrieved from nih.gov

Reed, L. S., & Handft, R. S. (1966). *National health expenditures, 1950–64.* Social Security Administration.

CHAPTER 2

Technological Advances Have Changed the Way Health Professionals and Patients Communicate

CHAPTER OBJECTIVES

- Identify key technological advances changing the way patients and providers communicate with one another.
- Discuss the Institute of Medicine's concerns for health information technology (HIT) and quality care.
- Discuss the relationship of HIT advances and the goal to achieve patient safety and quality patient care.
- Discuss how the use of HIT (e.g., electronic health records [EHRs], telemedicine, and self-service kiosks) could impact patient–provider communications in both positive and negative ways.
- Identify what is known about the implementation of HIT advances to enhance and protect communications between (1) patients and health care professionals and (2) between health professionals and health care facilities.

▶ Introduction

The number and kind of technological advances has grown in just about all industries, including health care. These advances enhance the knowledge of providers, patients, and families. Information technological innovations in health care almost always alter, at least to some degree, the ways health professionals communicate with patients and their families and with each other. They also play an important role in patients' access to health care, data gathering and assessment, care delivery, and evaluation of the efficacy of treatment. They include an electronic means of storing health information (HIT) and multiple opportunities to access health information on the Internet.

In July 2013, the Office of the National Coordinator for **Health Information Technology** outlined a detailed position on how health information technology (HIT) can impact patient safety (Health Information Technology Patient Safety Action and Surveillance Plan, July 2, 2013). This report drew attention to the Institute of Medicine (IOM) report *To Err is Human*, in that the failure of the health care system was criticized for the large number of avoidable medical errors harming patients. The major idea behind the support of HIT was that when HIT is integrated into the health care delivery system, improvements can occur both in the quality of care and patient safety. The report cited the following examples of potential positive outcomes:

1. Medication errors can be reduced, and clinical decisions about patient care are more likely to be evidence based.
2. Patient records can be centrally stored and would be accessible to a number of health care locations, available when and where needed as the patient moves between and within different health care organizations.
3. HIT can more efficiently report and track patient data within and across health organizations, improving management of hospital-acquired illnesses, population health, and the identification of widespread health threats.

Because HIT can also have potential drawbacks, the structure and design of these advances need to be monitored closely not only on the short-term but also on a continued basis. Potential drawbacks include loss of data about adverse events sometimes resulting from the design and execution of HIT systems.

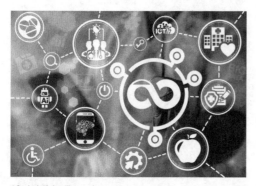

© Panchenko Vladimir/Shutterstock.

Consequently, the Office of the National Coordinator for Health Information Technology sets an objective to collect data and analyze HIT safety events to discover weak links and possible hazards in the implementation of HIT.

The role of communication in patient and health provider relationships is multifaceted; these communications (1) enhance or deter the formation of a working relationship and trust among patients, families, and providers; (2) influence what clinical data is obtained and consequently what data is available to assess and manage health conditions and corresponding care; (3) impact how and to what degree medical regimens are understood; (4) effect the degree to which providers are able to engage patients and families in their care; and (5) provide data germane to care beyond the initial patient–provider alliance.

The following discussion addresses key HIT approaches that have particular consequences for patient safety and quality care by altering the way providers and patients communicate with one another. There are a wide number and variety of HIT devices available to patients and their families.

These advances play a role in patients' access to health care, data gathering and assessment, care delivery, and evaluation of the efficacy of treatment. This discussion also identifies potential drawbacks of these advances. Each of these advances has implications for (1) how and when patients, families, and providers communicate (e.g., immediately

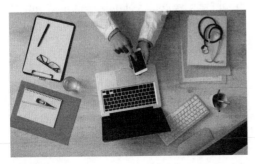

© Stokkete/Shutterstock.

and directly or indirectly); (2) what they communicate about (e.g., brief comments about how they are feeling or elaborate tracking of disease-monitoring data); and (3) where these communications occur (e.g., in face-to-face interactions or remotely).

▶ Electronic Health Records

The primary types of HIT drawing considerable attention are electronic health record formats. There are three types of electronic record keeping to be aware of: electronic medical recorders (EMRs), electronic health recorders (EHRs), and **personal health records (PHRs)**. We discuss them here and compare and contrast their similarities and differences.

Electronic medical records (EMRs) were actually the first system put in place by clinicians with the specific purpose of digitalizing and storing information about a patient's diagnosis and treatment seen in their medical practice. Otherwise, they contained the standard medical and clinical data gathered in one provider's office, but only in this one provider's office. They took the place of sometimes very cumbersome patient paper charts that included lengthy accounts of medical histories, diagnoses, medications, immunizations, and allergies. They were beneficial because they allowed providers the option of tracking treatment data over time, identifying in advance who was due for health promotion/disease prevention visits or screenings, and monitoring for ongoing concerns (e.g., vaccination history and health screenings).

As previously indicated, EMRs played a significant role not only in coordinating the patient's care, but also included records from a single provider or health care institution and were exclusively medical in nature. Furthermore, these records were a digital version of the paper charts in the clinician's office that were not shared with other providers outside this practice who could have had a significant role in managing a patient's care. They were used by providers chiefly to communicate diagnosis and treatment plans within the provider's practice group, but were not designed to be used outside the practice of the individual provider or provider group. Data was electronically collected, monitored, stored, and maintained typically in the provider's office. The ability to synthesize this data in a digitalized format, rather than relying on a bulky paper trail, provided easier access and in a timely manner. EMRs were thought to improve the overall quality of care in the provider(s) medical practice.

But, sharing patient information outside the provider's practice was difficult, and often patient records had to be printed out and faxed or mailed to other health providers, including specialists and other treatment facilities. The limitations of EMRs were significant and problematic in that health information exchange among physicians rarely occurred. Providers were not sharing data with other physicians, but they also did not share data with health facilities and hospitals outside their organization.

Electronic health records (EHRs) are now the most utilized method to store and transmit patient health care information. EHRs go beyond the data collected in EMR data-based office systems and include a more comprehensive health care history. They are digital health care information databases that are stored, potentially throughout the patient's lifetime, with the objective to support continuity of patient care.

The 2009 Health Information Technology for Economic and Clinical Health (HITECH) Act accelerated the adoption and meaningful use of EHR technology by U.S. physicians and hospitals. By 2014, the Centers for Medicare and Medicaid Services (CMS) EHR Meaningful Use program had distributed over billions of dollars to eligible health providers to

support providers' meaningful use of certified EHRs (CMS, 2016).

Additionally, the Office of the National Coordinator for Health Information Technology (ONC) funded regional centers located throughout the country to help health care providers implement EHR systems and demonstrate their meaningful use. Furthermore, ONC (2011) established standards for structured data that EHRs are required to meet to qualify for use in the CMS EHR Incentive Programs. CMS regularly updates guidelines specifying criteria all professionals and hospitals must meet to participate in the incentive program, and these updates are found on the CMS Incentive Program Basics website.

As previously explained, EHRs go beyond the data collected in just one provider's office and include a fairly comprehensive overview of the patient's history. They are centralized databases containing a collective and comprehensive medical history, and related information that can be shared across different health care systems (e.g., between a primary care provider and medical specialist or between a hospital and primary care provider, namely all providers involved in the patient's care). This form of communication between professionals and across institutions provides the opportunity for channeling communication in ways to better coordinate patient care.

EHRs can be very helpful in coordinating care because they tell the provider exactly what records to retrieve and where to get them. Additionally, they alert providers to who should receive copies of information about the care the patient is currently receiving. Because they are electronically initiated, they can potentially save considerable time and effort and, at the same time, reduce risks of errors in communication. Typically, these records include a variety of health-related information from many health professionals including primary care providers, hospitals, and clinic services.

The IOM has developed a comprehensive list of information that should be found in the EHR. These requirements are categorized in four groups: (1) clinical documentation (e.g., physician notes, problem lists, and medications); (2) test and imaging results (e.g., laboratory reports, radiologic reports, and other diagnostic test results); (3) computerized provider-order entry that includes orders for laboratory tests, medications, and nursing orders; and (4) decision support (e.g., clinical guidelines, drug-allergy alerts, and drug–laboratory interaction alerts). Hospitals that have only a partial list of functionalities are not considered comprehensive, but are considered to have a basic EHR system.

Early on, even though EHRs had clear benefits, it became clear that adoption of EHRs by both physicians and hospitals on a wide scale might be problematic. Published in 2009, a study by Jha et al. (2015) in collaboration with the American Hospital Association (AHA) found that hospital adoption of EHRs was insufficient. In their survey sample of 2,952 hospitals (excluding federal hospitals), they reported that only 12% of hospitals surveyed adopted a full range of EHR features. Still, 75% of these hospitals reported adoption of electronic laboratory and radiologic reporting systems. At the time of this survey, adoption of EHRs in U.S. hospitals looked bleak since very few had a comprehensive electronic system, and only a small number had even a basic system.

With benefits being significant and the problems in adopting EHRs on a wide scale becoming more evident, the U.S. Department of Health and Human Services (HHS) instituted policies and support for adoption of EHRs across the board. In a publication by the U.S. Department of Homeland Security (DHS) in 2014, it was reported that significant increases in the use of EHRs had occurred among office-based physicians and hospitals.

In a report from the National Center for Health Statistics (Hsiao & Hing, 2012), almost 8 in 10 (78%) physicians surveyed reported they had adopted some type of EHR system, with about half of those reporting saying they had adopted a system with advanced functionalities, doubling the 2009 rate. Hospital data indicated that about 6 in 10 (59% of those surveyed) had adopted an EHR system with certain advanced functionalities (quadruple the percentage for 2010). However, this study, as did the 2009 study, points out that more needs to be done to achieve widespread health information exchange. After the CMS instituted the EHR Incentive Program, many more hospitals joined the ranks and have achieved meaningful use.

In summary, EHRs are better replacements because not only do they do all the things EMRs were intended to do, but they also do more, a lot more. EHRs focus not only on all aspects of the medical care of patients, but also focus on the total health needs of patients. They are also designed to be shared across provider groups, including laboratories and specialists. Because of this, they have the potential to consolidate a vast amount of information from specialist visits, hospital stays, after care and rehabilitation, and nursing homes. Additionally, the information can be transmitted across the states and even outside the United States. Just as important, this information is designed to be shared with patients themselves. The term EMR is sometimes used interchangeably with the term EHR, but they should not be interchangeable.

Proponents of the system strongly believe that quality care results from the effective communication across and between all those involved in the care of the patient, including patients themselves. This enables all members of the professional team and the patient to engage in interactive exchange and effective communication on behalf of the patient and the patient's family.

Health providers and administrators are recognizing the advantages of EHRs and the benefits of having patients' digital health information follow them across the care continuum, especially as it promises improved provider–provider and provider–patient communication. Still, HIT experts warn that the system is only as effective as the operations supporting the technology; otherwise, if the operations are flawed, implementing EHRs may not achieve the desired goals and may be costly in both setup and maintenance and, in some cases, may be wasteful. Feedback from all participating team members is critical if EHRs are to reap benefits of improved communication and coordination of health care.

With every advancement in technology comes the possibility of problems. It should be noted that some clinician feedback suggests that electronic records can place the provider in front of a computer screen that takes more time away from direct patient care. They claim it is harder to interact with patients, and especially harder to maintain eye contact and establish empathy.

While not negating this possibility, recent research about physicians' allocation of work time on a daily basis suggested that providers balance time spent at their desks and direct contact with their patients. However, Tai-Seale et al. (2017) reported that results were mixed. Physicians were found to divide their time equally between seeing patients and desktop medicine—3.08 hours on office visits and 3.17 hours on desktop medicine each day. They also reported that over time, physicians showed a reduction in time spent with patient office visits and an increase in desktop medicine. They did not report on the time spent per patient during an office visit that would indicate the extent to which computers interfered with the amount and quality of time in direct face-to-face encounters. Desktop medicine consisted of communicating with patients through a secure patient portal, responding to their online requests for prescription refills, medical advice, ordering tests, sending staff messages, and reviewing test results.

Others suggest that care delivery may have been compromised by the rush to buy any system that supported the recommended format. In a recent review of the literature reporting the facilitators and barriers to the adoption of EHRs in the United States, 25 facilitators and 23 barriers to adoption were identified, which indicated that beyond the recognition that access to and transportability of data was perceived as facilitators, a continued preoccupation with cost remained. Limited financial backing and outdated technology were common barriers frequently cited in literature that was reviewed (Kruse, Kothman, Anerobi, & Abanaka, 2016). This criticism is targeted at how the systems were put in place, not their usefulness. Still, EHRs have gone a long way in improving communication channels and promoting coordinated patient care.

Personal health records (PHRs) bear some similarities to EHRs but are different from both EHRs and EMRs. Generally, a PHR is an electronic application used by patients to store and manage their own health information. Different from EHRs, patients themselves setup, access, and edit their PHRs. PHRs can include comprehensive information about the patient's health or issues related to the patient's health and welfare, entered by the patient or even someone helping the patient (e.g., a close friend or family member). A format for the PHR is described in detail on the website Medicare.gov (**EXHIBIT 2-1**).

Although something like this could be kept in a folder or paper file by patients and families, increasingly these records are kept secure with different computer programs that can be used to store health data for their personal use. Predesigned PHR programs give patients a unique user ID and password, providing the patient control over who sees it. Even health providers cannot access it without the patient's permission.

Patients can use their PHR to keep track of information from their visits to health care providers or treatment centers, record their health-related information, and link to health-related resources (service centers, websites, self-help programs). Most information that is in the patient's EMR or EHR can be downloaded to their PHR. Some providers

EXHIBIT 2-1 Basic Information Included in PHR Formats

- Identifying information such as name, birth date, address, emergency contact information, and religious affiliation
- General medical information such as the family history of chronic/life-threatening illnesses
- Date of the last physical examination performed and the name of the provider who performed it
- Current list of active medications and treatments (which includes the doses of patients' medication and when these medications were prescribed)
- A list of allergies to medications
- A list of any supplements or over-the-counter drugs the patient is currently taking

- A complete list of major illnesses and surgeries (including the names of the doctors and the dates of the procedures)
- A list of infections and injuries and the corresponding treatment plan (including the name of the provider and when the treatment occurred)
- Results of the most recent lab tests and screenings (e.g., EKG, EEG, or MRI) and dates of the tests/screenings
- General treatment information and insurance information such as the health insurance plan and the name of all providers currently treating the patient (names, phone numbers, and addresses)

and hospitals will offer patients ways to view their medical records and download the information to their own PHR.

The PHR is user-friendly in that it lets patients keep their health information in one place. This makes it easier for them to find information about both past medical services and recent health care whenever they need it, or when they are curious about their current health or progress over time. They can build a chronological list of services and changes in their treatment plan if they are being seen and followed for a chronic illness. Data in a PHR is also useful to providers, but patients have full control over the data stored and shared. Some patients may even use their PHR to record their impressions of the quality of care they are receiving and questions or doubts they have, as well as a list of questions they need to ask their health provider. Usually, patients will include emergency contacts in their PHR in case this information needs to be shared with the police or emergency medical technicians. PHRs are also user-friendly in that patients' caregivers and family members, with approval, can help patients record and update important information.

As previously noted, a PHR format is provided on various official websites, one being the Medicare.gov website (myPHR.com). Another resource is the U.S. Surgeon General's Office personalized health record. This tool is a family health history record (*My Family Health Portrait*) that can be shared with other family members and one's health care provider.

Also, some providers and health plans offer them for free. Furthermore, independent vendors create and maintain PHRs. Some will actually create and maintain the patient's PHR if the patient gives them permission to access health information from health providers. Medicare.org recommends the site: myPHR.com. This format has a number of helpful tabs (e.g., for medications, health conditions, allergies, insurance).

In summary, the use of EMRs, EHRs, and PHRs has significantly transformed communications among patients, families, and health providers and across health care institutions. Whereas patients and their families were previously less aware of plans for patient care and health status information, the advent of these electronic record formats have increased their health care knowledge and subsequently their readiness and capability to engage with their health care team. Additionally, the ability to transmit data quickly from patient to provider and across providers and health centers enhances coordinated care. These technologies allow providers to use patient information about health status and ongoing treatment for any condition the patient has making it possible for this information to be known to all those caring for the patient, even though they could be miles apart.

There is an additional aspect of electronic records that has revolutionized communication between patient and provider. This is the ease in removing discrepancies in the records. A major barrier in the treatment of patients is the inconsistency between what medical records report and what is actually occurring. A case in point is the discrepancy between what medications the provider thinks the patient is taking and what the patient is *actually* taking.

In the case of medications, does the patient's list match what providers think they are taking, and are they taking the medications exactly how they were prescribed? The provider's list, for whatever reasons, may be invalid because it does not reflect accurately what the patient is doing. Medication names, doses, when they were prescribed, and if they were discontinued should match. The number of errors in medication lists is significant and common. The kinds of discrepancies may include:

- Medications that are current versus those that have been discontinued,
- Dates medications were modified and what modifications were made, or
- When new medications were added to the list of prescriptions or discontinued.

The lack of fit between the provider's plans for a patient and what the patient is doing has, in the past, been a "black box." Otherwise, providers often did not know that discrepancies existed, and in some cases, these discrepancies were the answers to why a prescribed treatment, such as a medication, was not working. Not only do electronic record systems facilitate communication, but they can also significantly reduce miscommunication about the treatment plan.

In a perfect world, we would find no discrepancies between what the patient is doing and what the provider recommended or thinks the patient is doing. But, providers are working in a complex health care system that is often over-burdened with data and with many more patients than can be adequately tracked. With the advent of electronic storage and transmission of data, the provider's database has increased. Careful management and monitoring of these systems to ensure that benefits are maximized and risks are minimized are critical.

▶ Patient Portals

Patient portals constitute a form of HIT that gives patients access to their electronic medical and health records managed by their health care organization which can be a single provider, provider group, hospital, or other health care institutions. A patient portal is defined as "a secure online website that gives patients convenient 24-hour access to personal health information from anywhere with an Internet connection."

(HealthIT.gov; last updated: Monday, November 2, 2015)

Patient portals are not PHRs; instead, they are managed and owned by the provider, while personal health records are owned and managed by the patient. In some cases, they may share similar or copies of the same documents (e.g., if the patients download information from their PHR to their provider's patient portal, or the reverse, data from the patient provider's patient portal is downloaded to the patient's PHR).

The patient's health information is electronically entered and stored online in the patient portal and includes not only accounts of patient health information but also lab test results and even graph trends in lab findings. These systems also provide patients the opportunity to message their provider, refill a current medication, request an appointment or referral, and find information about a previous visit and upcoming appointments. There is no charge for this service. Patients can pay their bill online through this service, find a provider, and read about research and clinical trials at the center. It is confidential and allows patients' access to this information any time and any place.

The history of patient portals in some ways parallels that of EHRs. Like EHRs, patient portals were linked to the 2009 HITECH Act. Requirements that emerged in defining what was categorized as Meaningful Use (MU) included the notion that patients should have access to their health records, and this could be achieved with a patient portal, owned and managed by health care institutions or provider(s). Increasingly, private medical groups and public medical centers operate elaborate electronic systems that perform a wide range of information functions, and these systems update health records that can be made available to patients through a secure website.

It was believed that not only could these portals provide the patient access to health information, but also that these portals could enhance patient–provider communications, improve adherence to treatment, promote self-management of disease, and increase

patients' disease awareness. The logic behind improved communications stemmed from the idea that patients and physicians could enter and access the information almost simultaneously through the online patient portal system that connected them and promoted information exchange and interaction online. In fact, entries from the provider could include past and current medical records, the results of lab tests, a summary of the last office visit, and a list of current health problems the provider is treating.

From the patient, entries could include the results of home monitoring (e.g., blood pressure [BP] or blood sugar levels or the inclusion of test results not previously known to the provider). Additionally, patient portals can facilitate the exchange of emails between patient and provider about a number of issues relating to the treatment planned (e.g., clarifying the providers' opinions about the care planned and how the patient is progressing). Heretofore, such discussions could have occurred through telephone exchanges, but were more likely only when the provider and patient were face-to-face during an office visit.

Patient portals can potentially enable the patient to be actively engaged in their care and thus, promote their knowledge and insight into their health condition and its treatment. In some cases, patients may detect problems such as from posted lab results or even errors faster than their provider. Then, it is the patient who is actively identifying a need even before the provider notices it. In this way, issues of both quality of care and patient safety are addressed through the features of the patient portal.

The expectations associated with patient portal use may or may not be realized. One review of the 1990–2011 literature summarizing studies of patient portal use suggested that although the idea of empowering patients and improving quality care was discussed in the literature, there was insufficient evidence supporting the assumption that patients were more empowered and patient care was

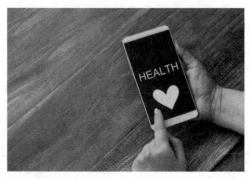

of a higher quality (Ammenwerth, Schnell-Inderst, & Hoerbst, 2012).

In a follow-up review of the literature on the effect of EHRs and patient portals on quality care since the initial report in 2011, Kruse, Bolton, and Freriks (2015) stated that more health care organizations now offer features of a patient portal which meets the intent of CMS MU guidelines (urging patients to be able to view their health information electronically).

While an increase in quality care in terms of patient satisfaction and retention was reported, there were only weak results supporting any improvement in medical outcomes. Irizarry, DeVito, and Curran (2015) summarized literature on adoption of patient portals and the factors that may influence sustained utilization. These authors concluded that patient portal use is associated with patients' interest and ability to use them and is strongly influenced by such factors as age, culture, ethnicity, education level, health literacy, health status, and the role of a caregiver.

It is suggested that some groups and communities (e.g., minorities and indigenous populations) may not have the abilities to or interest in using these forms of communication. As in the case of the impact of EHRs, more evidence of patterns of use across multiple populations and communities, and the positive impact and potential drawbacks of using patient portals on health care outcomes is needed.

▶ m-Health (Mobile Health)

m-Health, or mobile health, is a generic term that applies to the use of devices to collect and transmit health information, frequently with the use of health-related applications (apps). The most common m-Health apps are possibly fitness trackers. Other m-Health devices will collect data and monitor heart rate or asthma and diabetic clinical markers. m-Health apps are frequently used by persons with chronic

diseases (diabetes, cancer, cardiovascular disease) to self-manage their complex treatment plan.

A number of apps are also provided to young adults with chronic illnesses. Any condition requiring long-term management with frequent monitoring and/or many medications may benefit from the m-Health apps. These apps can use a variety of approaches, including medication alerts, symptom monitoring, and even communication connections with health care providers.

Advances in m-Health occur at a simple level, such as with the use of phone calls between the provider and patient, to the more robust system of using a digital platform to assess patient needs and appropriate medical treatment. These include the advantage of being free of wires and cords and enabling patients and providers to check on health needs and care planned on-the-go through the use of smartphones. Smartphones and tablets allow health providers to more freely access and send information. For example, providers can access the health records and lab results of patients without having a paper copy mailed or faxed to them. This access can occur during a face-to-face patient visit or outside the traditional medical visit format.

Providers can use m-Health for accessing or sending medical orders, documentation of health problems, or to simply access the Web to rule out potential patient diagnoses. They can also electronically send their evaluation of the patient's health needs to other providers or health care systems, thereby improving the coordination of patient care.

Initially, m-Health applications were used by a narrow range of patients, usually the most knowledgeable, younger, and health-literate populations. Recently, with the advent of further sophistication in apps (e.g., easing navigation challenges), their usefulness to others (e.g., elder patients with chronic debilitating illnesses) has shown promise. Also, m-Health apps are finding their way into developing countries, not just in industrialized nations.

Given the expansion of mobile phones in developing countries, the advantages of this modality have spread to poorer, less educated populations, closing the gap between those who have limited access to health care services to those who have a full range of services localized in their residential areas.

In their critical review of the literature on the use of m-Health approaches in developing countries, Davey, Davey, and Singh (2014) reported that unlike m-Health technology in developed countries, the majority of m-Health initiatives in developing countries are focused on prevention and disease awareness campaigns. The effectiveness and success of these initiatives are largely moderate compared to what is known about success in developed countries, but the potential in developing countries is promising.

M-Health devices have raised concern due to the inability to ensure proper and reliable data from some m-Health apps. Additionally, the absence of hands-on clinical oversight raises ethical issues. Whether designed in and for developed countries or for developing countries, continuous evaluation of their impact on patient–provider relationships and communications is critical. Making data about the effectiveness of the apps for certain patients and conditions available will guide both patients and providers in identifying the best app for a particular patient.

▶ **Telemedicine**

Telemedicine and telehealth are terms used to describe processes of exchanging medical information from one site to another via electronic communications with the goal of improving a patient's clinical health status. Supporting devices to assist in the assessment and treatment process include two-way videos, email, smartphones, and wireless tools.

We usually think about the delivery of health care as a face-to-face exchange between the patients, families, and providers either in an office or hospital setting. This is the classical way needs for health care was assessed and the way medical care was delivered and evaluated. Telemedicine or telehealth is a valuable addition to addressing gaps in health care delivery (e.g., health care delivered to patients who may not have access to health professionals or specialists because of their distance from available health care centers).

Examples would be those patients who are home-bound and isolated or who live in rural areas versus cities where health care centers are found. Research has found that patients distant from these centers can be clinically treated with the use of videoconferencing and other wireless technology.

Telemedicine services are often part of a health care institution's investment in information technology and the delivery of clinical care remotely. This approach has contributed to cost savings for both the patient and provider as the patient receives a medical assessment or education about self-managing their illness through video consultations with a remote physician, nurse, or specialist.

Telemedicine is not necessarily new and has received both positive and negative reviews by both physicians and nurse practitioners. Physicians have expressed concern about some telemedicine efforts and are cautious about showing support uniformly because of the possibility of delivering suboptimal care. This concern differs from that about the use of m-Health devices.

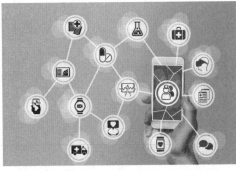

© A-image/Shutterstock.

M-Health is not to be used in place of direct observation of the patient, but telemedicine can be used in place of direct access. The organized provision of telemedicine or telehealth using video consultation with a patient and/or the treating local provider does not violate this ethic because the patient is visible to the provider or specialist and can be asked specific questions about what the specialist sees in the video chat with the patient or the patient and local provider.

Sophisticated home telehealth technology programs are particularly promising for bringing health care to distant rural areas. Luptak et al. (2010) described the potential usability of one program, Care Coordination Home Telehealth (CCHT), for medically complicated veterans in rural settings. Sometimes, a major treatment facility (e.g., Kaiser or the Veterans Administration [VA] health care centers) will offer a project or research study investigating the efficacy and cost savings of their specific telehealth program. A case in point is a study of the efficacy of the VA's Health Buddy program.

This effort helps patients be adherent to their treatment program, improve their health, reduce the severity of their medical condition, and avoid costly rehospitalization (Guzman-Clark, van Servellen, Chang, Mentes, & Hahn, 2013). This study revealed that measuring the successful use of such telemedicine is not easy and includes a complex interplay between the program and patient characteristics that impact patients' adherence to the use of the telemedicine system, in this case the Health Buddy.

The same conclusion was expressed in a study of routine telemonitoring for high-risk diabetic patients (Vest, Hall, Kahn, & Heider, 2017). This study explored the experience of implementing routine telemonitoring with high-risk diabetic patients in the context of primary care settings. The nurse researchers reported that effective communication between the clinical team and nurse telemonitor was essential. Furthermore, interviews revealed that the nurse–patient relationship was central to a successful telemonitoring experience.

Positive reviews included that telemonitoring was a useful tool in understanding patient social and economic factors and how these factors are likely to impact patients' health. It should be stressed that there are important differences between telehealth and m-Health. Health data derived from telehealth devices are considered reliable, and the industry is controlled with oversight provided through various regulating agencies (e.g., the Federation of State Medical Boards, Telemedicine Policies, and the American Telemedicine Association). On the other hand, m-Health devices are thought to not provide accurate enough information to guide clinical assessments, and currently there is no authority controlling or overseeing the industry.

In a recent statement from the AMA ethical guidance committee (AMA, June 13, 2016), telehealth and telemedicine were formally recognized as another stage in the evolution of new models that are shaping patient–physician interactions. It was stressed that even with new advances, physicians' fundamental ethical responsibilities remain the same.

Patients need to be able to put their trust in medical care that "place patient welfare above other interests, provide competent care, provide the information patients need to make well-considered decisions about care, respect patient privacy and confidentiality, and take steps needed to ensure continuity of care." Furthermore, providers are cautioned to

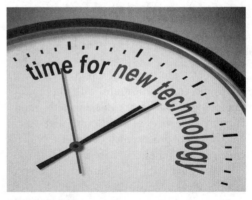

© Markus Gann/Shutterstock.

recognize the limitations of telemedicine in order "to make well-grounded recommendations for each patient."

▸ Self-Service Kiosks and Sensor Technology

Patient-managed self-monitoring tools are other forms of HIT and are available in the format of accessible **self-service kiosks** or new sensory technology, both of which offer up information not previously known by the patient. The classical example of simple kiosk use is monitors in pharmacies or drugstores to measure one's weight, BP, heart rate, and body mass index (BMI).

Sensory technology, rising in popularity, comes in the form of wearable watches to more formal assessment apparatus. Wearable watches inform patients about activity levels, heart rate, nutritional information about food consumed, and even vitamin deficiencies in food consumed in a given 2-hour period. Sensory devices can also monitor home-bound patient falls or problems in blood levels, which could activate a call to the provider for further assessment of the need for more information or assistance and even the need for more urgent care intervention. Another form of wearable **sensor technology** is simply alert sensors such as what is seen in wearable bracelets notifying others of a life-threatening condition or serious allergy to a medication.

Kiosk data and wearable technology are means to collect data on how one is doing. An added advantage are sensors that provide continuous data, making it possible to chart outcomes over time. These tools can prompt patients to be alert about something usual or a potential adverse health problem. Smart technology seems now to have no foreseeable limits, and as fast as technology advances, so does our ability to monitor our health and well-being.

Reported concerns include the potential drawback of the patient not receiving enough person-to-person discussion with a health provider. Typically, many formats used may warn patients to contact their health care provider— they do not connect the patient directly to a knowledgeable health provider.

▸ Self-Care Through Web Information Sources

Another technological development influencing patients' and families' access to health care communications and their self-care management of health and illness can be found on the Internet. Two decades ago, the online health care information revolution was estimated to include as many as 10,000 medically related websites, indicating that these were here to stay, and the number of people who access the Internet for health-related information was rapidly growing.

Internet Information and a Digital Divide

The growth in Internet use also drew concern for populations who do not have ready access to or who do not use the Internet. Namely, there is a *digital divide* between these two groups with disparate levels of knowledge as a consequence. That is, some populations have restricted access to Internet information, while others do not, and this phenomenon creates or accentuates differences in health illiteracy across communities. This *divide* may create disparate levels of health based upon differences in Internet source used and the specific sources accessed. Otherwise, those who use Internet sources may be more informed and able to prevent illness and enhance health while those unable to access internet sources may be less able to prevent illness and promote health. But, the quality of sources accessed also influence how well the public is informed and capable of ensuring good health.

There is an overall concern that vulnerable populations have neither access nor capacity to use health information on the Internet. These populations include not only those typically known to have poor levels of health literacy but also other groups not previously recognized, such as persons with disabilities (deficits in sensory perception, mobility, mental, and emotional health). Persons with disabilities are generally known to have poor literacy because they are less likely to graduate from high school and obtain postsecondary education, which would better prepare them to access, understand, evaluate, and effectively use Internet information. Clearly this information is a resource that could benefit them.

Wide Variety of Information Sources

There is a wide variety of Internet information sources available if accessed and understood.

Users may access websites, bulletin boards, list-servs, chat rooms, webinars, videos, or medical and scientific articles and government reports. These sources provide a vast amount of advice and knowledge of human conditions, directed at prevention, treatment, and/or recovery.

Some of these websites give alerts or health announcements that are very important to the average person or family seeking answers about their condition or that of a family member. These include paid ads to promote particular medications or alternative treatments or public announcements that are derived from official sources (e.g., the National Institutes of Health [NIH] or Centers for Disease Control and Prevention [CDC]). But still other sources promote products that they claim have widespread health effects, cure many diseases, and do this quickly and/or inexpensively.

TABLE 2-1 provides a list of some resources that can guide patients and families in

TABLE 2-1 Tools to Use in the Evaluation of the Quality of Information on the Internet	
Resource	**Service Provided**
Health on the Web: Finding Reliable Information (American Academy of Family Physicians)	Available in Spanish
How to Evaluate Health Information on the Internet (NIH: National Cancer Institute)	
User's Guide to Finding and Evaluating Health Information on the Web (Medical Library Association)	
Ten Things to Know about Evaluating Medical Resources on the Web (NIH: National Center for Complementary and Alternative Medicine)	Available in Spanish
Ten Tips for Evaluating Immunization Information on the Internet (Centers for Disease Control and Prevention)	
Understanding Risk: What Do Those Headlines Really Mean? (NIH: National Institutes of Health)	
Online Health Information: Can You Trust It? (NIH: National Institute of Aging)	

evaluating the quality of information they find on the Internet.

It is known that patients and families use this Internet information for a wide range of health-related issues: information about diet, fitness, medications, health insurance, specific diseases or illnesses, and recommended treatment for their conditions, including the availability of clinical trials. They also access data about available providers as well as preferred treatment centers and hospitals. Some patients and families access the evaluations and reviews of certain providers to help decide on the best provider that also accepts their insurance. Use of the Internet changes the potential questions patients and their families might ask of providers, and more time may be needed to address what they found on the Internet.

Impact of Patients' Internet Data and the Provider–Patient Relationship

When the patient or patient's family member(s) brings data to the provider that they gathered in searching the Internet, another aspect of the relationship is interjected. How providers react to this "*third party information*" will determine whether communication will be enhanced and successful or whether the trust and rapport that was previously established be disrupted in any way. What is typically found from the studies on why patients use the Internet is that patients might be missing something from their relationship with their provider. They may be dissatisfied with their communications with their providers, have ineffective communications, or their emotional needs may not have been sufficiently addressed. Sometimes, patient and families obtain information faster through the Internet than they would from contacting a provider.

In a study by Bylund et al. (2007) of patient and provider responses, patients described as challenging were those who used Internet information for self-diagnosis or self-treatment, or to test the provider's knowledge. Some physicians stated that they had limited Internet skills and attributed this to being too busy to improve on their computer skills. Even if the provider disagrees with the information the patient has found on the Internet, there is still the feeling that the provider is taking the information seriously—and this improves patients' satisfaction with the interaction. This study also revealed that providers' responses are associated with the strategies that patients use in presenting the data they found. Otherwise, when the patient was more assertive and used a less face-threatening approach, the provider was more likely to engage them in positive dialogue.

Given the opportunity for Internet education, would patients and their families be more satisfied with Internet use than direct communications with their provider? The answer is probably no. In a national telephone study by Hesse et al. (2005), it was found that while the use of the Internet for health care information was increasing, patients are still likely to trust and prefer information from their health care professionals who know them and their particular condition.

Patients' Needs for Guidance in Using Internet Information

Clearly the U.S. government is interested in the value of the Internet to educate patients and their families. The document *Healthy People 2010* (U.S. Department of Health and Human Services, 2000) recognizes the importance of patient–provider communication and the value of the Internet to facilitate access to a wide array of health information and health-related support services, and the extension of health communication. Objective 11.1 of this document urges the increase in the proportion of households with access to the Internet at home, with a target of 80% and baseline of 26%. While there is general endorsement for the use of the Internet for health information, there is equal or more interest in helping patients and their families to use Internet knowledge appropriately.

While there are several sources of information on the Internet, health care providers need to guide patients and their families on the use of this information. Caution is important in the use of any website information that does not appear to be official or reliable. It is not always apparent who is providing the information and whether the information is valid or not. Patients and their families vary in their knowledge and trust of Web-based information, particularly if it differs from what is told to them by their professional health care providers. Because patients may find it difficult to determine the credibility of the information they read online, it is important for health professionals to ask patients about what they have read, how they are understanding this information, and even give them additional and more reliable resources to answer their questions.

The NIH advises that any posting that is identified by ".gov" or ".org" is likely to be official, and generated from official government data sources. Also, never use Web information as an alternative to seeking professional medical help either to formulate a self-diagnosis or a treatment approach. Patients are encouraged to become informed and to discuss what they have learned with their medical care providers. Guidelines in talking to patients about information they have found on the Internet are listed as dos and don'ts. **TABLE 2-2** provides a list of dos and don'ts that are helpful when discussing information patients and their families have retrieved from the Internet.

Schwartz et al. (2006) studied family medicine patients who used the Internet to find how many of these users attempted to verify the source or information they retrieved. They reported that 90% attempted to verify the information they found, and the majority had discussed website information with their physician. This study concluded that physicians need critical appraisal skills to determine whether the information found by the patient or family is actually relevant to the patient's condition, and is based on the best available evidence. The following RED FLAG BOX illustrates the need of patients and their families to be cautious not only about the information they retrieve, but also how they use the information.

TABLE 2-2 Do's and Don'ts in Discussing Internet Information with Patients and Their Families	
Do's	**Don'ts**
Show interest in the content and source of the information.	Dismiss an invitation to discuss Internet information as invalid.
Interpret their use of Internet information as a positive attempt to engage in more informative conversations.	Interpret the gesture as a direct threat to your authority or medical judgment.
Direct patients to sources of good-quality consumer health information, including health-related Internet sites, but be aware of the educational level of the patient and whether he or she is likely to understand the information that will be provided.	Refer patients to medical sites that the provider has not personally reviewed both for content and ease of comprehension for the patient.

Be aware that in the course of searching the Internet, the patient may have become frustrated or fearful about what they read, and may have abruptly discontinued but may still harbor some misconceptions.	If the patient does not raise the issue of discovery of information on the Internet or other health-related information, do not assume that he or she has not been exposed to this information.
Instruct the patient about how to do his or her own evaluation of the quality of the Internet information.	Assume that the quality of Internet data is at least acceptable; the quality of information on the Internet is quite variable.
Be aware that patients may be using aspects of online interactive sites to gain support and/or to obtain information for a friend or family member.	Assume that the patient is using the Internet solely to gain information and that this seeking is directly related to their own health or condition.

 RED FLAG BOX: Self-Diagnosing and Choosing Treatment with Web-Based Information

The example is a patient searching the Web to find medical information about the neck (cervical) pain the patient is having and what treatment is needed. Neck pain for a variety of reasons is a very common complaint. The likely first step someone relying on Web-based information might take is to search the term "neck or back pain." Then they would likely be directed to identify the pain symptoms including duration and location in the neck and/or back where the pain is felt.

Since the patient is also interested in treatment, depending upon what the patient and the patient's family reads, they may be quickly linked to treatment for cervical back pain. A list of options might appear and include a conservative approach (e.g., exercise and spinal adjustment), medication (e.g., over-the-counter [OTC] analgesics or muscle relaxants), or surgery (e.g., spinal cord compression). They will also be interested in what is said about the accompanying pain and disability, or impaired functioning associated with these choices for treatment.

If the patient knows someone who has had surgery or has read about this type of surgery, the next concern could be "Which surgery is best for me?" Depending upon how knowledgeable the patient and family are, and discussions they have or have not had with health professionals, they may find the options are cervical spinal fusion or artificial disc replacement.

At this point or at any point in the process, the patient and family could decide, based upon the information on the Web, that they prefer the more conservative approaches. Without seeking a professional diagnosis from their primary care provider and/or consultation from a specialist, a reputable orthopedic surgeon, they could begin a rather long and unproductive trial on OTC medications and/or an exercise routine. While these options might help, at least initially, they might not be what their physician or specialist would suggest.

Discussion

Is the patient at risk by self-diagnosing and choosing a more conservative treatment without consulting a *bona fide* health professional? While the answer is rather obvious, it is important to understand why this use of Web-based information can lead to negative consequences that could impair patient functioning and quality of life for some time to come.

(continues)

⚑ **RED FLAG BOX: Self-Diagnosing and Choosing Treatment with Web-Based Information**   *(continued)*

The advice of a primary physician is needed because this physician can determine whether there is a need for a specialist. Any decision about appropriate treatment would take into account many different aspects of the patient's current condition (e.g., character and duration of symptoms, how the disabling the condition is, and how painful it is, as well as other existing chronic health problems or conditions [treated or not treated] the patient has). With the help of health providers, these factors can be assessed and a suitable treatment plan can be proposed. Most importantly, the patient's choice of treatment might not be the best option. While patients may select the conservative option, the process of delaying necessary surgery could limit the surgical options available to the patient at a later time.

Patients' Use of Support Group Activities on the Internet

There is another kind of information that may be on the Web that is worth noting. Of particular interest are the virtual communities that patients and families can join where they can share (even worldwide) similar interests and concerns about their disease or illness. These interactive communication options include chat rooms, discussion groups, support groups, and email exchanges. Sharing experiences has the effect of multiplying, many times over, advice and opinions. The sheer magnitude of potential information presents a challenge because providers are at a loss to really know what the patient has been exposed to and how this exposure might influence patients' and families' health-seeking and disease-management behaviors.

These virtual communities serve the purpose of providing information, but also social support. The opportunity to communicate with others in the same situation is a critical contribution. When confronting an acute or chronic condition, especially a life-threatening illness or injury, individuals frequently feel the need to talk to other people who have had or are currently in the same position.

Participation in a virtual community or chat room might be the only alternative to satisfy patients' and families' needs. Not only do these activities meet patients' needs for support, but they also direct patients as to how to find and evaluate what they have learned on the Internet about available services, providers, and treatments. Patients without medical knowledge may learn a great deal from others who themselves are not medical professionals. A great deal of self-help information is generated on the Web through organized social media sites (e.g., Facebook and Twitter). While the information shared may not be helpful or even reflect what the patient should do, it may be perceived to be of value because it provides a source of support. This kind of support is valued in the absence of enough clinical contacts that could address patients' needs.

Patients who may be coping with their illness alone may feel less isolated when they read the Internet postings of others. Rather than learning the specifics about the disease or illness, they may be more interested in reading the stories of others who have faced the same or similar health challenges. Still, patients and their families need to recognize that any information they gather through social media is not likely to be medically or scientifically based and should be shared and validated with their health professional.

There seems to be no single motivation that always drives Internet users to seek health information; there are many reasons behind the information-seeking behaviors of Internet users. Patients and families may be arming themselves with information not so much to challenge the provider's assessment, but to cope with and manage their condition and to prepare themselves to communicate with health providers in ways that will more fully answer their questions.

▶ Summary

Advances in HIT will continue to grow exponentially even to uncharted domains. HIT approaches almost always alter, at least to some degree, the ways health professionals communicate with patients and their families, between themselves, and across health care institutions. They impact how, when, where, and what is communicated, and play a significant role in patients' and families' access to health care and health care choices.

As noted by major professional organizations advocating for HIT and evaluating its use, important changes in health care delivery and health status can be positively impacted by advances in HIT. The impact can be seen in the quality of communication and in-depth discussions patients and their families have with providers. Others have suggested that HIT has the potential to cut the costs of care by curbing rehospitalization rates, reducing rates of disease morbidity and mortality, and improving provider–patient satisfaction with the care delivery process. However, there are several reasons why each of the technological advancements discussed in this chapter might fail to live up to their potential and/or present barriers to patient–family–provider communication.

First, and very important, not all HIT advances should be adopted in their current form. Designing and disseminating new technologies has been recognized as a profitable investment opportunity, and the number of new proposals, tested or not, are increasing.

They include several forms of alert technology, adherence support, and remote collecting and monitoring of the patients' vital signs. For example, one proposal is an alert technology system to send physicians to the patient's home, office, or hotel within 2 hours to treat urgent care needs.

Another new device allows patients to help in conducting their physical exam through a handheld telemedicine device. The device allows physicians to remotely examine patients and gather important medical vital signs. This particular device includes a way to transport the data to a secure patient record. Such proposals offer up some important benefits by securing access to care and promoting timely communication between patient and provider. But, like all innovations, it needs scrutiny at all levels.

It is also clear that patients differ in their readiness and capability to use HIT. The underlying principle here is that *the advantages and disadvantages differ across patients and health care systems*. In other words, the usability of any technological advancement is subject to the specific characteristics of the patient, provider, and health care institution. For example, EHRs have been widely adopted across both large and small health care institutions, and there are many benefits associated with this innovation. There were inherent problems in adopting EHRs. Early on, they were effective only if the institutions could launch them appropriately, and consequently, hospitals and health care centers were ill-equipped to provide a problem-free transition. Some hospitals invested in complicated systems that could result in more problems than advantages.

When implementing a particular HIT approach to improve patient–provider communication (e.g., EHRs), there are many kinds of hidden barriers. They include the vendor's product (the ability of the product to achieve its purpose and to do it reliably), patient characteristics, provider knowledge and acceptance, and system support for adoption of the change. For example, not all persons will use these innovations; in fact, we can predict who will use them and who will not on the basis of age, education, gender, socioeconomic status, and health status. Likewise, these advances may be available, but health professionals and health care institutions may not be equipped to use them because providers have not had the necessary education or training or lack the time to employ them effectively.

Some providers have criticized the patient portal communication and paperwork required to complete EHRs because the time and effort takes away from the very valuable time they need to truly listen to patients tell their health care story. Additionally, there may be institutional failure in rolling out these innovations in a timely and cost-effective manner. True, these innovations offer a number of important benefits to patients and their families, providers, and interinstitutional communication, but there are important potential drawbacks that still need to be addressed to bolster the widespread adoption and continued use of these technologies.

The role of HIT innovations is in its beginning stages, with many new proposals quickly appearing on the horizon. It is now possible to collect enormous amounts of patient and health care data, and this database has several uses. Not previously mentioned is the access to large data sets by compiling and sharing information about disease and its treatment. It is believed that such data sources will advance our abilities to predict illness and tailor patient care reflecting the aggregated information in these electronic records.

This aggregation of data from the patient over time and from other persons afflicted with the same illness or disease increases the possibility of predicting future illness through generations. An important area of science is genomic intelligence, which includes, for example, the study of cancer. Large datasets not only promote the prediction of cancer in future generations but also allow careful targeting of the best type of treatment for a particular form of cancer. There is no doubt that this area of science can improve the diagnoses, treatment decisions, and care outcomes needed to fight chronic and life-threatening diseases. Finally, and this can be said of all HIT, these advances need to be evaluated and monitored fully and over time as they are modified.

🔍 CITED STUDY: Possible benefits of E-Tools for Patient Medication Use

Many have questioned the benefits and possible drawbacks of e-tools in patient care management. The vast majority of patients being seen over time take at least one medication, if not several simultaneously. Are there benefits to patients who choose to use these apps? For example, do apps and other e-tools make it easier for patients to understand their medications, accept them, and continue to use them as they were prescribed? And, what are the risks if these apps are not used appropriately?

This area of research is addressed in the following paper:

Van Kerkhof, L. W. M., van der Laar, C. W. E., de Jong, C., Weda, M., & Hegger, I. (2016). Characterization of apps and other e-Tools for medication use: Insights into possible benefits and risks. *JMIR mHealth and uHealth, 4*(2), e34. doi:10.2196/mhealth.4149

The aim of this study was to identify characteristics of e-tool use along with the possible risks and benefits to patients with diabetes using these tools. The authors identified 116 apps or e-tools that dealt with using medications for diabetes. They concluded that many apps were available that offered simple functionalities (providing information/education, assisting users with therapy adherence, and helping users monitor the effects and possible side effects of their medications).

These researchers focused on apps for monitoring blood glucose levels and surveyed members of the Dutch Diabetes Association (May–June 2015). They found that the majority of the e-tools were downloaded less than 5,000 times worldwide, but this did not represent actual usage. The majority of the e-tools were not intended to be used by health care professionals, but only by patients taking these medications. The authors suspected that some apps might be used in place of health care professional communication or advice. Whether the e-tool could be used incorrectly and lead to incorrect patient decisions was also assessed. The researchers concluded that the majority of the apps for medication use were considered to be a quick source of information and conveniently available with perceived benefits of improving health and self-reliance. A minority of the apps had potentially high risks. Although how personal data was stored could be a concern, the respondents did not particularly list these risks as problems.

Discussion

1. What are the most important technological advances influencing communications between patients and health care professionals?
2. How might these advances impact patient safety and the quality of health care?
3. Give some specific examples of how these advances impact communications between health professionals and patients and corresponding treatment facilities.
4. What potential problems or drawbacks could be associated with the implementation of these new advances?
5. Are there certain steps that could be (or are being) taken to counter the potential drawbacks of these advances?

References

American Association of Medicine. (2016). *AMA adopts new guidance for ethical practice in telemedicine.* Retrieved from ama-assn.org

Ammenwerth, E., Schnell-Inderst, P., & Hoerbst, A. (2012). The impact of electronic patient portals on patient care: A systematic review of controlled trials. *Journal of Medical Internet Research, 14*(6), e162. doi:10.2196/jmir.2238

Bylund, C. L., Sabee, C. M., Imes, R. S., & Sanford, A. A. (2007). Exploration of the construct of reliance among patients who talk with their providers about internet information. *Journal of Health Communication, 12*(1), 17–28. doi:10.1080/10810730601091318

CMS.gov. (2016). *Medicare and medicaid EHR incentive program basics.* Retrieved from http://www.cms.gov/Regulations-and-Guidance/Legislation/EHRIncentivePrograms/Basics.html

Davey, S., Davey, A., & Singh, J. V. (2014). Mobile-health approach: A critical look on its capacity to augment health system of developing countries. *Indian Journal of Community Medicine: Official Publication of Indian Association of Preventive & Social Medicine, 39*(3), 178–182. doi:10.4103/0970-0218.137160

Guzman-Clark, J. R., van Servellen, G., Chang, B., Mentes, J., & Hahn, T. J. (2013). Predictors and outcomes of early adherence to the use of a home telehealth device by older veterans with heart failure. *Telemedicine and e-Health, 19*(3), 217–223. doi:10.1089/tmj.2012.0096

HealthIT.gov. (2015). What is a patient portal? Retrieved from www.healthit.gov/providers-professionals/faqs/what-patient-portal

Hesse, B. W., Nelson, D. E., Kreps, G. L., Croyle, R. T., Arora, N. K., Rimer, B. K., & Viswanath, K. (2005). Trust and sources of health information: The impact of the internet and its implications for health care providers: Findings from the first Health Information National Trends Survey. *Archives of Internal Medicine, 165,* 2618–2624. doi:10.1001/archinte.165.22.2618

Hsiao, C. J., & Hing, E. (2012). *Use and characteristics of electronic health record systems office-based physician practices: United States, 2001–2012* (NCHS Data Brief

No. 111). Hyattsville, MD: National Center for Health Statistics.

Irizarry, T., DeVito Dabbs, A., & Curran, C. R. (2015). Patient portals and patient engagement: A state of the science review. *Journal of Medical Internet Research*, *17*(6), e148. doi.org/10.2196/jmir.4255

Jha, A., DesRoches, C., Cambell, E., Donelan, K., Rao, S., Ferris, T., ... Blumenthal, D. (2009). Use of electronic health records in U.S. hospitals. *New England Journal of Medicine, 360*, 1628–1638. doi:10.1056/NEJMsa0900592

Kruse, C. S., Bolton, K., & Freriks, G. (2015). The effect of patient portals on quality outcomes and its implications to meaningful use: A systematic review. *Journal of Medical Internet Research, 17*(2), e44. doi:10.2196/jmir.3171

Kruse, C. S., Kothman, K., Anerobi, K., & Abanaka, L. (2016). Adoption factors of the electronic health record: A systematic review. *JMIR Medical Informatics, 4*(2), e19. doi:10.2196/medinform.5525

Luptak, M., Dailey, N., Juretic, M., Rupper, R., Hill, R. D., Hicken, B. L., & Bair, B. D. (2010). The care coordination home telehealth (CCHT) rural demonstration project: A symptom-based approach for serving older veterans in remote geographical settings. *Rural and Remote Health (Internet), 10*, 1375. Retrieved from http://www.rrh.org.au/articles/subviewnew.asp?ArticleID=1375

Office of the National Coordinator for Health Information Technology (ONC). (2013). Health Information Technology Patient Safety Action and Surveillance Plan. Retrieved from https://www.healthit.gov/sites/default/files/safety_plan_master.pdf

Schwartz, K. L., Roe, T., Northrup, J., Meza, J., Seifeldin, R., & Neale, A.V. (2006). Family medicine patients' use of the internet for health information: A MetroNet study. *Journal of the American Board of Family Medicine, 19*, 39–45. doi:10.3122/jabfm.19.1.39

Tai-Seale, M., Olson, C. W., Li, J., Chan, A. S., Morikawa, C., Durbin M., ... Luft, H. S. (2017). Electronic health record logs indicate that physicians split time evenly between seeing patients and desktop medicine. *Health Affairs, 36*(4). doi:10.1377/hlthaff.2016.0811

U.S. Department of Health and Human Services. (2000). *Healthy People 2010*. Retrieved from http://www.healthypeople.gov/document/HTML/Volume1/11HealthCom.htm

Vest, B. M., Hall, V. M., Kahn, L. S., & Heider, A. R. (2017). Nurse perspectives on the implementation of routine tele-monitoring for high-risk diabetes patients in a primary care setting. *Primary Health Care Research & Development, 18*(1), 3–13. doi:10.1017/S1463423616000190

CHAPTER 3

Problems in Access to and Availability of Health Care Intimately Linked to Patient–Provider Communications

CHAPTER OBJECTIVES

- Describe the reciprocal relationship between access to health care and a population's health and well-being.
- Discuss the connection between access to health care and availability, affordability, accessibility, and acceptability of health care services.
- Describe the patterns of disparities in access to health care services across communities and groups in the United States.
- Identify the importance of navigating the health care system in patients' gaining access to needed health care services.
- Analyze the likelihood that access to health care can ensure effective communications between patients and providers.

KEY TERMS

- Access to health care
- Affordability of health care
- Availability of health care
- Disparities in access to health care
- Usability (utilization) of health care
- Effective health care communications
- Health care reform
- Navigating the health care system

▶ Introduction

Limited **access to** and **availability of health care** is linked to patient–family–provider communications, and the link is quite clear. Without access to and availability of health care, patient–family–provider communications are limited, if existent at all. Limited access to relationships with health care providers can mean unmet needs for health promotion and disease prevention in addition to inadequate treatment for existing health conditions.

An increase in access and availability is the hope and goal of the U.S. health care system. To this end, **health care reform** has and is legislated to impact increased access and availability of health care services, and this legislation is expected to change on a wide scale communications between patients and providers.

In this chapter, we discuss the phenomena of access to care, disparities in health care services, and the context for health care reform. We will address the need to navigate the complex health care system in order to truly access quality health care. Finally, we also make the point that mere access and availability is neither a guarantee of good communications nor a promise of high-quality health care.

▶ Reciprocal Relationships: Health Care Access and Better Outcomes

It is a widely known and accepted fact that **access to health care** in the United States is not what it should be. *Access* here means the overarching concept describing entry into health care services. Access, by its very nature, is multifaceted and the result of several overlapping determinants (e.g., patient and family characteristics, provider distribution, and costs of services). For example, some patients and families will try hard to access health care services, while others will dismiss the need and go without them. The availability of different kinds of providers and specialists also influence the accessibility of services. Finally, the out-of-pocket costs of care impact which groups will and will not be able to access care.

It is generally assumed that *access* to health care affords individuals: better health, protection from disease, detection and treatment of a wide array of health conditions, injuries, disabilities, and a higher quality of life, as well as a longer life. Having both a usual and ongoing source of care leads to better health outcomes (AHRQ, 2008).

Access to health care, then, is defined as access to a service, provider, or institution as needed. Without access to health care, a wide range of health concerns can be overlooked or treated inappropriately. If access is not ensured, the consequences include not only the absence of better health but also an array of negative health care delivery outcomes, including delays in receiving appropriate assessment and medical treatment, and the likelihood of unnecessary hospitalizations if the health condition is not addressed early on.

Bierman and colleagues (cited in HealthyPeople.gov) emphasize that access to care entails the following steps: (1) gaining entry into the health care system, (2) accessing a health care location where the needed services are provided, and (3) finding a health care provider with whom the patient can communicate and trust. Disparities occur in different populations impacting individuals as well as communities. **Disparities in access to health care** services refer to unequal access balance across individuals and societies. Succinctly, this means unmet health needs for individuals and families.

By virtue of the fact that access can ensure freedom from disease and a higher quality of life, disparities in health care services disrupt the balance across individuals and communities where chances of a desired standard of living and higher quality of life are not equal. Historically, disparities were linked to racial and ethnic minorities, but the issue is far broader than what on the surface it appeared to be.

The causes of disparities in health care access are multiple and include a host of individual-level and system-level factors, including a lack of health insurance, lack of financial resources, irregular source of care, legal obstacles, structural barriers, lack of health care providers, language barriers, and age-related barriers (e.g., impaired mobility and poor health). Access tends to be very limited in a variety of groups, particularly the poor, disenfranchised, less health literate, regionally isolated, and uninsured or underinsured populations. Some groups are resistant to seeking traditional medical care services, adding still another potential barrier.

The reasons are multiple and can be compounded because these reasons also cluster. For example, some populations are at risk due to poverty, illiteracy, and lack of insurance. Others are at risk due to illiteracy, regional isolation, and uninsured status. Whatever the reason, or cluster of reasons, it is generally believed that barriers to accessing care can lead to important inequities and result in unmet health needs, delays in receiving appropriate care, inability to receive preventive services, and hospitalizations that could have been prevented (AHRQ, 2008).

A term sometimes used interchangeably with access is *availability*, but availability is not synonymous with access. Availability refers more narrowly to factors impacting the proximity to services (e.g., place of residence, location of services, hours of operation, or mechanisms for accessing a single provider or health center). In this way, services may be accessible (providers are located near the patient and patient's family), but not available (health services are conducted in ways that do not accommodate the patient and family's needs). Openings and closures of health care facilities impact access to care because they make services more or less available to the community.

▶ Interlocking Concepts Shaping Health Care Policy

Over time, the determinants of disease incidence and health care outcomes have been conceptualized to include multiple interlocking or interdependent factors. The concepts of *accessibility* and *availability* have already been defined and discussed. It is understood that without accessibility, disease remains uncontrolled and health care outcomes appear worse than they need to be. To reiterate, access to health care refers to access to a service, provider, or institution as needed, and availability refers more narrowly to factors impacting patients' use of services (e.g., place of residence, location of services, hours of operation, or mechanisms for accessing a single provider or health center).

In classical health care policy statements, access to care is a product of the interplay between related, but different, concepts. In a health care policy statement in Wyszewianski's article entitled Access to Care: Remembering Old Lessons (2002), *five* related concepts were identified and discussed (These concepts are displayed in **FIGURE 3-1**). In addition to the concepts of accessibility and availability already discussed, they include **affordability of health care**, accommodation, and acceptability. In this paradigm, *affordability* is the ratio of health care charges versus the ability of the patient to pay for these services. *Accommodation* is the extent to which the available health care services meet the needs, constraints, and preferences of the patient. And finally,

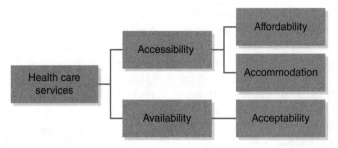

FIGURE 3-1 Interlocking Concepts Explaining Access to Health Care.

Modified from Wyszewianski, L. (2002). Access to Care: Remembering Old Lessons. Health Services Research, 37(6), 1441–1443. http://doi.org/10.1111/1475-6773.12171.

acceptability refers to the extent to which characteristics of both provider and patients are aligned in ways to provide a comfortable working relationship. An example would be the age, culture, religious beliefs, and ethnicity of each. Patients and families who receive care from providers of like characteristics may be more satisfied with these services. The idea is that this combination would promote a good relationship and higher quality communications.

In an Agency for Healthcare Research and Quality (AHRQ) update of the future directions for the National Healthcare Quality and Disparities Reports (Chapter 3), four quality of care components were identified. They include access, efficiency, care coordination, and a supportive health care system. Also in this report is clarity on the issue of what constitutes barriers to care.

Summarizing the literature on **health care utilization**, the report also clarified the relationship between utilization and quality care. In summary, barriers to care that result in differences in health care utilization may have a more significant impact on quality of care than other factors (e.g., insufficiencies in the health care workforce).

It has long been known that health care utilization is sensitive to patient-perceived health care needs and preferences. For example, despite the availability of some disease-prevention campaigns if the public does not see the need, care that is deemed to be of high quality will not occur. Furthermore, the report stated that greater utilization (use of health

care services) does not necessarily assure quality care. The report drew from the example that high use of inpatient services (hospital or emergency care) may be an indicator of poor access of outpatient services (clinics and care by primary care providers).

▶ History of Health Care Reform and Access to Health Care

Limited access and availability of health care is and has been the focus of health reform initiatives in the United States for a very long period of time. The history of health care reform is predicated on the idea that (1) too many citizens lack access to care and (2) poor access to care leads to low rates of health promotion and disease prevention, as well as early mortality rates. All this plays out in the context that **effective health care communications** between patients and providers are lacking.

Without access communications with health providers are severely curtailed. Poor access also means that assistance from providers is lacking; without this assistance (communication and intervention) patients and families are at the mercy of chronic illness, acquired injuries, and infectious diseases. Poor access and no or poor communications with providers equal delays in diagnoses and delays in timely and necessary medical intervention.

The challenges in U.S. health care delivery are poignantly outlined in national rates of morbidity and mortality in general and within high-risk groups. Heart disease, cancer, and chronic lower respiratory diseases were the leading causes of death in 2014, followed by accidents (unintentional injuries) and stroke. Heart disease and cancer together accounted for half of all deaths in the United States in 2014 (CDC, 2015) and remain the leading causes of mortality today.

Limited access and availability of health services are perceived, in part, to distinguish communities in the United States, meaning that some populations and communities are at greater risk for health disparities than others. For example, recent reports indicated that American and Alaska Natives born today have a life expectancy that is 4.4 years less than all other races in the United States (Indian Health Service: Disparities, 2017). While American Indians and Alaska Natives are at risk for mortality from heart disease and cancers, they also continue to die at higher rates than other Americans from many other diseases.

Considerable attention has been given to health care delivery trends and the potential impact of poor access. The National Center for Health Statistics (2012) reports changes over time in key health indicators. In a little over a decade (1997–2010), the annual costs of care increased from 11% to 15%. Furthermore, the percentage not receiving prescription drugs due to cost nearly doubled, and the percentage not receiving dental care due to cost also

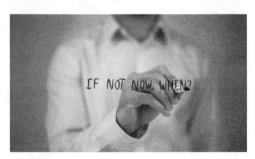

© Stockbakery/Shutterstock.

rose significantly. These statistics, rather than showing declining rates, have shown significant growth in costs of care.

While costs of care have climbed, and despite clear evidence that poor access to care prevails, especially in some high-risk groups, access to care has improved and has improved the health of millions of people in the United States. Major diseases have been prevented, and disabilities and injuries have been helped through access to health care. Furthermore, technology to perform early diagnoses of illness and treatment have improved the quality of life and longevity of patients. Recovery and improved quality of life and longevity have been shown in persons already experiencing key leading causes of death in the United States.

Still, our health care system is not helping enough. Despite improved medical technology, medical errors are the third leading cause of death in hospitals. Drug reactions are the fourth leading cause of death after heart disease, cancer, and stroke. Survival is unequally distributed across our population with deaths from major diseases varying by ethnicity and poverty level. Those impoverished and less advantaged are dying in greater numbers from these diseases than many of their more socially and economically privileged counterparts (National Center for Health Statistics).

The idea of gaps in health care to some communities in the United States resulting in disparities in health outcomes is closely related to accommodation and acceptability, and has been an ongoing concern and a subject of scrutiny. Explaining disparities in health care is complex. What is clear is that gaps in health care are evidenced in both the incidence and outcomes of disease.

The American Heart Association, in a policy statement about the future of cardiovascular disease (CVD) in the United States, raised the issue of disparities in incidence and outcomes stating that disparities are found in different socioeconomic groups and across geographical areas (Heidenreich et al., 2011).

Furthermore, it was emphasized that the existence of *primary* and *secondary* prevention of CVDs is less common in disadvantaged individuals and communities lending support to the concern that primary prevention is an issue and needs to be addressed through public health strategies. These public health strategies include arming all health providers with the tools to effectively communicate the need for prevention and a healthy life style.

With the backdrop of new vital statistics about health disparities and problems in access to care, renewed interest in universal health care reached a peak in the last decade and continues to be a focus of concern. It should be remembered that promoting universal health care has a long history.

There were, in fact, many attempts to secure access to health care dating back to the early 1800s. Following WWII, President Harry Truman called for support of universal health insurance. It was defeated in Congress. Another major milestone in supporting national health care reform occurred during the Clinton administration in 1993–1994. This plan required every U.S. citizen and permanent resident alien to become enrolled in a health plan. It specified both minimum coverage and maximum out-of-pocket costs. People below a certain income were to pay nothing. Like other health reform proposals, the idea was to support national health care while controlling the cost burden on citizens and permanent residents. This bill was met with opposition from both Republicans and Democrats as alternatives were put forward. In 1994, the compromise Democratic bill was declared dead in the Senate.

Next in line was the Patient Protection and Affordable Care Act (PPACA). This proposal, barring Congressional support, was signed into law on March 23, 2010. The Affordable Care Act (ACA) and PPACA are the same. The ACA was designed to address major deficits in the U.S. health care system. The problem of inadequate access for all

and insurmountable health care costs were the driving forces behind the reform. The expansion of the ACA evolved over the years postapproval, and certain care standards were put into place requiring everyone, excluding undocumented immigrants, to have health insurance coverage either through individual employer-based or government plans or to pay a penalty on their federal income tax. The limitations of the ACA have come center-stage as Congress struggles to replace the ACA with an alternative affordable option.

With any of the former attempts to establish universal coverage, the objective was not only to provide broader coverage but also to target poor care quality. The obvious was apparent: universal coverage is one thing, but more importantly, the effectiveness of care available to individuals was extremely important. Since the new legislation was enacted, several medical organizations and specialty groups weighed in on the potential impact on their selected practices. While support was expressed, the potential to increase health provider workloads with growing numbers of patients and concurrent increases in record keeping raised concerns. The fear was that these increases might take away from valuable time to have quality interactions with patients.

While the intentions behind health care reform were and continue to be needed and desired, the rollout has proven to be

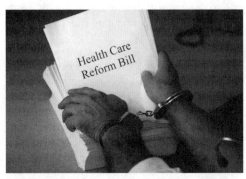

© Mikeledray/Shutterstock.

cumbersome and problematic. Growing reports of a lack of choice in insurance plans, unreasonable deductibles, and high premiums surfaced and led to concerted efforts to make major changes. One can understand that all of these results (lack of choice, unreasonable deductibles, and exceedingly high premiums) defeated the original intent of the ACA to guarantee access to health care to everyone.

▶ Disparities in Health Care Access

Despite any advances made in providing universal access to health care, disparities remain. Disparities in access refers to differences across individuals, communities, and countries in opportunities to access health care. The results are sometimes blatant inequities in access with the understanding that without opportunity and access to health care services the health and well-being for the less privileged will suffer.

The example of health disparities in American Indians and Alaska Natives in the United States was previously cited. Not only are these groups at risk for mortality from heart disease and cancers, but they also continue to die at higher rates than other Americans in many categories, including chronic liver disease and cirrhosis, diabetes mellitus, unintentional injuries, assault/homicide, intentional self-harm/suicide, and chronic lower respiratory diseases. A lower health status in these communities has been attributed to inadequate education, disproportionate poverty, discrimination in the delivery of health services, and cultural differences.

It should be no surprise that those who are less privileged may also be those who do not use advance technologies, such as patient portals and EHRs. For example, in a study focusing on disparities in EHR patient portal use in a large sample of patients attending nephrology clinics, older age, African American race, Medicaid status, and lower neighborhood median household income were associated with patients not accessing patient portals (Jhamb et al., 2015). It is possible that eHealth-use disparities could result in lower health status and greater health care disparities (Gordon & Hornbrook, 2016).

Recognizing both the consequences of disparities in access, the U.S. Department of Health and Human Services (HHS), AHRQ issued the National Healthcare Disparities Report (NHDR) (AHRQ, 2008). This report is a follow-up of the initial NHDR report in 2003. The NHDR 2008 is a 290-page report. The report is the product of an extensive collaboration among agencies at HHS and focuses upon differential access to care among subpopulations in the United States, identifying priority populations across many dimensions of care, including health care effectiveness, patient safety, timeliness of health care delivery, and patient centeredness. The purpose of the NHDR, mandated by Congress, was to identify differences and gaps and to track changes in these gaps or differences over time.

Data from core measures guided the analysis and formulation of the report on the quality of health care pertaining to a wide range of diseases and conditions—cancer, diabetes, end-stage renal disease, heart disease, HIV and AIDS, mental health and substance abuse, respiratory diseases, and care provided in nursing homes, home health, and hospice care. All age-range groups were addressed from children to older adults; furthermore, outcomes of care across racial and ethnic minorities, low-income groups, and residents of rural areas are compared and contrasted. Special emphasis was placed on "priority populations" defined as women, children, older adults, rural residents, and individuals with disabilities or special health care needs.

An alarming highlight of this report was that Americans too often not only do not receive needed care, but also may receive care that harms them (AHRQ, 2008, p. 1). The point was made that some receive worse care than others, supporting the idea that the quality of health care is different for different people and groups. Facilitators and barriers to health care was a specific focus of the report and was said to include a wide range of differences in patient, provider, and service-level factors. These include access to care differences, provider biases, poor provider–patient communication, and poor health literacy.

Although it is difficult to summarize even the entire Highlights section of the AHRQ, 2008 report, it is important to describe some examples of important findings. Several noteworthy findings summarized areas showing improvement and others showing that disparities remained the same or had gotten worse. For example, the following results indicated a decline in disparities.

- From 2000 to 2005, there was a decline in hospital discharges with complications for African Americans.
- From 2000 to 2005, the percentage of Asian women aged 40 or older reporting on having a mammogram in the last 2 years improved, resulting in a smaller gap between Asian and white women.

However, some data revealed disparities staying the same or getting worse. Those areas with the same or worsened outcomes included the following.

- Disparities increased in the percentage of adults 50 and over who received tests for colorectal cancer in four subgroups from 1999 to 2006.
- The number of African American and Hispanic patients experiencing a major depressive episode in the last 12 months who received treatment for depression in the same time period showed increased disparities.

- Additional disparities were noted in African American and Asian groups having worse disparities in receiving pneumococcal vaccinations for adults 65 and over.
- Disparities worsened in reports of adults receiving patient-centered care as an aspect of patient and provider communication, with African Americans and Asians showing worse disparities.

Historically, a series of reports and policies (Healthy People 2000, 2010, and 2020) all identified health disparities as a target for change, to reduce health disparities (Healthy People 2000), to eliminate health disparities (2010), and to achieve health equity and eliminate disparities (2020). On the horizon is the national report Healthy People 2030. The direction and aims of the report are briefly outlined and are available on the Office of Disease Prevention and Health Promotion (ODPHP) website, HealthyPeople. gov. A focus on equity and disparities is also a consideration in the Healthy People 2030 report, and the Federal Interagency Workgroup (FIW) is in place to guide the development of the framework for this report.

▶ Access Includes Navigating the Health Care System

Getting the best health care possible requires patients and families not only to have access to health care services but also have the ability to effectively navigate the health care system. Assuming some funding for access to care is in place, **navigating the health care system** is the next step in enabling patients to receive the care that is accessible.

Navigating the system presumes that there are not only facilitators to gaining access but also barriers or difficulties. Finding one's way through the system is essential, and difficult in the current complex and often fragmented system of care. For some time, guiding the patient to navigate the health care system was in the hands of the provider or provider group. The task is challenging and overwhelming in the context of the health care services these professionals already provide: health promotion and disease prevention, clinical assessments, diagnosis, treatment, and the management of treatment and recovery over time.

From the patient and family perspective, navigating the health care system is like making one's way through a maze, and this maze has several twists and turns. Not only does one have to navigate one's way through the basic insurance eligibility phase, but also through one's eligibility for the needed treatment and/or rehabilitation. The transition from hospital to home is a critical time when extra support and guidance is critical.

In an interesting study exploring the experiences of women who had survived ovarian cancer, system-based challenges were enumerated (Long et al., 2016). The authors explained that navigation of a complex ever-changing health care system can cause stress and could be detrimental to women's psychosocial well-being. The authors concluded that there was a need for a consistent, accessible care team and efficient delivery of resources. For these women, provider consistency, personal touch, and patient advocacy positively impacted their care experience. Their negative experiences were conceptualized as "little big things," which included system-based barriers or challenges (e.g., medical visit scheduling, wait times, pharmacy, transportation, parking, financial, insurance, and discharge).

In this publication, the recommendation of an accessible care team was emphasized. The continuity of patient–provider relationships in mastering the challenges of navigating the health care system has been previously recognized. *Nurse navigator* is a new role, not available on a wide scale, but has been shown to be helpful in assisting patients and families

navigate the complex health care system and selected health care settings. A nurse navigator generally plays the role of advocate and educator for the patient and patient's caregiver. Their primary focus is to remove barriers the patient and caregiver may experience during the course of the patient's illness. They will also monitor and coordinate patient care services. They are also prepared to give emotional support as well as tangible advice.

While nurse navigators can be found in most medical specialties, they are frequently assigned to cancer treatment centers with the understanding that the course of cancer treatment is complex and confusing. This care may be peppered with fears and concerns taxing patient and caregiver abilities to cope with the many decisions throughout the cancer care experience. In some cases, nurse navigators have also assisted patients with using health reform insurance exchanges. They may also be used to help consumers learn about their options and to purchase an insurance plan.

While the role of nurse navigator may be very helpful to patients, the role also presents challenges to effective communications between health professionals and patients, and subsequently for care coordination and continuity. Adding the navigator when there are numerous other social work and clinical professionals sometimes doing similar things can add to the patient's confusion and potentially can build a barrier between the patient and the patients' medical staff. This result is highly problematic, and nurse navigators are aware of this kind of result and work to minimize it.

Currently there are no guidelines to provide standards of care for nurse navigators. Where guidelines and supervision is absent, the need to oversee and manage the role is important. Additionally, if the navigator is not an official member of the clinical team and lacks professional qualifications, the advice given to patients could be problematic, and these problems may be missed by the clinical team.

Navigating effectively includes knowing how the system works, what will be asked and why, and who is available to assist the patient at each juncture of the care-giving process.

▶ Access No Guarantee of Effective Communication

Assuming we are able to ensure high rates of access to care and the availability of health care services (systems, institutions, and providers), is this a guarantee that effective communications between patients and providers will occur? The following is a discussion of this question.

As clearly described in the 2008 NHDR report, disparities in the quality of patient–provider communications exist across groups receiving health care services. Along these lines, it is important to understand that access is not a guarantee of effective patient–provider communications.

In the NHDR report, data were summarized from measures asking patients to evaluate communications on the dimension of "patient-centeredness" of their patient–provider communications. In a document describing the process of envisioning, the National Health Care Quality Report (Hurtado, Swift, & Corrigan, 2001), patient-centered care was defined as care respecting not only patients' needs but also their wants and preferences. It was also stressed that patients should have the education and support to participate in their care and in making decisions about their care. Patients surveyed were those that already had access to some level of health care service. They were asked about their perceptions of their care and the level of patient-centeredness of this care. The NHDR summarized the varying levels of self-perceived patient-centered care across different ethnic groups. For example, the perceptions of African Americans and Asian patients indicated that patient-centeredness in the context of patient–provider communications was deficient, and disparities were worse than previously reported.

In a paper reporting on interventions to promote patient-centered approaches to clinical consultations, Dwamena et al. (2012) stated that communication problems may be a result of health providers focusing on diseases and their management, rather than on the patient, their lives, and their health. In their extensive review of 43 randomized controlled trials, they summarized the effects of interventions aimed at promoting patient-centered care.

Reported positive effects of these interventions included greater clarity of patients' concerns and beliefs, better communication about treatment options, higher levels of empathy, greater patient perception of providers' attentiveness to them, and their concerns as well as their diseases. The results of these interventions, however, showed mixed findings, especially with respect to any possible effects on certain outcome measures (e.g., patient satisfaction, health behaviors, or health status).

A patient-centered communication approach to health care is a long-standing value in health care delivery systems and in the education of health providers across the board, no matter the specialty (general medicine, oncology, health promotion, or dental care). Patient-centered communication is linked not only to patient satisfaction and adherence to treatment but also to patients' levels of trust and engagement in the treatment process.

Having a primary care provider (PCP) as a source for care is an important indicator that access to care has been, at least in part, achieved. In fact, one survey question frequently asked to measure access to care is: "Do you have a primary care provider?" It is also thought that once assigned to a PCP, the patient will rely on this provider to help him or her gain access to other aspects of care (e.g., referral and assistance in getting access to a specialist, urgent care center, and health promotion programs). Otherwise, the PCP becomes the hoped-for-navigator in charge.

🚩 RED FLAG BOX: Access to Care Not a Guarantee of Effective Communication

The principle that access to care is not a guarantee of effective communication is an important one. The following example of a patient with a potential ankle fracture illustrates this phenomenon. The patient tries to explain her experience, but providers do not listen carefully.

A 37-year-old woman in good health takes her dog for a walk on a rainy day up a steep grade. She slips and slides down the hill and is unable to get up and walk on her left leg. The emergency medical team (EMT) is called to the site and transports the woman to the nearest hospital emergency room (ER). On her trip to the ER, she hears the EMT offer the comment: "It isn't a fracture you have no swelling." She arrives at the hospital and is seen by the ER nurse on duty and an on-call physician who conducts a brief interview. She explains her symptoms and what happened to all staff who approach her. She keeps repeating her story in hopes the staff will see the seriousness of her injury. She is left alone in the exam room to wait for the on-call physician. The nurse on duty prepares a splint to support a sprain.

Discussion

The woman has access to care and at least two professional health providers trained in emergency medicine. The ER physician decides to take an X-ray and discovers a fracture. The physician says: "You're lucky. If there was more than one fracture, we would have admitted you (to the hospital)." The discharge nurse prepares a stabilizing splint and gives the patient crutches and directions to come back within 3 days to the orthopedic division of the hospital for follow-up. She has never used crutches.

She calls for a follow-up appointment, and there are no available appointments for a week. She explains that she has a doctor's order to be seen before that, but the receptionist emphatically states there are no available appointments. Based upon her experience, how would this statement be received and how much trust would this woman have in the care she has received thus far? Now the patient is experiencing the disjointed nature of the communication between the ER and the hospital's Orthopedic outpatient department. In addition to feeling not being listened to, she is facing problems in navigating this complex relationship between the ER and Orthopedic division.

Feeling concerned and frustrated, the patient talks to a friend, and the friend tells her that it sounds worse than a simple fracture. Her friend takes her to an orthopedic specialty outpatient center where more X-rays were taken and a second fracture was discovered, making it a bilateral, double-fracture. Surgery was scheduled immediately.

Now, the nature and degree of disjointed care becomes clear. Communications at many levels, patient to EMT, ER staff to patient, and the referring hospital's Orthopedic department to patient, may not initially appear problematic. However, the ultimate outcome illustrates the role of ineffective communications that can be detrimental.

It can be argued that having a PCP is the first line of defense in warding off illness and promoting health, but it can also be argued that being assigned a PCP is not enough. PCPs can develop trusting sustainable relationships with their patients while providing health care services. However, as is true in all patient–provider communications, the quality of communication between the PCP and patient is critical and is directly linked to the likelihood that patients will receive appropriate and safe patient care services (Daker-White et al., 2015).

There is a good deal of literature describing effective communications between the patient and their families and health providers, and this literature will be addressed in several other chapters of the text. Most importantly, the emphasis on patient–family-centered communication in the literature is pervasive. An important insight underlying the support for patient–family-centered communication is the notion that patients' access to health care does not ensure that patients and their families will take advantage of the availability of these health care services. This is an issue of patient *utilization* of services.

It is important to understand that in addition to the several potential barriers within health care (e.g., cost, available resources, and institutions), patient factors influence whether these services are accessed. These factors include health literacy, perceptions of health and illness, social support, as well as demographic characteristics (e.g., age, gender, and cultural and religious beliefs).

Beyond these inherent potential barriers to navigating health care is the potential positive impact effective communications between the patient and health care provider can have. While this might be communications between any provider interfacing with the patient, the idea of the power of effective communication is based chiefly on an understanding of the potential outcomes of a sustained patient–provider relationship with one's PCP. Universal health care coverage is associated with the idea that every individual has an equal chance of having a sustained relationship with a PCP, and thus an equal opportunity for effective patient–provider communications.

🔍 CITED STUDY: Community-Based Breast Health Navigation Program

Access to community services as adjuncts to routine medical care has been studied for their positive effects on access to health care screenings. Adjunctive community services are important because they offer additional outreach to underserved populations and provide the messages (communication) needed to enable these communities to navigate the health care system and achieve the best health outcomes possible. These added services may be particularly helpful to people living in areas with minimal access to medical facilities. The following study examined the impact of a community-based mammogram programs on women's breast cancer screening behavior in St. Louis, Missouri.

Drake, B. F., Tannan, S., Anwuri, V. V., Jackson, S., Sanford, M., Tappenden, J., … Colditz, G. A. (2015). A community-based partnership to successfully implement and maintain a breast health navigation program. *Journal of Community Health, 40*(6), 1216–1223. doi:10.1007 /s10900-015-0051-z

The authors of this study emphasize that a breast cancer screening with appropriate follow-up and treatment reduces breast cancer deaths. The program caring for women in clinics providing mammography screening services found that women may not receive their annual exam and can be lost to follow-up, putting them at risk for untreated diseases. Based upon this knowledge, the clinic designed and implemented a patient navigation program in a partner clinic. Their objectives were to identify women overdue for a mammogram and increase mammography utilization.

The program identified and worked around patient-reported and system-level barriers to receiving a mammogram as well as follow-up post-screening visits.

Nearly all women participating in the program completed mammography. Cost was the commonly cited barrier to mammography. The authors concluded that such outreach programs were necessary to remove structural and financial barriers for accessing these preventive services.

▶ Summary

Wide-scale access to and the availability of health care services is critical to the health and well-being of our population as a whole, and our communities in particular. Access and availability directly impact patient–family–provider communications. The most obvious example of this is the idea is that without access and availability, patient–family–provider communications are nonexistent. Both directly and indirectly through quality patient–provider communications, access and availability are strong predictors of health, well-being, and longevity.

As detailed in this chapter, other key concepts are related to the constructs of access to and availability of care. These are affordability, accommodation, and acceptability. An increase in access to and availability of health care to all has been a longstanding goal of U.S. public policy. To this end, health care reform has and is legislated to impact increased access to and availability of health care services. This legislation is expected to change on a wide-scale communications between patients and providers by affording persons the opportunity to have a PCP and second, by ensuring they have support for navigating the complex health care system.

In this chapter, we discussed the context of health care in our evolving national health plan and made the point that mere access and availability is neither a guarantee of good communications nor a promise of high-quality health care for everyone. Despite any advances made in providing universal access to health care, disparities remain. Disparities in access refers to differences across individuals and communities in opportunities to access health care. The results are sometimes blatant inequities in access with the understanding that without opportunity to access health care services, the health and well-being for the less privileged will suffer.

Finally, providing patients and their families the support they need to effectively navigate the health care system is important but not easily achieved. For example, patients and their families need support and guidance in navigating the complex health care system, and this function frequently rests on the shoulders of the clinical provider team. Such responsibilities can overwhelm professional health providers assigned to deliver clinical care, and because of this, may be lacking or only periodically addressed.

If providers cannot help the patient and patient's family navigate the system, *real* access to care may be significantly impaired. Access at a very basic level then becomes unachievable despite universal access to health care that is affordable. This curious phenomenon, access but not accessibility, is concerning and significantly impacts those who have long histories of suffering health care disparities (particularly the poor and illiterate).

With this in mind, new roles have been designed (e.g., that of the nurse navigator). While there is a need for this new role, a number of concerns surround its implementation. Adding another role can add to the complex, confusing delivery system. This is particularly concerning if there is no direct line of communication between the navigator and the professional health care team. If there is a lack of coordination between the navigator and the health care team, the navigator may go outside the boundaries of the role and even recommend something that is counter to what the clinical team is striving to do. Additionally, the role may build still another barrier to the direct communication between the health professional and the patient and/or patient's family.

Finally, if and when the national health care delivery system is able to ensure high rates of access to care and availability of health care services (systems, institutions, and providers), there is no guarantee that effective communications between patients and providers will follow. A patient–family-centered communication approach in the delivery of health care has long-standing support from health care delivery systems and in the education of health providers across the board, no matter the specialty (general medicine, oncology, health promotion, dental care, etc.).

Patient–family-centered communication is linked not only to patient and family satisfaction and adherence to treatment but also to their level of trust and engagement in the treatment process. Finally, a patient–family-centered communication approach has been associated with positive treatment outcomes, improving not only the health and well-being of patients but also their functional and social capacity. In the next section of this text, Health Care Communications: Foundations for Understanding Communications in Health Care Settings, the relationship of patient–provider communication and quality care is discussed, further emphasizing the importance of the art and science of communication in achieving national health care policy.

Discussion

1. What is the difference between *access* to health care and *availability* of health care services?
2. How can limited access and limited availability of health care services impact patient–provider communications?
3. According to the Institute of Medicine, what three distinct steps are important in the access to health services?
4. Is it possible to ensure access to care to everyone when the availability of health care services is lacking?
5. Does access to and availability of health care automatically mean that patient–provider communications are effective?

References

Agency for Healthcare Research and Quality. (AHRQ). (2008). *National healthcare disparities report 2008.* Chapter 3, Access to healthcare. Washington, DC: AHRQ. Retrieved from http://www.ahrq.gov/sites/default/files/wysiwyg/research/findings/nhqrdr/nhdr08/nhdr08.pdf

Centers for Disease Control and Prevention. *Center for health statistics including data on chronic disease prevention and health promotion*, CDC, USA.gov.

Daker-White, G., Hays, R., McSharry, J., Giles, S., Cheraghi-Sohi, S., Rhodes, P., & Sanders, C. (2015). Blame the patient, blame the doctor or blame the system? A meta-synthesis of qualitative studies of patient safety in primary care. *PloS ONE, 10*(8), e0128324. doi.org/10.1371/journal.pone.0128329

Drake, B. F., Tannan, S., Anwuri, V. V., Jackson, S., Sanford, M., Tappenden, J., ... Colditz, G. A. (2015). A community-based partnership to successfully implement and maintain a breast health navigation program. *Journal of Community Health, 40*(6), 1216–1223. doi:10.1007/s10900-015-0051-z

Dwamena, F., Holmes-Rovner, M., Gaulden, C. M., Jorgenson, S., Sadigh, G., Sikorskii, A., ... Olomu, A. (2012). Interventions for providers to promote a patient-centered approach in clinical consultations. *Cochrane Database System Reviews, 12*, CD003267.

Gordon, N. P., & Hornbrook, M. C. (2016). Differences in access to and preferences for using patient portals and other eHealth technologies based on race, ethnicity, and age: A database and survey study of seniors in a large health plan. *Journal of Medical Internet Research, 18*(3), e50. doi:10.2196/jmir.5105

Heidenreich, P. A., Trogdon, J. G., Khavjou, O. A., Butler, J., Dracup, K., Ezekowitz. M. D., ... Woo, Y. J. (2011). Forecasting the future of cardiovascular disease in the United States: A policy statement from the American Heart Association. *Circulation, 123*, 933–944. doi:10.1161/CIR.0b013e31820a55f5

Hurtado, M. P., Swift, E. K., & Corrigan, J, M. (2001). *Envisioning the national health care quality report.* Washington, DC: National Academies Press.

Indian Health Service, U.S. Department of Health and Human Services. (2017). *Fact sheet: Disparities.* Retrieved from his.com

Jhamb, M., Cavanaugh, K. L., Bian, A., Chen, G., Ikizler, A., Unruh, M. L., & Abdel-Kader, K. (2015). Disparities in electronic health record patient portal use in nephrology clinics. *Clinical Journal of Social Nephrology, 10,* 2013–2022. doi:10.2215/CJN.01640215

National Center for Health Statistics (US). (2012, May). *Health, United States, 2011: With special feature on socioeconomic status and health.* Hyattsville, MD: National Center for Health Statistics (US). Retrieved from https://www.ncbi.nlm.nih.gov/books/NBK98752/

Long, R. K., Angarita, A. M., Cristello, A., Lippitt, M., Haider, A. H., Bowie, J. V., ... Tergas, A. I. (2016, December). "Little Big Things": A qualitative study of ovarian cancer survivors and their experiences with the health care system. *Journal of Oncology Practice, 12*(1), e974–e980. doi:10.1200/JOP.2015.007492

U.S. Department of Health and Human Services, Office of Disease Prevention and Health Promotion. (2008). *Healthy People 2030: Healthy people overview.* Retrieved from http://www.healthypeople.gov

Wyszewianski, L. (2002). Access to care: Remembering old lessons. *Health Services Research, 37*(6), 1441–1443. doi:10.1111/1475-6773.12171

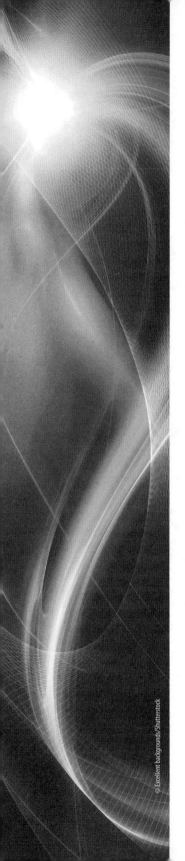

PART II

Foundations for Understanding Communications in Health Care

Part I of this text introduced *the context* of health care communications describing important national and global needs and goals in health care driving changes in the way providers communicate with patients and with each other. This discussion provided meaning to the circumstances facing the design and implementation of programs and strategies to improve communications to achieve quality patient care and effective communications across and between health care teams. Part II of this text turns to *concepts* and *principles* giving definition and description to the unique aspects of human communications.

There is much to know about the phenomena of human communication in health care. Interpersonal communication not only one of the most important of the basic life skills, but also one of the most important in achieving therapeutic goals with patients and their families. Patients and providers are humans first and differ by roles they perform. Patients request help, inform providers, and share thoughts and feelings with providers. In turn, providers enlist help from patients to achieve therapeutic outcomes, educate and inform them, and convey perspectives and predictions about expected outcomes of therapy and treatment.

Successful professional role development in the health professions depends on our knowledge and understanding of communication concepts and our competence in using interpersonal communication skills in a wide variety of health care settings. In few professions are interpersonal communication skills more important than in the health professions. As such, they have been studied extensively in health care delivery systems. Knowing principles and concepts of communication are generic and critical to patient–provider relationships.

Chapter 4, *Principles of Human Communication*, addresses the *anatomy* and *physiology* of human communications. The sensory modalities, information processing functions of the brain, and the role of memory and concentration are reviewed. The verbal and nonverbal dimensions of communications; the meta-communicative value of messages; and the basis for deficits in perception, processing, and transmittal of messages are discussed. Patients have a wide range of strengths and deficits in communicating effectively. Patients exhibit many strengths in human communications, and providers can engage these strengths when assessing their health status and educating them about medical treatment.

Still, for many, significant deficits exist and can impair their ability to communicate. These deficits may be a function of their health condition. For example, those suffering a stroke on the left side of the brain might have impaired speech and language (aphasia). Aphasia does not affect intelligence, but does influence patients' ability to verbally express their thoughts and feelings, and their speech is frequently jumbled, fragmented, or impossible to understand.

Chapter 5, *The Nature of Therapeutic Communications*, addresses an essential quality of health provider communications with patients. Communication must be *therapeutic* rather than being *nontherapeutic*. This chapter defines and compares and contrasts these two phenomena. Using therapeutic response modes and resisting nontherapeutic responses, which are frequently feeling-based and ill-planned, are addressed. Therapeutic response modes elicit elaboration and engage patients in active decision-making. In contrast, nontherapeutic response modes can cause patients to withdraw and clamp down and can lead to patients' withdrawing from treatment or passively resisting the provider's advice and guidance. Examples and the rationale behind the use of therapeutic response modes are presented.

Chapter 6, *Cultural Similarities and Differences and Communication*, addresses the need to avoid cultural blurring and improve effective communication in cross-cultural contexts. In this chapter, the importance of *cultural competence* is stressed. In a larger context, this includes *speaking the language* of the patient. Patients seeking health care may have limited English proficiency, but beyond their English language skills, their cultural beliefs and values may differ from Western medical and health care practices. Examples of specific responses are discussed because they can potentially carry different interpretations across groups. Communication fluency across groups is presented as a continuum, with cultural incompetent behaviors at the negative end of the spectrum and cultural competence at the valued opposite end of the spectrum.

It is not necessary to deliberate very long about the importance of communication to our roles as providers. What providers generally do not comprehend is that communication is both a science as well as an art. It is inconceivable that any text on applied communications would ignore the basic principles and concepts that have been culled from years of study of human communication.

CHAPTER 4

Principles of Human Communication

CHAPTER OBJECTIVES

- Identify and describe the sensory modalities and how sensory modalities transmit messages to the brain.
- Describe the process of sensory awareness and sensory receptivity.
- Describe ways in which perceptions affect the emotional experience of individuals.
- Explain how learning is a stimulus-processing activity.
- Discuss the interpersonal aspects of communication and how interpersonal communication may be either symmetrical or complementary.

KEY TERMS

- Analogic communication
- Autonomic nervous system (ANS)
- Bilateral symmetry of the brain
- Coding
- Corpus callosum
- Decoding
- Digital communication
- Encoding
- Limbic system
- Multidimensional communication
- Optical illusions
- Parasympathetic nervous system
- Principle of multidimensionality
- Reception
- Selective attention/selective inattention
- Sensory modalities
- Sensory modality strength
- Sensory transduction
- Split-brain
- Symmetrical or complementary communications
- Sympathetic nervous system

▶ Introduction

Human communication is the product of a combination of numerous physiological, psychological, social, and environmental influences. Patterns of communication are indeed difficult to understand without knowing the origins and intricacies of communication in their relationship to not only neurological functioning—particularly the workings of the central nervous system, but also the dynamics of communication in the interpersonal context.

The purpose of this chapter is to introduce concepts and summarize principles that enable us to better understand the process of human communication. From the standpoint of biophysiology, these include how sensory **reception** of information occurs, the basis for distortions of sensory experience, the processing function of the brain, and sensory and feedback mechanisms and learning. Axioms of human communication that address the origins of communication in interpersonal interactions are also discussed.

▶ Sensory Awareness and Sensory Receptivity

The Sensory Modalities

Recognition that sensory awareness and sensory processing is critical to understanding human communication leads us to consider basic concepts and principles about **sensory modalities**. There are five sensory modes: sight, smell, taste, touch, and hearing. In addition to these senses, humans also have the capacity to use the sense of balance, pressure, temperature, pain, and motion. While all senses play a role, the most salient sensory modalities to further our understanding of human communications in health care are the visual, auditory, and kinesthetic (helping

to control and coordinate activities such as walking and talking) modalities. Some individuals are particularly adept with the use of one modality (i.e., are better at picking up visual rather than auditory clues); others are multimodal, exhibiting strength in more than one modality. People are not exactly the same, and their capacities are capable of changing over time and in the context of our experience. To a certain degree, providers can train themselves to be more adept in using our senses.

Studies of the relative strength of one modality over another such as reported in the classical work of Gazda, Childers, and Walters (1982) suggest that age and maturation influence whether individuals are strong in only one modality or have mixed **sensory modality strength**. Several of the classic investigations in modality use and preferences have occurred in the field of education because identifying student strengths and limitations in the use of sensory modalities is important in designing educational programs that will be effective with students. Modality strengths refer to the channels of communication most efficient for processing information. Modality strengths can occur with a single channel or involve two or more channels. Conversely, modality weaknesses are those channels least efficient for processing information and learning. The most frequently reported strengths are visual acuity or mixed modality.

Our preferences for one modality over another can change over time and in relation to our health and previous and current experiences. For example, primary grade school children may learn better with auditory rather than visual channels, but entering middle school their strengths shift and vision becomes the dominant modality. These changes are addressed in a landmark theory about the development of modality strength (Barbe & Milone, 1981). Children have shown a developmental sequence of modality strengths with well-defined

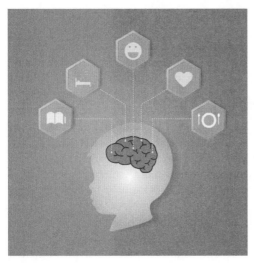

© Kan2d/Shutterstock.

auditory strengths in grade school. As they progress through elementary school, their modalities become mixed and interdependent, shifting toward the visual and kinesthetic. By adulthood, many people have mixed-modality strength.

Other researchers, however, contend that vision is the dominant modality of the species. But to conclude that vision dominates our experience may be a simplistic notion. Schifferstein (2006) points out that this idea implies that people always experience the world based on the visual information they receive. Such an interpretation is likely to discount the task at hand or activity in which people are involved, objects encountered, or the context of the situation. Schifferstein adds that people are more likely to use their sensory abilities differently depending on the task, such as driving a car or having a massage. Schifferstein's study revealed when asked to evaluate products vision was the most important sensory modality, but for half the products evaluated the importance of vision was lower than for one of the other sensory modalities (e.g., touch, smell, audition).

Countering the idea that vision is dominant across the board is also addressed in studies of individuals, groups, and societies. Modality preferences have been shown to vary as a function of age and societal influences, but not as a matter of gender, race or ethnicity, or primary language spoken. Mixed modality strengths are found more frequently in adults than in children. Those in less industrialized societies may differ in sensory modality preferences, but it is unknown whether age is a more significant determinant than societal influences. The debate continues, with some researchers claiming that adults are primarily visually oriented versus multimodal. While age might make a difference in our sensory strengths, it might be the same for all people across gender, race, ethnicity, and primary language spoken.

Of course, in the process of communication, all modalities work together to influence self-expression and our understanding of objects, tasks, and environment. A clear delineation of the strength or weaknesses within a given person may be difficult to establish. Still, researchers, particularly educators, are interested in the issue of modality variability and dominant modality in hopes of being able to predict and engage patterns of communication and patterns of problem solving when teaching different age groups.

While auditory modality strength is apparent in primary grade school children, teachers use multiple means to reinforce learning in this age group. They tap into both auditory and visual sensory modes and may explain that for this age group, both modes are used to reinforce a learning task because children forget what they are told and benefit from visual demonstration of facts and ideas.

Perhaps one of the most misunderstood aspects of sensory awareness is the assumption that the purpose of our sensory apparatus is to give us complete information about all the stimuli in our environment. In truth, our sensory capabilities are not designed to give us information in this way; the major purpose is to give us a very select range of feedback that is most useful to us at the moment. From studies of nonhumans (e.g., bees and other insects, as well as bats), it is known that some sights and sounds that are perceived by other species are not available to us. And, like many animal species, humans tend to be sensitive to only a certain range of stimuli—the stimuli most useful to our way of life. What distinguishes humans from other species is that humans can generally access a wider range of stimuli, and these stimuli are unique to our way of life.

Even humans, however, have been shown to have selective perceptual abilities despite a broader range of stimuli to select from. For example, people can taste the sweetness in certain foods and the bitter taste of some poisons (at low concentrations), but fail to discern other tastes that are neither harmful nor helpful. Our sense of smell is highly attuned to many gases, but insensitive to others such as nitrogen. In short, our capacity to perceive through our senses is biologically regulated, and these capacities are largely determined by the information that would be most helpful to us.

This principle of utility also applies to how and why one becomes selective throughout their lives. Utility for certain information changes as people grow. Consider for a minute an infant's capacity to perceive separation from a nurturing figure. While other stimuli are not meaningful, distance or nearness of the nurturing figure is critical to the infant. Our training and occupations can also influence our perceptual range. Law enforcement professionals are keenly aware of, and even exceedingly perceptive about, certain environmental threats. These capacities are not found in adults who work in other fields.

Repeated exposures to environmental cues influence our awareness of our surroundings, and repeated exposures to life-threatening conditions reinforce the need to accurately and quickly perceive environmental clues that may suggest danger. Providers' keen awareness of a patient about to experience a life-threatening change due to a significant decline or injury is a function of exposure to these situations and why some people become more acutely aware of the patient's physical and emotional cues through repeated experience. It also explains why lack of exposure to patients is likely to make providers more acutely attuned but less knowledgeable about how to interpret what they see.

Another important example of selective perception among groups of humans is that of pain. Pain is a perceptual phenomenon (Gregory et al., 2013). It arises from information gathered by pain receptors in tissue, modified by spinal and supraspinal mechanisms, and integrated as a discrete sensory experience (Gregory et al., 2013). People assign emotional meaning in the brain. The sensation of pain has strong motivational properties. In general, pain is to be avoided. Still, the perceived intensity and quality of pain varies a great deal. Pain stimuli can be the same, yet affect people differently. It is known from observations of athletes that serious injuries may be experienced with little pain. There are still other people who report extreme levels of pain when the injury or illness does not seem to justify the level of complaint. Does this also mean that some patients will require more medication than others with the same pain stimulus? This question is answered by the fact people experience pain differently, but also that the same pain stimuli can be perceived differently by the same person, depending on time and context, even when the stimulus for pain has not changed at all.

In a compelling review by Grahek and Dennett (2011), the distinction between pain without painfulness and painfulness without pain is made. They explain that the experience of pain is complex and not the same for everyone. It comprises sensory-discriminative, emotional-cognitive, and behavioral components which operate together but may be disconnected and exist separately. That is, one can experience pain but not feel in pain.

In patient care situations, providers commonly ask their patients to describe and rate their experiences of pain. It is expected that patients can answer with the needed information to determine a course of action. Health providers ask them, for example, to rate the level of their pain on a scale from 1 to 10, with 10 being the worse pain they have ever had. But, is our assumption faulty when patients are experiencing pain but not painfulness? If it is true that they have lost their access to cognitive and sensory-discriminative components, they may be unable to answer our question because they do not associate their pain with painfulness.

It is also known that health care professionals can alter patients' experiences of pain by changing their perceptions of the stimuli. When dentists say to a patient, "You're doing fine—just a little more (drilling)," or "this is going to 'sting' a little" (numbing the gum), they are swaying the patient's perception of the character of the stimuli. If a provider suggests that a pain experience is "a tug," "a needle prick," or a "dull" sensation, the patient's experience of the character of the sensation of pain might change. Additionally, the suggestion that pain will subside and relief is soon, it affects patients' perception of whether the pain stimulus is overwhelming or uncontrollable.

Understanding that the pain is temporary and/or within their control enables them to relax. Furthermore, relaxation reduces the negative experience of pain. Fear is a mediating cognitive appraisal that, when eased through relaxation or reassurance, will influence the patients' experiences of the sensation of pain. Most providers understand their role in helping patients manage discomfort and pain and will use the power of suggestion in helping their patients cope with pain stimuli.

Patients themselves are thought to be able to alter, at least in part, their experience of pain and other distressing emotions by altering their perceptions of thoughts and feelings. In the arena of cognitive psychotherapy, examples of reframing one's interpretations of situations have relevance here. One can perceive his or her life or relationships as "hopeless." Feelings of hopelessness generally increase anxiety and depression related to this observation and interpretation. However, if the perception of one's life situation is changed (e.g., a challenge is not hopeless), negative feelings of depression and anxiety seem to lessen, and one is able to adopt a more positive approach to problem solving life circumstances. The idea is that if cognitions, assumptions, and beliefs can be modified, one can change one's emotions and behaviors accordingly. Critical to a full analysis of the role of perception is knowledge of how stimulus awareness is processed in the brain.

▶ Processing Stimuli and the Brain

Through the Sensory Modalities to the Brain

When physical energy such as light, sound, heat, or cold reaches the sensory organs, it must be converted to a form that can be processed in the brain. The information processing that goes on within the brain has three distinct steps.

The first step is simply *reception*, the absorption of physical energy. **Sensory transduction** is the second step and refers to the conversion of physical energy to an electrochemical pattern in the neurons. Finally, **coding** takes place (**FIGURE 4-1**).

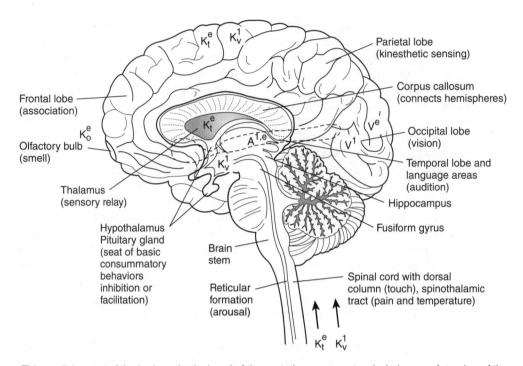

This medial aspect of the brain and spinal cord of the central nervous system includes a surface view of the temporal lobe, with language areas illustrated in dotted lines. Projection sites for receiving information through the sensory modalities are plotted with the following abbreviations:

$A^{1,e}$ = auditory input, both internal and external.

V^e = visual input in the occipital lobe, external.

V^1 = visualization in the deeper striate layers of the occipital lobe or temporal lobe.

K_o^e = kinesthetic input from sense of smell, external.

K_t^e = kinesthetic input from touch, external. The nerve signals move up the spinal cord in the dorsal column, are relayed through the thalamus, and are projected to the sensory cortex of the parietal lobe.

K_v^1 = kinesthetic input from pain and temperature, internal, visceral. The nerve signals move up the spinal cord in the spinothalamic tract, are processed in the hypothalamus, and are projected to the sensory cortex of the parietal lobe.

FIGURE 4-1 Medial View of Brain and Spinal Cord.

Reprinted from G. M. Gazda, W. C. Childers, and R. P. Walters, *Interpersonal Communication—A Handbook for Health Professionals*, p. 30, © 1982, Aspen Publishers, Inc.

Coding is the one-to-one correspondence between some part of the physical stimulus and some aspect of the nervous system. For example, light rays that strike retinal receptors (reception) are converted due to a change in the receptors' membrane polarization (transduction). The resulting train of impulses in the optic nerve has a frequency that increases as the intensity of light increases. This is evidence of coding. It should be remembered that sensory information is coded so that the brain can process it, and, interestingly enough, it may have little resemblance to the original stimuli. The idea that what is perceived is not exactly what may be, at least in the eyes of others, is an extremely important principle of human communication. The proverb "Believe half of what you see and nothing of what you hear" has some basis when one considers the fact that one always perceives selectively, and these perceptions were chosen among many.

It is possible, for example, to create **optical illusions**. Optical illusions exist because what is perceived is actually different from what is actually there. One very common example of an optical illusion is provided in **FIGURE 4-2**. When looking at one line with one eye and the other line with the other eye, the illusion is apparent. This optical illusion, the Müller–Lyer illusion, suggests that one line may be longer than the other; usually line B is reported to be longer than line A. In fact, these lines are of the same length. Various theories used to explain optical illusions generally agree that what causes optical illusions is within the brain, not within the sensory organ (eye). To experiment with your own response to optical illusions, online examples are available through the Web (search for keywords *Illusions* and *Paradoxes: Seeing Is Believing*).

The important principle to understand is that our perceptions are not the same thing as the stimuli that are picked up by our sensory receptors. An important line of study is the appearance of hallucinations in individuals experiencing mental illness (e.g., schizophrenia). Hallucinations are involuntary and can occur in the absence of any external stimuli. Thus, a person sees or hears something that is not there. How is this possible? Early on, Silbersweig and Stern (1998) explored these questions in human auditory neuroimaging studies. They were able to gather information about normal and abnormal conscious and unconscious brain states. Their work was important in understanding how the brain can literally create its own reality—it can be conscious of something that is not even there. This raises the issue of whether and how the brain responds to internal stimuli versus an external stimulus.

Using the example of faulty perceptions in persons with schizophrenia, the intrinsic deficit in their perceptual abilities can be understood. Schizophrenia is a severe psychiatric disorder, which includes not only perceptual impairment termed *positive symptoms* (delusions, hallucinations, and disorganized thoughts), but also negative symptoms (apathy, lack of motivation or avolition-apathy, and speech disturbance or alogia) as the disease progresses.

Cognitive deficits impacting memory also appear and are considered to be core symptoms in schizophrenia. Although studies of schizophrenia have typically focused on deficits in higher-order processes such as working memory and executive function, there is an increasing realization that deficits can be found throughout the cortex and are manifest even at the level of early sensory processing (Javitt & Sweet, 2015, p. 535). This is reflected in either impaired sensory precision, which would indicate neural dysfunction without sensory temporal regions of the brain, or increased distractibility, which would indicate impaired prefrontal function.

Cognitive dysfunction is a common, significant, and enduring feature of schizophrenia. These researchers found that sensory processing dysfunction, specifically in patients' ability to match auditory tones even

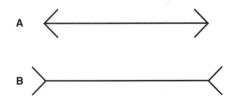

Müller-Lyer Illusions
Which Horizontal Line Segment is Longer: A or B?

FIGURE 4-2 Optical Illusions Perceptions Are Not Direct Reflections of Stimuli.

without distracting stimuli, were impaired. This dysfunction was particularly severe in a subgroup of patients who had poor treatment outcomes and who were more likely to need residential treatment. Recent reports on computational modeling of functional brain networks in functional magnetic resonance imaging (fMRI) indicate that understanding of higher cognitive functioning in schizophrenia is possible and reveal disruption in cognitive functioning in these patients (Dauvermann et al., 2014).

The human brain is a complicated system. Information processing starts with input from the sensory organs or modalities which transform physical stimuli such as pain, cold, loud noise (sound waves), or light. When sensory information reaches the brain, higher and more complex processing takes place. The human brain consists of as many as 100 billion neurons varying in size from 4 microns (0.004 mm) to 100 microns (0.1 mm) in diameter. Neurons are cells that send and receive electrochemical signals to and from the brain and nervous system.

These neurons are not haphazardly arranged. They are assembled in discrete areas of the brain, and these areas have their own specialized function. Still, people have the experience of unity. Thus, although their brains are divided into many parts, each containing many neurons, their consciousness is as one. The unity of consciousness comes from the many connections between various brain parts.

The **bilateral symmetry of the brain** provides that sights and sounds, which bring information in from the external environment, are processed by using both cerebral hemispheres together. The two hemispheres are connected by the **corpus callosum** for the transfer of information. In the normal brain, it appears that any information reaching one hemisphere is communicated regularly to the other, largely to corresponding regions.

Until the early 1950s, the function of the corpus callosum was not known. In the past it was, on occasion, cut by a neurosurgeon (e.g., to treat epilepsy or to reach a deep tumor in the pituitary gland). Scientists and researchers have reported anatomical, physiological, and behavioral discoveries about the specialization of the cerebral hemispheres. Experimental research findings followed to support the conclusion that if an individual is involved primarily in attending to internal visual images and fantasies, the person is less likely to be accurate in detecting external visual cues. And, if internal processing is primarily oriented around auditory fantasies (i.e., imagined conversations or music), then the person is less likely to be accurate in detecting external auditory signals.

Individuals look to the side or down to eliminate visual stimuli, especially the meaningful and reinforcing face of another person that might interfere with a train of thought. Dilts, Grinder, Bandler, DeLozier, and Cameron-Bandler (1979), in their landmark book *Neurolinguistic Programming*, illustrated the eye positions for visual, auditory, and kinesthetic accessing of information. They also identified each eye position with its particular body posture, breathing pattern, and hemispheric specialization (see **FIGURE 4-3**).

The right movements of the eyes access the left cerebral hemisphere for visual constructed (V_c) images, for visualization of novel and abstract patterns, or for auditory constructed experiences (A_c), putting an idea into words. The eyes looking down and to the right access an awareness of body sensations and kinesthetic information, including the kinesthetic visceral, tactile, and olfactory (K_{vto}). The left movements of the eyes access the right cerebral hemisphere for visual remembered (V_r) images, for visualization of eidetic patterns from past experiences, or for auditory remembered (A_r) experiences, and sounds and tape loops of messages from past activities. The eyes looking down and to the left are

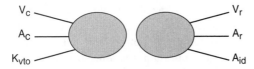

FIGURE 4-3 Eye Positions for Accessing Information. Visual accessing cues for a normally organized right-handed person: V_c = visual constructed; A_c = auditory constructed; K_{vto} = kinesthetic visceral, tactile, or olfactory; V_r = visual remembered; A_r = auditory remembered; A_{id} = auditory internal dialogue.

representative of an auditory internal dialogue (A_{id}), talking to oneself, probably in short cryptic commands and suggestions and simple sentence messages (see Figure 4-3).

The left cerebral hemisphere is associated with the development of speech and language. The temporal lobe is larger on the left side than on the right in about two-thirds of the brains examined. The left side is best developed in the brain of the fetus and newborn infants, suggesting that asymmetry does not result from environmental or developmental factors after birth. Electrophysiological experiments using auditory (click) and visual (flash) stimuli were designed to measure the evoked responses in the brains of both adults and 5-week-old infants. The results showed that auditory responses are significantly greater in the left hemisphere and visual in the right. It appeared that the fundamental auditory neurocircuitry needed for the growth of speech and language is biologically and asymmetrically designed for both initial acquisition and further development.

Early research indicated that the right ear may outperform the left ear in hearing and identifying competing digits, a reflection of left-brain dominance for language. The right ear has better access to the left cerebral hemisphere because of the crossed auditory pathways. While the right ear connects directly to the left cerebral hemisphere (language area), the left ear's route to the same area first must go to the right cerebral hemisphere and then cross over to the left side and the language area.

It was evident from studies with patients who suffered brain damage to the right cerebral hemisphere that the right brain makes an important contribution to human performance, having functions complementary to those of the left cerebral hemisphere. The right side of the brain probably processes information differently from the left, relying more on visual imagery than on language. The right cerebral hemisphere of the brain specializes in perceiving and remembering faces, unfamiliar and complex shapes for which there are no ready names, and drawings of incomplete gestalts in which parts are missing. Its importance is to spatial orientation and visuospatial relationships. It is thought to provide the neurological basis for the ability to take fragmentary sensory information and convert it to a coherent organization of the outside world.

Ordinarily, the left and right cerebral hemispheres exchange information when each hemisphere has access to the information that passed initially to the opposite hemisphere. All this occurs through the large bundle of fibers, corpus callosum, as well as several smaller bundles of fibers. What happens if the corpus callosum is injured? Clearly, any damage to the corpus callosum will result in impaired exchange of information. It is known, for example, from those who have had surgery to interrupt severe epilepsy, that epileptic seizures can be limited to only one side of the body. This is a positive outcome of the disruption in information flow. When seizures are so severe that they cannot be controlled by customary antiepileptic drug treatment, surgery has been performed to cut the corpus callosum. This results in preventing seizures from crossing from one cerebral hemisphere to another. Thus, when seizures occur, they are less severe because they affect only one side of the body. Interestingly enough, these surgeries have brought unexpected positive results because the seizures not only occur with less severity, they also occur less frequently.

The marvels of coordination between right and left cerebral hemispheres are also seen in other cases where **split-brain** phenomenon was observed. Observations of the roles of right and left cerebral hemispheres have led to many speculations. For example, is one sphere more important or more dominant? When it was first determined that the left cerebral hemisphere controls speech, the right sphere was viewed as subordinate. Its role was seen as one of support to the left sphere. Through further research, however, particularly with studies of patients whose corpus callosum was damaged (commonly referred to as split-brain patients), it became clear that the right cerebral hemisphere is capable of many more functions than was first thought. For example, the right cerebral hemisphere does understand simple speech, although it cannot control speech. It can also perform certain functions better than the left hemisphere, such as the control of emotional expression.

It has been shown that after damage to the right cerebral hemisphere, people not only have trouble forming facial expressions that depict emotions, they also have trouble understanding others' emotions. Also, people who have suffered damage to the right cerebral hemisphere speak with less than normal amounts of inflection, suggesting impairment in emotion. Also, the right cerebral hemisphere seems to be specialized for complex visual and spatial tasks. For example, people who have damaged their right cerebral hemisphere have difficulty finding their way from one place to another.

Perceiving to Emoting

Does everyone have emotions, even if they appear to have none? Let us say you have been asked to care for young children, 7–12 years of age, who, you have been told, possess "inhuman destructive capabilities." They seem to have superhuman powers and tell you they are on an important mission. They have been placed on Earth for the specific purpose of destroying the existing social structure so that a new social system can be established. Their eyes are opaque; they have platinum hair, and they look alike. Although they have faces, they have no recognizable facial expressions. Do they have emotions? Are they aware of feelings?

The question is not whether they have emotional experiences similar to other humans, such as anger, happiness, or sadness. You cannot know what it feels like to be like them. Indeed, they may not have any conscious experience of feelings. You are looking for familiar behaviors that suggest that they have emotions. Emotion, for you, is defined as temporary changes in inflection or in the intensity of behavior. Thus, from your point of view, if they attack another person and increase the intensity of their behavior to do this, they are showing emotion. Movement, which shows no change in intensity, is, for you, lacking emotion. You observe that they attack people, but the intensity of their movements stays the same. This scenario may sound like a script from a science fiction movie; still, the question is relevant: how do people know whether this group of children (or any human beings, for that matter) has feelings and emotions, and experience them in ways like themselves?

Emotion has been studied as a function of autonomic arousal. The intensity of behavior is largely governed by the functions of the **autonomic nervous system (ANS)**. The ANS has two systems: the sympathetic and parasympathetic processes. Both regulate the involuntary processes of the body. The ANS is named as such because it is thought to operate autonomously. There are many feedback loops in the body, and these continually send and receive information about individuals' experience.

Wilhelm Reich perceived the reciprocal action of sympathetic and parasympathetic systems (Buhl, 2001). Essentially, these two parts of the ANS function reciprocally. The sympathetic system controls arousal and the fight–flight mechanism, and the **parasympathetic nervous system** involves relaxation. The parasympathetic system comes into action after stimuli have been acted upon. It allows us to wind down while the sympathetic system governs arousal that occurred initially. Otherwise, the **sympathetic nervous system** prepares the body for intense vigorous response while the parasympathetic system increases digestion and other responses associated with relaxation.

The most compelling reason for the arousal of the parasympathetic system is frequently the removal of a stimulus that excited the sympathetic system in the first place. The example of people fainting after intense arousal illustrates this point. When something life-threatening happens (e.g., almost getting run over by a car), the sympathetic nervous system is excited. When the threatening stimulus is removed, a rebound effect—overactivity of the parasympathetic system—occurs. Thus, some people might collapse or faint after this initial intense sympathetic nervous system response.

Reaction from the sympathetic nervous system occurs not only because of initial stimulus to the sympathetic system but also as a result of the individual's interpretation of the stimulus. Individuals' interpretations of the stimulus are critical. This is why it is difficult to predict reactions when people perceive a threat or challenge. For example, predicting stress levels by simply counting stressful life events may be highly unreliable.

More accurate measures are those that factor in a valence or the perception of the stimulus. For example, changing jobs is generally regarded as stressful. Just how stressful can vary a great deal from one person to another, based on their perception of the change. They may not even regard it as a significant event.

Because of this, other methods are needed to explain how they perceive the change—for example, on a continuum from +7 (being extremely positive) to −7 (being extremely negative). To have a total hysterectomy may be perceived as very traumatic and threatening to some women but not to others. Would it be an error then to approach all women having this surgery with expressions of concern and sympathy? The surgery itself may not be the stressor; rather than the surgery, the confinement and separation from their children might be most worrisome. By discovering the unique distressing elements, one can respond more appropriately.

In the previous section, the importance of being able to alter perceptions of events was alluded to. The power of individual interpretations of stimuli has been described in certain cognitive approaches to counseling (e.g., cognitive behavioral therapy [CBT]). Questions about the neurocognitive effects of psychological counseling have been explored. Some researchers have suggested that CBT has the potential of modifying certain dysfunctional circuitry associated with, for example, anxiety disorders. The implications are that this form of counseling can functionally "rewire" the brain. In a systematic review to investigate neurobiological changes related to CBT in anxiety disorders, Porto et al. (2009) stated that despite the methodological limitations of studies reviewed, these neuroimaging studies revealed that CBT was found to change dysfunctions of the nervous system. Otte (2011) substantiated these conclusions that CBT is effective in the treatment of anxiety

It is believed that the mammalian brain continually rewires itself, suggesting that the brain is undergoing change many times within a single day. Do persons have the capacity to rewire their own brains? In the field of psychology, attribution theory suggests that when stimuli or events are perceived to be negative, but also judged to be global (affecting many parts of one's life), the experience can be more emotionally painful.

Recurring or enduring stimuli produce feelings of hopelessness. Conversely, when these same events or stimuli are perceived as manageable, they elicit feelings of hopefulness. It is known that the way in which stimuli or events are interpreted has a great deal to do with the way people respond. People who engage in actions of "mind over matter" are using their abilities to master challenges by reinterpreting the meanings of the stimuli. Making the stimuli (perceptions of the stimuli) less threatening is their way of modulating stress-related reactions. Thus, any given event or stimuli may produce a great deal of sympathetic nervous system arousal, a moderate amount, or very little. It depends on the individual's interpretation of the event and the way he or she processes the perception of the stimuli.

For a long time, it was thought that it was impossible to exert direct control over stress, including heart rate and other biologic processes affected by the ANS. With scientific advances and the practice of various versions of biofeedback, it has been found that people can control their responses to stress by progressively relaxing their skeletal muscles—as their muscles relax, their emotions become calmer. Voluntary control over responses like heart rate does not seem to be possible; however, indirect effects through the process of the progressive relaxation of skeletal muscles—possibly with biofeedback—do seem to reduce stress and promote calmness.

Emotions and the expression of emotions depend largely on an area of the brain called the **limbic system**. MacLean's early work (1970) used the concept to refer to this area of the brain; "limbic" comes from the Latin word *limbus*, which means border. Parts or structures of the limbic system form a border around certain midline structures of the brain. The brain area most important for emotions and emotional expression, *the limbic system*, is a circuit that includes the amygdala, the

hypothalamus, parts of the cerebral cortex, and several other structures.

MacLean (1973) identified this enlarged lobe as the connecting structure between the visual system and the limbic system of emotional behaviors. He suggested that the fusiform gyrus gives rise to the weepy feelings that people may experience upon witnessing an altruistic act. Altruism depends not only on feeling one's way into another person in the sense of empathy. It also involves the capacity to see with feeling into another person's situation.

Emotional behavior may be understood in part by studying the behaviors that are necessary for self-preservation and procreation. One list of such behaviors (modified from Denny & Ratner, 1970) is resting, eliminating, water balance, thermoregulation, feeding, aggressive–defensive behaviors, sexual behaviors, and care of the young. Animals, including humans, fulfill their basic needs in cycles that include an appetitive phase, a consuming phase, and a postconsuming phase. Even under the most normal circumstances, there is a rise and fall in body activities (e.g., brain, digestive system, senses of taste and smell, etc.). This cyclical rise and fall is referred to as facilitation or inhibition, respectively. Emotional behavior may be represented as exceptional states of facilitation or inhibition. Each of the several basic consuming behaviors has its own normal range of arousal and may also show a range of over-reaction (extreme facilitation) and under-reaction (extreme inhibition). The language used to describe feelings and emotions usually refers to these extremes. Examples of inhibitory words for under-reaction are *depressed*, *helpless*, *lonely*, and *discouraged*. Facilitation words for over-reaction are *excited*, *angry*, *panicked*, and *passionate*.

The limbic system is said to consist of the structures in the brain that are essential to emotion. The visual structures of the brain have connections to the limbic system in the prefrontal cortex and in the occipitotemporal lobe and the fusiform gyrus. There is evidence that these connections function to help individuals gain insight into the feelings of others—to see with feeling.

Autism is a condition previously believed to be related in part to damage in the limbic system. Because the limbic system is in charge of emotions, the lack of the emotional response characteristic of these children was thought to be limbic system-related. However, more is known about autism today, and rather than just a few regions of the brain, many structures are involved, including the amygdala, cerebellum, and other structures of the brain (Amaral, Schumann, & Nordahl, 2008), hinting at wide range maturation deficits impacting brain connectivity.

Accordingly, autism is a developmental brain disorder characterized by three distinctive behaviors that are not just emotional regulation. Autistic children have difficulties with social interaction, have problems with verbal and nonverbal communication, and exhibit repetitive behaviors or narrow, obsessive interests noticed by parents in the first 2 years of the child's life. Scientists are not certain what causes autism, but it is likely that both genetics and environment play a role.

New and exciting diagnostic testing suggests that autism may be diagnosed very early in childhood (NIMH, 2017).

Neuroimaging techniques, functional connectivity magnetic resonance imaging (fcMRI), have shown how brain regions are connected and synchronized in infants. These tests have recently demonstrated the possibility to predict autism in high-risk, 6-month-old infants (the National Institute of Mental Health [NIMH] reporting on a study published by Emerson and colleagues in *Science Translational Medicine*, 2017). Also, brain enlargement has been observed, but the timing and relationship between autism and autism spectrum disorder and the appearance of behavioral symptoms are unknown. Study findings have demonstrated that early brain changes can be detected during the period when autistic behaviors first appear (Hazlett et al., 2017).

Individuality in response processes is well studied. Each individual learns to depend on one sensory system or another, functioning well or not, as a means of perceiving and understanding the world. This dependence on particular sensory modalities is characteristic of human beings and generates patterns of experience that differ between and within individuals.

All humans have essentially equivalent sensory organs and structures, both anatomically and physiologically. The neurological pathways that serve the senses are presumed to be similar in all human brains. So, what makes for the individuality? As previously discussed, despite similar "equipment," no two individuals understand a particular occurrence in exactly the same way because of the differences that are learned through **selective attention** to sensory input channels, and with variations of experience with the senses.

"Selective attention to sensory input" means that at any time individuals usually attend to (are conscious of) one, or possibly two, of their sensory channels, and their immediate memory and attention is limited to only several "bits" of information. Immediate memory imposes severe limitations on the amount of information people are able to receive, process, and remember. Thus, the process of **selective inattention** explains in part why some information may not be perceived or attended to when individuals are faced with information overload. *Relearning* is recognizing something similar to what one knew previously. Thus, relearning a subject, say, a foreign language (French) that was previously studied is easier and more rapidly retrieved than learning a completely new subject. Although there are similarities between present experiences and memories, there are always differences.

Interference can occur if the mind gets confused about the similarities and differences between memories of previous experiences and these new experiences. Using the example of learning unfamiliar languages, attempting to learn two new languages at the same time, alternating back and forth, will tend to confuse you in areas in which the two languages are similar. Imagine that you are trying to learn Spanish and French at the same time. You previously understood French after 2 years of college-level French. You would be relearning the French you knew before and learning Spanish for the first time. Would this be more confusing than only relearning French or only learning Spanish for the first time?

The study of how much information can be processed and retained is interesting. "Bits" and "chunks" of information have been measured and quantified by several researchers to ascertain how much individuals can know at any one time. Much discussion has centered around the idea that the amount, while varied, is fairly constant. The number 7 (e.g., the number of bits of information [7 ± 2]) is constant for the absolute judgment of inputs into one sensory channel. It is known, however, that there may be quite a bit of variance in what is processed and retained. The ability to focus attention is thought to be important in protecting the brain from the bombardment of too much information, which results in confusion rather than retention of new information.

Learning from internal sensory representations includes how to pay attention to the feeling states of emotion, the visceral and proprioceptive cues for breathing and digestion, and the visual imageries of day and night dreams. Individuals "listening," so to speak, to their own bodies are knowing themselves through internal kinesthetic sensory information. Along these lines, people in states of meditation can pay selective attention to the responses occurring in the deeper recesses of the brain. They can monitor the rise and fall of emotional responses, particularly aggressive–defensive or sexual behaviors. They can identify "gut reactions" and catching the breath as kinesthetic sensory responses to stimuli.

So, one reason individuals have different experiences despite similar genetic endowments of the brain and body and despite similar environments is that, characteristically, each one attends to different aspects of the

self and of the environment. Several factors affect any one individual's attention and processing of stimuli. Some of these factors have been mentioned previously, including damage, injury, or even irritation such as that caused by epileptic seizures. However, both drugs and diet can have an effect as well, and because they can decrease the synthesis or release of serotonin, they are potentially mood-altering substances. This is one reason drugs and diet are seriously considered when explanations of violent outbursts, anxiety, and the inability to experience pleasure are studied.

Learning: A Stimulus-Processing Activity

Sensory information taken into and processed by the brain may have both short- and long-term effects on our behavior. Still, are all aspects of sensory information retained? One's memories have a lot to do with knowledge of the world and what actions are needed. Memory, however, is fragile and does not always serve people in the way that they need it to. As do young school children, adults forget, and our recall of information is not always as accurate as it needs to be to function properly. What is generally meant by memory is what scientists call *explicit memory*. This is our conscious, intentional awareness, of previous experiences that come to our conscious awareness in our everyday living.

How do patients, for example, remember to follow advice exactly as they are instructed? Their memories may be faulty; thus, providers may need to provide a number of recurring stimuli to help activate more accurately what was said. In the case of medication adherence, providers can distribute pill boxes, refrigerator magnets, timers, pictures, and medication logs. Hopefully, these aids enhance conscious recollection of previous experiences with the provider during the time they were given instructions. And these recollections will trigger a memory of what they heard providers say or what was shown to them.

Over the course of the study of the mechanism of memory and response, many theories of learning have been put forth. Perhaps one of the most renown is Pavlov's theory of higher nervous activity (Chilingaryan, 2001). Pavlov's classic theory of conditioning emphasizes the role of reward. Underlying this theory is the notion that the learning process is successful because it increases the probability of a desired outcome.

Pavlov proposed that learning consists of transferring a reflex from one stimulus to another. In this way, a stimulus that would normally elicit a response could be replaced with a new stimulus that would, in turn, elicit the same response. This theory, merely an inference, suggested that pairing a conditioned stimulus with the unconditioned stimulus caused the growth of a new or strengthened connection between a conditioned stimulus center in the brain and an unconditioned stimulus center in the brain. However, neither Pavlov nor his colleagues could actually observe this hypothesized growth of connections in the brain.

Pavlov's theory, like those of many other theorists of the time, was overly simplistic in many ways. First, it presumed that learning about stimuli was not related to those stimuli (i.e., learning about tastes is the same as learning about temperatures). Second, the immediacy of the learning experience was viewed as important, but was not examined in the context of the situation. It is known that certain learning (e.g., eating certain foods and getting sick) happens with a single instance. It does not take several trials to realize you should avoid this food. Also, learning to avoid the food that caused you to become sick can happen even if the taste of the food and illness are separated by short or long durations. In summary, learning can occur differently, depending on what is to be learned.

It is generally believed that during learning, some change must take place in the neurons in the brain. But, this change could take many forms, from the growth of a new axon, to new connections among neurons, to increased or decreased release of synaptic transmitters, and so on. And, it is generally believed that the mechanisms differ, depending on the particular learning task. That is, the mechanisms are not the same for all instances of learning.

In summary, learning is often attributed to changes made over large areas of the nervous system. No matter how much of our brains participate in the process of learning, what is always required is change at the cellular level. For learning to occur, cells (neurons) must change their properties. Studies that address single-cell changes attribute the changes to biochemical changes. Impaired learning is often associated, then, with chemical deficiencies in the brain. Theories of this kind have demonstrated that certain drugs might impair or improve learning through different biochemical processes. Studies of memory, for example, suggest that certain proteins must be synthesized. Some drugs and hormones have been shown to facilitate memory, and while the specific action is not known or well understood, the biochemical transmission at synapses is the focus of attention.

As has been shown in this discussion of the neurophysiological basis for communication, several processes and structures are involved, ranging from small, molecular changes to larger regions of the brain and the entire central nervous system. These dynamics, in and of themselves, are exceedingly complex and are addressed in a great deal of depth in other discussions of brain topography and brain chemistry.

The reader is encouraged to explore the fascinating world of neurophysiology and the progress that has occurred in understanding perception and learning. Neurolinguistics is a specialized science that studies how people receive information through the senses, process the information in neurons and neural pathways in the brain, and express the information in language and behaviors. Still to be described are the interpersonal and relationship principles of communications that come to us largely from the behavioral science fields.

▶ Interpersonal Foundations for Human Communication

Communication has been labeled the *conditio sine qua non* of human life and social order in the classic studies of Watzlawick, Beavin, and Jackson (1967). Communication (see **FIGURE 4-4**) occurs on three levels—intrapersonal (or that which goes on within an individual), interpersonal (referring to that between individuals or within groups), and mass communication (that which is transmitted publicly). It is also clear that from the beginning of their existence, people are not only refining their neurophysiological capacities to communicate, they are equally engaged in the process of acquiring the social rules of communication. Historically, much of what is known from science comes from the study of communication as *a one-way phenomenon.* Knowledge of communication was largely gleaned from studies of speaker-to-listener communication; communication as a function of the process of interaction was virtually ignored.

Now providers operate with a much higher level of understanding about communication. They no longer think of communication as a simple process of **decoding** (the process of interpreting a single message) and **encoding** (creating a message to be transmitted). Human communication is interpersonal in nature and thus much more complex. They think of communication as a series of messages (interactions) and as patterns of interaction (transactions). The principles and concepts presented in this discussion will address aspects of communication that are interpersonal and interactive.

Human communication is of two types: digital and analogic (Gazda et al., 1982). When someone is referring to something by name, they are employing **digital communication**. The same object can also be described as a representation or likeness, and represents **analogic communication**. The following example may help differentiate these two types. When one is visiting a foreign country, and listens to people speak, they may not understand any of the language. However, if they watch the people while they are speaking—for example, their intentional movements—it is easier to understand at least some of what the communication is about. This latter form of communication, which often includes the nonverbal content and the context of the interaction, is analogic communication.

Humans are the only species known to use both digital and analogic communication. Although people rely heavily on digital communication, there are times in which they rely almost exclusively on analogic communication. With messages that people perceive and send to define relationships, they predominantly use analogic communication. Some say that emotionally disturbed children and animals are keenly aware of analogic communication. The special intuition that these groups are believed to possess makes it very difficult to deceive them. Because people use and receive both types of communication, they are constantly translating from one to another. It is like having two languages—Spanish and French—and, as sender or receiver, having to flow between them. One's abilities to translate from one mode to another is vital. To talk about one's relationships, one must translate largely analogic data to the digital form (e.g., by choosing words to describe feelings towards another person).

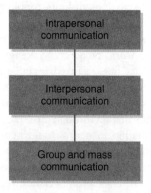

FIGURE 4-4 Human Communication Contexts—Within, Between, and Across People.

And when translating from the digital to the analogic, one risks the loss of information that cannot be communicated symbolically.

The Principle of Function or Utility of Communication

As in the biological sciences, the study of communication in the social sciences has led to understanding communication by the identification of its *function*. This is to say, what people perceive and express is influenced by their need to perceive and express.

Everything one learns, for example, is relative unless it has a point of reference. The point of reference may be described as human needs. For example, survival and, from an interpersonal standpoint, security are basic needs. What is generally agreed upon is that this principle of function holds true for virtually all perceptions and expressions. Sensory and brain chemistry suggest that only relationships and patterns of relationships can be perceived and that these form the basis of human reality.

So, in one way or another, functionality is dominant in human communications; one does not just perceive an event, rather an event is scanned to look for meaning related to one's needs. In this way, objects or people are not the target of our perceptions, rather they are functions. This is an important principle because it depicts the fact that perceptions are not random events, but are organized around one's perception of meaning. Thus, it is possible to say that one's initial awareness, and any subsequent rectification of this awareness, is highly influenced by their awareness of themselves and the needs they experience.

There are implications for teaching patients about their health needs and treatment approaches. For example, patients do better when they understand their health condition and the need for treatment. Our role is frequently one of identifying whether they perceive a need to know and working with shaping their perception of need to know. When counseling adolescents about the need to use an inhaler to treat asthma, providers might explain that exertion on the football field without using an inhaler can impede their ability to play well. What interests the patients gives clues about what they will want to know and how they might understand their condition. Actually, this approach is used frequently with a wide range of chronic illnesses to improve patient adherence to treatment.

The Principle of Process

The second major concept of human communication in an interpersonal context is that of *process*. When one thinks about how communication occurs in relationships, it is understood that no statements can accurately reflect a communicative exchange if not first analyzed from the standpoint of function, and then analyzed from the standpoint of an ongoing and ever-changing process. Messages sent and received are products of a continuous process; they are not independent of other stimuli in the interpersonal environment. Communication, then, is a mutually interdependent activity among two or more individuals in a changing environmental context.

The interpersonal communication process consists of a dynamic exchange of energy among two or more individuals within a specific sociocultural context. Literally, communication is a process in which individuals share something of themselves, whether it is feelings, thoughts, opinions, ideas, values, or goals. This process, when it happens in effective interchange, helps make individuals feel more human, more in touch with reality, and more capable of social intimacy. Also, the ability of individuals to influence one another and thereby exercise power, and even control, should be considered an important impetus for interpersonal communication. The communication process has frequently been depicted in a linear fashion, but has now been replaced by more complex conceptual models. **FIGURE 4-5** illustrates this phenomenon.

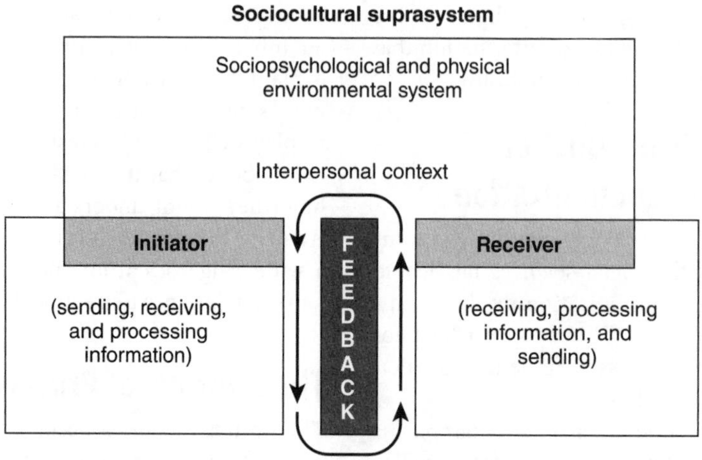

Sociocultural suprasystem

FIGURE 4-5 Functional Components of the Communication Process.

A concept critical to understanding communication as a process, then, is that of *feedback*. Feedback is a series of responses that depicts change. It is not a linear chain of events (e.g., event A affects event B, B affects C, C, in turn, affects D, and so on). Rather, D leads back to A. Therefore, the process is circular and dynamic. Feedback plays an important role in establishing, modifying, and stabilizing relationships. The concept of feedback is frequently addressed as a loop. That is, in relationships, the behavior of each person affects, and is affected by, the behavior of each other person.

Systems that engage in feedback are distinctively different from those that do not; they generally display higher degrees of complexity. In open systems theory, open systems are generally differentiated from closed systems by the process of fluidity and permeability achieved to a great extent through the process of feedback (see **FIGURE 4-6**).

It is known that some very *closed systems* (e.g., cults) restrict feedback, both within the system and between the system and the larger suprasystem—society-at-large. Perhaps the reasons cults restrict feedback exchange is that feedback and the exchange of information across the boundaries of the system would result in the disruption of the system. Thus, to maintain homeostasis, the cult (system) disallows open exchange with the external environment. There is virtually no feedback exchange process. This scenario can be contrasted with *open systems*. An example of open system feedback can be found in families that function well.

Functional families can display intricate levels of feedback and information processing. Family decisions may require members to voice their preferences to one another in ongoing, continuous ways. These decisions are a direct result of multiple views, not the opinions of one or two members. Decisions occur as a result not only of people voicing their views but also because these views are reactions to the views of others. *Fluidity* is one characteristic of these systems, and information can flow easily from member to member and between the family and its external environment. This process is *transactional* because individuals in an interaction affect others and are affected by themselves.

Theories of causality may not fully appreciate the dynamic process of information exchange between individuals. In theories of causality, it is appropriate to speak about the beginning message or statement and the results (at the end of the chain). When applying the principle of the feedback loop, this explanation is faulty—A may not cause B; the

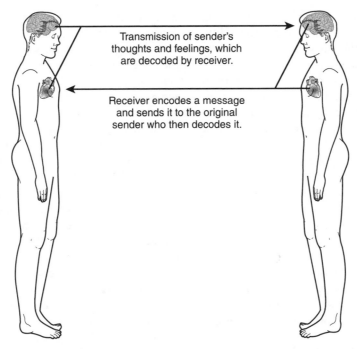

Sender-receiver

The sender encodes his thoughts and feelings into words and gestures and transmits them to the receiver via sound, touch, sight, and smell. At the same time, the sender is receiving messages from the person with whom he is communicating.

Receiver-sender

The receiver deciphers the sender's transmission. He determines what request the sender is making of him after he decodes the sender's cognitive and affective messages. Simultaneously, the receiver is sending messages to the other person.

Feedback
Feedback refers to the circular process by which
Sender and Receiver influence one another.

FIGURE 4-6 The Reciprocal and Circular Nature of Interpersonal Communication.

Data from S. Smith, *Communications in Nursing*, 2nd edition, p. 5, © 1992. Mosby Yearbook.

beginning is arbitrary and depends on where one enters the loop.

The Principle of Multidimensionality

A third important principle of interpersonal communication is that it is *multidimensional* (see **EXHIBIT 4-1**). What does **multidimensional communication** mean, and what are the dimensions? Usually when speaking of the multidimensionality of communication, what

EXHIBIT 4-1 Multidimensionality of Human Communication

- The content dimensions
- The feeling or emotional dimensions
- The relationship dimensions

is meant is that communication has two distinct levels: (1) the content dimension and (2) the relationship dimension. The classic work of Watzlawick et al. (1967) revolutionized ways of looking at communication, describing to the **principle of multidimensionality**. Previously, one thought of communication as the simple exchange of content. Otherwise, A informs B about something, and in turn, B may respond to this transmission or content level. This notion was by the idea that communication is more than the exchange of content or information.

Watzlawick and colleagues drew attention to the fact that communication is much more than the simple exchange of content or information. Recognizing that communication has at least two dimensions (content and relationship aspects), suggested that one cannot fully understand communication until something is known about both aspects. One reason why the content level of messages was easier to understand was that the relationship aspect may be more hidden, while the content aspect more transparent.

The idea of multilevel communication was further refined by clinicians' descriptions of three levels, not two: (1) the content level, (2) the feeling or emotional level, and (3) a level that describes the perceived relationship of one communicant to another. This model incorporates the idea that every message has a separate emotional quality that further clarifies both the content and the relational levels of the communication. Regardless of whether one differentiates between two or three levels, it is clear that communication is used not only to exchange information (e.g., facts or ideas), it is also used to address the interpersonal relationship dimension.

Consider the command: "Take this pill now with this water." The explicit message, or content aspect of this expression, is the obvious: you need to take the pill. However, suggested here, through both verbal and nonverbal clues, is evidence about the relationship and even what feelings the provider has about the patient. The command communicates authority: one person (provider) perceives herself/himself in an authority relationship

with the other (patient or client). One has power over the other, and this is enacted in the exchanges that occur. Somewhat subtle is the underlying attitude: *I have expectations of you, and if you do not do as I say, you will let me down.* Furthermore, *my expectations are legitimate.*

Said in a somewhat different way, one aspect of a message conveys information—this is synonymous to the content of the message. It may be about anything regardless of whether it is true or false, valid or invalid, or even indecipherable. The command quality of the message, however, describes how the message should be received and, therefore, describes the relationship of the communicants. Putting these relationship aspects into words, they would say: "This is how I see myself in relationship to you, you in relationship to me or how, at least, it should be."

Consider these two expressions that seemingly communicate the same directive: "Take this pill with water—it'll be easier," and "If you refuse the water, you won't be able to take this pill." While these statements communicate approximately the same content (i.e., you need to take this pill with water), they define somewhat different relationships with the patient. The first example suggests a more supportive, facilitative relationship, while the latter suggests a supervisorial, somewhat skeptical relationship.

Sometimes the distinction between levels of communication are depicted in descriptions of *meta-communication* and *meta-information*. Meta-communication is a term frequently used to identify communication about the communication. It is communication about how a message is supposed to be received. The report aspect of the communication conveys the data. The command (meta-communication or meta-information) describes how this communication should be taken. "You better take me seriously" is one verbal translation of the meta-communication in this message: "If you think I'm going to take out the garbage, you're

Verbal
• Verbal message
• Speech
• Tone of voice and voice inflections
• Sequence, rhythm, and cadence of words

Nonverbal
• Facial expression
• Posture
• Movement or gestures
• Body position
• Spatial dimensions

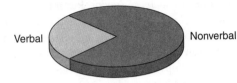

Verbal   Nonverbal

FIGURE 4-7 Categories of Verbal and Nonverbal Communication.

crazy!" The relational or meta-communicative aspects can also be expressed nonverbally by frowning or piercing looks, or through the context of the encounter, as when people criticize each other in front of strangers.

Communication about the relational aspects, or feeling dimension, sometimes occurs at the nonverbal level.

This brings us to still another important axiom of human communication: Communication is both *verbal* and *nonverbal* (see **FIGURE 4-7**). Sometimes verbal communication is the term used to describe the content level of a message. Otherwise, what did the sender say? This is the information or direct message intended. Nonverbal aspects of communication—facial expressions, gestures, positioning—are perceived by those who receive our messages and are considered part of the communication or interaction. Nonverbal aspects frequently disclose the feeling or relational dimension of the communication as evidenced in photographs of individuals' facial expressions (see **FIGURE 4-8**).

Can you imagine being in a relationship where you cannot have access to the nonverbal content of the interaction? Facial expressions, posture, and movement would not be available data. In the case of patients who suffer impairment in vision, how are they able to understand beyond the content of messages? Otherwise, how would they draw conclusions about the emotional and relational

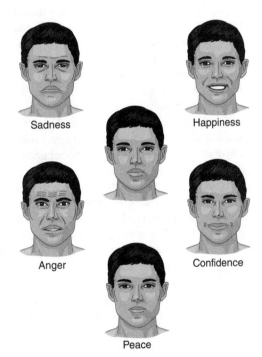

Sadness   Happiness

Anger   Confidence

Peace

FIGURE 4-8 Humans Rely Heavily upon Nonverbal Aspects of Communication (e.g., Facial Expressions).

aspects of the interaction? They would need to rely almost exclusively on the spoken word, together with evidence of inflection, pace of speech, and tone of voice, to establish the other person's feelings about them. Would they be secure in their judgments or satisfied with this data? Most likely the answer is, not really. Under the circumstance that patients have both significant vision and hearing loss, health providers resort to other ways of communicating relational aspects of messages. What do you think they would do? If you say that they would use touch you are right. But, they might couple touch with other strategies such as talking more slowly and louder.

What is characteristic of human communication is that meta-communication (communication that classifies the relationship) is extremely important. A great deal of what is communicated through nonverbal channels is symbolic. Facial expressions or body movements are symbolic representations of the nature of the relationship between communicants. Not only do humans rely heavily on nonverbal aspects, but they are also trained to use these aspects to communicate more effectively and efficiently.

Discrepancies between verbal and nonverbal communication (messages) are generally picked up in human dialogue. Discrepancies can occur in many ways, for example, in different verbal reports or in differences between verbal and nonverbal messages. Consistency in communication is important because it provides a foundation for trust. Should communication be inconsistent or two opposing messages be delivered, there is reason to mistrust the other person and the relationship. In most relationships, one does not look for or search for inconsistencies across verbal messages or between verbal and nonverbal messages. However, if given a reason to mistrust someone, people have the capacity to fine-tune their perceptions and be observant of mixed messages whether they are blatant or only somewhat apparent.

The Principle of Communication Inevitability

The idea that communication occurs on both verbal and nonverbal levels brings us to the next important axiom of interpersonal

communication: the impossibility of not communicating, or communication inevitability. Watzlawick et al. (1967, p. 48) first referred to this idea as a major property of behavior. In other words, there is no such thing as *nonbehavior*. Putting it in simpler terms, *one cannot not behave and one cannot not communicate*. If we understand communication as behavior, then we can also say that no matter how much a person tries, they cannot not communicate.

Drawing from the previous discussion of nonverbal and verbal communication, we find that words or silence, activity or inactivity, all have message potential. They influence others, and therefore, others, too, cannot not respond to these communications. To express this idea in brief: we are always communicating whether we are exchanging words or not. The health professional who looks straight ahead and avoids eye contact when passing by a patient's family, or reads the patient's chart, moves in front of another provider to return it, and checks his beeper without acknowledging anyone's presence are both communicating— even though no words are exchanged.

The mere absence of talking does not mean communication has not occurred. In both cases, what is communicated is that the providers are busy and do not want to speak to anyone or be spoken to. Family members and staff, respectively, usually get the message and behave, in turn, by leaving them alone. Is this any less of an interchange of information than the most animated conversation?

It is also true that communication may not be intentional. Much of what is communicated is, in fact, unintentional, unplanned, and even unrealized. When we understand that messages are multileveled and include nonverbal behavior, this idea is quite plausible. Consider, for example, that a health provider has a particular negative attitude about another provider. Nothing said can substantiate this suspicion. Nonetheless, it is understood, and if people around them were asked about their relationship, they would confirm this assumption: "Yes, they have problems communicating."

Still, there are no data, or is there? The data is largely in the nonverbal communication that is exchanged between the providers. Therefore, when we think of communication units, we do not mean simple verbal messages but rather multifaceted occurrences in which several factors are involved—verbal, tonal, postural, and even contextual aspects. Likewise, these factors have varied ways of affecting communication as well as several permutations.

Permutations and variance can often be a function of cultural differences. At other times, it is a reflection of the mental or emotional stability of the sender. Some of these permutations appear in behaviors of the mentally ill or the functionally impaired. A case in point is an emotionally disturbed patient who is mute and whose withdrawal and immobility express anger at those around him. Some people intentionally avoid verbal exchanges to sever commitment. A sequence of avoidance behaviors may also be interlaced with a willingness to communicate. Because human relationships are complex, the explicit and implicit use of communication, which includes both verbal and nonverbal dimensions, is also very complex. Many impasses in communication relate to the complexity of relationships and the involvement of communication channels.

The Principle of Punctuation

The complexity of human relationships is also reflected in the cause and effect patterns that communicants claim exist. This notion is especially observed in communications in which conflict exists. The principle of *punctuation* and *sequence of events*, although not a major communication principle, is relevant to our understanding of the circularity of communications. When we ask two or more people to report on the patterns of their communication, we may get two very discrepant stories.

Looking in from the outside, we would say that the communication we observe, from A to B to C and to D, is an uninterrupted series of exchanges. However, to those participating in the dialogue, there is a beginning, a middle, and an end. The participants see a cause-and-effect relationship and behave as though this is reality. They may punctuate their remarks at any one time in the series to depict their believed status or their desired status. These perceived beginnings, middles, and ends depict a pattern of responses that communicates something about how one communicant sees themself in relation to another, such as on issues of power, control, and intimacy.

The process of sequencing responses is inherent in all humans and is neither bad nor good. It serves the purpose of organizing behavioral events and is vital to ongoing relationships. Tendencies to organize interactions can display the specific rules of a culture. For example, if males were dominant decision-makers and females predominantly followers, the interpretation of a sequence of events A to D would illustrate this cultural prerequisite. That is, we would judge, and others would confirm, that the interaction begins with A directing B to do something. It would not be concluded that B decided to do something and A simply reiterated the objective of the action after it was first initiated.

Interpretations of the inner workings of arguments further illustrate this point. With a couple who argues, who starts the argument? And, does party A withdraw because party B insults A, or is party B critical because party A withdraws? Who initiates and who reacts—party A or party B? Depending on what patterns these communicants see in their relationship, the reported sequence of events will be different. Both parties may be guilty of distorting aspects of the argument, and this further complicates the situation. Finally, depending on the cultural orientations of the participants, the beginning, middle, and end may be very different from what we perceive as outside observers, or even what each party thinks is occurring. It is clear then that the nature of a relationship is played out in the perceived punctuation of the segments of communication.

The Principle of Symmetrical or Complementary Communication

A final axiom of interpersonal communication that is key to understanding human communication is that communication (in relationships) is either **symmetrical or complementary**. People take either symmetrical or complementary roles in relationships and communicate accordingly. In the first case (symmetry), communicants tend to mirror each other's behavior. In the second instance (complementary), one party's behavior complements the other's. In the first case, the differences between the respondents are minimized—both parties pull toward their common base. In the second type, maximizing differences is important.

If we studied the pattern of communication among and across multiple dyadic relationships and across ethnic and cultural groups, what would we find? Is the principle of symmetry or complementary universal? Also, what impact does the individual's role play in this process? Although not entirely known, it might be true that these patterns exist and are universal. We know that individuals' roles play a part. Classic examples of complementary communication are the parent–child, boss–employee, and leader–follower dyads. Usually these dyads participate in socially defined ways to depict superior–inferior and primary–secondary roles. Distinctively different are dyads that interact as if both parties were equal. This may be seen in some colleague and marital relationships, but might not be the case across various subgroups and cultures. What is obvious is that communication that depicts these arrangements will generally hold true regardless of the contexts or circumstances. Boss–employee interactions, for example, usually reflect superior–inferior status, even if the parties interact outside their professional roles. No matter the intentions to behave as equals, they are aware of the underlying hierarchal arrangement prescribed by their roles.

▶ Summary

In summary, human communication is indeed complex. The neurological, biochemical factors impacting the information received and the neural activity by which we process this information are fascinating. Our abilities to utilize communication in patterned ways to initiate, modify, and maintain relationships distinguishes us from all other species. These processes are put forward in this chapter as axioms or concepts and principles substantiated by evidence and observation. In translating science to pragmatics, we run the risk of overgeneralizing or minimizing details.

It is not the intention of this chapter to synthesize all scientific data. Rather, the objective is to discuss key concepts and principles from both the neurobiological and behavioral sciences on the subject of human communication—functional and dysfunctional. The objective was also to summarize what is known about therapeutic and nontherapeutic approaches in health care. The chapters to follow build on the evolving evidence accrued through time. Much of ongoing research evidence can be translated into clinical practice, and there is important new evidence to demonstrate its utility in understanding the functions of the brain and communication processes. An example of new research making a significant difference are advances in the science of rejuvenating memory and improving sensory awareness among our aging and impaired populations.

Discussion

1. Identify the sensory modalities and how sensory modalities transmit messages to the brain.
2. Explain how it is possible to understand what is seen or heard, but not be able to verbally describe what is seen or heard.
3. Perceptions affect the emotional experience of individuals. Can you identify any illnesses or conditions in which perceptions are impaired?
4. Give examples of ways learning occurs through the stimulus-processing activity and explain how children with autism or autism spectrum disorders may have difficulty with tasks of learning.
5. Discuss the differences between functional and dysfunctional communication.

References

Amaral, D. G., Schumann, C. M., & Nordahl, C. W. (2008). Neuroanatomy of autism. *Trends in Neuroscience, 31*(3), 137–145. doi:10.1016/j.tins.2007.12.005

Barbe, W. B., & Milone, M. N. (1981, February). What we know about modality strengths. *Educational Leadership, Modality, Instructor,* 44–47.

Buhl, H. S. (posted 2001). Autonomic nervous system and energetic medicine. *The Science of Wilhelm Reich.* Retrieved from http://www.orgon.articles/article1.htm

Chilingaryan, L. I. (2001). Pavlov's theory of higher nervous activity: Landmarks and developmental trends. *Neuroscience and Behavioral Physiology, 31*(1), 39–47. PMID:11265812

Dauvermann, M. R., Whalley, H. C., Schmidt, A., Lee, G. L., Romaniuk, L., Roberts, N., ... Moorhead, T. W. J. (2014). Computational neuropsychiatry—Schizophrenia as a cognitive brain network disorder. *Frontiers in Psychiatry, 5,* 30. doi:10.3389/fpsyt.2014.00030

Denny, M. R., & Ratner, S. C. (1970). *Comparative psychology: Research in animal behavior.* Rev. ed. Homewood, IL: Dorsey Press.

Emerson, R. W., Adams, C., Nishino, T., Hazlett, H. C., Wolff, J. J., Zwaigenbaum, L., ... Piven, J. (2017). Functional neuroimaging of high-risk 6-month-old infants predicts a diagnosis of autism at 24 months of age. *Science Transitional Medicine, 9*(393), pii:eaag2882. doi:10.1126?scitranslmed.aag2882

Gazda, G. M., Childers, W.C., & Walters, R. P. (1982). *Interpersonal communication: A handbook for health professionals.* Gaithersburg, MD: Aspen Publishers, Inc. (Epigraph from pp. 141–142).

Grahek, N., & Dennett, D.C. (2011). *Feeling pain and being in pain.* Cambridge, MA: The MIT Press.

Gregory, N., Harris, A., Robinson, C. R., Dougherty, P. M., Fuchs, P. N., & Sluka, K. A. (2013). An overview of animal models of pain: Disease models and outcome measures. *Journal of Pain, 14*(11), 1255–1269. doi:10.1016/j.jain.20133.06.008

Hazlett, H. C., Gu, H., Munsell, B. C., Kim, S. H., Styne, M., Wolff, J. J., ... Piven, J. (2017). Early brain development in infants at high risk for autism spectrum disorder. *Nature, 542,* 348–351. doi:10.1038/nature21369.

Javitt, D. C., & Sweet, R. A. (2015). Auditory dysfunction in schizophrenia: Integrating clinical and basic features. *National Review of Neuroscience, 16*(9), 535–550. doi:10.1038/nrn4002

MacLean, P. D. (1970). The limbic brain in relation to the psychoses. In P. Black (Ed.), *Physiological correlates of emotion* (pp. 129–146). New York: Academic.

MacLean, P. D. (1973). *A triune concept of the brain and behavior.* Toronto, ON: University of Toronto Press.

Otte, C. (2011). Cognitive behavioral therapy in anxiety disorders: Current state of the evidence. *Dialogues in Clinical Neuroscience, 13*(4), 413–421. PMID:22275847

Porto, P. R., Oliveira, L., Mari, J., Volchan, E., Figueira, I., & Ventura, P. (2009). Does cognitive behavioral therapy change the brain? A systematic review of neuroimaging in anxiety disorders. *Journal of Neuropsychiatry and Clinical Neuroscience, 21,* 114–125. doi:10.1176/jnp.2009.21.2.114

Schifferstein, H. N. J. (2006). The perceived importance of sensory modalities in product usage: A study of self-reports. *Acta Psychologica, 121*(1), 41–64. doi:10.101/j.actpsy.2005.06.004

Silbersweig, D. A., & Stern, E. (1998). Towards a functional neuroanatomy of conscious perception and its modulation by volition: Implications of human auditory neuroimaging studies. *Philosophical Transactions of the Royal Society B: Biological Sciences, 353*(1377), 1883–1888. PMID:9854260

Smith, S. (1992). *Communications in nursing* (2nd ed.). St. Louis, MO: Mosby Yearbook.

Watzlawick, P. J., Beavin, J., & Jackson, D. D. (1967). *Pragmatics of human communication.* New York, NY: W.W. Norton & Company, Inc. (Epigraph from p. 13)

CHAPTER 5

The Nature of Therapeutic Communications

CHAPTER OBJECTIVES

- Compare and contrast functional and dysfunctional interpersonal communication.
- Discuss disturbances in perception, processing, and expression.
- Identify therapeutic interviewing skills, and differentiate them from nontherapeutic approaches.
- Discuss nondefensive communication that inevitably leads to functional and therapeutic encounters.
- Complete the personal inventory for nontherapeutic interviewing.

KEY TERMS

- Disturbed communication
- Extrospective and introspective tendencies
- Functional communication and dysfunctional communication
- Therapeutic communication
- Therapeutic interviewing skills

▶ Introduction

The idea that provider communication can be more or less helpful is not a new idea. Providers' abilities to create therapeutic effects through communication have been at least partially addressed in all the health care professions. Communications between health providers and patients deemed therapeutic share the following at the very least: help patients to cope, form strong interpersonal relationships built on mutual trust, and enable patients to successfully deal with health needs and adapt to illness restrictions.

On the contrary, those communications that are nontherapeutic can create divisiveness between patients and providers, cause patients to respond defensively, and rather than providing support, leave the patient feeling judged, or even rejected. The idea of communication being either therapeutic or nontherapeutic is put forth in idealistic terms, where meanings of *good* and *bad* are ascribed to various provider–patient encounters. Thus, it is important as to whether interaction is *therapeutic* or, conversely, *nontherapeutic*, and how **therapeutic communication** can be maximized, and nontherapeutic communication can be minimized.

This chapter discusses several important assumptions about therapeutic communication—some that can be substantiated, others that reflect biases about communication and the nature of the helper–patient relationship. The overall premise is that providers need to make communication the central component of care delivery and structure it in a patient-centered manner.

▶ Therapeutic Communication Defined

Therapeutic communication in the patient–provider relationship is interpersonal exchange, using verbal and nonverbal messages, that culminates in the patient being helped. Health care providers need to be able to elicit responses from patients and families that are in some way beneficial to them. Therapeutic communication is communication that expresses support, provides information and feedback, corrects distortions, and provides hope.

If one considers that humans have an inherent need to be heard and understood, any interchange that leaves patients feeling

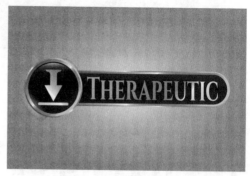

© Artist_R/Shutterstock.

heard and understood is, at some level, therapeutic because it provides for this basic human need. Patients are much more likely to be satisfied with their care when they participate in therapeutic encounters and establish rapport with their health care providers (Baumann, Baumann, Le Bihan, & Chau, 2008). Along with this is the patient's need to gain information about their symptoms and treatment, ask questions, and discuss ideas. Therapeutic communications with their providers help them feel the comfort of a partnership with those who will help them.

Humans, to some degree, need and want effective communication exchange. Self-expression, for example, can be therapeutic if it evokes acknowledgment and understanding from another person. The basic need to express oneself and to be heard and understood has been met. Despite that this need is prevalent to all humans does not mean that it is defined and valued equally across groups. Even the importance of being heard and understood plays out differently as a function of age, gender, ethnicity, socioeconomic status, education, and cultural.

As is therapeutic communication, nontherapeutic communication may be received differently as a function of these basic characteristics. Consider several of the patient complaints described in the *Introduction* to this text. For example, patients talked about these aspects of their communications and relationships with health care providers and explained:

> [What is difficult is] "wanting to speak to someone who really cares (and not having anyone)." I'm lonely and isolated. Somebody recognize that I need someone to show they really care about me.
>
> "People come into your room without permission. They come in and don't identify themselves. I feel like a guinea pig." How can I tell if they should be here or not? What are they going to do to me?
>
> "Not always understanding doctor's answers to my questions. I ask a question and get a *nonanswer* for an answer. I am supposed to be satisfied with that?" Do they think they are really helping by treating me this way?
>
> "I go for my annual checkup and my doctor keeps talking about his special projects. Finally, I had to say to him 'what about *me* doc?'" Maybe I don't have any major problems but still I want my doctor to ask me about my health and any concerns I have even though he might not think I have a problem.

Is it possible that these comments reflect expectations that are not shared by all individuals and groups? The complaint about feeling isolated and alone might be expressed differently if this patient was a young adult male, or perhaps not be something a young adult male patient might express. Feeling like "a guinea pig" may be something an educated person might experience and would say. Not getting answers that are clear from health care providers is universal. But, would a middle-aged migrant woman of Middle Eastern descent feel as concerned as those from Western industrialized societies where some patients engage in shared decision making. Finally, the complaint that the health professional is not concerned about them and is focused on other interests is very commonplace. Still, would a young teenage girl say this?

The idea that it can be generic to all persons, but valued differently, is discussed further in this chapter. Therapeutic communications must take into consideration multiple and often different views of both patients and their families.

Distinguishing the Use of Therapeutic Approaches When Used by Providers, Not Lay Persons

An important assumption about therapeutic communication is that it can result from a number of helping relationships, beyond that of patient and health care provider exclusively. Therapeutic communication is not a skill practiced exclusively by health care professionals. In actuality, therapeutic communication can be practiced by anyone. Whether informal spontaneous interchanges between friends, or purposeful interaction such as between provider and patient, it is assumed that one communicant is more able or ready to respond in a helpful manner, and that this occurs over a series of exchanges of messages. It is true that providers care much about the impact of their communication with patients. It is also true that the average person may care and is also capable of being therapeutic.

Therapeutic encounters are either isolated events or occur spontaneously as a product of ongoing relationships. The behavior most associated with the therapeutic effects of friends and family is providing positive support and strength to patients. In fact, the average person may be a valuable source of support and communicate in supportive ways for long periods without realizing it. Patients, also recipients of support, may gain from the dialogue also without knowing it. Besides providing tangible support cooking, transport, and providing home care, family and friends are capable of dealing effectively with worry and sadness and correct misperceptions that cause the patient stress. More appropriately, it is important for providers to tap into and use the natural therapeutic potential of friends and family.

What differentiates the provider who practices therapeutic communication and the average person who does the same? There are some distinct differences:

1. The provider consciously intends to influence the patient in a therapeutic manner.
2. With this intention, providers usually have a professional goal or objective in mind. They are not using this approach to achieve personal gain. In other circumstances, outside the health provider–patient relationship, this is not the case. For example, politicians say hopeful things to gain votes and salespersons make people feel good in order to increase sales. Providers have the intention of helping the patient for the patient's sake. The patient's well-being, not the provider's personal gains, is the driving force behind the words used, and how they are expressed.
3. Providers will perceive deficits in patients' perception, processing, or expression of ideas and information. Providers attempt any deficits they encounter in therapeutic relationships. Providers will focus on ill-expressed thoughts and feelings, breakdowns in expression, and distortions in perception. It is not by chance that deficits in perception, processing, or expression are addressed. Rather, providers purposefully attempt to improve the communication capabilities of patients (see **EXHIBIT 5-1**).

In summary, therapeutic communication can be practiced by many, not just by providers, in very specific healer–patient circumstances. Therapeutic messages and communication

---

EXHIBIT 5-1 Differences in Provider and Layperson Use of Therapeutic Communication

Health Providers Communications Display

- Conscious intention to achieve a therapeutic purpose.
- Professional aims or goals guiding messages.
- Intentions to help patients "feel better" or "get better."
- Attempts to correct deficits in patients' communications through asking questions or seeking clarity.

Layperson Communications Display

- Spontaneous, sometimes thoughtless responses.
- No particular therapeutic purpose, known nor intended.
- Intentions to help people "feel good" may be secondary to achieving another purpose (e.g., selling an idea or product, or winning an argument).
- Attempts to improve others' communications may or may not be the intention.

can be very spontaneous and occur under ordinary circumstances without much fore-thought or planning. Understanding the universal nature of therapeutic communication can create optimism about the human potential, as well as the natural helping resources that are available to patients and their families.

Currently there are a number of professional organizations which inform nonprofessional caregivers or laypersons, frequently family members of patients experiencing some form of chronic or serious illness, about how to communicate with patients. Many patients with chronic illnesses engage their families (spouses, children, parents, or siblings) during difficult times when patients are feeling vulnerable or situations are difficult and challenging. Many of these guides can be found on the Internet, such as those for speaking to patients with alcohol and drug abuse problems, mental illness, and eating disorders. Guidelines generally advise one or more of the following:

1. Let the patient know that you are there for them and committed to helping them get better.
2. Show that you are listening, and if you cannot help them, you will find someone or some resource that can.
3. Help them to find trustworthy information and offer to go with them to medical visits.
4. Encourage them to seek help beyond what you can offer, such as support groups for patients with the same illness or condition.

There are particular instances in which the role of patient–caregiver communication is being examined for the effect upon patient outcomes (Fisher & Nussbaum, 2015; Mallinger, Griggs, & Shields, 2006; Shin et al., 2016). Fisher and Nussbaum explained that

family communication is an important means of adapting to stress, coping, and successful aging in older persons dealing with cancer and called for an integrating family communication into care.

Approaches might include asking patients to bring in a family member to appointments where care decisions and test results are being considered and providing support services geared to both the patient and family members. Mallinger et al. addressed the needs of breast cancer patients and the benefit of open and supportive family communication. In their study, they found that open family communication was associated with better mental health outcomes in women coping with survivorship and overcoming the stress of living with a cancer diagnosis. In the study by Shin et al. (2016), national survey data to examine the interactions and communications between family caregivers and patients concluded that the promotion of family intervention to enhance openness to communication about patients' cancer may benefit patients considerably.

Continued communication between patient and caregiver is more likely because cancer has become a chronic disease entailing long-term management. It was suggested that the mental health and quality of life for patients as well as their caregivers could be improved. Studies such as these help us understand that the role of nonprofessional caregiver communications is a significant one and will continue to be.

Functional and Dysfunctional Communication Patterns

While some providers will be engaged in restoring patients' health, both directly and indirectly, such as by overseeing medications, treatments, or surgical procedures, all providers manage patients' ongoing communication capabilities. In the counseling professions, this responsiveness to and management of communication is focused in-depth on the form and content of patients' communications. Although patients need to be functional communicators, they are not always good communicators.

Functional Communication Prerequisites

Functional communication is characterized by an absence of disturbances in perception, processing, and expression of thoughts and feelings. Functional communication is often associated with signs of health. When communication is functional, one presumes a basic level of health, however, when dysfunctional poor health is suspected. As put forth in the chapter on the anatomy and physiology of communication, sending, receiving, and processing messages is complex and disruptions can occur in one or more areas.

Not all individuals are accustomed to expressing thoughts and feelings through expressive language. At a very minimum (1) persons need capabilities in perceiving appropriately, (2) learning the language and symbolic and metacommunication systems that prevail in their community, (3) acquiring and correcting information in order to maintain an appropriate view of self and the world, (4) integrating experiences into a comprehensive whole and the resolution of contradictions, (5) learning by imitation or experience the means by which one can achieve desires and influence others, and (6) sorting out and eliminating interferences from internal and external noises.

Depending on the age, health status, educational, cultural, and socioeconomic characteristics of the individual, a command over all these tasks may not be possible. When a provider recognizes that patients have deficits in these functionalities, not only are they judging the patient's stage of

EXHIBIT 5-2 Summary of Necessary Prerequisites for Functional Communication

- Perceive appropriately.
- Learn the prevailing language and symbolic systems.
- Acquire and correct information when necessary.
- Integrate experiences into a comprehensive whole, resolving contradictions when and where they occur.
- Sort out and eliminate interference from internal and external environmental "noise."

growth and development, they are referring to many other factors that are affecting their current communication behavior (see **EXHIBIT 5-2**).

Signs of Dysfunctional or Disturbed Communication

Patients may not only be impaired in their communication capabilities, but also they may exhibit patterns of **disturbed communication**. The concept of disturbed communication was first addressed in the classic work of Jurgen Ruesch (1961). Subsequent to its earlier uses, disturbed communication has come to be used to describe a wide range of problems. These include pathological communication in persons with formal thought disorders (unusual or dysfunctional ways of thinking), such as that found in schizophrenia (NIMH, 2016) and autism spectrum disorders (Solomon, Ozonoff, Carter, & Caplan, 2008), or in brain connectivity disorders exhibiting problems in information exchange, such as those patients with Alzheimer's disease (Thomas et al., 2014).

Disturbed communication can occur episodically or appear as a more stable phenomenon. Unlike those individuals whose capabilities have not yet been fully developed due to, for example, learning a new language, people with disturbed communication could have regressed in their usual ability to communicate effectively. Changes in abilities can come on quickly (e.g., in the case of a stroke), or slowly (as in the case of acquired impaired vision or hearing loss). Of particular concern is the increasing incidence of vision difficulties in the U.S. population. Varma et al. (2016) reported on increases in visual impairment and blindness reporting that in 2015 over 1 million people were blind and over 3 million had visual impairments. These statistics and others raise concern not only for the health of these individuals but for their capacity to function and effectively communicate.

The reasons patients exhibit disturbed communication are many, including normal aging, brain disorders, injury and trauma, emotional disturbance, poor health status, learning disability, and relational stress. **Dysfunctional communication** is diagnosable through the observations of verbal and nonverbal behavior. When "diagnosing" disturbed communication, one is also interested in "why" and "what" needs to be restored or enhanced.

As a Function of Patient Environment

It must be said that disturbed communication may also be a function of the interaction of the patient with environment, as in the case of intensive acute care psychosis. This is a phenomenon observed, particularly in older persons, when hospitalized in medical or surgical intensive care units (ICUs). ICU delirium and psychosis are increasingly prevalent conditions and may occur at any time during recovery from an acute illness.

Delirium results from a number of factors and is a disturbance in consciousness and impaired abilities to receive, process, store, and recall information. Patients in the ICU are particularly at risk for delirium. Assessment of delirium in these patients is made difficult by the fact they are mechanically ventilated and cannot communicate (Ely and colleagues, 2001). Delirium and inability to communicate can often occur in patients with mechanical ventilation in the ICU. In acute care psychosis, the patient usually shows significant disorientation or irritability and may even have auditory and/or visual hallucinations. This acute brain failure is frequently associated with dehydration, low blood oxygen, and infectious states. Although impairment in processing information is significant, the occurrence does not seem to reflect a more substantial psychiatric disorder. Rather, it is a temporary shift in cognitive capacity and thought to occur in many patients whose stay in the ICU exceeds 5 days. Causative factors include sensory deprivation, sleep disturbance, lack of orientation to time, date, and place, and noise from medical monitoring machines that also disturb sleep in the ICU.

Despite the fact that the commonly seen syndrome, ICU psychosis, was initially observed to be temporary and largely devoid of long-term consequences, Wesley et al. (2001) emphasized that all is not known about this kind of delirium in the ICU because of a lack of valid measurement, and ICU delirium is more than a short-term ICU psychosis. In fact, there is evidence of long-term deficits for a significant percentage of patients, with patients continuing to demonstrate symptoms of delirium after discharge. Furthermore, Wesley et al. (2003) demonstrated that delirium in the ICU was an independent predictor of higher 6-month mortality and longer hospital stays, documenting its importance as a form of organic function.

As a Function of Dyadic Relationships

Forms of disturbed communication can have an early origin in early childhood development and continue through adulthood. One form is *incongruence*. Communication is more or less congruent or incongruent. Much interest has been directed at the importance of congruence and our ability to recognize and learn from congruent versus incongruent messages, both as children and adults.

When one thinks of *congruent communication*, what is usually meant is that the verbal statement is consistent with behaviors associated with its content. For example, when patients are speaking about the uncertainty of their diagnosis, they frequently demonstrate worry in their tone of voice and physical gestures. They may appear tense, mildly agitated, or confused. These nonverbal components are generally consistent with being anxious, uncertain, and worried about one's diagnosis. Sometimes patients will exhibit these behaviors but express confidence or denial about the uncertainty of their diagnosis. When this occurs, their communication is incongruent because their verbal message is inconsistent with their nonverbal responses. Similarly, providers can communicate with incongruence. Say, for example, you as a provider are delivering some very bad news and simultaneously smile. Your nonverbal communication is not congruent with the message you are giving. Even if the smile is a nervous response, it is confusing to the patient.

Incongruence is an important quality of communications not only because it suggests impairment or disruption, but also because of its association with prevention and treatment.

A particularly interesting but exploratory study of problems with incongruence and children's adherence to diabetic diets makes this point (Chisholm et al., 2014). In a study of the effect of incongruence in communication between mothers (the primary caregiver) and young children (ages 6–8) with type 1 diabetes,

incongruence was correlated with poorer child adjustment problems. That is, higher levels of maternal incongruent communication correlated with poorer dietary adherence. Conversely, positive mother–child communications was associated with better adjustment outcomes. Underlying reasons could include the fact that incongruent messages are confusing for children and foster ambivalence, for example, eating foods with high sugar content becomes confusing when mothers' verbally express "we should do it" but nonverbally show negative attitudes about the choice such as punctuating the statement with a frown.

Signs of Faulty Communications in Patients Communications with Health Providers

Do providers always identify impaired communications in patients? In part, this depends on their level of emotional intelligence or their ability to perceive the emotional impact a conversation might have on a patient or the patient's family. Rather than employing emotional intelligence, many providers use the patient's spoken message to understand what the patient is saying without examining the meaning for the patient behind the message. For example, if patients react to a serious diagnosis by laughing or shrugging their shoulders, does this mean they have no feelings about what the provider just said? The likelihood is very small that patients do not have feelings about a serious diagnosis. They may not, however, have immediate access to these feelings, and therefore are unable to address the meaning this diagnosis has for them.

There are *give-away* signs of impaired processing and expressing of thoughts and feelings. Easily recognizable clues would include any one or more of the following behaviors: messages might be too long, too short, or ill-placed. The patient's capacity to communicate effectively is hampered, and while this may be a temporary situation (as in the case of shock and extreme stress), it may be indicative of more pervasive communication difficulties (as in the case of injury or trauma).

Other clues that the patient is having difficulty can be picked up from patients' nonverbal responsiveness. Patients' nonverbal behavior can indicate problems in perceiving and processing information. The acoustic dimensions of the patient's voice (e.g., the intensity of speech, punctuation or emphasis, intonation, and speed) can also depict disturbed states as well.

Can providers get clues through voices? What is a *healthy voice*? People who are under stress speak differently. Actual changes in muscle contraction, as well as in the rhythmical patterns of breathing, and in the functions of the vocal cords occur when individuals are stressed. Therefore, a healthy voice might be one that displays harmonious tones, smooth transitions, and calm, composed rhythms. But, one might also argue that some people disguise their emotional state and mimic these characteristics to convince others that they are "OK," "fine," or "well," when in fact they are not functioning up to par. There is a way to differentiate between feigned functional communication and actual *healthy* communication. First, look for the general patterns. A sense of well-being may be initially expressed, but within minutes, patients' level of functioning and how they are feeling might change. Also, observations of inconsistencies in verbal and nonverbal messages is another way to determine how well the patient is doing. Look for incongruences.

Another way to conceptualize and assess disturbed communication is to take each functional aspect of communication behavior and identify the system that is most defective. As previously discussed, disturbed communication can occur in the realms of perception, evaluation or processing, and expression (see **EXHIBIT 5-3**). These systems overlap, and it is extremely important to understand how disturbances are both independently and interdependently manifested. Health care providers

EXHIBIT 5-3 Categories of Disturbed Communication

- Disturbance in perception of stimuli/messages.
- Disturbance in processing stimuli/messages received.
- Disturbance in expression of messages.

continually assess patients' level of communication and any changes that might occur. Some patients are able to effectively receive, process, send messages, and respond appropriately to our questions, but others may only be able to send or receive a message—some may not be able to do either.

If a total-system approach is applied, one would understand that even though these elements (perception, evaluation, processing, and expression) can be separated out, it would not be possible to understand human communication without considering their interdependency. That is, a malfunction or disruption in one (e.g., in perception) has implications for the others. For example, a disturbance in perception will most likely have implications for how one processes and evaluates input. This, in turn, may affect expression—at least, the appropriateness of the expression.

When, for example, perception is distorted, judgments about input will be faulty. Faulty judgment, in turn, has implications for the appropriateness of expression. Finally, if expressions are faulty, then a disruption may occur in further evaluative and perceptive functioning. In summary, problems in any one dimension will result in problems in another. The relationship between these systems or channels is complex, and while the principle of interrelationships applies, there is probably more to the interaction than what can be deduced in a causal inference, or even from the standpoint of a feedback loop. The human brain and how it interprets the senses is exceedingly complex.

One could say, for example, that a patient pulls away from the physician's hand because the child or adult fears pain or discomfort. The provider is not there to induce pain, so is this reaction a result of a distortion of reality? One's brain is capable of making its own reality. Humans are affected by both internal and external stimuli. What seems illogical to us may make sense to the patient. Former memories of pain come to bear on the patients' current perceptions. A complex array of stimuli impacts the patient from a variety of sources, including the data derived from the process of evaluation and expression. If one were to pinpoint the primary system that is disturbed, one would also have to recognize that this is only part of the larger picture.

Disturbed Perception and Sensory Impairments

The primary role of perception is to enable us to obtain information from the environment. This function is accomplished through sensory neurons which communicate about physical phenomenon in our environment. Sensory neurons have nerve endings embedded in tissues that serve to pick up and transmit characteristics such as light, sound, smell/taste, and pressure. Certain aids are specially designed to compensate for impaired sensory capacities. These include hearing aids, visual aids that magnify objects or the written word, and even medications that improve a sense of smell for patients experiencing persistent sinus inflammation and infection.

Disturbances in *perception* or perception as the primary source of pathology are studied by many professional disciplines. The neurobehavioral, psychosocial, neuropsychiatric, and neurophysiological sciences study the exactitudes of human perception, and many of these scientific principles have been alluded to in a previous chapter of this text. The problems of selective inattention, sensory deprivation, sensory distortion, and the inability to balance between sensory input (from internal and external sources) are examples of problems in perception. The classical example of selective inattention occurs when a person ignores significant details of events, perhaps to avoid unpleasant feelings, but in doing so, negates the importance of certain details.

Not all treatments for selective inattention would be called humane. In fact, a former common practice of treating people who experienced a condition called *hysterical blindness* was to shock them (e.g., by slapping them in the face). This jolted the patient's awareness and restored the patient's full vision. As stated in the reports of treatments of patients, "Give chloroform, make the patient mad, or a sharp slap on the skin will often cure the case. No medicine is needed" (State of Missouri, 36th Annual Session, 1893). It was thought that the blunt directedness of this action forced the patient to reconstitute his or her line of vision and to respond to a greater number and/or kind of stimuli.

Can you imagine such a practice in health care today? What has evolved as current practice is much different from those primitive methods. The former condition referred to as *hysterical blindness* has been recategorized and labeled as a conversion reaction, or disorder. Although this condition can be accompanied by illness, the symptoms cannot be explained by medical illness, injury, or by medical evaluation, and usually begins after a stressful event. Typically, patients lack control over their symptoms. Their symptoms cannot be turned off or lessened by them on their own.

Other approaches are reported to be effective with functional visual loss not due to physical injury or illness and include stress management and psychotherapy. Techniques sometimes include confrontation in the context of supportive psychotherapy. The idea is that the provider can awaken patients to a wider scope of stimuli by observing astutely (patients' nonverbal and verbal communication) and mirror back or confront patients with facts they have ignored. But caution is needed because in some cases these conditions are linked to stressful events, and patients' growing recognition may trigger painful memories. In summary, interventions must be performed by qualified professionals in the context of a supportive therapeutic relationship. This does not require the jolt of a slap, using chloroform, or making patients mad.

Sensory distortion is another form of sensory disturbance and can occur in other ways akin to selective inattention. *Selective inattention* refers to the blocking out of stimuli and results in distortions of perception, but other behaviors also contribute to perceptual distortion. For example, some people misinterpret others' communications because they apply stereotypic interpretations, or they generally experience things differently. They may even have an intolerance for the ideas or behaviors of others. They may also be unaware of the specific social or cultural context of their interpersonal situations. Sometimes, they are so highly adapted and trained at picking up some stimuli that they fail to see others. These are all examples of selective inattention and perceptual distortion resulting from societal influences, not medical conditions.

While sensory distortion occurs due to personal deficits, sensory acuity can simultaneously reflect strengths, not weaknesses. Consider the fact, for example, that some people are oblivious to inner cues. Emotional feelings—fear, sadness, and anger—may be out of their range of awareness; or physical sensations—pressure, tension, and even pain—are not perceptible. These individuals may, however, be very proficient at perceiving stimuli outside themselves from environmental clues or subtle shifts in the moods and behaviors of others. To some extent, health care providers may fit into this latter category. They may be very good at perceiving others' needs (**extrospective**) but much less aware when it comes to sensing their own needs (**introspective**). *Introspectively* handicapped persons can transform their natural tendency to

focus outside themselves into a skill. However, the result may be dysfunctional perceptivity.

In contrast, *extrospectively* handicapped persons can easily recognize internal stimuli but miss or neglect signals and signs from the external world. To some extent, young children fit this category. They are attuned to their internal feelings of hunger, pain, and fear, but they will misjudge external stimuli. They may purposefully disregard external clues, or because they are ill equipped, they may not attend to all external stimuli. In fact, a major role of adults in our society is and has been to protect children from their underdeveloped abilities to perceive and judge external stimuli. Whether or not individuals are strong at picking up internal, or external, clues, the imbalance is important. To help these individuals, the weakest stimulus capacity needs to be strengthened while protecting and nurturing the strongest stimulus capacity.

Sensory deficits, another category of perceptual dysfunction or impairment, can be of several kinds. The most commonly observed sensory impairments are those of hearing or vision. Reports based on standard hearing examinations estimate than an outstanding 1 in 8 people in the United States aged 12 and older (13% or 30 million) has hearing loss in both ears (NIH, NIDCD, 2016).

In 2015, 3.2 million Americans had visual impairment due to having 20/40 or worse vision; another 8.2 million had vision impairment due to uncorrected refractive errors, for a total of 11.4 million people (NIH, 2016). Visual impairment and blindness cases in the United States are expected to double by 2050. Rates of hearing and vision loss are also expected to double by 2050 due in part to the baby boomers aging.

Vision and hearing loss may be congenital and permanent, or temporary, requiring no significant long-term adaptation. Defects in vision will affect expressive behavior. For example, many blind people do not speak with punctuation or intensity. Their speech tends to be bland, due in part to the fact they cannot perceive, and therefore react to, the nonverbal expressions of the other person. Likewise, disturbances in hearing will affect the development of speech. Other disturbances in sensory awareness include equilibrium and tactile capabilities. These disturbances also impede individuals' perceptions.

Disturbed Processing and Cognitive Impairment

Disturbances in processing of information obtained from the senses are many, and include the capacities to cognitively and emotionally deal with stimuli. Decision-making and memory are frequent outcomes of the capacity to process and evaluate perceived stimuli. If providers say that someone is having difficulties in decision-making, for example, they may be suspicious of some deficit in the area of cognitive and emotional processing. Is this a state condition (dependent on current circumstances) or a trait condition (a more lasting characteristic)?

Methods of codification and the ability to assess probabilities are part of the decision-making process. To evaluate by using probabilities ensures individuals of safe and proper actions. When one cannot or does not assess events using probability, or when they cannot remember what happened to choose and apply a probability model, they are at risk for evaluating stimuli inadequately. This problem may be more or less serious. Take, for example, dieters who choose to have just one bite of chocolate cake or candy or just one sugar drink. Having been at the mercy of passion for sugars and sweets such as chocolate cake and candy or drinks laced with sugar in the past, this is risky behavior. One bite of cake can lead to a piece, one piece to a second piece, and so on. If one cannot remember what it was like to be "seduced" by chocolate cake, or cannot assign a probability to the chance of eating more than they should, one's processing of data is defective.

Moods, feelings, and attitudes also influence judgment and decision-making. As a matter of fact, these factors have a great deal to do with our decisions. One could conclude, for example, that the reason they fell into the "just have another bite" situation was that feelings or moods influenced their desires to avoid using the concept of probability. Capacities to make decisions also depend on one's ability to scan information that is held in one's memories, to consider this information, to modify any considerations, and to act. Having determined that "good sense" would mean one should avoid even the sight of chocolate cake, it is as if one short-circuits good sense to get to the pleasure. At this point they have defaulted on applying probability principles.

The result of acting requires us to make a choice and to regulate our behavior based on our choice. This process can be affected by our abilities to scan, to arrange experiences in an orderly way, and to draw on stored information. Our strengths and abilities in these areas are influenced by many circumstances. Aging has an effect on memory, but it also transforms our abilities to scan for relevant information and establish risks. Some memory disturbances occur when individuals remember experiences but cannot apply what they experienced and learned to new situations. Each time that they are presented with the problem, they approach it as if they had never experienced it at all, a brand-new event does not elicit lessons learned. One carries out the same problem-solving steps that one used during the first encounter with chocolate cake, or a similar urge they had when they first encountered the problem. Disturbances in processing information are important, despite the heavy emphasis on abilities to perceive and express.

Disturbed Expression and Impairments in Sending Messages

The overriding function of our ability to express ourselves is the opportunity it affords us to participate in interpersonal relationships. Without the ability to express ourselves, and this involves many facets of our central or peripheral nervous systems, including various motor capabilities, one simply cannot relate to others or get confirmation or acknowledgment of one's ideas or actions. In short, there is limited ability to make an impact on others.

This condition affects not only enjoyment of relationships but also one's self-concept and self-esteem. People who have speech impairments, for example, will exaggerate their associated facial expressions and postural responses. The purpose is to establish enough meaning in their messages to trigger a definitive response from others—but, the response that they desire, not one that is hurtful. Disturbances of expression can include inhibited, exaggerated expression, or the absence of expression altogether. There are also motor defects that can affect our abilities to express ourselves.

Because communication is highly influenced by the interpersonal context, communicants who display an absence of speech or inhibited or exaggerated expression may be reflecting their perceptions of the interpersonal dynamics in which the encounter occurs. One might say that some adolescents are speechless not because they have a permanent disability but because they are reacting to some stimulus in their social or interpersonal encounter. Stuttering and repetitive speech can occur when children and teens are "nervous" or fear speaking in front of their peers. But, is this the case when the teen cannot clearly tell his parents the results of his exam? Both instances describe a social context for poor expressive language, but the roles and reasons differ.

With peers, there is a fear of being ostracized or shunned, of being embarrassed or teased. With parents, the fear may be more of worrying about disappointing their parents. Fearing disappointment may lead to incomplete messages or ambiguous descriptions to avoid a complete lie. Problems of expression can either be biologically induced or reflect social and interpersonal relationship dynamics—at least the individual's views of the relationship and what might damage this relationship.

Many of us have seen several cases in which there are defects in expression that are a result of motor impairment. People with nerve lesions, muscular disorders, or other impairments that affect weakness or paralysis of the muscles in the face, tongue, or throat usually suffer expressive deficits. This group also includes patients whose expressions are complicated by the involuntary movements of tremors and tics. Essentially, the specific defect alters the character of the person's expression. These deficits are usually permanent, and individuals learn to compensate for the defect. If one carefully listens and observes these communications, it is possible to identify (1) the immediate effect of the defect on speech, (2) individuals' compensatory response to the defect, and (3) patients' responses to their own perceptions of the reactions others will have.

Expressive language disorders are found in school-aged children. These disorders are conditions in which a child has a lower than normal ability to use vocabulary, use complete sentences, and remember the words to use. These children have difficulties getting their meaning or message across to others, even parents and teachers. Despite these expressive language difficulties, the same child might have normal language skills to understand others' and written communication when they read messages. The cause of these disorders is not well-understood, but the causes may be due to a number of factors—malnutrition, damage or injury to the brain (cerebrum), or even genetic factors.

Autism in children is a special category and is characterized by deficits in expressive communication. A recent summary of the problem of autism spectrum disorder in children, and their problems in using expressive language are explained in NIH, NIDCD, 2016. Problems in expressive language skills are multiple and include repetitive or rigid language, narrow interests, and exceptional abilities. These children may be unable to carry on a conversation and display uneven language development. These latter symptoms can be misjudged to be a result of a hearing problem or poor nonverbal conversational skills. Without an ability to use meaningful gestures or nonverbal expressions to support their speech, they may become frustrated and act out their frustration with vocal outbursts or inappropriate behavior [NIH Pub. No. 97-4315, October 2016].

Sending messages, and our skills in doing it effectively to get the response desired, is highly tied to one's ability to function in roles of employee, boss, parent, spouse, or friend.

At the workplace, one knows that they will do better if they speak clearly and simply, speak loud enough to be heard, and be consistent in what they say. Messages are sent using both verbal and nonverbal behaviors. One's nonverbal behaviors should be congruent with the spoken word. Nonverbal gestures or body language can express a great deal and influence whether one's messages will be received as intended or will be misinterpreted. Persons who have speech deficits sometimes have trouble in matching their verbal statements with their nonverbal gestures.

Sending messages is clearly influenced by technology and social media. Social media sites and the rapid exchange of emails and voicemails introject another element. With recent communication technology, including the sending of text messages, emails, and voice

messages, one is confronted with a number of choices to amplify one's messages and punctuate the meaning of the messages. This occurs with the use of balloons and confetti, bold and italic remarks, and the addition of icons and pictures.

In summary, disturbances in communication run the gamut of perceptual, processing, and expressive functions. They may be temporary and contextual, or they may reflect a long-standing motor deficit. The exact origin and nature of the problem is important but not always critical to our understanding of how to communicate effectively with these individuals. The most important aspect is that providers are able to recognize the source and nature of the communication deficit(s) and persist in their attempts to not only understand the basis of the symptoms, but also ways they can support patients' communication.

It is not the purpose of this chapter to address at length the medical conditions that affect communication, which are numerous and include specific neurophysiologic and neurochemical deficiencies that are found in a variety of patient populations. They include the variety of language and speech disorders, developmental delays, and specific motor deficits. These conditions are extremely important to the study of disturbed communication, but the exact medical explanations are not a topic for this general review nor the focus.

Before leaving the topic of disturbed communication, it is important to address the phenomena of *dysfunctional* communication. While disturbed communication connotes a specific defect, dysfunctional communication suggests a process that is highly linked to the interpersonal context of relationships. For example, when family therapists describe dysfunctional communication behaviors in family members, they are usually suggesting that *patterns* of dysfunctional communication are associated with larger-scale family dynamics and difficulties. Therefore, they attempt to change interpersonal or family dysfunctional communication patterns with a variety of approaches, depending on their training and theoretical persuasion.

Some theorists have clarified problematic communication by differentiating dysfunctional communication from the functional type. For example, expressive communication that is too much or too little, too early or too late, or tangential (in the wrong place) is said to reflect dysfunction. Dysfunction, here, not only refers to the explicit communication behavior but also to the nature of the encounter as a whole.

Perhaps the most important understanding of dysfunctional communication patterns is found in the historical work of certain theorists' studies of family dynamics (Satir, 1967; Watzlawick, Beavin, & Jackson, 1967; Watzlawick, Weakland, & Fisch, 1974). Satir (1967), for example, explicitly defined the characteristics of a dysfunctional communicator. According to Satir, dysfunctional communicators overgeneralize; assume that others share their feelings, thoughts, and perceptions; assume that their perceptions or evaluations are complete; and assume that what they perceive or evaluate will not change. These individuals assume there are only two possible alternatives (they tend to dichotomize or think in terms of African American or white): (1) that what they attribute to things or people are actually a part of those things or people and (2) that they can get inside the skin of the other person (not only to act as a spokesperson for that person, but also that others can do the same with them).

Individuals who exhibit functional communication, as opposed to dysfunctional, are more likely to use qualification and clarification. These individuals tend to clearly state their case, are ready to clarify or qualify their remarks, and ask for feedback. They are also receptive to feedback when they receive it. Providers who establish effective communication with patients will not only exhibit functional communication, they will also be model communicators. They exemplify clear communication and also teach patients how to achieve it. To do this, they must spell out the rules for communicating accurately, emphasizing checking out the meanings of messages and correcting invalid assumptions.

Providers need to be very clear in their own messages, showing a willingness to repeat, restate, and carefully explain how they reached conclusions. It is hoped that through both the providers' modeling and their capacity to interrupt dysfunctional communication, the patient will be encouraged to move toward more-effective communication styles. Therapeutic communications with patients require specific knowledge and skill sets. Among these are the abilities to engage the patient in therapeutic interviewing, to assist the patient to communicate more effectively, and to avoid the traps of dysfunctional communication.

▶ Therapeutic Interviewing Skills

Much has been written about the principles and practices of therapeutic interviewing. In this text, specific techniques of therapeutic communication and therapeutic interviewing (referred to as critical competencies) are described in detail in the next section of the text. The purpose of this discussion of therapeutic interviewing is to provide general groundwork for the principles and practices to be discussed later on in the text.

Therapeutic interviewing has very specific objectives. Generally, *therapeutic interviewing* is established to accomplish one or more of these aims:

■ Elicit full descriptions from patients about their health care condition and concerns.

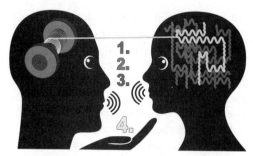

© Sangoiri/Shutterstock.

- Create an interpersonally safe place for patients to talk about themselves, and be able to explore their problems in detail.
- Reduce any acute emotional distress associated with patients' immediate condition.
- Offer support and reassurance.
- Establish an expanded list of patients' primary and secondary health care problems.
- Engage patients in a problem-solving process that demonstrates the collaborative aspects of the provider–patient relationship.
- Prepare patients for self-management of their health and illness.

Therapeutic Communications and Therapeutic Interview Encounters

The specific types of questions and responses used to accomplish the overall goal of establishing a therapeutic encounter are many. With regard to even one therapeutic response, such as asking open-ended questions, the approach can be used again, can be modified, or can be discontinued based upon the reactions received. For example, the provider can use a question, can reask the same question, can refer back to it later, or can replace it with a more appropriately worded question to effectively engage patients in conversations about an important related topic (see **EXHIBIT 5-4**). Using a series of open-ended questions about different topics is

---

EXHIBIT 5-4 Therapeutic Response Modes

- Using silence.
- Offering acceptance, empathy, and compassion.
- Acknowledging and giving recognition (e.g., verbalizing the unspoken but implied message).
- Offering broad openings.
- Making and offering observations and summarizing.
- Reflecting one's own perception of the patient's thoughts, feelings, and reactions.
- Focusing the patient, and at other times, prompting exploration.
- Translating thoughts into feelings and feelings into thoughts.
- Encouraging evaluation or appraisal.
- Validating the patient's perceptions and/or beliefs.

---

an equally effective approach. Or, providers can switch between using open-ended and closed-ended questions depending on their appraisal of how well the interview is going.

These response modes are discussed in considerable detail in chapters to follow. There are many responses that achieve the overall aim of the therapeutic encounter. In chapters to follow, specific therapeutic response modes are discussed in detail with explanations of why and when they are appropriate.

Nontherapeutic Communications

Just as there are various recommended responses to maximize therapeutic encounters with patients and their families, there are those to avoid because they do not foster therapeutic relationship building, and may even impose barriers to an effective working relationship. Earlier in the "Introduction" to this chapter, several different kinds of complaints that might be voiced by patients when they are dissatisfied with their care, their provider, and their relationship with the provider and system of care, were identified. Here are a few to review in the context of nontherapeutic response modes:

> **False reassurance:** "I'm afraid my health provider (doctor) is not telling me the truth (cancer diagnosis)." I can't trust what he or she says.
>
> **Scolding or moralizing:** The health provider (nurse) got mad when I told her I couldn't take my pill with water." Why is she mad at me? Doesn't this ever happen with other patients?
>
> **Lack of appreciation of what problems mean to patients:** "Not always understanding the health provider's (doctor's) answers to my questions. I ask a question and get a *nonanswer* for an answer. I am supposed to be satisfied with that?" Do they think they are really helping by treating me this way?
>
> **Belittling and defensive responses:** "I had some legitimate questions, but the nurse got defensive…was demeaning, she raised her voice and called me: 'Dear', 'Sweetheart', 'Honey' …that just made me more frustrated, and I thought it was very inappropriate. She didn't speak English very well. I just wanted concrete answers and she contradicted herself." When I ask questions, I think I deserve an answer.

Notice that each of these examples demonstrates specific ways communications may not foster therapeutic encounters. These responses frequently impose barriers to an effective working relationship.

EXHIBIT 5-5 is a list of nontherapeutic communication responses. At one point or another, most of us have fallen into communication

that "missed the mark." You are encouraged to evaluate your past use of these modes and how you might go about correcting your approach. Nontherapeutic phrases and gestures impose barriers to effective working relationships because they limit patients' verbal expressions, cause negative reactions, or even make patients feel threatened.

These responses are usually nontherapeutic, but not always. There are appropriate ways and times to use advice, to probe, and even confront patients. However, for beginning providers, it is helpful to know that most of these responses are problematic and result in negative patient–provider encounters. There is the assumption that therapeutic communication requires time, and this time is not always available. Popa-Velea and Purcarea (2014) explained that the answer is not necessarily more time but the "a better use of time." They also maintain that the most efficient way to implement and sustain providers' positive attitudes is the standard integration of communication and practice in the concept of a bio-psycho-social model of care.

The Positive Context of Therapeutic Encounters

The positive context of therapeutic interviewing is extremely important. *Context* refers to the specific strengths and deficits of patients in communicating effectively (including inherent medical problems impacting communication capabilities), the physical environment, the goals and skills of providers, and the focus of the encounter. Positive context refers to the combination and interplay of all factors to achieve supportive and effective encounters with health providers.

Providers as facilitators of positive communications: As suggested in several areas of the text, providers work to facilitate communications of patients, many of whom may exhibit

EXHIBIT 5-5 Nontherapeutic Response Modes

1. **Scolding or moralizing:** Inferring that patients' behaviors are wrong or "not okay." This tends to inhibit expression and cause patients to get upset.

2. **Judging, criticizing, or labeling:** Similar to moralizing are the tendencies to judge and criticize patient behaviors which also impede understanding and trust.

3. **False reassurance:** Stating that patients will feel better soon when they will not is an example of false reassurance. It can be confusing and tends to cut short patients' explorations of their concerns.

4. **Closed-ended questioning:** Only asking questions that can be answered in one to three words limits the ability to explore patients' thoughts about what they say or ask.

5. **Summarizing:** Summarizing what patients have said can be helpful, but when done too early could have the effect of limiting patients' discussion about important topics as does using only closed-ended questions.

6. **Using stereotypic responses:** Using phrases like "that's bad" (meaning "good") to express understanding or an attempt to impress patients. The use of some stereotypic responses may not be understood by all patients and can appear phony and out of place in a professional–patient relationship.

7. **Belittling or defensive responses:** These replies diminish the significance of patients' experience and can lead to anger. Patients' experience many fears and concerns, and some of these may differ from opinions of health providers. Explaining to a patient who would rather die, rather than face pain, "Oh, those are common feelings of people in your position…you'll get over it," is belittling because it implies weakness in the patient.

8. **Interrupting responses:** Interrupting patients, and particularly if followed by introducing an unrelated topic, breaks the flow of patients' conversation before they can complete thoughts or ideas and can shut off patients' exploration of important health topics.

9. **Lack of appreciation of patients' problems:** Denial of the significance of patients' problems can be perceived as treating patients' concerns in a cavalier manner.

10. **Giving approval or disapproval:** Communicating approval or disapproval explicitly or subtly limits patients' feelings of freedom to communicate without fearing judgment.

11. **Open disagreement:** Responding by openly disagreeing with patients puts providers in opposition to patients. It can result in patients not disclosing important related information, for example, having discontinued a medication without notifying their provider or wanting a less aggressive treatment.

12. **Advice giving:** Although providers commonly advise patients about a course of action, advice-giving is not always helpful. In certain instances, it can cause patients to feel incapable of being self-directed and competent in self-management of their health conditions.

13. **Probing questions or statements:** Directing a line of inquiry is important, but when this becomes excessive, it may give the experience of unnecessary probing.

14. **Challenging questions or statements:** Challenging is a clear and present danger to patients' expression. It tends to make patients feel that they have to prove what they say—they generally become defensive.

15. **Socializing responses:** Engaging in chitchat or revealing personal data while "break-the-ice" is not therapeutic. In social dialogues, participants share talk-time more equally. When used in patient—provider conversations, it generally calls for equal time for the provider to self-disclose. This decreases the patients' time to self-disclose.

dysfunctional communication patterns. Their dysfunctional communication could be a result of a transient state (e.g., pressure or stress), or it may be long-standing, resulting from ongoing communication deficits. Frequently exhibited disturbances in perception, processing, and expression are as follows:

- Verbalizing too much or too little.
- Verbalizing inappropriately to the context of the events.
- Using incomplete sentences or thoughts.
- Behaving as if they have communicated clearly when they have not.
- Misperceiving environmental stimuli.
- Exaggerating certain meanings of a message, ignoring other aspects, or attributing different connotations to an event than what is intended.
- Overgeneralizing or undergeneralizing, and failing to access stored information.

Because the majority of patients experience some difficulties in communicating, an important role of the provider is to identify, manage, and modify these deficits. This context of therapeutic interviewing is extremely important—it includes the social and environmental context for the provider's communication with the patient.

The purpose of therapeutic interviewing is to build or maintain an effective patient–provider relationship and to assess the patient through the patient's disclosure of thoughts, feelings, behaviors, and experiences. Because interviews require patients to communicate something personal, and even threatening, the interviewer must establish rapport and trust with the patient. This includes creating a safe place for the patient to disclose. A place that is protected from intrusions and interruptions is important for two reasons: (1) a protected environment is likely to make patients feel comfortable and (2) in order to collect data adequately—this includes the multiple levels of patient communication (verbal, nonverbal, and metamessages)—the provider must have a "noise-free" environment.

The data from an interview reflects the context of the interview. It is important to understand how patients communicate based on the content of the interview and characteristics of the interviewer. It is known, for example, that patients are less open about certain issues, typically when addressing issues of nonadherence to treatment, ill-advised drug and alcohol use, and risky sexual practices. Patients respond differently to providers based upon the providers' age, gender, and their professional role. This is why providers can elicit different reactions, both positive and negative, from patients. Who you are and what you are like may influence what the patient does or does not tell you.

Patients also react to the particular physical environment in which they are asked questions. They may be rather close-mouthed in settings that lack privacy. Patients also react to their most immediate life circumstances, crisis, and symptom status. Finally, patients react to the provider's approach—the specific way in which the provider formulates questions. All successful interviewers take these factors into account when planning to approach patients.

One's style of interviewing and choice of questions should be influenced by the perceptual, ethnic–cultural, and educational characteristics of the patient. The adage "begin where the patient is," is a good one. Basically, providers can never push patients further than they can go, nor expect them to adapt to our stylistic peculiarities. It is inappropriate to use complex medical jargon with patients who are incapable of understanding the meaning of even the simplest medical phrase. It is also inappropriate to require patients to endure lengthy interviews of 2 hours if their anxiety levels or attention spans cannot meet the challenge. Sometimes knowing and using the jargon or language of the specific ethnic or cultural group is likely to increase patients' willingness to communicate problems.

Regardless of the circumstances, providers must always demonstrate respect and concern for patients. Showing interest, concern, and understanding indicate that providers regard the patient as worthy, and helps to reduce the fear and anxiety surrounding the illness and its treatment. The affective tone that the provider uses with the patient is extremely important and can make or break the interview no matter how sophisticated the provider is in using techniques.

▶ Preparation for Avoiding the Traps of Dysfunctional Communication

Avoiding the traps of dysfunctional communication is certainly possible, but this requires knowledge, skill, and practice. Providers need to be able to communicate effectively and therapeutically with their patients, and this is an ongoing learning requirement. This seems so straightforward but so many times ignored. Still, the techniques of effective communications are being taught everywhere, and providers, once trained in effective communication, go back for "booster shots." Booster shots come in the form of course work, employee training, and continuing education programs. The goal, *we can always improve our communications*, is a standard the business and consulting industry knows well. Billions of dollars are poured into (and made) helping employees and administrators communicate with clients and each other.

Training in Interpersonal Communications

Training in interpersonal communications is helpful to health providers because it improves their ability to communicate as well as their ability to help others. The purpose of effective interpersonal communication is to help others learn about themselves, and make decisions based on this knowledge. Another purpose of communication is to foster self-learning—people can learn about themselves by sharing with others and by monitoring their own words and actions.

One of the biggest entanglements that a provider can experience is the trap of engaging in defensive communication. Defensive communication in providers is generally indicative of a perceived threat, and its corresponding feelings of anxiety, fear, and guilt. The consequence of defensive communication is generally that messages will be misunderstood, and that back and forth communication will reach a standstill. This is to be avoided at all costs because disruptions in communication are tantamount to disruptions in care.

Identifying Defensive Communications

Defensive communications are rather obvious. But, it is important to identify and name them to interrupt the process. The following is a list of behaviors that are generally indicative of a defensive posture:

- Labeling
- Interrupting
- Judging
- Using tunnel vision
- Advice giving
- Preparing rebuttals

Notice how many of these behaviors are also mentioned in the list of nontherapeutic responses (interrupting, judging or showing disapproval, advice giving, challenging, or preparing rebuttals). While there are many other indicators of defensive communication, these are most commonly observed. People communicating defensively usually use more than one of these responses. Not only is it important to be aware of specific responses, but also of clusters of defensive responses, as they are problematic.

To illustrate this idea, consider someone who is reacting negatively and defensively. They may label or blame, interpret others' behaviors, judge others, and develop rebuttals sometimes simultaneously. When this defensive posture is executed with high intensity, it can be likened to a "machine gun." This machine-gun approach has one result—everybody gets out of the way. No one wants to get caught in the cross-fire, so observers are also likely to exit the encounter. The end result is that no one fully understands, and the communicants have a decidedly negative view about the prospects of being heard and understood by the other person.

The alternative, nondefensive communication, enhances the possibility that not only our needs for information but also those of the patient for support and counseling will be met.

It is exceedingly more esthetically pleasing. Nondefensive behaviors observe and report, share information, and engage others in mutual problem-solving processes. They generally produce an increased mutual understanding and encourage communicants to continue their dialogue beyond any initial exchange.

From a diagnostic standpoint, all patient–provider interviews can be judged on a relative scale—more or less therapeutic. Establishing the degree to which one uses nontherapeutic interviewing with a single patient or group of patients can be measured if one analyzes patient encounters and establishes potential problem areas. Personal inventories help providers establish which, if any, of the common nontherapeutic responses they are using (see **EXHIBIT 5-6**). The assumption of this self-inventory is that nonproblematic provider responses are those that maintain focus and guide both the provider and the patient's learning, while problematic responses short-circuit the therapeutic process.

EXHIBIT 5-6 Personal Inventory for Nontherapeutic Interviewing Skills

On a scale of: 1 (all the time) to 8 (none of the time), how frequently might you do the following when interviewing patients?

I. Switch off problem-centered data by talking about:
- Unrelated focus
- Incidental material

II. Maintain superficial discussion by:
- Avoiding elaboration
- Switching to unrelated superficial focus; denying the significance of the patient's stated problems
- Asking closed-ended questions

III. Intervene personally by:
- Giving opinion to life situations of the patient without exploring
- Giving unsolicited personal comments or opinions
- Giving personal information or socializing responses
- Expressing approval or disapproval
- Moralizing, belittling, or challenging
- Seeking agreement from the patient/disagreeing with the patient

(continues)

EXHIBIT 5-6 Personal Inventory for Nontherapeutic Interviewing Skills *(continued)*

IV. Close off exploration by:
  - Prematurely giving an interpretation
  - Prematurely advising solutions
  - Prematurely giving reassurance
  - Prematurely closing the topic
  - Using judgmental stereotypical responses
  - Interruptive responses
  - Excessive probing

V. Introduce or follow illogical content by:
  - Changing key words without validating change
  - Following vague content or referent as if it is understood
  - Introducing vague content or referent
  - Questioning on different topics or levels without waiting for a reply
  - Speaking to questions or statements of the patient in conflicting ways
  - Ignoring questions from the patient

Frequency of use: Pattern I.
                     Pattern II.
                     Pattern III.
                     Pattern IV.
                     Pattern V.

Use of the tool: (1) Identify each provider's response; (2) mark NP = nonproblematic, or P = problematic; (3) total P responses using tool.

Assessing one's therapeutic and non-therapeutic communication responses with patient encounters is only the first step. It is, however, an extremely important step because no real change can occur until such identification and assessment is completed. These assessments can occur formally, for example, through feedback from coursework, professors, supervisors, or peers. Much of this assessment, conducted on a continuous basis, must be carried out through individuals' commitment to the process of personal self-assessment.

Self-assessments include, but are not limited to, an analysis of encounters that turned out poorly, especially those that produced conflict and tension. Changing communication patterns is not always easy, but if providers believe in the importance of functional and therapeutic communications, they will understand the need and accept the responsibility for self-examination and continual improvement.

▶ Summary

Therapeutic communication is not altogether confined to providers—others less well-trained in medical care can communicate therapeutically. Providers differ, however, in that they deliberately employ therapeutic communication skills and knowledge. The therapeutic provider communicates with patients whose communications are potentially dysfunctional. Patients' communications can be dysfunctional for many reasons and have both transitory and permanent causes.

Providers not only model functional communication, they modify the dysfunctional patterns of others' communication. Therapeutic interviewing is clearly within the domain of every provider's role. **Therapeutic interviewing skills** tend to focus the patient and increase learning, whereas nontherapeutic communication tends to inhibit communication, especially the processes of feedback, clarification, and qualification. Practicing therapeutic communications requires the provider to conduct ongoing self-assessments in which patient–provider encounters are analyzed on the basis of therapeutic-nontherapeutic dimensions. While formal peers' and/or superiors' evaluations are critical, providers' personal commitment to conduct self-assessments and gather feedback from their patients is essential to maintaining a therapeutic approach.

Discussion

1. Can disturbed perception impact expressive language? Explain the reasons behind your answer.
2. What is meant by the terms functional and dysfunctional communication?
3. List three examples of provider–patient communications that would be classified as therapeutic or nontherapeutic.
4. Describe defensive communications, and the specific behaviors associated with defensiveness.
5. Is it correct to say once you have mastered therapeutic interviewing you will be able to handle all interpersonal relationships with patients? If not, why not?

References

Baumann, M., Baumann, C., Le Bihan, E., & Chau, N. (2008). How patients perceive the therapeutic communications skills of their general practitioners, and how that perception affects adherence: Use of the TCom-skills GP scale in a specific geographical area. *BioMedCentral Health Services Research, 8,* 244–245. doi:10.1186/1472-6963-8-244

Chisholm, V., Atkinson, L., Bayrami, L., Noyes, K., Payne, A., & Kelnar, C. (2014), An exploratory study of positive and incongruent communication in young children with type 1 diabetes and their mothers. *Child: Care, Health and Development, 40,* 85–94. doi:10.1111/cch.12004

Ely, E. W., Inouye, S. K., Bernard, G. R., Gordon, S., Francis, J., May, L., ... Dittus, R. (2001). Delirium in mechanically ventilated patients: Validity and reliability of the confusion assessment method for the intensive care unit (CAM-ICU). *JAMA, 286*(21), 2703–2710. doi:10.1001/jama.286.21.2703

Fisher, C. L., & Nussbaum, J. F. (2015). Maximizing wellness in successful aging and cancer coping: The importance of family communication from a socioemotional selectivity theoretical perspective. *Journal of Family Communication, 15*(1), 3–19. doi:10.1080/15267431.2014.946512

Mallinger, J. B., Griggs, J. J., & Shields, C. G. (2006). Family communication and mental health after breast cancer. *European Journal of Cancer Care, 15,* 355–361. doi:10.1111/j.1365-2354.2006.00666.x

Missouri State Medical Association. (1893, p. 182). *Transactions of the 36th Annual Meeting of the Medical Association of the Missouri State Medical Association* held at Sedalia, Missouri, May 17, 1893. (Dr. A.D. Williams response to the paper presented by Dr. Thompson).

NIH. (2016). *Visual impairment.* Retrieved from www.nih.gov/

NIH, NIDCD. (2016). *Quick statistics about hearing.* Retrieved from https://www.nicdcd.nih.gov/

NIMH. (2016). Schizophrenia. Retrieved from www.nih.gov/

Popa-Velea, O., & Purcarea, V. L. (2014). Issues of therapeutic communication relevant for improving quality of care. Journal of Medicine and Life, 7(Special Issue 4), 39–45. PMID:27057247

Ruesch, J. (1961). *Therapeutic communication.* New York, NY: W. W. Norton. (Epigraph from p. xiv)

Satir, V. (1967). *Conjoint family therapy.* Palo Alto, CA: Science and Behavior Books.

Shin, D. W., Shin, J., Kim, S. Y., Yang, H.-K., Cho, J., Youm, J. H., ... Park, J.-H. (2016). Family avoidance of communication about cancer: A dyadic examination. *Cancer Research and Treatment: Official Journal of Korean Cancer Association, 48*(1), 384–392. doi:10.4143/crt.2014.280

Solomon, M., Ozonoff, S., Carter, C., & Caplan, R. (2008). Formal thought disorder and autism spectrum: Relationship with symptoms, executive control and anxiety. *Journal of Autism and Developmental Disorders, 38*(8), 1474–1484. doi:10.1007/s10803-007-0526-6

Thomas, J. B., Brier, M. R., Bateman, R. J., Snyder, A. Z., Benzinger, T. L., Xiong, C., ... The Dominantly Inherited Alzheimer Network. (2014). Functional connectivity in autosomal dominant and late-onset Alzheimer's disease. *JAMA Neurology, 71*(9), 1111–1122. doi:10.1001/jamaneurol.2014.1654

Varma, R., Vajaranant, T., Burkemper, B., Wu, S., Torres, M., Hsu, C., ... McKean-Cowdin, R. (2016). Visual impairment and blindness in adults in the United States: Demographic and geographic variations from 2015 to 2050. *Journal of the American Medical Association, Ophthalmology, 134*(7), 802–809. doi:10 .1001/jamaophthalmol.2016.1284

Watzlawick, P., Weakland, J. H., & Fisch, R. (1974). *Changing a system*. New York, NY: W.W. Norton and Company, Inc.

Watzlawick, P. J., Beavin, J., & Jackson, D. D. (1967). *Pragmatics of human communication*. New York, NY: W.W. Norton & Company, Inc. (Epigraph from p. 13).

CHAPTER 6

Cultural Similarities and Differences and Communication

CHAPTER OBJECTIVES

- Describe current key health care disparities in the United States and provider–patient communications' contributions to resolving disparities.
- Discuss and define the concepts of culture, cultural differences, acculturation, and culturally competent health care.
- Discuss the influence of subgrouping on communication.
- Describe the hypothetical continuum of cultural destructiveness to cultural proficiency.
- With at least one other individual, discuss your own cultural programming.

KEY TERMS

- Acculturation
- Culture
- Cultural competence

- Cultural competence continuum
- Cultural identity
- Multicultural environment

▶ Introduction

There is evidence that all people are influenced by cultural programming. While **culture** is an ambiguous term, it generally refers to values, beliefs, knowledge, art, morals, laws, and customs acquired by individuals and groups. It is generally believed that individuals and groups acquire patterned ideas and behaviors while residing with others. When individuals and families move from one culture to a new culture they experience **acculturation** or the transfer of values and customs from one cultural group to another. Cultural programming, a sort of built-in "software," influences our perceptions, ways of processing and interpreting data, and our expression of ideas and feelings. Once providers recognize what their own cultural programming is, they have the capacity and responsibility to explore more fully the communications of others.

In the practice of health care, both one's personal and professional culture affect how they perform their roles with patients and patients' families. Providing culturally appropriate education and self-awareness training is critical to improving care and eliminating health disparities. It is essential to understand the role of the patient–provider communication interchange in such important outcomes as health disparities, either contributing to or resolving health disparities. It is appropriate to launch this chapter with some background on our multicultural society and factors that influence access to health care across groups in the United States. Following this discussion is a review of basic tenets of culture awareness.

▶ Our Multicultural Environment

Providers in the United States live in **multicultural environments**. One's diversity is depicted in several specific, yet overlapping categories—language spoken, cultural orientation, and religious affiliation. There are other distinctions, such as age, gender, race and ethnicity, education, economic status, and residence that reveal one's unique presentation. The following discussion describes the diversity of our make-up given with respect to language, culture, and religion, and details the profile for the world as a whole and the United States in

particular. Can our diversity divide us? Does it unite us? What divides? What can do both—divide and unite? And, most importantly, what is the impact of cultural diversity on the use of health care services and quality care?

Language diversity: There are over 7,000 languages in the world, but this does not account for linguistic differences. In fact, this figure is difficult to determine because it is not always clear whether a language is a language and not a dialect. There are instances in which Chinese and Arabic are considered single languages and also language families that house several different dialects. Part of what has emerged is the opportunity for a second language.

So, among those that speak a single language such as English, it is difficult to know whether for this group it is not the only language, there may be a second language spoken. Then there are the nationalities of these English speakers that impact how and when they speak one or more language. Despite the fact that over 7,000 languages are spoken throughout the world, only 23 of these languages account for more than half the world's population (Simons & Fennig, 2017). Linguistic homogeneity is often a path to widespread acceptance and understanding.

Cultural diversity: Cultural diversity in our U.S. population is evident in a number of ways including, age, gender, racial and ethnic background, values and beliefs, and languages spoken.

It is known that across the world and in the United States, not all residents speak English or know, understand, and accept the values and norms of behavior ascribed to by most Americans. The number of cultures in the United States and around the world is difficult to determine in part because culture is not a stand-alone concept. Culture is a composite of racial, ethnic, religious, and social groups. There are over 7 billion people in the world and nearly two-thirds of them are Asian living on less than one-third of the regions of the world. The United States makes up just over 320 million people or approximately 4%–5%

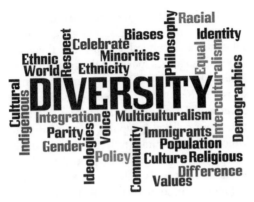

© Rob Wilson/Shutterstock.

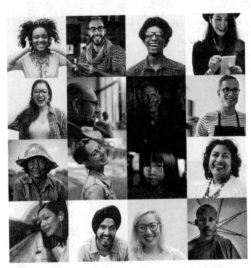

© Rawpixel.com/Shutterstock.

of the world's population. It is ethnically and racially diverse, sometimes referred to as *a melting pot*; and has acquired this standing through large-scale migration from many countries.

Those that study cultures in the United States explain that there are essentially six cultural groups—primarily Western, African, Native American, Asian, Polynesian, and Latin American. The primarily Western orientation has been strongly influenced by other groups immigrating to the United States throughout its history. However, this orientation is shaped by many social and historical events, and these events in some cases are associated with health disparities.

A case in point is the health disparities in health status and access to care among endogenous populations, particularly American Indian and Native Americans in the United States. These groups have been significantly affected by cultural programing based upon historical and ongoing marginalization and cultural dislocation. These factors have contributed to a lack of trust in traditional public health campaigns and health service approaches which they feel know little about their beliefs, practices, needs, and health disparities.

While the United States was previously viewed as a *melting pot*, it has recently been referred to as a *salad bowl*, meaning that it is culturally diverse. *Culture* is a term used to describe identifiable integrated patterns of human behavior that include customs, beliefs, values, behaviors, and communications. Culture is said to be passed from one generation to another and can be observed in racial, ethnic, religious, and social groups. The ideas people have about health and the language they use in encounters with health providers are related to their culture. Just how health literate they are is also related to their culture, as is the circumstances in which they seek health care and communicate about health (CDC, 2017).

Religious diversity: Culture encompasses religious affiliation. Some cultural beliefs, values, and behaviors also have roots in religious affiliation. There are an estimated 4,200 different religions in the world, and these are generally classified into several main religions—Christianity, Roman Catholicism, Islam, Hinduism, Buddhism, and Judaism. In the United States, according to a 2015 Pew Research Center report, there is an important shift taking place, namely a rise in the number of people who are religiously unaffiliated, from 16% in 2007 to 23% in 2014. Also, among U.S. religious groups, there is considerable range in racial and ethnic diversity (Lipa & Pew Research Center, 2015).

One's sociocultural heritage is not necessarily a true picture of their **cultural identity**. *Cultural identity* refers to the extent to which individuals subscribe to a given culture. Everyone is said to have a cultural identity. More often than not, individuals have several cultural identities due, in part, to the fact that one's cultural heritage is rich. One can come from a particular sociocultural background but not identify with this heritage. One's culture is in fact the orientation to which they subscribe.

The United States was previously described to have a significant number of different social, religious, and cultural groups, and there are multiple languages spoken in the greater United States. The country is diverse; formerly referred to as *a melting pot* but currently described as *a salad bowl*. The term *cultural diversity* is descriptive of our cultural groupings. It is the extent to which group identities (reflective of individuals' age, gender, ethnic, and social group, etc.) differ. Cultural diversity is reflected in every society, but more so in some societies than others.

🔍 CITED STUDY: Delays in Seeking Health Care among Muslim Women

Delays in seeking care are critical to quality health care outcomes. Postponing has been linked to poorer prognosis and even higher mortality rates. A number of factors have been shown to be associated with delays in seeking care across a wide range of patient groups and include poor access to care, costs of care, and lack of health care insurance. However, there are also psychosocial and cultural factors impacting delaying care.

In an exploratory study assessing the relationship of religion-related factors and delays in seeking care, 254 Muslim women were surveyed in Chicago. The ethnic-racial distribution of the sample was balanced and included African Americans, Arab Americans, and South Asians (those from Pakistan and India). The researchers hypothesized that religiosity, fatalistic beliefs, perceived religious discrimination in health care encounters, modesty, and the use of complementary alternative medicine and worship practices for health would impact health care-seeking practices in this sample.

Vu, M., Azmat, A., Radejko, T., & Padela, A. I. (2016). Predictors of delayed health care seeking among American Muslim women. *Journal of Women's Health, 25*(6), 586–593.

Results of the study indicated that higher levels of religiosity and modesty levels were related to delays in care seeking. Having lived in the United States for more than 20 years was negatively associated with care-seeking delays. The researchers confirmed their hypothesis that many women delay seeking care due to a perceived lack of female clinicians, and concluded that there was a need for gender-matched provider–patient assignments. Otherwise, delays in seeking care might be reduced if female Muslims received care from female health providers.

🔍 CITED STUDY: Masculinity and Race Impacting Health Help-Seeking among African American Men

Delays in health-related help-seeking are important for men and women, but factors impacting men to seek health care may be complex. The researchers in this study examined factors such as race and ethnicity, history with discrimination, and the extent to which men prescribe to traditional masculine roles as predictors of their health help-seeking. In a study of the relationship of masculinity and race among a cohort of community-residing African American men, data from 458 study participants were analyzed.

The researchers examined the importance given to traditional masculine norms (e.g., a high sense of control, emotional toughness, and independent coping, and also everyday experience with racial discrimination which has been shown to be associated with resistance to help-seeking in health care settings).

Powell, W., Adams, L. B., Cole-Lewis, Y., Agyemang, A., & Upton, R. D. (2016). Masculinity and race-related factors as barriers to health help-seeking barriers among African-American men. *Behavioral Medicine (Washington, DC), 42*(3), 150–163. doi:10.1080/08964289.2016.1165174

The researchers found support for conceptualizing African American men's diminished health help-seeking as reactance, or an attempt to restore autonomy, freedom, and sense of control in the face of persistent social identity threats. However, results suggested that diminished health help-seeking is not only a reaction to perceived threats to masculinity. They found that African American men face a number of race-related threats that may work together with their sense of masculinity to impact their health behavior.

The researchers concluded that health disparities and inequities among African American men is dependent upon enhancing health help-seeking. However, if the goal is to improve disparate health outcomes among African American men, everyday racial discrimination experiences that chip away at help-seeking motivations need to be addressed.

▶ Disparities in Health Care and the Role of Provider–Patient Communications

Foundations for Cultural Competence and Removal of Disparities

The underlying principle behind culture, health care communication, and effective health care service is the idea that communication effectiveness can be increased when health care providers and organizations *recognize and bridge cultural differences that may contribute to miscommunication* (CDC, 2017). Ineffective communication brought on by cultural differences can lead to health care disparities. In 2002, an important and landmark document provided a convincing review of existing literature on racial and ethnic disparities in health care. This document was the Institute of Medicine (IOM) report titled *Unequal Treatment: Confronting Racial and Ethnic Disparities in Health Care* (IOM, 2002). According to this report, a significant body of research and literature indicates that a lack of cultural competent care is directly related to poor patient outcomes, reduced patient compliance with treatment, and increased health disparities, regardless of the quality of services available.

Wide dissemination of this report raised awareness of the magnitude of the problem in the United States and resulted in several health care initiatives and subsequent literature representing many areas of medical practice that called for action to reduce these disparities. The need to expand existing evidence of disparities by examining the role of poor provider/patient communication as a contributor to health care disparities among minority patients was raised (Diette & Rand, 2007). The IOM report examined the extent to which certain racial and ethnic minorities receive a lower-quality of health care than nonminorities. Considerable attention was given the need to ensure *health equity*.

Among the many reasons given for these disparities resulting from patient–provider communication were (1) patient stereotyping,

(2) culturally related communication barriers, and (3) provider biases. Patient *stereotyping* can affect the quality of communication, especially if perceived as distancing and as a lack of respect. Following this important IOM report, other reports and initiatives paved the way for creating **cultural competence** in the health professions. Reports were in some cases also backed by research data.

Crawley, Ahn, and Winkleby (2008) studied patients' perceptions of medical discrimination and screening rates for colorectal and breast cancers in a large California database. They found significant relationships between perceived racial- or ethnic-based medical discrimination, and women's rates of screening, with perceived discrimination associated with lower rates of screening. Subsequent studies did not look at perceptions of medical discrimination but did find a relationship between perceived discrimination in general and cancer screening rates. Sorting out whether medical discrimination or general discriminatory experience is the stronger predictor is difficult. Both types of discrimination need to be examined for their impact on health screening, particularly when screenings can make the difference between surviving from such diseases as cancer and dying due to late cancer detection.

Culturally related communication barriers can result in some groups refusing diagnostic tests and treatment because of fear, mistrust, confusion about the health care system, and beliefs about harm that are not grounded in fact. An increase in the proportion of providers coming from under-represented minorities and effective training of all providers in the tenets of cultural competence has helped address these concerns.

Healthy People 2020 followed the IOM report and clearly laid the foundation for promoting cultural competent care. As stated by *Healthy People 2020*, vulnerable populations "have systematically experienced greater obstacles to health based on their racial or ethnic group; religion; socioeconomic status; gender; age; mental health; cognitive, sensory, or physical disability; sexual orientation or gender identity; geographic location; or other characteristics historically linked to discrimination or exclusion." This document outlined the national health promotion and disease-prevention goals and objectives with 10-year targets and includes an emphasis on health equity and the elimination of health disparities revealed in the IOM report.

Additionally, the 2010 Patient Protection and Affordable Care Act (PPACA) was designed to support the development of model curricula for cultural competency, and inclusion of cultural competency and health literacy training in primary care, dentistry, and dental hygiene training programs (Maryland Department of Health and Mental Hygiene, Office of Minority Health and Health Disparities, 2013).

Dynamics of Health Care Communications and Cultural Competence

Health provider exposures and encounters with diverse populations vary. Some providers have considerable breadth and depth of experience with diverse groups—others encounter more homogeneous groupings. The breadth and depth of experience is a function of the region of the country, and whether providers are practicing in a rural, urban, or suburban area. Exposure to wide-scale diversity can promote cultural competence and respect and acceptance of diversity, but this is not always the case.

Communication barriers between health care providers and patients can occur regardless of wide-spread exposure to a diverse group of patients. Communication barriers are often of a sociocultural nature. As described by *Healthy People 2020*, vulnerable populations "have systematically experienced greater obstacles to health based on their racial or ethnic group; religion; socioeconomic status; gender; age; mental health; cognitive, sensory, or physical disability; sexual orientation or gender identity; geographic location; or other characteristics historically linked to discrimination or exclusion." *Health Equity* will serve as a primary resource for organizations and individuals who serve these populations at the community, state, regional, tribal, and national levels.

As detailed in the IOM report, providers' conscious and subconscious beliefs and perceptions about their patient can impact the type and effectiveness of the care and treatment given. Specifically, there is a negative association between racial/ethnic minority status and both the quality of health care received and positive health outcomes, even after accounting for treatment site, insurance status, and other patient characteristics. These barriers can be due to differences in culture, language, race or ethnicity, gender, and social class, or they can be due to generational differences among individuals within the same culture. Providers are often most aware of the power of sociocultural diversity when they are confronted with individualizing a medical regimen to meet patients' unique personal circumstances.

In communicating with patients and their families, it is critical that clinicians understand and respect the cultural patterns that influence patients' perceptions of their problems, their usual ways of responding to and coping with health concerns, and their willingness to accept the treatment they will be asked to follow. Of particular importance are those groups who may harbor long-standing resistance to Western medicine, or whose views and beliefs of their health problems, what has caused them, and how to treat them, differ from traditional medical approaches.

It is hardly ever simple to interact with patients and their families when value systems and cultural backgrounds are unfamiliar. The

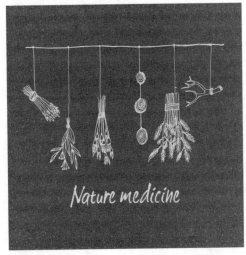

Nature medicine

© Tasiania/Shutterstock.

situation becomes even more complicated when language barriers also exist between the providers and patients. Differences in values and the inability to understand the communications of others are important because they can produce social distancing.

Social distancing in patient–provider relationships is detrimental to learning more about the patients, and inhibits the development of a therapeutic patient–provider relationship built on mutual trust and respect. Additionally, perceived social distancing can affect whether a patient will accept or even return for treatment. Crawley and colleagues (2008) studied the relationship of perceived medical discrimination and cancer screening behaviors in racial and ethnic minority adults. Discriminatory behaviors or perceived discrimination has been shown to be a major causal factor in health disparities in minority populations. Perceived discrimination was significantly associated with the likelihood that minority women and men would not be screened for certain kinds of cancer, breast and colorectal and colorectal, respectively.

In summary, perhaps nowhere is it more crucial to be able to understand and speak another person's language than in the health services arena. Whether in an outpatient or inpatient setting, and across all levels of illness, the patients' and families' ability to express needs and feelings and to know that they have been understood is important. Within health settings, uncertainty and fear are naturally occurring responses to an actual or perceived threat of illness and injury. These fears can be accentuated by the awareness that no matter how hard one tries, the provider may not really understand the patient's expressed thoughts and feelings and care for him or her in the way they need to be cared for.

▶ The Influence of Sociocultural Factors on Perceiving, Processing, and Self-Expression

Our sociocultural affiliations, as well as religious and ethnic influences, contribute to our unique programming. Health care providers have still another source of unique programming and orientation toward health and health care services. It is important to appreciate this aspect as well as our other group affiliations. As members of a health care culture, providers have a distinctively different language (including medical jargon), norms, beliefs, and values not usually shared by people who are not health care providers.

In encounters with patients, it is important to keep in mind one's unique programming, but most importantly, strive to understand how patients' sociocultural background influences the way they perceive our communication, process what we tell them, and express to us what concerns them.

Patients' sociocultural orientation, religious affiliation, race and ethnicity, age, and gender can all give clues to patients' perception of health and illness and how they will engage in encounters with health care professionals. The

following are examples of how sociocultural affiliations impact communication processes.

Cultural Affiliations and the Encounters with Health Care Providers

Culture is an important component of behavioral determinants of health. That is, the customs, practices, and traditions as well as the beliefs and values of individuals, families, and communities influence their health status (Eckardt et al., 2017). Although culture is only one factor among many that influence individuals' health status, it is important. Cultural and religious beliefs can influence adoption of health behaviors and recognition of existing health problems.

Patients may have many affiliations that influence their behavior as well as their acknowledgment of problems needing medical attention. These include, but are not limited to, culture and religious affiliations. Examples of how cultural and religious affiliations can influence the experience of illness and the descriptions of symptoms, is outlined in detail in a literature review by Hollingshead, Ashburn-Nardo, Stewart, and Hirsch (2016).

In their review of pain experience in Hispanic/Latino Americans, these researchers grouped study reports addressing pain experience, response to pain, and seeking and receiving pain care. Their reported findings are noteworthy. They cited literature indicating that Hispanic Americans report fewer pain conditions compared to non-Hispanic whites or African Americans. Still, they experience more severe chronic pain, acute postoperative pain, and acute fracture pain.

The authors also described literature that indicated in traditional Hispanic cultures, pain and illness are viewed as disharmony with or punishment from God. Another important cultural belief is the *hot and cold* theory of disease which plays a significant role in whether Hispanic Americans choose

EXHIBIT 6-1 Dialogue Box: Hypothetical Scenario

(James) is a 60-year-old African American male, married with six children and four grandchildren. He has a college education and is a member of the Mormon religion. He is employed part-time as a public school teacher making $50,000 a year and has a part-time job as a tennis instructor. His place of birth is Boise, Idaho, but he currently lives in a small town in the suburbs of Salt Lake City, Utah. This patient's cultural heritage and programming is rich and depicts many possible sociocultural orientations.

Any predictions about what he says and how he responds to communications with health care providers would best be made with all these facts in mind. Until providers know what aspects of his *cultural programming* are most influential in the context of the interaction, it is not possible to fully understand his communication. Added to this picture is the fact that he occupies the role of patient as he is about to be hospitalized for surgery to correct a deviated nasal septum. His surgeon is White, in his late 60s and is a well-known and successful doctor in the community. On the day of admission, he engaged with his surgeon in the following conversation:

PATIENT:	"Play any tennis lately?"
SURGEON:	"I was in a doubles match Saturday!"
PATIENT:	"Oh, how did you do?"
SURGEON:	"James, I need to get you set up here. You remember what I told you in my office?"
PATIENT:	"Yes."
PHYSICIAN:	"Good, I'm going to order your pre-op medications. I'll be back later."
PATIENT:	"Okay, Doc—you're the boss, boss!"

From the content of his communication, one would say that James's affiliation with tennis is a dominant aspect of his programming. Still, when this exchange is evaluated further, it appears that social inequity is an issue, and showing deference to the surgeon is an aspect of this interaction. While James attempts to relate to his surgeon as one tennis player to another, his surgeon shifts to a professional doctor–patient relationship.

Further, James acknowledges the hierarchy by replying in essence "You're the doctor, I'm the patient—I'm here to follow your orders (boss)." While the surgeon may have good intentions about establishing a participative and collaborative patient—physician relationship, the outcome of this transaction appears to be a certain amount of interpersonal distance: "Let's stay within (the boundaries) our roles." Social distancing seems to occur as there is a need to separate roles between the patient and physician.

There are numerous reasons for James's communication about power differences, and they are worthy of consideration. One possibility is that James is responding to differences in social status as a function of role differences—doctor versus patient. Another possibility is that James is sensitive to racial differences and replies in the context of discrimination against African Americans (historically) and comments about an inferior status in the eyes of whites. What enables the provider to better understand James's communication is his choice of words and the intonation of those words. Still, without knowledge of his specific cultural programming, judgments about his responses are, at best, tentative.

cultural remedies or seek medical care. The perspectives raised in this review inform providers that the experience and expression of symptoms are indeed influenced by patients' cultural programming.

The role of deference in patient–provider encounters illustrate the culturally held beliefs that patients come from a place of less social power and influence compared to health care professionals. The following patient–physician dialogue illustrates important points about socio–cultural influences on patient–provider communications (**EXHIBIT 6-1**). In this scenario, a patient is discussing his surgery and preoperative instructions with his surgeon.

▶ Changes in Social Ethnic Grouping in the United States

It is safe to say that what prevailed as mainstream culture (including race and ethnicity, language, and religion) in the United States decades ago do not prevail today. In fact, the usefulness of describing *majority* (mainstream) culture in today's world is questionable. Previously the United States was likened to a *salad bowl*. While the United States is culturally, ethnically, and religiously diverse, there are differences across groups. Americans' identification with one or more minority groups has relevance in the United States.

According to the *Healthy People 2020* report, (ODPHP, 2020, HealthyPeople.gov), one-third of our population identifies themselves as belonging to a racial or ethnic minority group. The U.S. Census Bureau Report (2015) stated that by 2044, more than half of all Americans are projected to belong to a minority group (any group other than non-Hispanic white alone). The Census Bureau Report projecting characteristics of minority and majority groups noted that minorities by 2040 are estimated to make up 50.3% of all Americans (March 3, 2015, Report No. CB15-TPS.16). Additionally, 2020 projections of children under 18 years also indicate that non-Hispanic whites may no longer comprise over 50% of children, with 50.2% representing minorities. And by 2060, the nation's foreign-born population is expected to be nearly 19% (one in five) of the total population.

Within each ethnic–racial group there can be numerous subgroups. One's subgroup affiliations also influence their communications with health care providers and how they seek and receive care. For example, the Asian population has several main subgroups:

Chinese, Filipino, Indian, Vietnamese, Korean, and Japanese. Their subgroups are Pakistani, Cambodian, Hmong, Thai, Laotian, Taiwanese, Bangladeshi, and Burmese. These groups can be minority groups within the larger group—Asian. Hispanics/Latinos in the United States include persons from Cuba, Mexico, Puerto Rico, and South Central America, which are subgroups of the larger group—Hispanic.

The critical point about subgroups is that persons from subgroups may not share the values and perceptions of the larger "minority" or those of the "majority" group. Geographical region, heritage, nationality group, lineage, and country of birth can make a difference. While there are similarities between larger minority groups and their subgroups within the same geographical region, members can even feel suspicious and fearful of providers representing not only the majority group at the time but their larger minority group. They may view them as more powerful, and because they are from a racial–ethnic subgroup, view them as unable to act in their best interest.

Members of minority groups or subgroups of minority groups can frequently exhibit, at least initially, suspicion and fear of clinicians from either the majority group or larger minority group. In many instances, responses of minority patients to health providers or a different ethnic or racial group is immediately mistrust, followed by guarded communication. The role of trust in the provider and the use of preventive services among low income African American women is described by O'Malley and colleagues (2004). They concluded that stronger patient-provider relationships with high levels of trust may indirectly lead to better health in these women if it results in better adherence to screening recommendations. A special case of this phenomenon is racial–ethnic immigrant groups who have experienced severe abuse in the hands of a dominant culture and may not trust health providers or health care institutions.

Unsubstantiated Beliefs about Minority and Majority Groups

Providers, like many other social groups, may harbor attitudes or beliefs about both minority and majority groups with whom they come into contact with. These attitudes and beliefs may have basis in very little direct contact or from exposure to a subgroup within a minority or majority group. There is no question that they sometimes have *stereotypic views*. For example, common misconceptions include: all white Americans take health care for granted and are difficult to please, Asians are "stoic" and may not confide in you, and indigenous peoples practice complementary health care rather than seek medical care from established health centers.

Patients can have equally set views of providers. Some common unsubstantiated views are white male physicians feel they are superior, women physicians are more compassionate, minority group health professionals are undereducated, and Asian medical practitioners are "unfeeling." The standard for care regardless of patient–provider differences and similarities is building a relationship focused on effective communication based upon mutual respect, understanding, and openness—with a caution not to hold onto unsubstantiated assumptions when caring for patients and their families.

Subgroup Affiliations Shape Communication

As previously established, patient–health provider communications can differ across cultural groups and depend to a certain degree on matches or mismatches of providers and patients. This is also true for subgroups. The following example depicts differences within an ethnic category—Asian culture. In the Vietnamese culture, talking is customary. Silence may be uncomfortable, and unless one party is angry or upset, long silences are unusual. Likewise, in the Filipino culture, talking is enjoyed and silence is uncomfortable. The only time that talking is not approved is when an elder is speaking—then it is a sign of disrespect to talk. These patterns run counter to other Asian groups where silence is considered a sign of wisdom, and speech may be regarded as frivolous.

These tendencies, if accurate, are not universal for all Asian subgroups. An important distinction is the educational background and immigration experiences within and across subgroups. For example, some groups, such as the Japanese and Korean subgroups, value and acquire superior communication skills by virtue of higher education goals and achievement. Still, there are other groups whose ability and interest in engaging in health care discussions are more limited in part to their language deficits or customary responses to others, especially those in authority positions. Some Asian patients may expect health providers to learn of their health concerns in the context of a polite conversation which may not address directly the provider's questions: "How can I help you today?" or "What brings you in today?"

When health care providers intentionally shape their verbal and nonverbal behavior to be respectful of the patient's background, they are practicing with the intentions to be culturally competent. This commitment is a step toward removing cross-cultural barriers.

▶ Cultural Competence—A Developmental Process

In our multicultural society, we are all exposed in varying degrees to diversity. Just how much attention is paid to these differences depends on one's values, biases, type of exposure, and the attitudes of one's reference groups. If providers (1) value individuals as unique in their own right, (2) hold few fixed judgments about any individual or group, (3) have multiple exposures (especially quality exposures) to the differences of others, and (4) have reference groups which value cultural differences, it is more likely that they will be culturally competent in dealing with others. Within the health care setting, this means a heightened awareness and appreciation for patients' differences in self-disclosing, in interacting in the provider–patient relationship, and in perceptions of illness and risk of disease. In recent years, the need to become culturally competent with patient groups have extended beyond minority status due to race, religion, language spoken to patients with varying disabilities, older age, gender identification, and sexual orientation. Research has shown that these groups experience health inequities and are at risk for poor health care communication.

According to a report from researchers at Harvard and Cornell Universities and published in *The Commonwealth Fund* report (Betancourt et al., 2002), cultural competence in health care can be defined as "the ability of providers and organizations to effectively deliver health care services that meet the social, cultural, and linguistic needs of patients." Issues of cultural competency cross many segments of patient care, including end-of-life care (Curtis, Engelberg, Nielsen, Au, & Patrick, 2004).

Tong and Spicer (1994), in a classic description of differences across patient and provider groups raises the problem of the lack of familiarity and lack of tolerance. These authors described the basis for frustration between Eastern patients and Western caregivers, noting two distinct characteristics of which Western caregivers are unfamiliar. The first pertains to the fact that the family assumes the major role of decision-maker on behalf of the patient. The second relates to the Eastern belief of silence surrounding the discussion of

dying (and impending death) versus the Western orientation, which advocates openness and honesty.

By gaining a greater understanding of these cultural traditions and practices, providers can deliver more culturally competent health care. Patients often hold divergent explanations for their symptoms. By learning their explanations for their health problems, providers are ensuring a more culturally sensitive approach to patient care.

To better understand where one is in the process of becoming culturally competent, it is helpful to consider all the possible ways of responding to cultural differences. There is more than one approach to understanding the process of getting from cultural insensitivity to cultural competence. The most commonly used description identifies these important concepts—cultural awareness, cultural sensitivity, and cultural competence. But, between these steps, typically plotted on a continuum, there may be other steps that describe behaviors at different levels of **cultural competence continuum**. For example, *The Guide for Teaching Health Professionals Cultural Competency* defines a developmental sequence detailing the levels of novice, intermediate, and advanced cultural competency.

In the *Resource Map* for promoting effective communications, respecting patients' cultural beliefs, and listening nonjudgmentally to health beliefs are viewed as novice- or intermediate-level competencies. Expressing a nonjudgmental, nonshaming, and respectful attitude towards individuals with limited literacy (or health literacy) skills is considered an advanced cultural competency skill. These and other conceptual frameworks provide information supporting the idea that learning and developing cultural competency skills is a process.

In an early classic theory of cultural competence by Cross, Bazron, Dennis, and Isaacs (1989), the notion of a cultural competence continuum was addressed. However, this time, rather than positive descriptors of competency positions on the continuum, this theory included both negative and positive descriptors. These authors plotted competence on a continuum where the concept of *cultural destructiveness* is at one end and *cultural proficiency* is at the other. But, between these two points on the continuum, there are many possibilities. In applying this theory, it is important to keep in mind that individuals are not easily typed nor should they be pigeon-holed (assigned to a category that is too rigid or exclusive).

Providers are capable of a variety of responses, depending on the context of the situation and the persons involved. Some providers may display cultural competence in some contexts but not in all. Therefore, it is more useful and accurate to think about selected behavioral responses than it is to rigidly categorize individuals as one type or in one stage of development. Having made this point, it is important to clarify the various terms used to describe level-of-competence and behavioral responses using this classic theory of cultural competence continuum.

Cultural Destructiveness

Way at one end of the continuum and representing a negative position is "cultural destructiveness." Attitudes, practices, and communications that are "destructive" to cultures and, therefore, to the individuals who come from these cultures, are represented at this point on the continuum. Individuals and groups of individuals who participate in cultural genocide, boarding schools that removed Indian children from their homes, laws that restricted Asians from bringing their spouses to the United States, and assaults on African Americans by the Ku Klux Klan are perhaps the worse examples of cultural destructive behavior.

These actions were blatant attempts to deny people of their basic human rights. In the health care arena, services that have denied people of cultural practices of natural healers, removed children from their families based on

ethnic bias, or purposely risked the well-being of people of color through medical experiments without their knowledge and consent are examples of culturally destructive clinical practices.

Systems can also deny cultural differences by severely curbing individuals' rights to communicate in their native language. Demands that English must be spoken in major institutions (hospitals, clinics, schools, judicial departments) may not deny individuals their basic rights. Still, one could make the case that without choices, and with multiple pressures to relinquish one's native language, providers could be close to abusing human rights and cultural destructiveness. Individuals and institutions adhering to this extremely negative position generally believe that there is a majority culture, that the dominant culture is superior, and that subcultures or subgroups within or outside the dominant culture are inferior.

Bigotry (intolerance towards others who hold different opinions than oneself) translates into vast power differences that allow the dominant cultural group to control, exploit, and disenfranchise others. While not many examples are found in the health care system today, it is important to be aware that practices that disenfranchise subgroups may have been implemented and may be historically grounded in policy that is not apparent. Refer back to the study of African American men's delays in health help-seeking, and the subtle ways that the history of discrimination can impact help-seeking behaviors.

Blatantly or subtly, there are aspects of culture that are not obviously denied but may be shamed or prohibited. These include nonverbal communication, including gestures, body motion, and use of space. When shunned or shamed, these aspects of one's cultural orientation are inhibited and controlled.

Cultural Incapacity

Not as extreme, but still potentially detrimental in a multicultural society is "cultural incapacity." Cultural incapacity is influenced by beliefs of supremacy of one group, but unlike cultural destructiveness, it is not characterized by intentional behaviors aimed at eradicating the beliefs, values, and practices of minority cultures.

Rather than by intentional acts to control minorities, individuals who are displaying cultural incapacity may lack the vision and capacity to be effective due to long-standing exposures to bias in their social groups (e.g., their paternal and/or maternal posture toward minorities). Their attitudes reflect subtle racial biases which may not be immediately apparent to them. The following hypothetical clinical example describes how cultural incapacity may occur even though the provider is problem solving a clinical care issue (**EXHIBIT 6-2**).

By maintaining stereotypes, service in this setting will remain unhelpful. At the heart of the problem is a certain amount of ignorance and unrealistic suspicion and fear that may even permeate the health care facility giving unmarried young Hispanic mothers ("repeaters") feelings that they are not always welcomed, and are generally expected to be poor health care investments.

Cultural Blindness

Providers who experience *cultural blindness* also suffer from a lack of information (Cross et al., 1989). Unlike those in the former category, these individuals usually take pride in being unbiased. The problem, however, is that they are *blind* to their own cultural influences and do not fully understand the influence of culture in others' responses. Midpoint on the continuum, these individuals profess that all people are the same (i.e., equal), and culture or ethnicity makes no difference.

These providers, according to Cross, are participating in cultural blurring. Providers in this category believe that approaches used to provide health care services to people of the traditionally dominant culture suffice for all groups. In this instance, culture is invalidated by omission, and this problem is often compounded because services are not coordinated to reflect the unique needs of patients and their families.

Patients may be left to negotiate service delivery with more than one provider in a language they may not fully understand. While the service–delivery philosophy may appear liberal and unbiased, it has the tendency to make services so stereotypical and rigid that they are ineffective for all but the most assimilated subgroups.

An example of this tendency would be the application of family therapy for all groups whose family members have a serious mental

---

EXHIBIT 6-2 Di alogue Box: Hypothetical Scenario

Provider bias about the health care behavior of one mother is described in this scenario as a Latina mother and her young child. Ramona H., a 24-year-old Latina and an unmarried mother came to the dental clinic with her 6-year-old son, Alton. Her son needed to be seen for a dental checkup. While Ramona was there, she asked the dental assistant whether she could have her older sons, Javier (10 years old) and Juan (11 years old), seen as well. The dental assistant ushering Alton (of mixed African American and Latino races) to the examining room thought to herself "Why does this mother keep having babies out of wedlock? She's had so many boyfriends; doesn't she care about these children? She is a typical welfare abuser. They (Juan and Javier) look OK—I'm not going to let her 'use the system.' She'll just have to wait 3 months for their next regular visit." In turn, Ramona may notice the assistant's disapproval and think to herself: "That woman is treating me like dirt! She thinks I'm a bad person. I need to talk to someone else because she won't help me." The assistant's view that Latinas "use the system" and do not care about their children is a bias that, while not communicated verbally, is communicated nonverbally to this mother, and will no doubt cause some conflict between the providers and the patient.

illness. Despite good intentions and in the spirit of fairness that seems to characterize program planners, the model of care reflects a middle class, nonminority existence. Services and providers may ignore differences in views of health and illness, and the tendency for some families to keep problems contained in the family and private, even in family therapy. To expect some women to express open dissatisfaction toward their husbands in couple's therapy ignores the cultural tenets regarding traditional male–female roles in many subgroup minority populations. Culturally blind providers ignore cultural differences and encourage assimilation.

Cultural Precompetence

Unlike individuals who are culturally blind and disregard both the effects of their own and others' cultural heritages, *culturally precompetent* persons realize the limitations they have in providing culturally sensitive responses (Cross et al., 1989). They also attempt to improve their services to one or more subgroups. People in this group are growing and enhancing their cultural competence skills and knowledge. They may learn the languages, try culturally sensitive interventions, consult others from the culture, and initiate training in cultural competence for themselves and their colleagues. They may recruit minority individuals to serve on boards of directors of community health care planning programs.

Precompetent providers are clearly committed to delivering quality care through culturally sensitive programs. As such, their interest and commitment might be recognized by patients, and if they do not understand something, patients are likely to work with them cooperatively.

Cultural Competence

Toward the positive end of the cultural competence continuum is *cultural competence*. Cultural competence refers to a high level of

capacity to accept and respect differences (Cross et al., 1989). This requires ongoing self-assessment, careful attention to the dynamics of differences, and continuous expansion of cultural knowledge. A variety of responses are used to adapt health care practices for the specific needs of persons from minority cultures. Culturally competent providers are highly perceptive. They view minority groups as distinctly different from one another and distinctly separate from the dominant majority group. They understand that within any given minority group there are subgroups, each with important cultural characteristics. Providers in this category seek to engage minority staff, are committed to change, and are capable of negotiating a bicultural perspective. The goal for themselves and their colleagues is to become proficient in cross-cultural situations.

Cultural Proficiency

While cultural competence is a fluctuating, evolving, and changing capacity, the goal is to reach, at the far end of the continuum, *cultural proficiency*. The highest level, cultural proficiency within a multicultural society may not occur for all. This goal is not easily reached and requires a great deal of self-assessment, knowledge building, and consultation with others. Individuals at this end of the continuum hold cultures in very high esteem. They seek to research and develop culturally sensitive practices and health care programs. As such, they will be regarded by others as experts or specialists and may be called on to assist in restructuring health care services (Cross et al., 1989).

At each level in the culturally competency continuum, certain principles can be applied. Movement on the continuum relies on (1) valuing differences, awareness, and self-assessment, (2) understanding cross-cultural dynamics, (3) building cultural knowledge, and (4) adapting practice to reflect the patient's cultural context. The pathway to competence includes learning about one's culture, the culture of others, exploring the cultural orientation of patients and families, finding and using resources to help patients with a broad range of social, psychological, financial, as well as medical needs.

Cultural competence behaviors have been identified and described by a range of health practitioners since the original IOM report on inequities. Categories of personal qualities, knowledge, and skills are summarized below in list form (**EXHIBIT 6-3**).

▶ **Understanding Your Own Cultural Programming**

Health providers who are striving to develop or enhance their cultural competence are advised to conduct ongoing self-assessments. This means that providers should be able to

---

EXHIBIT 6-3 Personal Qualities, Knowledge, and Skills for Cultural Competence

I.   **Personal qualities:** Personal qualities refer to characteristics inherent or fostered that can facilitate culture competence:
   - The capacity to respond flexibly to a wide range of possible health care situations and solutions.
   - Acceptance of a full range of population differences—age, gender, education, sexual orientation, linguistic, cultural, race and ethnic, as well as regional differences among people.
   - A willingness and level of comfort working with culturally different characteristics, such as minority groups and subgroups.
   - The ability to recognize and describe their own personal values, stereotypes, and biases about their own and others' differences.
   - Recognition of how one's biases can lead to patient resistance and conflict with the health care needs of patients.
   - A personal ongoing commitment to become more culturally competent, changing biases, stereotyping, or prejudices.
   - Recognition of the history of their profession which may have unknowingly, but systematically, provided less care and concern for persons of different racial and ethnic groups.
   - Acknowledge and seek out colleagues from other groups, particularly members of minority groups, to refine one's thinking about health care to these groups.

II. **Knowledge and awareness:** Knowledge of the
   - Unique culture of patient groups and subgroups (including cultural practices, prevailing perceptions of health and illness, and past experience with health care).
   - Impact of patients' minority or majority status, and what this might mean in the context of help-seeking and adherence to health care regimens.
   - Any variations in help-seeking behaviors of patients, families, and communities.
   - Patients' language, speech patterns, and communication styles that will influence how to engage patients in their health care.
   - Impact of social service agencies and national policies on patients and their families, especially if they are immigrants to the United States.
   - Health care and social service agencies, persons, informal networks, and their own research capabilities) that patients typically use, and that might be utilized on behalf of patients and families. Collect resource information about relevant programs and services.
   - Ways in which professional values may conflict or seem to conflict with the needs of patients and families, and ways in which these values can be used in support of patients' needs.

- Any social or political affiliations or agencies interacting with the patient and family, particularly those in power positions, such as Immigration, Social Security, Social Services, Child Protective Services.

III. **Skills:** Skills may be in place or learned over time and practiced to achieve proficiency and include abilities to:
- Learn about and refresh one's learning about the cultures of patient groups and their families.
- Make health care assessments and care plans taking into consideration patients' background and culture.
- Communicate clearly and accurately about health care information to patients, families, and communities, and to engage and work with a translator when needed. Avoid the use of medical jargon. Many patients (especially those with lower socioeconomic status and education, those with disabilities, nonwhite racial and ethnic minority groups, and the elderly) have below basic health care literacy.
- Discuss any diversity issue, whether due to age, gender, race, racial and ethnic differences, and respond to culturally based cues patients and families provide.
- Identify stress and conflict that may arise in patients help-seeking experiences, and any current social or political issues impacting patients and families.
- Use interview strategies that respect and respond to any strengths or limitations in language facility in patients and families.
- Use theories of patient empowerment as they apply to the patients' unique culture.
- Engage patients and help them use social, educational, psychological, and medical resources in their communities.
- Recognize and address issues of racism, racial stereotypes, and myths in colleagues and the institution that impede the delivery of quality care to all. Promote access to quality care in high-risk populations, including refugees and immigrants.
- Evaluate the validity and applicability of culture competence techniques, research, and knowledge in working with ethnically diverse and underserved minority patients in your health care setting.
- Promote the incorporation of multicultural approaches within the traditional biomedical framework.
- Take an active role in facilitating coordination of care across health care agencies for at-risk populations.

Cultural competence, personal attributes, knowledge, and skills can be gained and refined through training and experience. Providers are encouraged to avail themselves of opportunities to polish their personal attributes and to build their knowledge and skill. Exposure to the positive aspects of different cultures, and even negative experiences, in helping relationships will facilitate learning, but for those who are more novice than expert, this learning is best done under the supervision of faculty and clinical experts.

assess themselves, their relationships, and communications, and develop a sense of their own cultural uniqueness. The premise is that as providers are able to understand how their own culture shapes their life views, beliefs, and communications, and it will be easier for them to establish how they may need to adapt in interacting effectively with individuals from other cultures. Individuals who are self-aware can anticipate barriers and minimize the negative effects of cross-cultural differences.

To appreciate cultural similarities and differences, providers need to recognize the influence of their own culture on how they think and act. In part, bias and stereotyping behaviors occur on an unconscious level. These unconscious responses toward patients may even be inconsistent with one's conscious beliefs and values (Burgess, van

Ryn, Dovidio, & Saha, 2007). Thus, a purposeful self-examination of one's own cultural influences can lead to a better understanding of oneself and the impact of culture.

What appear to be small differences can result in major misunderstandings. For example, when anticipating families' learning needs to prepare them to care for the patient at home, it is imperative that you understand what the patient considers what "family" and "family involvement" mean to the patient and the family. To the provider, family involvement may mean working exclusively with the spouse to enable him/her to perform caregiving tasks. To the patient, involvement could mean ignoring the spouse and involving the extended family (e.g., the patient's older siblings). Knowing one's own cultural biases can minimize the effects of cross-cultural misunderstanding.

Self-Recognition of Personal Programming

Understanding one's personal cultural programming is best arrived at by questions, provided the questioning mirrors back provider's personal programming. Sometimes questions administered in small groups of diverse people have a higher yield. The group discussion tends to stimulate one's own recall and recognition, and, at the same time, each member who hears another's self-assessment is learning something about cultural similarities and differences. **EXHIBIT 6-4** provides a list of general questions aimed at stimulating recognition of one's cultural programming.

Many providers do not recognize how their own cultural values have shaped their day-to-day experiences and how day-to-day behaviors have been reinforced by their family, peers, and social affiliations. For those who are still somewhat doubtful of the ability of culture to determine behavior, specific and detailed cultural analysis will reveal just how persuasive culture is. Remember, aspects of culture include (1) one's set of values and norms, (2) shared beliefs and attitudes, (3) relationship patterns, (4) communication and language patterns, and (5) prescribed daily activities, including dress and appearance, food preferences, and time consciousness.

Acknowledging Differences

Taking each one of these more-global aspects of culture, it is possible to generate a specific

---

EXHIBIT 6-4 Recognizing Your Personal Cultural Programming

- Establish your cultural heritage by identifying your place of birth, current affiliations, and religious and ethnic alliances. For example, are you from the United States or outside the United States? A small town or large city? Do you have a religious affiliation, or do you define yourself as spiritual but not religious?
- What reactions/curiosities do you have about your own cultural programming?
- Does any aspect of your cultural identity come in conflict with other aspects? For example, do you see yourself as assertive, but your culture does not support this behavior?
- What is the most influential part of your cultural programming?
- How does your cultural programming affect your communication? For example, are there things that you would share only with close family members? Are there things about your family that you would not share with providers?
- What do you know about the cultural programming of others (your superiors, peers, colleagues, patients, etc.)? If you do not know their cultural background, what would you guess it to be, and why? Does their communication give you clues about their cultural programming?

list of the ways in which cultures influence individuals but are different across groups of individuals. What is accepted in one culture may be considered inappropriate in another. The mainstream Anglo culture, for example, has been said to be characterized by individualism, self-reliance, action, and a sense of control over one's environment. These characteristics are most apparent in males, and can be seen in minority groups within the United States as well.

In contrast, Buddhist teachings adhere to a fatalistic view of life. Life is suffering, and suffering is caused by desire. In this context, suffering in pain may be considered to be simply a fact of life rather than a health emergency. Many Asians prescribe to the theory of three possible causes of disease—the physical, the supernatural, and balances (yin–yang). They rely heavily on forms of self-care that include offerings to spirits, dermabrasion, and hot–cold and herbal remedies.

There are 21 Spanish-speaking countries in the world whose people are called *Latino*. Latinos, however, are not monolithic. It is not possible to generalize and be absolutely accurate. Latino communities have been observed to value a present-time orientation, the extended family, the interdependence of family members, differentiation of sex roles, unconditional respect for adults, and deference to authority. Although Latinos have similar values, there may be a great deal of difference across their subgroups. Some Latinos are more formal in language and style. South Americans, for example, are said to be more formal than are Latinos from the Caribbean. Characteristics (e.g., gender, age, immigration status, religious affiliation, social status, and reasons for immigration) all play a role in the cultural programming of Latinos. In Latino communities, the chief barrier to accessing health care is usually the lack of insurance coverage, but in addition, there may be a general distrust of modern medicine. Many

Latinos believe in folk medicine and have great faith in their *courandaro* (or neighborhood healer). They feel that the courandaro always knows exactly what is wrong, while a physician does not. The Latino observes the medical practitioner asking many questions before offering a diagnosis, while the courandaro seems to recognize the problem immediately and knows how to deal with it.

There are other reasons patient–provider relationships with some Latinos might inhibit effective communications. Latinos generally show a good deal of deference for persons in authority, including the health care providers they see. Van Servellen et al. (2003) noted the importance of considering this cultural phenomenon in building medication adherence intervention programs. Deference to providers may, in fact, prohibit full disclosure of what is actually occurring in the patients' response to the treatment regimen. Are patients likely to say everything is "fine" in order to please the provider?

Knowing that patients' culture may deem certain behaviors or interactions more acceptable than others will assist providers in communicating more effectively. Aspects of culture that influence health care encounters are multiple. Values and norms, beliefs and attitudes, relationship patterns, communication and language, and daily activities are influenced by one's culture. Essentially, when aspects of culture are operationalized, the link between culture and patients' responses becomes clear. In the helping–healing process, awareness of the other's culture, and the differences that exist between the patient and provider, will enable the provider to anticipate misunderstandings and further sensitize providers in their interactions with patients.

While the first task is to raise one's conscious awareness of the impact of culture, this is not sufficient to secure cultural competence. Going beyond requires acknowledging cultural differences between yourself and the patient. Operating on the basis of differences

---

EXHIBIT 6-5 Analyzing Interactions in Which Cultural Differences Exist

Aspects of Culture

   I.   Values and norms
  II.   Beliefs and attitudes
 III.   Relationship patterns
  IV.   Communication and language
   V.   Daily activities

Patient's Cultural Reference: Formal

- Bows, embraces, handshakes, and kissing.
- Hierarchical destiny is predetermined by race, class, and gender inequality.
- Focus on the extended family. Loyalty and responsibility to the family of origin.
- Relational intimacy is less important.

- Implicit and indirect. Emphasis is on the context of messages.
- Religion may control how a person dresses. They eat when hungry. Value is on promptness and efficiency.

Your Cultural Patterns: Informal

- Handshakes. Egalitarian. Determinism.
- Individualized race and gender equality.
- Focus on the nuclear family. Independence from the family is valued. Interpersonal intimacy is desired.
- Explicit, direct communication. Emphasis on the content of a message.
- A wide range of dress/style is accepted. Eat at a social functions. Time is relative.
- Schedules are changed to accommodate relationships.

---

is as important, or more so, than acting on similarities. Furthermore, the ability to analyze interactions in which cultural differences exist is an important skill that is not easy, but may be a valuable long-term goal and commitment.

EXHIBIT 6-5 presents each of five previously identified cultural aspects and compares and contrasts a hypothetical patient and provider interaction. Differences in values and norms, beliefs and attitudes, relational patterns, communication and language, as well as the usual daily activities illustrate that these differences that exist between the provider and patient may be significant and potentially cause resistance and conflict. For example, the value placed on direct communication (provider) and indirect communication (patient) has the potential to generate uneasiness, conflict, misunderstanding, and mistrust. What seem to be of minor importance, can cause patient–provider communications to be out of sync. This apparent minor difference has

the potential for developing into something major; that is, there is a strong possibility that the patient will leave and not come back to see this provider again.

▶ Summary

By the year 2030, ethnic and racial minority groups in the United States are expected to increase to nearly 40% of the total population. The issue of health care disparities in these groups loom over the health of the nation. A facet of this problem is the contribution of internalized discrimination and inadequate patient–provider communications.

The cultural backgrounds of providers and patients are composed of learned norms, values, customs, and beliefs that are similar but different. If providers are to be as effective as they can be in providing holistic care to patients of culturally diverse backgrounds, their technical expertise and communications must be grounded in the knowledge of and respect for the various cultures they encounter in a broad range of health care settings. This is particularly true for situations in which providers are from cultural and ethnic backgrounds different from the patients for whom they are caring.

It is important to note that there is an emergent body of research that addresses discrimination and racism not only at the individual and dyadic relationship level but at the institutional level. Examples beyond the relationship level are noted by Smedley (2012), who explains health inequity as the result of racial disparities imbedded in inequitable distributions of societal power and social status. The case studies in this chapter highlight the interaction of gender and internalized racism which potentially create a unique challenge for minorities in the U.S. health care system.

What has emerged is a growing consensus that providers must look beyond the traditional understanding of racism as largely an individually mediated phenomenon to understand the health consequences of the lived experience of race in the United States, and how race intersects with other factors such as gender, socioeconomic status, and geography (Smedley, 2012).

Is the current health provider work force ready, willing, and able to provide culturally appropriate care? Sound cross-cultural practice begins with a commitment to provide culturally competent care. At the very heart of this commitment must be an awareness and acceptance of culturally different expressive behaviors, and an understanding of the dynamics of difference in the context of the patient–provider relationship.

Culturally competent health care providers not only acknowledge cultural differences, but also incorporate these differences in planning and implementing care. A culturally competent system of care acknowledges and incorporates—at all levels—the importance of culture, the assessment of cross-cultural relations, vigilance toward the dynamics that result from cultural differences, the expansion of cultural knowledge, and the adaptation of services to meet culturally unique needs. While cultural competence is a concept that can be applied to an entire system of care, it is also a concept useful in assessing the cultural practices of one's individual facility.

Cultural competence should be viewed as a goal toward which providers can strive. To be realistic, becoming culturally competent is a developmental process. Providers are all, at some point, on a continuum. One's behaviors and attitudes reflect their position on the continuum at any one time. It is important for providers to assess their own personal level of cultural competence with the understanding that it may be a long-term investment. Verbal and nonverbal expressive behaviors are influenced by one's cultural orientation.

Above all other circumstances, inattention to obvious and even subtle differences in expressive behavior may serve to alienate patients and their families. Health care providers must be sensitive to the differences in cultural perceptions about the role of the sick, the role of the family in health care, the roles of the young and old, the roles of women and men, and even the symbolic importance of foods and diet. Helping the patient comply with health care regimens requires knowledge about these and other cultural values.

A final word of caution is important. While it is imperative for providers to be culturally sensitive, too much attention to differences can inappropriately distant the provider from the patient. Beginning clinicians may be too willing to acknowledge these differences and act accordingly. Where language barriers exist, it is important to get assistance, and if the patient openly requests a different provider, then this request should be honored if possible. However, unnecessary accommodation, for example, by offering to get someone else to care for them can be problematic. This offer can be interpreted as a lack of acceptance or even rejection. Cultural differences are inevitable, and diversity training can equip providers in most situations to deal effectively with cultural nuances.

Advances in cultural competence education has gained momentum for a variety of reasons: emerging regulatory/accreditation pressures for undergraduate and graduate education, societal pressures, funding opportunities, and due to the increasing diversity within faculty, student groups, and patients. Several undergraduate and postgraduate programs offer substantial training to enhance the development of cultural competency in health care.

Many programs propose a combination of experiential and course content. Students evaluations after cultural competence training and education vary, and undergraduate students may not feel totally capable of delivering cultural competent care. In an evaluation of medical students enrolled in the first and fourth year of their undergraduate program, cultural competence was seen to increase, but students still reported feeling inadequately prepared and skilled in many important aspects of cross-cultural care (Green et al., 2017).

Low skillfulness ratings for counseling patients about their use of complementary or alternative medicine, and identifying religious beliefs and cultural customs that might affect clinical care, were apparent in students even in the last year of their academic program. Researchers expressed concern because these aspects of care are central to preparing culturally competent practitioners before they begin their medical residency.

High levels of cultural competence, a fluid process, does not eliminate all problems in communicating with patients and their families, but it does help reduce cultural insensitivity and conflict occurring in health care settings. A point well worth noting is that culturally competent care also requires an openness on the part of patients and families to resolve the barriers they face, and challenge and overcome their experiences of culture inequity and discrimination which might have very deep roots. Patients' interest in lessening these barriers in the presence of a culturally competent health practitioner and in the context of a culturally competent health care system might significantly impact existing health disparities and, in the long term, health inequities found too often among our ethnic and racial minority groups.

Discussion

1. Discuss the question: do cultural differences divide or unite people from dissimilar cultural groups?
2. Provide data to substantiate that the United States is a *mixed salad*, no longer *a melting pot*.
3. Define culture and discuss how one's culture might influence their access to and acceptance of health care in the current health care system.
4. Discuss the stages leading up to cultural competence, and identify your stage of cultural competence.
5. Discuss ways in which internalized racism, together with other population characteristics (e.g., age and gender), might impact help-seeking health behaviors and subsequent health disparities.

References

Betancourt, J. R., Green, A. R., Carrillo, J. E., & The Commonwealth Fund. (2002). *Cultural competence in health care: Emerging frameworks and practical applications*, Field Report. Retrieved from http://www.commonwealthfund.org/usr_doc/betancourt_culturalcompetence_576.pdf

Burgess, D., van Ryn, M., Dovidio, J., & Saha, S. (2007). Reducing racial bias among health care providers: Lessons from social-cognitive psychology. *Journal of General Internal Medicine, 22*(6), 882–887. doi:10.1007/s11606-007-0160-1

Centers for Disease Control and Prevention. (2017, March 22). Culture & health literacy. Reviewed from https://www.gov/healthliteracy/culture.html

Crawley, L., Ahn, D., & Winkleby, M. (2008). Perceived medical discrimination and cancer screening behaviors of racial and ethnic minority adults. *Cancer Epidemiology Biomarkers Prevention, 17*(8), 1937–1944. doi:10.1158/1055-9965.EPI-08-0005

Cross, T. L., Bazron, B. J, Dennis, K. W., & Isaacs, M. R. (1989). *Towards a culturally competent system of care*. Washington, DC: CASSP Technical Assistance Center, Georgetown University Child Development Center.

Curtis, J. R., Engelberg, R. A., Nielsen, E. L., Au, D. H., & Patrick, D. L. (2004). Patient-physician communication about end-of-life care for patients with COPD. *European Respiratory Journal, 24,* 200–205. PMID:15332385

Diette, G. B., & Rand, C. (2007). The contributing role of health-care communication to health disparities for minority patients with Asthma. *Chest, 132,* 802S–809. doi:10.1378/chest.07-1909

Eckardt, P., Culley, J. M., Corwin, E., Richmond, T., Dougherty, C., Pickler, R. H., … DeVon, H. A. (2017). National nursing science priorities: Creating a shared vision. *Nursing Outlook, 65,* 6, 726–736. Retrieved from www.nursingoutlook.org

Green, A. R., Chun, M. B. J., Cervantes, M. C., Nudel, J. D., Duong, J. V., Krupat, E., & Betancourt, J. R. (2017). Measuring medical students' preparedness and skills to provide cross-cultural care. *Health Equity, 1*(1), 15–22. doi:10.1089/heq.2016.0011

Hollingshead, N. A., Ashburn-Nardo, L., Stewart, J. C., & Hirsh, A. T. (2016). The pain experience of Hispanic Americans: A critical literature review and conceptual model. *The Journal of Pain: Official Journal of the American Pain Society, 17*(5), 513–528. doi:10.1016/j.jpain.2015.10.022

Institute of Medicine. (2002). *Unequal treatment: Confronting racial and ethnic disparities in health care (full printed version)*. Washington, DC: The National Academies Press. doi:10.17226/10260

Lipa, M., & Pew Research Center. (2015, August 27). *10 Facts about religion in America.* Retrieved from www.pewresearch.org

O'Malley, A. S., Sheppard, V. B., Schwartz, M., & Mandelblatt, J. (2004). The role of trust in use of preventive services among low-income African-American women. *Preventive Medicine, 38,* 777–785. doi:10.1016/j.ypmed.2004.01.018

Powell, W., Adams, L. B., Cole-Lewis, Y., Agyemang, A., & Upton, R. D. (2016). Masculinity and race-related factors as barriers to health help-seeking barriers among African-American men. *Behavioral Medicine (Washington, DC), 42*(3), 150–163. doi:10.1080/08964289.2016.1165174

Simons, G. F., & Fennig, C. D., (Eds.). (2017). *Ethnologue: Languages of the world* (12th ed.). Dallas, TX: SIL International. Retrieved from https://www.ethnologue.com/

Smedley, B. D. (2012). The lived experience of race and its health consequences. American Journal of Public Health, 102(5), 933–935. doi:10.2105/AJPH.2011.300643

Tong, K. L., & Spicer, B. J. (1994). The Chinese palliative patient and family in North America: A cultural perspective. *Journal of Palliative Care, 10*(1), 26–28. PMID:7518506

University of Maryland College Park School of Public Health and Herschel S. Horowitz Center for Health Literacy. (2013). O'Malley Brown, & Secretary, PRIMER—Cultural competency and health literacy: A guide for teaching health professionals and students. Retrieved from https://health.maryland.gov/mhqcc

U.S. Census Bureau. (2015, March 05). *New census bureau report analyses U.S. population projections* (Report No. CB15-TPS. 16). Retrieved from https:/.www.census.gov

Vu, M., Azmat, A., Radejko, T., & Padela, A. I. (2016). Predictors of delayed healthcare seeking among American Muslim women. *Journal of Women's Health, 25*(6), 586–593. doi:10.1089/jwh.2015.5517

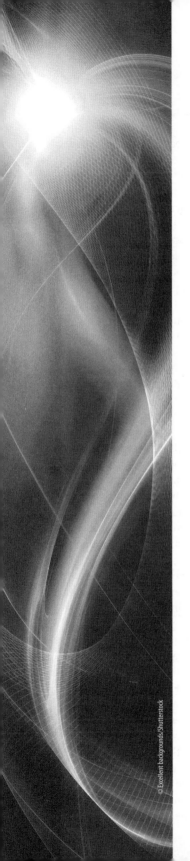

PART III

Critical Competencies in Therapeutic Communications

Good communication skills are not acquired by osmosis. Therapeutic communications in health care settings must be learned and practiced, and in many cases, relearned and even modified. Acquiring therapeutic patient-centered and family-centered communication skills can be time intensive, but these skills are critical elements in effective provider–patient interactions.

Patients and their families do and will react to providers' interpersonal skill strengths and deficits. They will not necessarily distinguish provider personal skill deficits from system barriers that make an otherwise compassionate provider appear cold, distant, and uncaring. All health providers need to take their fund of skills and competencies in therapeutic communications seriously. In the chapters that make up this part of the text, important therapeutic response modes are presented and discussed in depth, one at a time, allowing time to evaluate the unique contribution of each skill set.

Before launching this extensive discussion of specific therapeutic response modes, it is important to frame this discussion in light of an important communication principle. Therapeutic response modes must always be understood and used in the context of a patient–family-centered perspective—who is the patient and family, what is the patient and family experiencing, what does the patient–family need, and is the patient–family likely to be receptive to the response are all important considerations. Further, basic patient and family characteristics—age, gender, ethnicity, culture, socioeconomic status, level of education, preferred language, level of health literacy, and presenting health problems—cannot be ignored when choosing specific therapeutic response modes. Response modes are general and applicable to many patient populations; however, the choice and use of any response mode should reflect a patient–family-centered approach.

When using any of these response modes, it is absolutely essential that providers understand how each approach might be received and understood by different patients and their families and modify their approach accordingly. Along these lines, while attention to technique is important, it is equally essential that providers understand that using techniques should not discount the importance of authentic connections with patients and their families.

Over the last two decades, considerable attention has been given to alternative, less-formalized approaches that strengthen patient–provider communications and providers' ability to shape therapeutic encounters with patients and their families. These include listening to patients' stories and the conversational approach as opposed to the traditional focused interview. This is not to say that the topics covered in a formal interview are dropped, but an open, client-focused, less-controlled approach is used to begin or supplement focused questioning.

Masson (2005) suggests that emphasis is placed on listening to patient stories as a means to providing culturally competent care. Taking time to get to know the patient through stories, preferred language, even photographs can increase our ability to care for culturally diverse individuals and underserved groups. This alternative, more than the structured interview, is felt to produce an accurate shared understanding of the patient's health status. As indicated by Roter and Hall (1992), *talk* is the main ingredient of health (medical) care.

It is the fundamental way in which the provider–patient relationship takes form and the fundamental instrument by which therapeutic goals are achieved. While providers use a number of other tools and tests, talk is what organizes the patients' history, symptoms, and experiences. Several positive changes are advanced and are summarized in seven communication transforming principles (Roter & Hall, 1992). Communication:

1. Serves patients' needs to tell the story of their illnesses and the provider's need to hear it.
2. Reflects the special expertise and insight that patients have into their physical state and well-being.
3. Respects the relationship between patients' mental states and their physical experiences of illness.
4. Maximizes the usefulness of the providers' expertise.
5. Acknowledges and attends to emotional content.
6. Respects the principle of reciprocity in which the fulfillment of expectations is negotiated.
7. Overcomes stereotyped roles and expectations so that both the patient and provider gain a sense of power and the freedom to change within the encounter.

Interactions between providers and patients and their families vary in structure and intensity. The therapeutic response modes discussed in this section are relevant regardless of the mode in which provider–patient talk occurs. It is important to note that using client-centered talk approaches are not always received as positive by all providers, patients, and families.

Providers, for example, recognize that talk means time, and they may not feel they have or can afford to have the time to talk to patients. Formal interviewing appears to them to be more efficient in a busy health care system. Additionally, a talking approach may be perceived by providers, patients, and families to be incongruent with their cultural norms and values. For example, some providers, patients, and families may prefer a direct-controlled interview because they want to carefully measure and control what they give and receive. Just as this approach may be incongruent with one's cultural style and norms, we also know that much too structured interviews are usually devoid of patient particulars—their feelings, fears, attitudes, and expectations. There is data to show that for many patient populations, particularly those experiencing health inequities, formalized interviewing styles, when used exclusively, may miss the necessary information that customizes care and results in health care quality. This being said, the following chapters on therapeutic response modes will provide important skills and knowledge instrumental in client-centered care.

Chapter 7, "The Pervasive Role of Confirmation, Empathy, and Compassion," discusses the importance of a major element in helping relationships. The ability to more fully understand the experience of others, and reflect this sensitivity in helping encounters is critical. The process of formulating and delivering effective therapeutic empathic responses is discussed. Other concepts, confirmation and compassion, which are associated with empathic communication, are presented and discussed. Finally, the case is made that these three-sister modes—empathy, confirmation, and compassion—go together to achieve patient-centered communication and are extremely powerful in patient–provider relationships.

Chapter 8, "Communications That Contribute to Trust and Mistrust of Providers," addresses the basic role of trust in the process of assessing and helping patients. Without trust in providers, patients will not easily disclose their fears and concerns. So many issues in health care and disease prevention today include the discussion of difficult and sometimes embarrassing topics (e.g., drug and alcohol use, obesity, sexual practices, and poor adherence to treatment regimens). Each one of these topics is important to disease management and health promotion, but patients, as well as providers, may be hesitant to discuss them in patient–provider encounters, especially in primary care settings. Still, the majority of health care is delivered in primary care settings, and there is little room to be either shy or resistant. Because trust is critical in

promoting change in patients, it is vital to the helping process across a wide-range of health care settings. Mistrust can derail therapeutic interventions.

Trust, once established, can be broken. Understanding conditions under which trust is cultivated, and mistrust avoided, arms the provider with capacities to achieve and sustain meaningful in-depth relationships with patients and their families.

Chapter 9, "The Art and Skillful Use of Questions," discusses the use of questions as therapeutic response modes. Perhaps the most prevalent form of communication in the health care profession is the use of questions. In part, this is due to the assessment and diagnostic orientation of providers. Questions can vary—they can be closed-ended (such as eliciting a "yes" or "no" response or open-ended (asking for more detail about "what" and "when"). In short, questions are the primary means by which providers gather data. The format of the questions elicits different patient responses. It is important to understand the types of questions available to us, their use, and expected responses associated with them.

Sometimes questions fail to produce in-depth disclosure. Silence is a therapeutic response mode that is examined for its power to establish a comprehensive, in-depth gestalt. Chapter 10, "Therapeutic Use of Silence and Pauses," details ways in which this response mode enhances empathy, respect, and understanding.

Because silence and pauses can also be used in unhelpful ways (e.g., in withdrawing support it is important to understand the power of silence as it is used in both helpful and unhelpful ways). Silence also has a specific meaning in various cultural contexts and minority populations. Silence responses may be respectful or punitive; the actual interpretations are dependent on a multitude of interpersonal factors, including the cultural orientation of the patient.

In addition to questions and silence, providers can use self-disclosure to facilitate the aims of helping relationships. Chapter 11, "The Impact and Limitations of Self-Disclosure," discusses this important nondirective approach. Self-disclosure by providers frequently begets self-disclosure by the patient. This is because provider self-disclosure communicates authenticity, genuineness, and empathy that encourages, in turn, patient self-exploration and self-disclosure.

The key to provider self-disclosure, as is the case for many other response modes, is appropriateness. Appropriately delivered, self-disclosures will be met with matching responses. Inappropriately offered self-disclosures, such as those that are ill-timed, may lead to confusion and uneasiness in patients. Guidelines for the formulation and delivery of self-disclosures are discussed in detail.

Up to this point, the therapeutic response modes addressed are considered to be facilitative and foundational. There is yet another set of response modes that appear evaluative and judgmental if not used carefully. In Chapter 12, "The Proper Placement of Advisement," the skill of advice-giving is discussed. Providers issue advice on a regular basis on issues of health promotion of disease self-management; this mode is somewhat reflexive. The provider assesses or diagnoses a problem and follows with a solution. While advice-giving is common in patient–provider encounters, it is a poorly understood phenomena in interpersonal communication. Because advice-giving usually contains evaluative and judgmental components, like other modes, it works best when a strong relationship has been built through repeated use of facilitative dimensions like warmth, respect, and empathy.

If advice-giving does not provoke action, other approaches may. Chapter 13, "Reflections and Interpretations," examines how these distinctively different strategies produce self-awareness and change. While reflections merely paraphrase patients' expressions, interpretations provide additional information. Interpretations can be mild, moderate, or intense; the level of interpretation frequently designates the degree of threat the patient experiences when an interpretation is offered.

The maximum level of demand in health professionals' communications comes from the use of confrontations, orders, and commands. These modes are not comfortable for many providers, especially those who want to facilitate, not dominate, the patient's course of action. Were it a perfect world, we could settle for less judgmental, nonevaluative forms of communicating. But the fact of the matter is, it is not a perfect world; these response modes are necessary and cannot be supplanted by facilitative, nondirective approaches.

In the final chapter of this section of the text, Chapter 14, "The Judicious Use of Confrontations, Orders, and Commands," these approaches are addressed. Providers who utilize these response modes risk being evaluative, judgmental, and conditional. This risk is minimal if these strategies are employed when a strong relational bond exists between patient and provider. The probability of action toward problem resolution is frequently highest when patients are exposed to these strategies. Yet, like many of the other evaluative, judgmental modes, these response modes are most successful when a strong therapeutic alliance has been formed.

In therapeutic relationships, health providers must try to understand what health and illness means to the patient and the patient's family and create a therapeutic sense of connection in the patient–family–provider relationship. Several interviewing techniques can enhance such an outcome—rapport setting, connecting on an interpersonal level, respecting cultural implications, and communicating understanding can help providers enhance their sensitivity to subtle clues on which issues of meaning and connection often depend.

Therapeutic response modes are skills, and like all skills, they are to be practiced. It is important to exercise patience in the acquisition and perfection of these skills. It may surprise the reader to learn that the ultimate objective is to learn the skill but then to forget it. The mark of a seasoned clinician is knowing the skills, but blending the skills with their own unique interpersonal style.

Practicing these skills does not always result in perfect encounters. We need to know what to do if things do not happen the way we planned. There are always options to restate what we mean or want to ask. One option that can reverse our course and save our day is what I call, *The Eraser Option*, stopping the direction of what you have said, and starting again. An example would be: "You know that's not what I wanted to ask; what I think I need to know is…." Thus *Eraser* is just that, the opportunity to erase what you started to do, reverse course, and be successful.

It is understood that any attempt to use a therapeutic response mode might fall flat. But there are always options to redirect the conversation. Also, failure of a technique or approach is more the provider's concern than that of the patient or patient's family. In large part, it is providers caring and healing functions, not the enumerable strategies and skills they have at their disposal, that make the biggest difference.

CHAPTER 7

The Pervasive Role of Empathy, Confirmation, and Compassion

CHAPTER OBJECTIVES

- Distinguish between empathy and sympathy.
- Discuss how empathy is "emotional knowing" in a patient–provider encounter.
- Discuss the meaning of the statement that empathy, confirmation, and compassion are three-sisters with a common purpose.
- Identify and analyze outcomes expected when using empathy, confirmation, and compassion.
- Identify several barriers to being empathic with a patient or developing the capacity for empathy. Discuss client, provider, and environmental barriers.

KEY TERMS

- Active listening
- Avoidable suffering
- Compassion
- Confirmation
- Empathy
- Emotional knowing
- Identification

- Incorporation
- Increasing connectedness
- Inherent suffering
- Reducing alienation
- Reverberation
- Sympathy

▶ Introduction

Empathy is sometimes described as a cognitive process, and at other times an emotion expressed toward someone who is suffering. As a cognitive process, **empathy** is the understanding of another person; as an emotion, an expression of sharing feelings. The ability to feel empathic and to demonstrate empathy is dependent on one's ability to feel one's own feelings, to identify them, and to use this capacity to express **compassion**.

Health providers are possibly at their best in patient–provider communications when they can express empathy. Clinical empathy includes understanding the patient's situation, perspective, and feelings as well as their attached meanings; communicating understanding and checking its accuracy; and acting on that understanding with the patient in a therapeutic way (Platt, 1992 as presented in Kiosses, Karathanos, & Tatsioni, 2016). Empathic communication is universally accepted to be both a need and source of satisfaction of care across diverse racial/ethnic groups (Hohl et al., 2016).

Empathetic listening is showing empathy while listening in patient–provider relationships. Understanding the unique ways health status or a health condition affects individuals legitimizes patients' illness and suffering and contributes to feelings of connections with others. In the classic work of Carl Rogers, listening and empathetic responses are stressed, and can be found in health provider's assistance to help patients feel less alone and isolated for the moment; at least the patient is feeling "a connected part of the human race…" (1980, p. 150). Sherman and Cramer (2005, p. 338) stress that empathy is not only the ability of the provider to understand a patient's experiences and feelings, but "the capability of communicating this understanding."

The knowledge of patients is generally limited, but not always. Assessing what the patient does and does not know or understand is only part of the task. Knowing how the clinical knowledge or lack of it affects the patient is important. The lack of understanding can result in confusion and stress, and the empathic understanding from health providers can build hope and trust. The provider, then, must know the patient beyond the clinical data immediately available. That is, providers cannot wholly grasp subtle and complicated feelings and experiences except by emotionally knowing the patient.

Educational programs in the health professions have long stressed the importance of empathy in providing patient-centered, culturally competent, patient care; and while there are those who might dismiss the importance of empathy or take it for granted, professional organizations as well as policy makers and educators take it seriously.

The purpose of this chapter is to define and describe empathy and the nature of empathic responses. Second, the therapeutic value of empathy is described, and steps to achieve empathy are identified. Nonverbal aspects of communication as well as reflective statements and silence are discussed as they enhance empathic communications in the provider–patient relationship.

Finally, common barriers to empathic understanding are identified, and ways to overcome these barriers are described. This discussion also includes addressing the pairing of key interpersonal concepts—empathy, **confirmation**, and compassion. These concepts operate in supportive ways to achieve the overall goal of patient-centered, culturally competent health care delivery. The literature reports associations between empathy, empathetic interviewing, and empathetic response, and (1) patients' views that providers really care, patient satisfaction, and trust; (2) greater treatment adherence; (3) more accurate diagnoses of patients' conditions, and patients' abilities to process negative information about their diagnoses and treatment; (4) ability of the provider to shift patients' negative responses to some level of therapeutic value; and (5) lower the probability of medical malpractice claims.

▶ Definitions of Empathy and Empathic Response

The word *empathy* was originally coined "Einfrehlung" by German psychologist Teodor Lipps who, in 1887, used this term to refer to the experience of losing one's self-awareness, and fusing with an object. Today, empathy is described as an objective awareness of, and insight into, the thoughts, feelings, and behavior of another (including their meaning and significance). Kraft-Todd et al. (2017) define empathy as "a social-emotional ability having two distinct components: one *affective*: the ability to share the emotions of others, and one *cognitive*: the ability to understand the emotions of others."

Empathy has also been discussed in the context of *emotional intelligence*, which is defined as the awareness and management of emotions in self and others. According to Satterfield and Hughes (2007), in the context of the provider interacting with patients, this would include the provider's ability to work with emotions in oneself as well as in the patient for the benefit of both the provider and patient.

Empathy, or the capacity for "**emotional knowing**," is thought to humanize interpersonal interaction. For those who study empathy phenomenologically, empathy is a complex process describing a holistic experience of the patient. It involves a synthesis of human dimensions—conscious and preconscious awareness, subjective and objective views, and closeness but distance from the patient's experience. Physical, psychological, emotional, and cognitive processes—occurring simultaneously—achieve an empathic response.

Empathy is often confused with related concepts such as **sympathy**, pity, and identification.

Empirical studies of empathy emerged in the middle of the 20th century because of the influence of Sullivan (1953), and subsequently as a product of the efforts of Carl Rogers (1957, 1961). In recent times, the increased interest in empathy is found to be contextually relevant.

Satterfield and Hughes (2007) summarized the current state of affairs in health care that deter empathy. Essentially, providers are under increased pressure to see more patients, within no additional time periods and with less administrative support. As a result, patients frequently feel rushed, unsupported, disconnected, devalued, resentful, and distrustful. The consequences, along with provider fatigue and burnout, can be a vicious cycle with the potential of unprofessional behavior and further decline in both patient and provider satisfaction.

Perhaps the most significant work on the concept of empathy and its therapeutic value stems from the early writings of Carl Rogers in the 1950s. Rogers, in his client-centered approach to counseling, conceptualized empathy as a major factor influencing client (patient) growth and change (1957, 1961). Rogers's description of empathy stresses the importance of multiple facets. The empathic way of being with another person, according to Rogers, means entering the private perceptual world of the other and becoming at home in it.

Rogers further states that it is a process of being sensitive, moment by moment, to the changing experience of this person to a multitude of feelings—fear or rage, tenderness or confusion (whatever the person is experiencing). It also means checking with the other person the accuracy of one's sensing, and being guided by the replies and responses one receives. Rogers's model and assertions about the influence of empathic understanding stimulated considerable research aimed at measuring empathy and its impact on those seeking counseling. Truax and Carkhuff (1967) designed the first empathy scale, the Truax Accurate Empathy Scale, later revised by Carkhuff (1969).

From that time on there were a number of empathy scales developed, some of which were specific to the concept of clinical empathy. Scales that followed included the Jefferson Scale of Physician Empathy (JSPE), which is used in evaluating empathy in physicians, medical students, residents and dental students (Hojat et al., 2002), and the Consultation and Relational Empathy (CARE) (Kraft-Todd et al., 2017). The JSPE and CARE are discussed in more depth in the section about measures of empathy in clinical practice.

▶ Differentiation Between Empathy and Other Related Concepts

Differences Between Empathy and Sympathy

Perhaps the most confused notion and misunderstood idea is that sympathy is empathy. While sympathy does express feeling "with the patient," it is very different from the expression of empathy, which is the task of mentally putting one in the shoes of another, and then verbally conveying that one understands what it must be like. While empathy is a preferred skill, sympathy can be considered risky.

The actions of sympathy include the inclination to think or feel like another, but the crucial difference is that sympathy also includes the display of pity or sadness. People who sympathize are unable to separate their own feelings from those of the other. Empathic responses are not the equivalent of feeling sorry for another person; they involve appreciation for another's thoughts and feelings without displaying feelings of pity and sadness. There is the chance that patients and families will react very negatively toward sympathetic responses because, rather than bringing them

together, sympathy tends to set patient and provider further apart.

Sympathy and Emotional Knowing

With sympathetic responses, that which is usually missing is the emotional intellectual connection that guides the provider to articulate a reply. Without the ability to fully understand the perceived experience and feelings of the patient, an attempt to empathize may become a self-centered exercise in sympathy. Consider the following dialogue between a nurse health provider and a patient who is hospitalized and whose diagnosis is end-stage cancer. The patient has not seen her small children for two or more weeks. The nurse approaches her to assess her depressed mood and establish a relationship (**EXHIBIT 7-1**).

Sometimes providers are not ready to deal with the experience and feelings of the patient. They have feelings but their attempts to empathize become exercises in sympathy that actually make the patient feel worse.

In this dialogue, the nurse was probably feeling the helplessness that the patient projected in her emotional response. To recover from her own emotional pain, the nurse responds as if she were trying to make the patient feel better, giving bits of advice on how the patient could establish communications with her children. Believing she had "hit on a good idea," she pursued the idea of videotaping.

While videotaping may have been a good idea, what the nurse expressed made the patient feel that the nurse could not cope with or manage her feelings and the tragedy she faced. Thus, the patient apologized for her feelings. Then, in a feeble attempt to make the patient feel better, the nurse follows with a very sad commentary, "You don't feel that you are going to be around for your children much longer."

This may be true, but it may not be the most salient point for the patient; rather, loneliness and no one to talk to may be. And, while this is a critical issue, the way it is

EXHIBIT 7-1 Dialogue Box Illustrating Awkward Attempts to Be Empathetic

PROVIDER:	"Hi Mrs. _____. How are you doing today?"
PATIENT:	"Okay, I guess."
PROVIDER:	"You know, I've noticed that you have no pictures of your children in your room."
PATIENT:	"No…I don't."
PROVIDER:	"How would you like it if we called your husband and asked him to bring some in?"
PATIENT:	"Well, yes. That would be good!" (Silence)
PROVIDER:	"You know, better yet, we could make it possible to have you do a videotape for them—that way they could actually see you…see how you are."
PATIENT:	Looks at nurse, studying her response.
PROVIDER:	"What is good about a videotape is that they can keep it forever."
PATIENT:	Begins to cry. "I'm sorry…I guess I'm just upset."
PROVIDER:	"I can understand that you feel upset…You don't feel that you are going to be around for your children much longer."
PATIENT:	Nods. Silence.

approached tends to be rather cold and distant. Most observers would judge the nurse to be sympathetic. The reader may also judge the interaction as a self-centered gesture on the part of the nurse to find an easy solution, a quick fix. Sympathy is rarely purely altruistic; rather, it can be an exploitive function, and mask other feelings that may be inappropriate in the relationship. Frequently, sympathy can mask feelings of relief: "I'm glad I don't have your problem" or feelings of helplessness and powerlessness: "Sorry I can't help you…and I don't know who can." Providers may think that their verbal replies do not reveal these conflictual attitudes (let me help you with this; I can't help you); but the fact is, providers are rarely able to completely disguise their innermost thoughts and feelings.

Unwittingly, providers can reveal these attitudes in the choice of their words or nonverbal communication. Merely feeling what the patient is feeling or "suffering with" the patient may not give the provider the objectivity that is needed to fully comprehend the patient's dilemma. In the previous dialogue, the nurse lacked an awareness of herself and her ability to tolerate the patient's expression of pain.

This was not immediately revealed in her verbal comments, which appeared accurate, but rather it was more apparent in the direction that her dialogue took—her lack of anticipation of the effects of her statements and her attempts to "fix things." What the patient really wanted was someone to talk to, listen to her, and be present during her painful situation. When providers establish a high level of empathic responsiveness, feelings of pity and sorrow are irrelevant. Providers are able to sustain a recognition of the patient's pain, maintain separateness, but also prevent unnecessary distancing.

▶ Measures of Empathy in Clinical Practice

The interdisciplinary literature on empathy is vast, and gives additional insight into the concept of empathy and its meaning in a clinical setting. A wide range of health disciplines are interested in the importance of empathy in the clinical setting, and ways in which empathy can be taught and evaluated (**EXHIBIT 7-2**).

There are several assessments and surveys to measure empathy in the medical and social psychology literature; these scales have been used in measuring in physicians, medical students, residents, and dental students. All aspects of empathy are difficult to observe in its totality, and some researchers have opted to measure verbal or nonverbal empathy, or both. Whatever measure is used, it often captures an aspect of empathy from patients' perspectives

EXHIBIT 7-2 Therapeutic Benefits of Demonstrating Empathy

1. Communicates understanding, caring, and compassion
2. Enhances patients' and families' sense of being listened to and being fully understood
3. Enables patients and families to feel at ease
4. Provides patients and families opportunities to tell their stories
5. Enhances patients' engagement in and sense of control of their care and treatment
6. Improves the likelihood providers will understand the meaning of the patient's condition from the patient's point of view
7. Increases providers' abilities to help patients and their families based upon their enhanced perceptions of their needs and feelings

of their patient–provider encounter and students' needs in professional health education and training programs.

The two current and commonly used measures tap into either patients' evaluations of empathic encounters with health providers, or students' self-assessments of their use of empathic responses in their interaction with patients. The CARE, previously mentioned, is believed to be sufficiently reliable and validated. This measure is preferred by those evaluating empathy in clinical settings because of its reference to patient–provider relationships (Kraft-Todd et al., 2017).

Patients are asked questions about primary care visits and hospital interactions with a range of categories: (1) made to feel at ease, (2) allowed to tell one's story, (3) really listened, (4) treated as a "whole person," (5) fully understood their concerns, (6) showed care and compassion, (7) were positive, (8) explained things clearly, (9) helped them take control, and (10) helped to create a plan of action (Rakel et al., 2009). They are asked to rate their encounter with the provider on how well

they demonstrated these empathetic responses using a scale where 1 is poor and 5 is excellent.

The measure used to assess providers' perceptions of the extent they practice empathy skills is the JSPE that was also previously mentioned. In recent years it has been used in self-assessments of providers' tendencies toward empathic styles. For example, it includes positive-worded items such as: "I try to understand what is going on in my patients' minds by paying attention to their nonverbal cues and body language," "I try to imagine myself in my patients' shoes when providing care to them," and "I believe that empathy is a therapeutic factor in medical treatment" (Hojat et al., 2002).

Both measures, CARE and the JSPE, have been used extensively and, in some instances, in different countries where empathy is perceived to be an essential component of provider–patient relationships.

Expressing Empathic Responses

Empathic responses are facilitated by the process of "**active listening**." In most descriptions of the process of healing, it is clear that the provider of healing has taken some time and energy to learn about the experience of the sufferer's ailments or difficulties in the process of developing the basis for the plan of care.

Furthermore, early on it was felt that troubled patients yearn for an interested and concerned listener. Fleishman (1989), for example, recognized the need for persons to have someone to listen with nurturing attentiveness, grouped such yearnings with the need to be seen, known, responded to, confirmed, appreciated, cared for, mirrored, recognized, and identified. He described this need as a yearning for "witnessed significance."

Active listening enables providers to address this important need. Active listening is different from merely hearing and repeating what was heard. Active listening refers to a sensitive, discerning use of the sense of hearing akin to the classic concept of Theodor Reik (1951, pp. 144, 146–147, 150) "listening with the third ear." Reik, in describing the skill needed by the psychoanalyst, stated that analysts need "to learn how one mind speaks to another beyond words and in silence."

This process can reveal not only what patients are saying but what they are thinking and feeling. Active listening is also referred to as *empathic listening* or *reflective listening*. These concepts refer to ways to reach mutual understanding. In any case, the process is one of connecting emotionally while simultaneously connecting cognitively. Listening within the Rogerian client-centered framework captures both the active aspect of the provider, and the increased sensitivity to the world as the patient sees it. It is the provider's role to assume, in so far as he or she can, the internal frame of reference of patients; perceiving the situation as patients see it and patients as patients see themselves. In doing so, the provider must lay aside all perceptions from the external frame of reference. This process, an active, not passive activity, places providers at an advantage in fully understanding the patient.

In summary, active listening is a vehicle for empathy. Active listening increases the probability that providers will focus their attention on the patient. Without active listening, empathy cannot occur. We are not clairvoyant nor armed with the capacity to read patients' minds without attending to a wide range of clues. With active listening, providers take in data using all communication channels simultaneously—visual, auditory, and kinesthetic—to fully perceive the patient's needs and concerns. Providers who engage in active listening can be distinguished because they exhibit a variety of behaviors indicative of good listening. These behaviors are listed in **EXHIBIT 7-3**.

EXHIBIT 7-3 Behavioral Signs of an Empathic Listener

- **Eye contact.** Good eye contact does not mean that the provider is "glued" to the eyes of the patient. Rather, good eye contact may be given in spontaneous glances that express interest and a desire to communicate. Poor eye contact consists of never looking at the patient, of staring at patients constantly and blankly, or of looking away from patients as soon as they look at you. Cultural differences may also affect the level of eye contact appropriate for a given interaction. In some cultures, to demand eye to eye contact would be disrespectful.

- **Postural position.** Posture includes both body gestures and facial expressions. Supportive postural positions include sitting or standing with your body facing the patient, while communicating responsive facial expressions. Rigid body posture can be modified with flexible movements toward the patient, again, indicating a desire to be with and attend to the patient. Being preoccupied and in constant movement not related to the patient generally communicates disinterest. No facial expressions (stoicism) or too much inappropriate smiling, nodding, or frowning could, under certain circumstances, communicate a lack of authenticity.

- **Verbal quality.** Good verbal quality is as important as the words that the provider chooses to use. These qualities include a pleasant, interested intonation. The provider's speech is neither too soft nor too loud. It can reflect the context of the contact and reflect back any particular feeling state that is expressed by the patient. Speaking harshly to a patient who is crying is obviously inappropriate; still, expressing concern when there is no reason for concern is confusing. Patients may "read things into" verbal and nonverbal messages that are not meant nor factual.

- **Verbal messages.** Messages to patients can be worded to reflect the provider's understanding of the patient's experience. This may include choosing culturally relevant terms, the patients' own words for their experience, and analogies or paraphrases selected from patients' descriptions. However, providers' interpretations of patients' messages need to be clearly separated from the providers' own accounts of what the patient says or feels.

🔍 *CITED STUDY: Patients' Responses to Physician Empathic Responses*

Patient–physician encounters have been shown to result in better health outcomes and patient satisfaction. These researchers audio-recorded and coded the interactions between 40 primary care physicians and 320 of their overweight or obese patients. They assessed patient satisfaction and how much the patient felt the physician supported their need to change their behaviors.

Pollak, K. I., Alexander, S. C., Tulsky, J. A., Lyna, P., Coffman, C. J., Dolor, R. J., … Østbye, T. (2011). Physician empathy and listening: Associations with patient satisfaction and autonomy. *Journal of the American Board of Family Medicine, 24*(6), 665–672. doi:10.3122/jabfm.2011.06.110025

When physicians were rated by independent coders as more empathic, patients reported a higher rate of "excellent" satisfaction than when physicians were rated as less empathic. The authors felt that because empathy is defined as physicians' understanding patients' perspectives, this might make patients feel more understood, and thus more satisfied with their care. In the author's previous studies, empathy in patient–physician encounters was associated with patient behavior change. Furthermore, they cite another study that showed that when physicians expressed compassion for as few as 40 seconds, patients reported feeling better and less anxious.

Active listening requires providers not only to hear, but to listen; not only to see, but to perceive; and not only to touch, but to feel. Sensing without integrating data from these major communication channels can cause providers to come up short when expressing an understanding what patients' are experiencing. When it comes to integration, providers' must gather personal strength to see patients' conditions from patient viewpoints, no matter how tragic and painful it may be.

▶ The Relationship of Empathy and Confirmation

Empathy enables the process of confirmation or the feeling of being valued. It is through providers' capacity to empathize that confirmation is felt by patients. There has been a long-standing interest in humanity's basic need to be heard and attended to, relating to an inherent search for confirmation that one is valued. Confirmation can bestow approval and validation. These needs have been described by some to be as important as needs for personal safety. Without a sense of being seen and heard, most individuals may have difficulty trusting their interpersonal environments.

The need to be affirmed has been described in theories of growth and development, recommended to achieve viable work settings, in concepts of functional–dysfunctional relationships, and even in paradigms that predict conditions of escalating tension and dispute. Those who study the process of conflict resolution and mediation realize that the number one culprit in creating conflict is the absence of communication in which parties are not really listening nor paying attention to the messages of one another. It is the mediator's job to restore communication and set the ground rules that will enhance effective attending and listening behaviors in the disputants. It is presumed that this change will not only prepare the parties to negotiate their interests, but will also demonstrate parties' willingness to value one another.

Our need to be understood is a powerful motivating force, and is particularly important to patients when they encounter potentially life-threatening situations. Any attempt to ignore or belittle patients' needs to be understood is counterproductive to effective patient–provider encounters and relationships. Confirming responses convey that providers value patients as persons, respect what they have to say, and appreciate patients' perceptions and stories about their health needs and problems.

Confirming responses are promising signs that positive and effective patient–provider relationships and communications will occur, and may continue through the duration of a treatment episode (**EXHIBIT 7-4**).

EXHIBIT 7-4 Examples of Confirming Responses

- Acknowledgment by responding directly to what patients have said
- Statements of genuine concern and interest in patients' unique needs
- Agreement about judgments and direction for care when there is legitimate reason to summarize the directions for care, and patients' understanding and acceptance of care
- Supportive responses expressing appropriate reassurance and understanding of patients' experiences and expressions
- Attempts to clarify messages in order to better understand patients' words and stories
- Expression of positive feelings toward patients by complimenting them on their strengths and positive steps toward managing their health care needs.

Health providers should issue confirmation in their dialogue with patients as if it were a significant healing agent. Confirmation responses have the effect of making the patient feel worthy. Confirmation responses acknowledge the other's unique value as a person. These responses make a patient feel valued, and although the provider may not agree with everything the patient says or does, these replies demonstrate responsiveness that is necessary in a supportive patient–provider relationship.

On the contrary, disconfirming responses are opposite of confirming responses. While confirming responses strengthen feelings of being valued, disconfirming responses can threaten one's sense of self and of being valued (Stewart, 2006). Disconfirming responses in patient care settings include impersonal treatment of patients and what they have to say, being oblivious to what they need or say, or treating their responses as irrelevant.

Just as there are specific ways in which providers can confirm patients as individuals, there are certain response patterns that deny a patient's worth and tend to make patients feel less valued. Disconfirming responses are generally inappropriate or irrelevant. Not only do they express a lack of empathy, they generally suggest that empathic responses will not be forthcoming.

Disconfirming responses are typical in disputes, and are usually what anger parties and make resolution of differences next to impossible. Consider the case of two parties who express through their communications that the views, desires, and concerns of the other are not important or irrelevant. The negative results of this encounter mean that both parties interpret the attitudes to mean "you are not important or valuable." These interpretations fuel attitudes of mutual resentment and tend to fix each individual in a position—usually a position antagonistic to that of the other party. Interpersonal conflict results as each party is certain that the other is not to be trusted under any circumstances because no trustworthy person would deny another's views and, in essence, their existence.

Disconfirming responses in patient–provider relationships ignore or disregard the patient's spoken word as well as the intent of the patient, sometimes not allowing full expression of thoughts and feelings. While incoherent or incongruent messages may be confusing to the patient, the indirect effect suggests that the provider is not "in tune" with the patient. Disconfirming responses can be of several kinds (**EXHIBIT 7-5**).

Consider the following dialogue between a pharmacy technician and a patient who is asking to have a prescription filled.

PATIENT: "Can you fill this, please?"
PROVIDER: "Humm, Pru-Care; George is this thing working now?"

EXHIBIT 7-5 Kinds of Disconfirming Responses

- Making irrelevant replies leaving the patient to feel that what they said has nothing to do with the subject matter
- Interruptive remarks can stop patients from completing their thoughts and occur when providers introject comments, sometimes completing patients' sentences before the patient has had a chance to finish speaking
- Tangential comments show lack of respect for patients' statements by switching the subject of the conversation in midstream by beginning to acknowledge what the patient says but switching the subject
- Impersonal responses occur when providers give the impression that patients' stories are trivial, and they are oblivious to what the patient has said or means

PATIENT: Appears confused and concerned; is silent. (Provider is not answering patient's question)
PROVIDER: Turns to patient: "We've been having problems with this computer." (Again, tangential to the real question)
PATIENT: Looks expectantly as pharmacy technician and pharmacist talk behind the counter for about 5 minutes.
PROVIDER TO PATIENT: "It will be about 15 minutes."
PATIENT: "Will it really be 15 minutes?" (Noticing that there is no one else waiting)
PROVIDER: "I say 15 minutes; it might be less. This way patients don't get upset if I give them a high number and it is ready sooner."

Note that the beginning response to this patient was an irrelevant remark from the patient's point of view because the patient is asking to fill a prescription given to her by her doctor. At first it appeared that the patient did not get a direct answer—only a remark that ignored the need to know.

Although the issue of the computer being down was relevant to the provider, it was not relevant, at least initially, to the patient. In fact, it really was not until several minutes had passed that the patient's question was answered directly. Notice that the patient even questioned the response—"15 minutes?"—not totally convinced that the provider knew how long it would take. The provider made a vague reference to wishing to please the patient but implied that the provider was more interested in preventing the patient from getting upset than addressing his or her need for reassurance that the prescription could be filled, and that this would occur in a timely manner.

The following dialogue between a provider and a patient who is anticipating surgery is yet another example of how patients are commonly disconfirmed in dialogues with providers (**EXHIBIT 7-6**).

EXHIBIT 7-6 Dialogue Box Illustrating Potential Disconfirmation of Patient

PATIENT:	"You know…I'm kinda worried… It probably is silly to worry. I guess it's a minor surgery, certainly not a liver transplant or anything…heh heh!"
PROVIDER:	"There is nothing to worry about; you've got a good surgeon. Before you know it, you'll be in the recovery room." (Irrelevant remark)
PATIENT:	"Yeah, I guess you're right. It's stupid of me to worry about it." (Laughs nervously)
PROVIDER:	"I'll have the nurse come in and get you ready. In the meantime, try to keep your mind on how you're going to feel when you get out of here." (Irrelevant remark)

Here, again, is an illustration of what appears, on one level at least, to be an innocuous conversation. The provider is not critical—in fact, the provider comes across as friendly and somewhat helpful. However, the subtle underlying messages tend to ignore the patient's thoughts and feelings. The patient's fear of surgery is minimized. Through irrelevant and somewhat tangential replies, the provider succeeds in avoiding what is bothering the patient. The message, "your feelings are not important enough to discuss," will probably have a deleterious effect on further attempts by this provider to communicate effectively with the patient.

In short, as Northouse and Northouse (1992) suggest, it is painful if others respond in a disconfirming manner that neglects the receiver's own experience, and it is rewarding or satisfying if others affirm these experiences. Taken in the context of the patient–provider relationship, such responses can "make or break" the relationship.

▶ The Relationship of Empathy and Compassion

Compassion is considered to be a cornerstone of quality health care, and is recognized as so by patients, families, health care providers, as well as health policy makers (Sinclair et al., 2016). Recent concerns about suboptimal patient care and a lack of compassion have caused health care policymakers to question whether clinicians are adequately prepared to practice compassionate caring, that is, the preparedness of clinicians for the challenging environment in which they practice (Sinclair et al., 2016). Compassionate care is intimately linked to empathic encounters with patients and their families. Like feelings of confirmation, feelings of compassion stem from providers' capacities to empathize. Compassionate caring is acting with warmth while providing individualized patient-centered care.

Compassionate caring can help buffer the impact of stress on patients in a wide array of health care events from learning of unfavorable diagnostic test results, to diagnosis of a new illness, impairment from an unexpected injury, and the realization of declining health which is irreversible. All patients to some degree because of current or impending illness or disability are faced with the powerful experience of loss; loss of physical mobility, physical and emotional functioning, loss of body image, loss of social roles (parental, spousal/partner roles), and, in some cases, loss of employment. Inherent in these real possibilities or perceived threats are fears of loss of independence and declining self-worth.

Type of loss experience is a function of a patient's injury or illness. For example, fear of loss of physical functioning due to an accident or injury is very common. Women fearful that a breast lump will be cancerous are likely to experience not only a threat to life but also alterations in body image. Patients with a

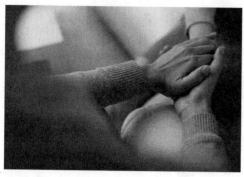

© Pressmaster/Shutterstock.

diagnosis of aggressive prostate cancer worry not only about the threat to life but the loss of sexual functioning. Patients with emphysema (chronic obstructive pulmonary disease) face the probably of a progressively worse condition limiting their ability to do everyday activities (e.g., walking up stairs). Those with depression and anxiety may worry about role functioning, and the loss of enjoyment from those things that previously provided satisfaction.

Adolescents living with diabetes may experience fear of exposure, loss of friends and social status, loss of favorite foods, and worry about the long-term consequences of diabetes on their life goals. Whether actual or imagined, mild or severe, loss due to injury or acute and chronic illness permeate many patient experiences. Providers who are capable of showing compassion in their encounters with patients and their families are desperately needed by some patients and their families, and appreciated by all.

Compassionate caring in health care represents an ideal way of interacting with patients entailing an active response to patients' suffering, distress, and discomfort. To fully understand compassion, it is important to explore the experience of suffering. Dempsey, Wojciechoweski, McConville, and Drain (2014) identify two sources of suffering—inherent suffering and avoidable suffering.

Inherent suffering refers to those experiences deriving from the medical condition or its treatment. For example, patients experiencing pain from a diagnosis of osteoarthritis

are experiencing inherent suffering in limbs affected by their arthritis. Since arthritis may also be associated with depression, lack of mobility and agility, these symptoms are also considered an inherent source of suffering.

In some cases, such as with a diagnosis of breast cancer, the patient may suffer pain, loss of appetite, fatigue, and emotional distress, all aspects of inherent suffering. But, the treatment given to patients can also constitute inherent suffering. This includes the pain and frightening aspects of surgery, chemotherapy, radiation treatment, breast reconstruction, and any necessary rehabilitation that follows. Even if health care was excellent and providers well qualified, the full effects of inherent pain may not be enough to eliminate this inherent suffering. Health providers can modify inherent suffering, such as with pain medication, and less invasive surgical procedures but it would be impossible to eliminate inherent suffering.

Dempsey and colleagues go on to differentiate inherent suffering from **avoidable suffering**. It is the role of providers to prevent avoidable suffering whenever and wherever possible. Avoidable suffering frequently occurs when care is suboptimal. Suboptimal care occurs when, for example, there is a shortage of staff and resources to respond to patients' needs. It also occurs when there is an absence of courtesy, unusually long waits to be seen, difficult to understand procedures and expectations, and poor coordination of care and teamwork. Both inherent and avoidable suffering needs to be addressed. Just how well this is done will make a significant difference in the level of patient suffering.

Studies of patient and health professional opinions of compassionate caring clarify its meaning and intention. Certain interpersonal and informational skills were seen to be associated with compassion in clinical communication; these include attentiveness, listening, understanding, confronting, and providing prognostic information in a sensitive and caring manner. Descriptors of compassionate caring included the following behaviors: noticing or sitting with patients, showing understanding, and nonverbal behaviors such as use of silence, making eye contact, smiling, listening, posturing, head nodding to indicate understanding and acknowledgement, and tone of voice.

Tierney et al. (2017) explain that compassionate care is not always something that can be achieved, especially with patients who seem unwilling or unable to engage with health care professionals. Still another barrier, as with empathic encounters, is having the time to tune to patients' difficulties and lack of resources or staff to respond in a therapeutic manner.

Difficulties in teaching and nurturing compassion during professional training are also seen as a barrier. Patient families recognize the importance of compassion especially when facing bereavement or impending death of a loved one. There is considerable discussion about whether the capacity for compassion is inherent in individuals or whether it is taught. Most agree that whether taught or inherent, compassion can be nurtured and grows or awakens when health care providers are exposed to clinical situations and their personal and family experiences with suffering (Sinclair et al., 2016).

Provider compassion is felt to be therapeutic for patients, families, and even health providers themselves. However, there is evidence that repeated expression of compassion in intense clinical situations may raise stress levels and burnout in health providers, particularly in nurses. Otherwise, *compassion fatigue* is a consequence of repeated exposure to emotionally intense patient situations. Duarte, Pinoot-Gouveia, and Cruz (2016) studied compassion fatigue and found that high levels of affective empathy could be a risk factor for compassion fatigue. They explained that self-compassion might protect nurses from compassion fatigue and should be taught, along with self-care skills, to help providers avoid compassion fatigue and burnout.

In summary, compassionate caring is intimately linked with empathy; being empathic enables providers to express compassion when patients are suffering. Compassion is shown in empathic encounters as providers respect human dignity, listen to patients, and show warmth in the process of acknowledging their suffering.

▶ The Therapeutic Value of Empathy

When the impact of empathy is put in very simple terms, it can be said that empathy allows the listener (provider) to heal. To the extent that providers' communications become the foundation of the relationship, the empathic response is central to more basic issues of trust and self-disclosure. Additionally, in clinical practice, empathy is the skill used by providers to decipher and respond to the thoughts and feelings of the patient in the provider–patient relationship.

Empathic understanding and empathic responses are critical to every phase of the patient–provider relationship. They are critical in capturing information to make an assessment in the early stages of the relationship, engaging patients in shared decision-making about their care, and long-term self-management of their care. As previously suggested, patients feel empathic providers can be trusted. When they trust providers, they are more likely to disclose important details about their condition, thoughts, and feelings and follow through on important self-management programs. Also, they are more likely to express high levels of satisfaction with their care. Specific ways empathy yields better patient outcomes can be explained by the following processes: **increasing connectedness** and **reducing alienation**.

Increasing Connectedness

In part, the impact of empathy is achieved through patients' feelings of connectedness with the provider. Feelings of connectedness are reinforced by confirmation, described earlier as a concomitant factor in binding the provider and patient together. In Rogers's model of client-centered therapy, empathy, together with unconditional positive regard and congruence, elicits important patient outcomes beyond facilitating the patient–provider relationship.

Rogers (1980) stated that through the use of these factors, the client (patient) will feel understood and be better able to cope. Rogers's method is said to build patient's self-esteem due to feelings of being cared for, no matter what. The providers' support for the patient, according to Rogers, is eventually adopted by the patient, who thus becomes more self-accepting and better able to cope.

While connectedness is frequently used to explain powerful patient–provider relationships, the concept itself is ambiguous (Phillips-Salimi, Haase, & Kooken, 2012). In an important effort to bring clarity to the concept of connectedness, these authors explored the term as it is used in the literature.

They found five distinct perspectives and seven attributes. These attributes were intimacy, sense of belonging, caring, empathy, respect, trust, and reciprocity. They added that although these attributes were salient, further research was needed to examine connectedness from the perspectives of patients and providers. They concluded with recommendations for provider practice which included raising an awareness of the importance of patient–provider connectedness and exploring its relationship to positive patient outcomes.

Reducing Alienation

According to Rogers (1980), empathic responses also reduce patients' feelings of alienation. Feelings of alienation can arise in patients for many reasons. Their condition, especially conditions that appear visually distasteful (e.g., scars from severe burns) or that trigger social judgment (e.g., HIV/AIDS), may cause them to feel stigmatized. Alienation can be self-imposed as certain patients distance themselves from others either because of their illness (e.g., with schizophrenia) or because of their recovery process (e.g., with common responses to grief).

Feelings of alienation can provoke loneliness and experiences of being alienated even from health care professionals whose role is to help them. People who feel alienated and socially stigmatized may not always pursue early treatment if they recognize that admitting to certain symptoms will make them experience even more social alienation.

Feelings of alienation can also cause patients to feel timid about being seen again or to work effectively on any health care challenges. Empathic responses respect patients as is, making them feel understood and accepted, thus directly countering the effects of any negative results of alienation. In this way, the patient is helped to seek advice, continue treatment, and endure, for the purpose of getting better.

During the early phase of helping, empathy is critical because without an empathic basis on which to understand the patient's world, there is no foundation for helping. Attempts to help can be perceived as insincere gestures, and advice may be felt as irrelevant. It is clear to the patient that empathy from the provider is an investment of time and effort. Providers who demonstrate their willingness and their ability to be empathic are perceived as trustworthy, capable of helping, and able to handle the task of caring. Under these conditions, patients can feel secure enough to enter into a relationship with the provider despite any concern about being stigmatized or judged due to an illness or health condition.

The following dialogue between a nursing student and a patient demonstrates how empathic responses can create the leverage needed to move the patient beyond initial dysfunctional responses to their illness (**EXHIBIT 7-7**).

During this somewhat lengthy discussion, the nursing student was able to establish the meaning that "pain" held for the patient. From the provider's initial assessment, physical pain was the issue. How to get this patient to accept more pain medication was the challenge. Yet, a

---

EXHIBIT 7-7 Dialogue Box Illustrating Effective Empathic Responses

PROVIDER: "Do you remember me? I came by to say hello yesterday…my name is…."

PATIENT: "I think so."

PROVIDER: "How are you doing today?" (Sitting down, maintaining eye contact)

PATIENT: "I'm better…my leg hurts a lot. It's difficult for me to be in bed all the time."

PROVIDER: "That is very difficult…I'm sure. You know, I'm concerned about your pain medication. Is your medication making it (the pain) tolerable?" (Empathic response)

PATIENT: "Well, I want to be fully awake. I don't like to be 'drugged up'; you can't think straight."

PROVIDER: "You have a valid concern." (Confirmation) "Have you had a past history of bad experiences?"

PATIENT: "No, not really. Well, I've heard what morphine does, the horror stories about being on medications like that."

PROVIDER: "What have you heard?"

PATIENT: "Oh, of people becoming addicted, being mean or just out of it…and saying things they don't really mean."

PROVIDER: "So you are really concerned that this might happen to you." (Empathic response) "And, I'm thinking that the pain you have now is more than you need to have."

PATIENT: "There's the emotional pain too."

PROVIDER: "Yes, would you like to talk about that—the emotional pain?" (Confirmation)

PATIENT: "I have a good husband. People, well they say, 'Oh my God, what happened to you.' I hide my legs a lot. I can't take it when they say those things."

PROVIDER: "Are you afraid I might react the same way?"

PATIENT: "No…"

PROVIDER: "You know you've kept the covers over your legs the whole time. Do you think you could show them to me?"

PATIENT: "Sure, I get upset with other people; I don't like to watch their faces; I feel like a 'circus act.' My legs are three times the normal size from my knees down."

PROVIDER: "Yes, well I can understand that your experience of what is happening is very painful to you, in more ways than just one." (Empathic response)

---

fuller understanding of the patient's experience leads the provider to understand the patient's concern about the effects of pain medication and feelings of shame and disgust. These aspects might be equal, if not more important, to the patient.

The empathic responses of the nursing student become the catalyst for discovery and for gaining insight. It is more likely that the nursing student will now address "the patient's world" as the patient perceives it, and integrate this knowledge along in an appropriate plan of care which should help the patient master the emotional pain associated with her disfiguring medical condition. It is also more likely that the patient will regard the relationship as helpful—not irrelevant. Under these conditions, the patient may be more receptive to taking the advice her physician and other nursing staff as well.

▶ The Empathic Process—Steps to Arrive at Empathy and the Capacity for Empathy

It is accurate to say that empathy is established through a series of steps that engage the provider's cognitive and affective capabilities in caring for patients. Individuals are not just empathic when they want to be, and it is not an inherent trait at birth. Individuals do have different capacities to be sensitive to others, and some people listen more carefully than others.

However, empathy is more complex than simply being sensitive to others' thoughts and feelings in the process of listening to them. Even though complex, empathy is a skill that can be learned and relearned. Later in this text, barriers to empathic communication are addressed. It will be clear that empathy cannot always be easily established, and an otherwise empathic provider may not be consistently empathic in all patient–provider encounters.

The process of establishing empathic communication has been described by various authors, some of whom describe empathy as consisting of both verbal and nonverbal components. There are various nonverbal behaviors that are usually perceived by patients as empathic. These are face-to-face positioning with direct eye contact and interest, and a receptive appearance conveyed with an absence of defensive postures (e.g., crossed arms and/ or legs). Various behavioral indicators were previously outlined in Exhibit 7-1.

Many have addressed the steps to take to become empathic and to express empathy toward patients. These recommendations include ways to combine cognitive and affective capabilities in providers in order for them to effectively express empathy. Satterfield and Hughes (2007), in speaking of emotional intelligence, describe attitudes, knowledge, and skill in using empathetic emotional intelligence in encounters and how these can be taught. An important landmark description was that by Katz (1964). Ehmann (1971) described the process of empathy as formulated by Katz. According to Katz, the empathic process is summarized in four basic steps.

Identification

The first condition or step is **identification**, stated as the need for the provider to first comprehend the situation and feelings of the patient. This step requires the provider to relax some self-control in order that the patient's situation seems real, rather than remote. In the previous example, the provider relinquished her tendency to advise the patient about appropriate dosages of pain medications in order to try to comprehend the patient's view: "Have you had a past history of a bad experience?" This question requires that the provider temporarily refrain from telling the patient what she needs to do. Additionally, it brings the very remote aspects of the patient's experience which includes a host of concerns and emotional responses in better proximity to the provider.

Incorporation

The second step or condition is **incorporation**. The process of incorporation means that the experience of the patient that is now known to the provider is taken into the self of the provider. Although the experience is recognizable as that of the patient, not of the provider, this step helps bring the patient's reality and its underlying meaning into the provider's awareness. In the dialogue between the nursing student and patient in **EXHIBIT 7-7**, the student commented: "So you really are concerned that this might happen to you." This comment is a verbal indication that the provider has allowed the patient's experience to penetrate the provider's awareness of the patient's condition.

Reverberation

Reverberation is the third step in the model by Katz. The provider's past experience interacts with that which is known to the provider from the patient. The student's innermost thoughts—the patient is afraid of becoming an addict—is noted. The provider also knows this will not happen but the patient feels that it could. This process is an example of reverberation which leads to further understanding of the feelings of the patient. Otherwise, the patient's words echo what the provider understands as being a fear that many patients have about taking pain medications.

Detachment

Detachment, the final phase in establishing empathy, refers to the provider's return to his or her own frame of reference. The results of the first three steps culminate with other objective knowledge of the patient (e.g., the patient's fear of addiction and her shame about her disfigurement). This information is then fed back to the patient so that the patient experiences the provider's capacity to be empathic. The student replies: "Yes, well I can understand that your legs are very painful to you—in more ways than just one." It is important to note that this feature of the patient's experience of physical and emotional pain is the basis of empathic understanding. And, the patient's experience will influence from this point on the approach the provider will take in addressing the patient's pain.

The original work by Smith (1992) is useful in identifying the steps taken to achieve empathic encounters with patients. These steps are useful for providers who struggle with empathy and are very practical. Smith first recommends that providers clear distracting thoughts and priorities from their agenda. Second, providers should focus on the patient; giving the patient full attention and communicating interest. Third, providers reflect on both the verbal and nonverbal aspects of the patient's communication.

With this as a basis, the next step is to pick out the predominate themes of the patient's experience (e.g., the fear of addiction to pain medications, the patient's desire to be cognitively intact, and the shame she experiences from perceived disfigurement). The fifth step is actually communicating or conveying to the patient an empathic response, reflecting some of the patient's key words to acknowledge her anguish and anxiety (e.g., "the emotional pain" you are feeling). The sixth and final step, according to Smith, is to evaluate the effectiveness of the empathic response. Because the purpose of being empathic is to reduce the patient's burden (e.g., the emotional pain about his or her legs), it would be important to assess whether the patient did feel better after disclosing her concerns and receiving acknowledgement and support from the provider.

While the dialogue between the patient and student did not include an appraisal of the results of the conversation, it is easy to suggest what this may have included. The dialogue could have gone like this:

PROVIDER: "I have a much better idea of what you are dealing with."

PATIENT: "Yes, I didn't know myself…I guess my real 'pain' is about how I look. The physical pain is important too, but not as important."

PROVIDER: "Oh."

PATIENT: "I feel better that I finally talked about this. I thought you would think it is silly, guess you don't."

PROVIDER: "I don't."

If the patient were asked directly what was helpful about the dialogue, she might reply, "feeling that the staff understands me better, knowing myself better, and realizing that the staff may not think that my feelings are silly."

These guidelines, identified by both Katz and Smith, are useful to providers who are attempting to acquire or improve on empathic responses. In addition, it is important to understand that empathy and nonverbal communication convey culturally specific meanings (Lorié, Reinero, Phillips, Zhang, & Riess, 2016). What is interpreted to be empathic in one culture may not be seen as empathic in another. In fact, there may not be a behavior or feeling that resembles empathy as we know it. The context for establishing empathic encounters needs to consider the cultural differences across groups, especially because empathy and nonverbal expressions of empathy play a significant role in fostering trust in patient–provider relationships. Empathy is multifaceted. What becomes clear in the discussion that follows is that in the current context of health care delivery, empathy and its necessary conditions must be executed in some instances under considerably negative odds.

▶ **Barriers to Empathy in the Provider–Patient Relationship**

As stated previously, empathy engages providers in multidimensional ways—cognitively, affectively, and behaviorally. The process of communicating empathically with patients and their families cannot always occur when there are internal or external barriers. In health care, these obstacles include provider, patient, and environmental or delivery system factors. The following discussion focuses on barriers originating from each of these three sources.

Provider Barriers

Beyond the simple intellectual barriers—not knowing how and why to use empathy—are the personal characteristics of providers that can inhibit their abilities to be empathic. These include various cognitive and affective capabilities. Empathy requires passion, and the development of skills is contingent on the importance placed on empathy, especially in the context of professional health care education. Empathy can be learned or acquired and then be left behind when science and detachment are valued and empathic responses are not.

As previously described, providers may have little to no control over distracting situations in their encounters with patients. Some providers are easily distracted by other pressing concerns. There may be pressures to complete a work assignment, to finish paperwork,

or to make it to a meeting. Other distractions of a personal nature (e.g., relationship problems, financial strains, minor health problems, and emotional distress) may contribute to the provider's inability to set aside competing concerns and demands and focus on the patient or patient's family. Some providers lack the ability to concentrate, which tends to be a trait phenomenon, not a state condition reflective of current stressors the provider is facing.

A second provider barrier is the inability to relax personal self-control sufficiently enough to experience the patient's circumstances. A condition also affected by provider stress is the tendency to regard the patient's condition in terms that are familiar to the provider, not the patient. This is a serious problem when it also includes the provider's unfamiliarity with cultural or religious beliefs that are important to the patient and family. Sometimes rigidity narrows the provider's focus to the extent that no new information or new insight is allowed in. When this occurs, provider control works at cross purposes to empathic patient encounters. Although provider control makes the patient encounter appear manageable to the provider, the truth is that nothing much is managed if the outcome minimizes feedback about the patient's experience.

Empathy also requires providers to incorporate the patient's experience in what they know about the patient. This is a cognitive activity. Providers who are unable to concentrate will not be able to complete this process. Also, providers who can make cognitive associations but not maintain objectivity can participate in reverberation, but they fail to remain detached and fail to complete the cycle by offering salient observations. Errors of this kind may be the result of provider stress but also reflect bad habits.

A final comment that pertains to provider barriers is difficulties in identifying and witnessing the pain and agony patients experience. As previously stated in this text, empathy is an emotional knowing of the patient. The sharing of unpleasant and sometimes painful thoughts and feelings can create an urgency to block this experience in order to alleviate these feelings. Providers vary in their abilities to witness patients' painful thoughts and feelings. Their capacities can also differ with the same patient over time.

Most health care providers choose health care professions to help patients overcome illness and promote health. It is probably not the case that providers lack this courage entirely, but that for whatever reasons, one's tolerance waxes and wanes. Obviously, if the provider exhibits a long-standing inability to be in the presence of patient agony, the specific work situation may not be the career of choice. For example, some providers may have difficulties caring repeatedly for terminally ill patients or children with life-threatening conditions. Less intense care settings such as primary care or well-baby clinic settings may compliment providers' unique skills and interests.

Before moving to patient–provider barriers to empathy some mention of the "burnout syndrome" is appropriate. *Burnout*, sometimes referred to as "the professional stress syndrome" refers to a cluster of behaviors intended to protect the provider from identifying too closely with patients. In those professionals in which burnout has continued unchecked, emotional exhaustion is followed by *depersonalization*. Depersonalization refers to the inability of the provider to experience patients fully; providers can develop a detached, callous, and even dehumanizing response to the patients they care for.

Patient Barriers

There are patient level barriers that may inhibit or limit the level and frequency with which providers can achieve empathic understanding. Patient characteristics including illness, cognitive capacities, age, gender, and cultural orientation can all impact patients' openness to and comfort with provider–patient discussions which raise fears, emotions, and difficult subjects.

Not all patients are open to in-depth exploration of their thoughts and feelings. Some groups of patients regard self-disclosing as a sign of weakness or as a betrayal of relationships with significant others. Cultural norms and beliefs can influence attitudes about self-disclosure. For example, some male patients may feel uncomfortable talking about fears and emotions. Females of certain ethnic or cultural groups may feel that talking about sexual concerns with their primary care provider is prohibited and violates a bond with their partner.

Patients of this type may not be willing to share their experiences on a more intimate level, even if they could be convinced of its merit. Still other patients may want the provider to understand their thoughts and feelings but fear disclosure opportunities. Disclosure for them may raise concerns about being rejected by the provider if they told the provider everything that they are or are not doing. For example, for the patient who is discarding medications instead of taking them as instructed, sharing their fears surrounding taking this medication may cause the provider to be angry and disappointed.

In this instance they may not risk discussing their medication fears if they think the provider will express disapproval. This disapproval may be viewed as more painful than not being fully understood in the first place. The patient's willingness to risk exposure is highly unlikely, and the provider may need to accept, at least initially, a rather cursory level of communication. With development of the patient–provider relationship, the patient's willingness to disclose important details may improve over time.

Some patients and/or family members accept and even welcome the opportunity to have in-depth discussions with providers but have difficulty communicating their experiences. This could be due to communication deficits due to illness, poor health literacy, and/or language differences between the patient and provider. In these instances, the provider may feel somewhat defeated, but as the patient and provider establish a common frame of reference with language that suits them both, empathy can improve. Unlike the circumstances previously described, patients who desire empathy but have difficulty expressing thoughts and feelings may not regard empathic responses as an infringement on their privacy. With this type of patient it is appropriate to try to establish grounds for improved empathy despite the obvious barriers that difference in verbal faculties and language present.

Environmental Barriers

Barriers to establishing empathic encounters do include provider and patient factors, but another important source of obstacles come from the health care delivery system itself. Some providers will tell you "It isn't me, it isn't the patient. It's the system!" And, in many cases they are correct. That so-called *something else* usually refers to the administrative, organizational, and physical constraints of the clinical setting. Specially, the something else includes poor staffing, distracting noises, lack of privacy, pressures to see more patients, and poor patient-centered care policies.

Recounting how a patient's experience fits the provider's knowledge of other patients' experiencing the same trauma requires time in order to piece together facts and observations. This time is not always available particularly in poorly staffed clinical settings. Active listening, a requirement in achieving empathic encounters, can be significantly stymied by distracting noises and lack of private places to talk. Identifying unique aspects of patients' circumstances requires attention to facts and features not easily derived from patient charts. When providers are pressured to see more patients than what they can reasonably care for or treat, bottom-line interventions can take first place over emotional needs of patients. All of these potential barriers can be further amplified by the lack of patient-centered care policies which would define the care more holistically. Providers are "behind the eight ball" because they frequently practice in environments that are full of distractions where time and individual attention to patients are at a premium.

There is no doubt about the fact that providers practice under challenging circumstances that raise stress levels. In part, this is due to the fact that patients and families experience extraordinary distress. Lack of time to attend to detail is extremely stressful under circumstances of maintaining safe care. Unsafe practice environments may exist that place increasing demands on providers to take professional risks that they are not prepared to manage. Beginning clinicians may be least equipped to manage such care complexities. Unsafe environments create high levels of tension and, of course, such situations are less likely to yield empathic responses from providers.

Consider the following circumstance in which a patient is experiencing excruciating pain and the environment is not conducive to empathic responses.

> The child (an 8-year-old girl) lies screaming in terror as the clinician proceeds to change dressings covering burns on three-quarters of her body. Noise from patients in the next room, the whirlpool, and providers' communications over the intercom compete with the frightening cries of the young patient. Several other clinicians stand by in silence, appearing numbed to the sounds of the young patient. No one speaks to the patient; they hardly speak to one another.

The barriers to empathic responses with this patient are more than those coming from the providers who are witnessing the patient's agony. They come from the patient's inability to express her fear and also from the circumstances. Debridement of wounds, especially burns, is very painful and can be very difficult to witness. Noise, machines, people trying to communicate, and failure to control the patient's distress all inhibit empathic responsiveness. These circumstances present a tremendous challenge to providers.

The circumstances are ones that are not likely to be forgotten. Left unexpressed, providers' feelings about many similar patient care encounters may influence them in the future. A chance to be brief and gain support on many levels can protect providers from avoiding future encounters, and strengthen their resolve in promoting empathic patient–provider interactions. The absence of empathy, regardless of its cause, hinders therapeutic outcomes, the ultimate goal of patient–provider interactions.

▶ Summary

Discussions of empathy are important in our concerns for humanizing patient care. It has been said that computed tomographic (CT) scans offer no compassion, and magnetic resonance imaging (MRIs) have no "human face." In the classic reflections of such scholars as Schatz (1995), only human beings are capable of empathy. This is not a message to discount the value and contribution of technical advancements; these screening devices help us see things we can otherwise not see.

However, empathy is another *diagnostic tool,* and it is frequently in the presence of skillfully executed confirmation and compassion. It is an essential part of our role as caregivers. Schatz warns that we must enhance this natural emotion that exists in each of us. Discussions of the roots of our need for detachment and equanimity go back to the classic writings of Sir William Osler. Lest the pendulum swing too far and recent trends in communication patterns reduce our abilities to "see within" another, we must protect our capacities for forming empathetic relationships.

In successful empathic encounters, providers are able to "stand inside the patient's shoes," participating in the world of the patient while maintaining sufficient objectivity. In more recent teachings, the skill of emotional intelligence depicts our need to assess emotional responses in both ourselves and our patients but focus on the patient's experience. Sympathy tends to be a reactive response, turning attention to the provider and away from the patient. If providers share the very same feelings and needs of patients, it is likely that they will be unable to provide any help in meeting these needs in patients.

Empathy is a complex phenomenon that involves cognitive, affective, and communicative components. The process of observing the world of another, feeling what it must be like to be that person, yet maintaining separateness from that world, is not a simple process. There are guidelines, steps to be completed and which build upon skills of attending to and concentrating on the needs of our patients and their families. Active listening involves the patient and ensures that patients' perceptions, needs, and concerns are articulated in provider–patient interactions. Rather than clinical detachment, empathy helps providers establish effective communication, which is important for accurate patient diagnosis and patient care management.

There are inherent challenges in achieving empathy. Barriers may come from providers themselves (e.g., their inability to witness difficult patient situations), or they may come from patients who are either unwilling or unable to permit the provider an inside view of their condition and concerns. Finally, barriers are inherent in many health care environments in which distractions are commonplace and time and attention to the unique aspects of patients are at risk due to poor staffing and pressures to see many more patients. Satterfield and Hughes (2007) warn that medical professionalism in providers is being challenged by these growing demands that may significantly erode patient–provider relationships.

Empathy can be fostered, and barriers can be reduced. If providers are willing to use this therapeutic response, there are no limits to one's capacity to heal—an outcome set in motion by active listening and the capacity to acknowledge and affirm the unique experience of the patient. Additionally, with empathy there is a greater capacity to modify the inherent suffering of patients, and the avoidable suffering that comes with a less than effective patient-centered health care delivery system.

Discussion

1. Using your own words, what does being empathic mean to you?

2. If empathy is necessary for therapeutic patient–provider relationships, why is sympathy likely to impede empathic responses?

3. Discuss the relationships between empathy, confirmation, and compassion.

4. Identify potential affects of empathy on patient–provider relationships.

5. List several barriers to empathic responses in the patient–provider relationship; then identify whether these are patient, provider, or environmental barriers.

References

Carkhuff, R. T. (1969). *Helping and human relations: A primer for lay and professional helpers, Vol. 1; Selection and training.* New York, NY: Holt, Rinehart, and Wilson.

Dempsey, C., Wojciechoweski, S., McConville, E., & Drain, M. (2014). Reducing patient suffering through compassionate connected care. *The Journal of Nursing Administration, 44*(10), 517–524. doi:10.1097/NNA.0000000000000110

Duarte, J., Pinto-Gouveia, J., & Cruz, B. (2016). Relationship between nurses' empathy, self-compassion and dimensions of professional quality of life: A cross-sectional study. *International Journal of Nursing Studies, 60,* 1–11. doi:10/1016/j_ijnurstu.2016.02.015

Ehmann, V. E. (1971). Empathy. Its origin, characteristics and process, *Perspectives in Psychiatric Care, 9*(2), 72–80. (Cited in S. J. Sundeen, G. W. Stuart, E. A. D. Rankin, and S. A. Cohen, *Nurse-client interaction—Implementing the nursing process.* St. Louis, MO: Mosby Yearbook, Inc., 1994, p. 176.)

Fleishman, P. R. (1989). *The healing zone: Religious issues in psychotherapy.* New York, NY: Paragon House.

Hohl, S., Molina, Y., Koepl, L., Lopez, K., Vinson, E., Linden, H., & Ramsey, S. (2016). Satisfaction with cancer care among American Indian and Alaska Natives in Oregon and Washington State: A qualitative study of survivor and caregiver perspectives. *Supportive Care in Cancer: Official Journal of the Multinational Association of Supportive Care in Cancer, 24*(6), 2437–2444. doi:10.1007/s00520-015-3041-x

Hojat, M., Gonnella, J. S., Nasca, T. J., Mangione, S., Vergare, M., & Magee, M. (2002). Physician empathy: Definition, components, measurement, and relationship to gender and specialty. *American Journal of Psychiatry, 159*(9), 1563–1569. Retrieved from http://jdc.je erson.edu/crmehc

Katz, R. L. (1964). *Empathy: Its nature and uses.* Oxford, England: Free Press Glencoe. doi:10.1037/h0094441

Kiosses, V. N., Karathanos, V. T., & Tatsioni, A. (2016). Empathy promoting interventions for health professionals: A systematic review of RCTs. *Journal of Compassionate Health Care, 3,* 7. doi:10.1186/s40639-016-0024-9

Kraft-Todd, G. T., Reinero, D. A., Kelley, J. M., Heberlein, A. S., Baer, L., & Riess, H. (2017). Empathic nonverbal behavior increases ratings of both warmth *and* competence in a medical context. *PLoS ONE, 12*(5), e0177758. doi:10.1371/journal.pone.0177758

Lorié, A., Reinero, D. A., Phillips, M., Zhang, L., & Riess, M. D. (2016). Culture and nonverbal expressions of empathy in clinical settings: A systematic review. *Patient Education and Counseling, 100*(3), 411–424. doi:10.1016/j.pec.2016.09.018

Masson, V. (2005). Here to be seen: Ten practical lessons in cultural consciousness in primary health care. *Journal of Cultural Diversity, 12*(3), 94–98. PMID:16320938

Northouse, L. L., & Northouse, P. G. (1992). *Health communication—Strategies for health professionals* (2nd ed.). East Norwalk, CT: Appleton and Lange.

Phillips-Salimi, C. R., Haase, J. E., & Kooken, W. C. (2012). Connectedness in the context of patient-provider relationships: A concept analysis. *Journal of Advanced Nursing, 68*(1), 230–245. doi:10.1111/j.1365-2648.2011.05763.x

Pollak, K. I., Alexander, S. C., Tulsky, J. A., Lyna, P., Coffman, C. J., Dolor, R. J.,…Østbye, T. (2011). Physician empathy and listening: Associations with patient satisfaction and autonomy. *Journal of the American Board of Family Medicine, 24*(6), 665–672. doi:10.3122/jabfm.2011.06.110025

Rakel, D. P., Hoeft, T. J., Barrett, B. P., Chewning, B. A., Craig, B. M., & Niu, M. (2009). Practitioner empathy and the duration of the common cold. *Family Medicine, 41*(7), 494–501. PMID:19582635

Reik, T. (1951). *Listening with the third ear: The inner experiences of a psychoanalyst.* Garden City, NJ: Garden City Books. (Epigraph from p. 144)

Rogers, C. (1957). The necessary and sufficient conditions of therapeutic personality change. *Journal of Consulting Psychology, 21*, 95–100.

Rogers, C. (1980). *A way of being.* Boston, MA: Houghton-Mifflin Co.

Rogers, C. R. (1961). *On becoming a person.* Boston, MA: Houghton Mifflin.

Roter, D. L., & Hall, J. A. (1992). *Doctors talking to patients/patients talking to doctors: Improving communication in medical visits.* Westport, CT: Auburn House. doi:10.1046/j.1369-6513.2000.00073.x

Safran, D. G. (2003). Defining the future of primary care: What can we learn from patients? *Annals of Internal Medicine, 138*, 248–255. PMID:12558375

Satterfield, J. M., & Hughes, E. (2007). Emotion skills training for medical students: A systematic review. *Medical Education, 41*, 935–941. doi:10.1111/j.1365-2923.2007.02835.x

Schatz, I. J. (1995). Empathy and medical education. *Hawaii Medical Journal, 54*(4), 495–497. PMID:7601673

Sherman, J. J., & Cramer, A. (2005). Measurement of changes in empathy during dental school. *Journal of Dental Education, 69*(1), 338–345. PMID:15749944

Sinclair, S., Norris, J. M., McConnell, S. J., Chochinov, H. M., Hack, T. F., Hagen, N. A., … Bouchal, S. R. (2016). Compassion: A scoping review of the health care literature. *BMC Palliative Care, 15*, 6. doi:10.1186/s12904-016-0080-0

Stewart, J. S. (2006). *Bridges not walls* (9th ed.). San Francisco, CA: McGraw-Hill.

Sullivan, H. S. (1953). *The interpersonal theory of psychiatry.* New York, NY: W.W. Norton & Co.

Tierney, S., Seers, K., Tutton, E., & Reeve, J. (2017). Enabling the flow of compassionate care: A grounded theory study. *BMC Health Services Research, 17*, 174. doi:10.1186/s12913-017-2120-8

Truax, C. B., & Carhuff, R. (1967). *Toward effective counseling and psychotherapy.* Chicago, IL: Aldine.

CHAPTER 8

Communications That Contribute to Trust and Mistrust of Providers

CHAPTER OBJECTIVES

- Define trust as a therapeutic element in patient–provider relationships.
- Distinguish between global trust and specific trust.
- Differentiate between trust and mistrust in provider–patient relationships.
- Discuss provider trust in patients and the potential for strengthening the patient–provider relationship.
- List at least three phases in the process of trust building in a therapeutic relationship.

KEY TERMS

- Genuineness
- Global trust
- Implementation phase
- Initiation phase
- Mistrust
- Respect

- Specific trust
- Termination phase
- Trust
- Trust in patient scale
- Trust–mistrust continuum

▶ Introduction

While relationship barriers do exist in every patient–provider and family–provider relationship, one that should not be ignored is a lack of **trust**. Studies of patients' trust in providers, and for that matter, level of trust health providers have in patients, directly and indirectly impact patient outcomes and utilization of health care services. In this chapter, the relationship of trust to patient outcomes, the definition of trust and **mistrust**, as well as barriers to trust building in health care delivery systems are discussed.

Trust is critical and a trusting relationship needs time to build. Although time is necessary, it is not sufficient. There are a number of trust-building strategies that can aid in trust building, even in the absence of long-term relationships. This fact is very important because many of the previously held beliefs about building trust over time are impractical in today's system of care that discourages continuity of relationships and perfect coordination across the health care team. Understanding trust and specific strategies to promote trust can assist health professionals to provide better care that can lead to better patient outcomes (LoCurto & Berg, 2016).

Critical to the feeling dimension in provider–patient and provider–family encounters is the phenomena of trust. While it is difficult to tease out the impact of any single communication skill because there is a great deal of overlap, establishing trust is felt to be the single most influential factor behind the patient's acceptance of provider opinion and willingness to engage in positive health-related behaviors.

Historically, there was unanimous support for the premise that patient trust in providers is a critical aspect of the patient–provider relationship (Pearson & Raeke, 2000) and "the cornerstone" or "the bedrock" of medical care (Tarn et al., 2005). Gopichandran, Wouters, and Chetlapalli (2015) add that trust is "the unwritten covenant" between the patient and physician that implies that the physician will

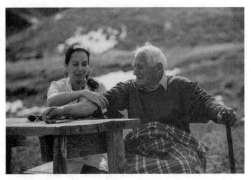

© Adriaticfoto/Shutterstock.

do what is in the best interest of the patient. This covenant also operates in most if not all health provider relationships with patients and patients' families.

The idea that a patient–provider relationship should be predicated on trust is not only a value, but has substance in what can be achieved if patients and providers operate in the context of a high level of trust.

For example, trust has been shown to promote important patient outcomes such as access to health care promotion and screening, utilization of health care services, improvement in patient adherence to medical regimens, and greater patient satisfaction.

LoCurto and Berg (2016) enumerate the various study findings reporting that trust is associated with more favorable attitudes toward providers, greater continuity of care, delivery of preventive care, adherence, and satisfaction with care. An interesting analysis of the relationship of trust and health suggested that the relationship between the two is circular in that generalized trust is related to health, but health also predicts trust (Giordano & Lindstrom, 2015). These researchers proposed that uncertainty/vulnerability associated with poor health lowers trust. Gopichandran et al. (2015) emphasized that patients' trust in health care is even more important given patients' vulnerability when they are ill.

Support for the findings of patient level of openness and provision of important clinical data were explained in part by the following observations—patient disclosure is more likely when trust exists, and this disclosure is also more complete if the patient trusts the provider. Trust, then, is important to successful patient–provider relationships. Trust also potentiates behavior change. Patients are more likely to experiment with and adopt new health-related behaviors (e.g., health screening and smoking cessation) and adhere to their new medical regimen if a climate of trust exists in their relationships with providers (O'Malley, Sheppard, Schwartz, & Mandelblatt, 2004; Thom, Hall, & Pawlson, 2004).

Finally, trust is particularly important to patients with illnesses and/or injuries that make them feel personally vulnerable. Feelings of helplessness, powerlessness, and hopelessness are eased when patients feel that providers can be trusted. Shenolikar, Balkrishnan, and Hall (2004) address this principle in their study of patient–physician encounters with vulnerable populations. In part, the unpredictability and uncertainty surrounding illness and treatment is lessened when providers can be trusted to behave in positive and predictable ways.

▶ Definitions of Trust and Trust-Based Relationships

To **trust** is to rely on the veracity and integrity of another individual. Thom et al. (2011) define trust as "an expectation that the other person will behave in a way that is beneficial, or at least not harmful, and allows for risks to be taken based on this expectation." They add, for example, patient trust in physicians provides the basis for risking disclosure of personal information.

People who trust others have confident expectations about the benefits of relationships with others without undue concern for lack of control. Halbert et al. (2006), among others, believe that patients experience trust when they believe that their welfare is placed above all other considerations. Patient trust, and for that matter family trust, in providers also includes their perceptions that providers' communication behaviors are reliable and trustworthy. Evidence of trust occurs in patients' perception that providers are sincere, honest, benevolent, and credible in what they do (Berry et al., 2008).

Trust Is Better When Mutually Felt

The literature on patient–provider trust has largely focused on patient trust of the provider. Otherwise, it was important that patients trusted providers, and less emphasis was placed upon providers' trust of patients. Recent research examines providers' trust of patients and the interaction of patient and provider trust or lack of trust.

Early on, Rogers (2002), in an insightful expose of doctors' trust of patients, argued that it was *morally important* for doctors to trust patients. Implied here is that providers' trust of patients is the foundation for medical relationships which support patient autonomy and leads to a better understanding of patients' interests. Mutual trust may be as important as patient trust in providers, and this is the approach used by Thom et al. (2011) in developing a measure of physicians' trust in patients.

These researchers developed and validated the **Trust in the Patient Scale**. This scale assesses, for example, the extent to which providers have confidence in patients about whether they will provide them all the information they need, answer questions honestly, follow the treatment plan as instructed, and let them know when there has been a major change in their condition.

The scale also included items about whether the provider felt the patient respected their time and did not manipulate the relationship for personal gain. The researchers added that the assessment of clinician trust in patients could allow for examination of the consequences of trust when it is mutual or when lacking in the provider. These consequences—mutual trust or limited trust—could be studied for their link to care processes or patient and patient–provider relationship outcomes. For example, how would poor continuity of care impact mutual trust, and what effect might low levels of provider trust have on the quality of patient–provider interactions. And, is there a causal link; otherwise, when patients distrust providers, will they withhold information, and will this lead to providers not trusting patients.

Types of Trust

In their classic work describing relationship potential, Northouse and Northouse (1992) differentiate between two types of trust—general and specific. According to these authors, *general trust* is the trust that individuals have of other people in a global sense. This kind of trust is consistent much like a trait characteristic. People who generally trust others would be categorized as having a high level of general trust.

Specific trust, the second type of trust, is the trust an individual has of another person in a specific relationship. Patients and families who mistrust a particular provider would be categorized as possessing low specific trust. Trust of this kind depends on the specific interaction in the here-and-now. This distinction is important because individuals can manifest high **global trust** and low specific trust simultaneously. They may also exhibit low global trust and high specific trust.

Trust is not something that is just absent or present. It is a complex phenomenon that is manifested differently in interpersonal relationships and can change when an individual is involved in specific relationships, in particular situations. In provider–patient relationships, trust occurs when two conditions are met:

- Patients perceive that providers have their best interests in mind.
- Patients perceive that these same providers are capable and competent to help them.

For patients to truly trust a provider, both criteria must be met. Consider the contrary. A patient perceives a certain provider to have his best interests in mind but this provider is judged to lack competence. The patient might withhold trust but it depends on whether the patient perceives the provider's lack of clinical competence. Otherwise, the patient and family may not feel sufficiently knowledgeable to evaluate the provider's level of competence.

Consider the case when patients perceive the provider to be technically competent but judge the provider to be disinterested in their concerns and care preferences. In this situation, the patient may withhold trust but for different reasons. The question is, do patients' perceptions of clinical competence override feelings that providers do not care? Is the patient likely to seek out providers that exhibit both qualities or remain with a provider that they judge to be disinterested but competent?

High levels of trust are associated with beliefs that events are predictable, and that providers are both sincere and competent to address whatever arises. It follows that beliefs to the contrary might evoke suspicion, fear, and mistrust. A list of patient perceptions, beliefs, and attitudes associated with patients' mistrust of providers is contained in **EXHIBIT 8-1**.

Trust, Respect, and Genuineness

Trust encompasses respect. All patient–provider encounters, if they are to be therapeutic, must be based on respect and genuineness. **Respect** means acknowledging the value of patients and families, and accepting their individuality as well as their unique needs and rights. Communications of this type include listening to patients, acknowledging patients' preferences, giving choices where possible, and treating patients with dignity. **Genuineness** refers to a provider's ability to be open and honest with the patient. Providers who are genuine are congruent in their communications. Their verbal statements are congruent with their nonverbal behaviors.

EXHIBIT 8-1 Patient Perceptions, Beliefs, and Attitudes Associated with Mistrust of Providers

- You won't like me or approve of me, especially when you get to know my problems.
- You won't be there when I need you.
- You don't really care about me, my condition, or my care; your expression of caring is meaningless.
- You are more concerned about making money (from tests, procedures, etc.) than being honestly interested in me and the care I need and prefer.
- To you I am a guinea pig, a burden, unimportant (compared with other patients you see, things you do).
- You won't really be able to help me or my condition, and you are not telling me this.
- You appear to be helpful, but something will go wrong and I will not get the care I need.
- You can't possibly know or understand how I feel.

Genuineness is often achieved by self-disclosures; providers' self-disclosures can lead to greater closeness with patients. Providers can be observed to say things like "I have had several patients tell me that" or "a friend of mine has had the surgery you will have." There are various versions of this type of self-disclosure, and the objective is the same, communicating familiarity and promoting patients' feelings that the provider is genuinely concerned about their well-being. While provider self-disclosures generally demonstrate genuineness, this response mode warrants careful use. Some self-disclosures can actually create the opposite effect and result in patients' feeling that providers are preoccupied with their own concerns, not those of the patient. Further discussion of the response mode "use of self-disclosures" is provided in Chapter 11.

A critical factor affecting patients' and family members' trust of providers is the distancing behaviors that communicate disinterest and lack of concern. Providers' nonverbal communications—for example, avoidance of eye contact, lack of facial expression, physical distancing, and hesitancy to be in patients' presence for any significant length of time—can create feelings of distance that might lead to distrust. But this depends upon the patient's preference for these gestures. For example, direct and prolonged eye contact can make some patients and providers uncomfortable.

These behaviors do not send messages about providers' lack of clinical competence, but they do communicate to patients a lack of concern and caring. While interpretations about providers' behaviors or statements are not always accurate, the behaviors just cited can have indelible effects on patients' attitudes toward providers. Providers who conduct themselves in ways to raise concern might not be convincing in their roles as patient advocates or will they easily persuade patients to alter poor health habits.

The Trust–Mistrust Continuum

Trust, like many other aspects of interpersonal relationships, is best viewed on a continuum as a **trust–mistrust continuum**. That is, patients can exhibit a very high level of trust or a very low level of trust. Somewhere in between are those individuals who exhibit a healthy appropriate level of trust. A concept of importance is *blind trust* which is trusting with insufficient reason. One's position on the continuum of trust and mistrust depends on many factors, including past experiences with trust and mistrust and, current exposure to situations and/or relationship that evoke trust.

While it is true that trust is "earned," providers' are often in encounters with patients and their families where they feel they must prove their trustworthiness. It is also true that some individuals may have difficulty trusting under any circumstances and under care of a wide range of health providers.

Patients' personal health and social histories will reveal clues about their level of trust and the likelihood that trust will come easily. Patients who have been traumatized as youth, those who have been abused as children or adults, and those who experience cognitive impairment may be particularly cautious or guarded because it is difficult to suppress past experience or evaluate the behavior of the provider. They may be suspicious and need to question the motives and/or the behaviors of providers.

Just as trust is earned, it can also be broken. Providers who behave in nurturing ways with their patients and their families initially ignore their needs in the next encounter and show inconsistent attitudes and responses. If trust requires consistency, then inconsistency will deter experiences of trustworthiness. It is difficult for patients to trust providers if they think they cannot depend on them. Dentists who promise their patients, especially children, pain-free extractions and actually cause pain can evoke confusion that may result in mistrust. Energy that could or should be directed toward coping with the procedure and pain is eroded if patients need to assess or reassess the provider's true level of caring and trustworthiness.

Trust and Mistrust

Patients and families who mistrust typically behave differently than those who trust. They might communicate with defensiveness. They might be guarded in their speech or be altogether noncommunicative. They might exhibit caution and even suspiciousness. In contrast, patients and families who have high levels of trust are generally more open and responsive. They are likely to communicate hope and faith in their provider and their proposed plan of care, and are willing to take risks under provider guidance.

The early origins of the psychosocial concept of trust stem from experiences of relationships in infancy. The classical work of Erik Erikson (1993) details the first of eight stages of psychosocial development as—trust versus mistrust. Trust versus mistrust is the first stage that humans encounter throughout their lifetime. Basically, Erikson's theory was that early patterns of trust (or mistrust) development are powerful, and help individuals come to terms with trust or mistrust for the remainder of their lives.

People first learn trust based on what they see, hear, feel, and experience in social encounters, primarily with infant caregivers. Beginning feelings of confidence and faith stem from learning that they will receive what they need and have behaved in certain ways to get what they need. Parents and caregivers perform these functions early on; but, in time, self-confidence results from perceiving that one is both self-reliant and trustworthy.

The process that patients go through in becoming confident in their abilities to render self-care parallels this primary experience. That is, trust in providers is felt, and with it comes a growing trust in one's own abilities to get what is needed. Identification with the provider and the helping relationship enables patients to experiment with and become adept at aspects of self-care management.

Patients who look back on learning self-care measures (e.g., giving themselves intramuscular injection medications, cleaning wounds or irrigating procedures, or caring for their colostomy) may comment that they never thought they would be capable of these tasks. Through trust in the provider or provider team, patients learn to cope with their limitations, master skills, and resolve problems and frustrations related to their health conditions even when these problems and tasks initially felt overwhelming and unattainable. Thus, positive outcomes arise from trusting relationships. Trust creates a climate of support. It also produces feelings of comfort and security. Additionally, because it reduces defensive communication, it generally yields more complete and honest disclosures. Because of this, the process of establishing trust is taken very seriously.

Mistrust of medical establishments and health care providers is real and present more often than one would expect. The health provider can act as a barrier or enabler of trust. If their relationship with a patient and family member is not based upon trust, the patient is not likely to rely on these providers and the probability of patients changing unhealthy behavior is lower (Moreno-Peral et al., 2015).

Mistrust is the opposite of trust—the belief or experience of providers not respecting their best interests is a basis for patient mistrust. There is ample evidence of patient and family member mistrust of health providers and health care institutions, and this evidence is now readily available to the public through social media including websites (e.g., yelp.com).

Previously, patients and patient families had few opportunities to obtain provider reviews by former patents and few opportunities to express their experiences leading to question the trustworthiness of health care providers and health care institutions.

The following examples represent actual comments from patients but have been altered to protect the identity of the patient and/or family member expressing these opinions. The examples of comments are not intended to evoke a discussion about: who was at fault or is it true or not. Rather, the examples illustrate how patient and family experiences can result in feelings of mistrust (**EXHIBIT 8-2**).

EXHIBIT 8-2 Patients' and Family Members' Comments About Mistrusting Health Providers

Example: Family Member Experience with a Hospital Nurse Manager

"Nurse Manager X on the Medsurgical unit was disrespectful and unprofessional toward my very ill grandfather. My family was humiliated and deeply hurt by her comments and rudeness. Later, she apologized when confronted and said she was having a bad day, seriously? You are the manager of the unit, how unprofessional! Other nurses were very kind and compassionate, can't thank them enough...."

In this example the nurse manager is acting disrespectful toward the family member's grandfather, and the family reacted very negatively toward the way the nurse manager acted. Further, the family member does not accept the apology and reasons because the behavior goes beyond what would be expected, even when one is "having a bad day." The family expressed the attitude that nurses in leadership should be capable of rising above their personal experiences and exercise leadership. They note that other staff were very respectful and seemed to have their best interests in mind despite the poor role modeling by the nurse manager.

Example: Patient's Experience with Office Procedures in a Visit to the Podiatrist

"It is so sad to find doctors who seem so much more interested in making money than helping people. I went in to get some treatment on my toes. Not much engagement...just a sales pitch and making sure to run my credit card before any treatment. (What am I going to do, run out of the office after my laser treatment before payment?) The whole vibe in the office is off, but I can handle that if the treatment would work. I wish I just trusted that voice inside that didn't trust..."

Patients can be sensitive to what they perceive to be the motivation of health providers. As in this situation, the patient feels the provider is more interested in getting paid well for the visit instead of really focusing on helping the patient. The patient adds that not only does the provider not have his or her best interests in mind but also delivers care that did not work, a reflection of problems in clinical competence.

(continues)

EXHIBIT 8-2 Patients' and Family Members' Comments About Mistrusting Health Providers *(continued)*

Example: Family Member Describing Mistrust of an Oncologist Care Provider

"Doctor X is a self-serving doctor with a "god complex" and extremely horrible bedside manners. He isn't that smart and the experiments he runs on patients are silly. Really really silly. Not to mention, his reputation among his peers is very low. Prior to seeing, another oncologist told my father and me that we should not see him…her words were, "he will kill you." Dr. X used my father for his radical silly treatments, and kicked him to the next doctor when his liver was no longer useful.…I know my dad would've had 5 years more in reasonable comfort…."

In this example, family member criticism is levied at both the oncologist's bedside manner and lack of clinical competence, again two aspects inherent in satisfying trustworthiness from the standpoint of patients and family care givers.

▶ The Process of Establishing Trust

Concerns about provider trust surface in the beginning with patients and their families. Patients' trust in providers usually evolves over time as the patient tests both competence and respectfulness of the provider. Along these lines, it is important to understand the formation of trust in the context of building a therapeutic relationship.

Does trust mean different things to different patient populations? For example, do minority populations report lower levels of trust of physicians, and health providers in general? Otherwise, the process of establishing trust might vary as a function of age, race, sociocultural differences, and socioeconomic status.

Halbert et al. (2006) reported that trust of health providers were lower in African Americans compared to whites. While fewer quality interactions were associated with low trust in health providers for both African Americans and whites, usual source of medical care was only associated with low trust among the African Americans surveyed. Because the cause of low trust might differ across patients and families, providers' attempts to establish trusting relationships among different minority populations should consider what unique and culturally appropriate steps would enhance trust.

In general, the emotional climate of initial encounters may be guarded. Patients and their families may avoid risking self-disclosure until they observe that providers are acting on their behalf. When we speak of the process of establishing trust, we are referring to the establishment of a good relationship based on mutual trust. Trust specific to a relationship is not arrived at quickly.

The phases of a therapeutic relationship in which trust is forming can be described in several ways. These phases are usually conceived of in three stages; however, some models contain four or more stages or substages. The model presented here addresses the specific issues of self-disclosure and trust. For a relationship to be therapeutic, respect, honesty, and consistency are critical; but, the essential variable of trust and the beliefs congruent with a trusting relationship are even more essential to provider–patient interactions.

The Initiation Phase

The first phase in relationship building is termed the **initiation phase**, also referred to as the introductory or orientation phase. This phase consists of the very first contact between provider and patient. Whether through a telephone conversation or an actual face-to-face encounter, this contact sets the tone and climate for the relationship.

Initially, the provider's demeanor, attentiveness, and responsiveness give patients an idea of what to expect. But, as Doescher, Saver, Franks, and Fiscella (2000) explain, this is only a rough indicator of how the relationship might evolve as the patient and provider become more acquainted. The essential importance of this initial contact with respect to trust is that the potential for trust is scrutinized. Patients in this phase are likely to project onto the provider attitudes from former relationships that may have been positive, neutral, or, in some cases, negative.

The expectations of patients and their families are based on previous experience and begin to be confirmed or altered. Providers too may have developed preconceptions about the patient and/or family, and these impressions are validated and/or revised in this initial phase. Additionally, providers may project onto the patient attitudes and experiences with former patients that may or may not share common characteristics. Some providers develop preconceptions of patients that include expectations that the patient cannot be trusted, will be unreliable in following directives, and will lack faith in the treatment plan. The provider's own preconceptions must be tested in this initial phase.

In these initial interactions, it is the provider's obligation to establish a climate that is conducive to trust. This climate includes expressions of respect and caring in a context of genuineness and consistency. These elements, sometimes referred to as a supportive relationship, enhance or foster the possibility that a trusting relationship will result. Any preinteraction expectations that have negative effects on trust should be changed or revised for the patient.

Initial encounters that display understanding and caring for the patient and/or family are important because they help dispel anxieties and fears. The supportive, nonthreatening aspects of this encounter make it easier for patients and their families to share their fears and concerns. Beliefs that patients have

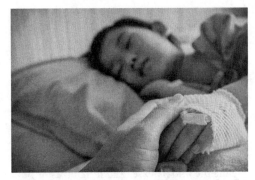

© Kdshutterman/Shutterstock.

that contribute to mistrust must be countered with factual information or sequential positive experiences. Sometimes these beliefs depict patients' overall global perspectives on relationships. Whether they reflect global or specific attitudes, they are potentially problematic to building the therapeutic relationship.

Putting the patient at ease is not only achieved by the general tone or climate of the encounter, it is also achieved by specific communication strategies. One very common strategy is the use of "small talk." Small talk is helpful in building trust with adults but also with children and teens. Small talk could include weather, time of day, or something about the patient's everyday life experiences.

It could also include comments about any difficulties finding the clinic or office, or about the waiting period. Small talk has the potential for putting the patient at ease because it reveals the humanness of the provider—that providers are people and are affected by the same earthly events or conditions that impact patients. Sometimes this small talk includes humor, which also seems to reduce initial tension.

Not all providers are comfortable with small talk. There are some pitfalls in engaging the patient and/or family superficially. First, the patient or family may judge the provider's comments or attempts as superficial and insincere. Even more problematic is the patient's interpretation that the provider is not open to serious discussions. For these reasons, small talk is frequently replaced by nonverbal expressions of caring and more direct commentary about how the provider envisions this initial encounter. Small talk can also be problematic for providers because the shift to more important health issues may be difficult to bridge once this superficial tone has been established.

Trust, then, begins with an initial testing of preconceptions and early attempts to place the patient at ease. These steps are not sufficient, however, either in establishing trust or in completing the initial phase. Recall that trust is built on the perception that providers are reliable. It follows, then, that an important aspect of creating trust is the task of clarifying the purpose and procedures in any patient–provider encounter.

While the purpose of contact is usually clear, the procedure or process to meet the treatment aims is not. For example, patients may understand that the purpose of their visit is a physical exam. The exact steps they must take and when and if they will need X-rays or lab work is not always specified. Additionally, the relationships between these procedures and the original purpose may be unclear. Patients may understand that they are having a follow-up exam but be unclear about how a certain test gives evidence of their recovery. It is always important to give patients and/or their families sufficient time to ask questions and to obtain enough feedback to put them at ease. Their inability to obtain clarification in a timely manner will serve to be a significant barrier to their trusting providers.

Although this is changing, patients generally think that providers are powerful and know everything. If providers do not reveal what they know, providers are suspect. They may be regarded as insensitive, uncaring, or unable to understand them. Any one of these scenarios creates mistrust. And, once in place, it is difficult to convince a patient of the contrary. Providers sometimes try to "cover their tracks" but this can be seen as giving weak and inadequate excuses. Refer back to the definition of a trusting relationship—patients want to be convinced that they take priority over other considerations.

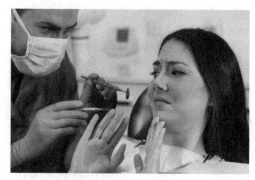

© Antonio Guillem/Shutterstock.

Explanations about what to expect and what procedures will occur will provide additional structure to the encounter—structure that gives meaning to the actions that are to follow. Eliciting patients' willingness to participate, however, is a separate intervention, albeit following naturally as a consequence of providers' description of the purpose.

In many provider–patient contacts, this agreement is taken for granted (i.e., the patient is assumed to accept and be willing to follow providers' directives). Consider, for example, that patients are generally expected to accept such things as lab work and X-rays without needing clarification or even without giving their explicit consent. What underlying assumptions operate to suggest that patients have, in fact, agreed? We would say that if patients objected, they could register this objection. However, there is an implied contractual arrangement between provider and patient that is important to understand.

Provider and patient roles are, in fact, social roles. Complementary role behavior in most provider–patient interactions consists of the helper (provider) doing something to help the helpee (patient). It is understood that once an encounter has occurred, professional responsibility dictates the performance of role behavior. Appropriate complementary role behavior includes patients' responsibilities to accept the care that is presented to them by providers who are recognized as clinical and professional experts. Unless otherwise cued to be more assertive, they might be hesitant in expressing their objections.

Informal contracts are generally replaced with specific mutually agreed-upon plans of action. In health care, these plans are communicated verbally and in writing in the patient's medical and health records. A mutually agreed-upon plan of action depends on goals that are clear and fully communicated. All plans for care should elicit patient consent. The mutuality behind goal formulation, by definition, implies that the care plan is not imposed on the patient. Rather, it is based on collaboration between the patient and the provider.

A level of mutually agreed-upon care planning would seem to be impossible without sufficient trust. First, mutual goal-setting requires patient self-disclosure. This level of revelation occurs under conditions of trusting attitudes. Second, for any patient to explicitly agree on a plan of action, he or she must be convinced of the provider's competence and goodwill. Thus, it is safe to say that provider–patient relationships will falter at the point of a mutually agreed-upon plan if trust has not sufficiently been established beforehand.

There are specific problems in communicating about plans of care that do not enlist patients in the decision-making process. While these problems may not reflect a lack of trust, they will affect the level of trust that will emerge in provider–patient relationships. When providers spend time communicating, but patients and/or their families are unable to understand the information they are given, there is concern. Low literacy, fear, anxiety, or some other factor (physical or emotional) can limit their ability to grasp and understand what they are told. This can lead to mistrust or blind trust. Problems of no trust or of inadequate trust in the initial phase have significant implications for the treatment or **implementation phase** that follows.

The Implementation Phase

Implementation of a course of action, whether it is a structure for assessing health, treating disease, or referral, it is ideally grounded in a relationship of mutual trust. During this phase, assuming that trust is in place, the provider and patient are mutually engaged in confronting and working on health problems.

A major role of the provider in the implementation phase is to help patients cope with and master threats to their health. This includes instruction in health-related changes as well as giving provider feedback from clinical assessments that will help evaluate the success of the medical regimen. Otherwise, the provider needs to be reassured that patients will report back to them any changes in their condition or their use of prescribed medications or treatments.

As a rule, this phase does not proceed free of disruption and barriers. The first barrier is reluctance. To put a plan into action, the patient must accept the authoritative opinions of the provider. If the patient is not convinced of the provider's competence, then forward movement will not occur, even if the patient expresses commitment to the treatment goals and needs the help of the health provider.

A common problem that also relates to patients' faith in their treatment is that the plan of action may not result in expected and desired outcomes or not in the time frame expected by patients. Failed treatment approaches are sometimes interpreted as provider incompetency. Failed plans can also be internalized, and patients may blame themselves for failed attempts. For example, "if I had only taken my medication according to the instructions, the results would be different."

If patients fail to comply and not inform the provider or deliberately fail to follow directives, then feelings about personal failure may be appropriate. However, patient guilt about treatment failures can be irrational much of the time for several reasons—they do not understand that the lapse in medication taking would not have made a difference or both patient and provider are responsible because the provider failed to give clear directions and explanations.

Whether the provider's competence or the patient's responsibility is perceived to be at the crux of the problem, the experience of failed treatment can threaten mutual trust in subsequent therapeutic encounters. It is advisable to discuss the results of interventions fully and completely, pinpointing reasons these actions fell short of expectations. Providers who are trustworthy are willing to discuss failures and successes. Trust, if damaged, can be restored. However, failed treatment can result in patients' failure to return and must be addressed openly and honestly early on.

An important component of trust building and maintenance in this phase is the process of assisting patients to manage the impact that illnesses or the threat of illness may have on them. Providers who not only address disease but also the impact of disease will convince patients of their caring and concern. Appropriate patient supportive self-management is critical.

The Termination or Closure Phase

If all goes well, the helping relationship that is initially established will survive the course of an illness or several illness episodes. This includes the ups and downs of treatment where plans are not always successful and barriers to trust have not always been dealt with adequately. The **termination phase** is that point in time when the therapeutic relationship is closed.

Closure occurs because goals have been accomplished, and there are no further apparent needs for care from the current provider. However, many patient–provider relationships end abruptly or before the current care planned is no longer necessary. Patients may require referrals to specialists, may leave the geographical area, or their health may deteriorate to the point that a different level of care is required. When patients are referred to a specialist, it is generally understood that they will return to their primary care provider to resume treatment or for follow-up.

The primary principle behind a successful termination is prior planning and preparation. This means that providers should discuss termination of care and discharge issues with patients from the start in the initiation phase.

While the major issue is the appropriateness of the closure, the major task when this issue is resolved is to draw the lines of separation. Officially, termination means no longer being responsible for treatment decisions. It is extremely important that the patient fully understands the conditions of this phase and that beyond a particular point or point in time, the current provider will not be responsible for future health care services. It is unwise for a patient to be accepting care from two or more providers simultaneously unless this was planned.

Patients, particularly those who have learned to trust and value the provider, may have difficulty relinquishing their emotional ties to the provider. This reluctance is an important signal to providers to specify and clarify the meaning of ending the relationship.

One difficulty that may occur and that is potentially detrimental to patients is the patient's assumption that the provider is still very much in a provider role with them. Sometimes they will not complete a referral because they think that they can return to discuss their health concerns with their original provider. In some instances the plan may include returning to the original provider, but if not, patients need to be given clear directives about the appropriate means of getting the care they need.

Final encounters, sometimes referred to as discharge planning sessions, summarize the current episode of care for the patient and/ or family. In this meeting, the care plan and course of treatment, including discussions of successes and failures, will not only provide perspective but will also reaffirm the professional aspects of the relationship. Terminations of treatment are always accompanied by written documentation to the patient, with copies going to the medical records, regardless of whether closure occurred in a face-to-face encounter or not.

Problems associated with terminating care can include:

- Providers' failing to communicate clearly and fully the conditions of closure.
- Providers' reluctance to handle the patients' emotional responses to terminating the relationship.
- Providers inappropriately continuing relationships despite the advisability of closing treatment.
- Patients' assumptions that they can return to the original provider even when seeing a new provider for the same health concern.

In summary, each one of the several phases of the provider–patient relationship is affected by patients' trust in providers and providers' trust in patients. Therapeutic alliances are believed to proceed through these phases. Trust is a factor that can sufficiently affect the speed and quality of progression, and without trust, chances for a therapeutic alliance can be seriously derailed. Progress, whether it includes gathering patient data for a comprehensive assessment or persuading patients to change health-related behaviors, will not be possible.

▶ Trust-Evoking Behaviors

As previously indicated, one dimension of trust is patients' observations that providers have their best interests in mind. It was also suggested that without satisfying this element, trust would not occur. Provider competence is only one part of the picture. A listing of provider-based behaviors and specific communications that can evoke trusting responses from patients are found in **EXHIBIT 8-3**. Acknowledging the value of patients is a necessary part of conveying concern for their best

---

EXHIBIT 8-3 Provider Behaviors That Evoke Trust Through Confirmation

Basic Provider Characteristics and Behaviors

- Honesty
- Consistency
- Respect and caring, openness, and genuineness
- Reliability, adequate follow-up, and follow-through
- Congruence between verbal and nonverbal communication

Specific Communications Which Evoke Trust and Show Confirmation

- Direct acknowledgment and appreciation of patient's uniqueness
- Informing about and clarifying expectations
- Continued supportive responsiveness
- Verbal expressions of positive regard, including respect, warmth, and caring
- Active listening
- Nonverbal expressions of positive regard—smiling, appropriate eye contact, warmth in tone of voice, and approachable body posture

---

interests. However, confirmation is a distinct way of communicating acknowledgment and acceptance. It plays a unique role in patient–provider communication. The therapeutic response mode—confirmation—was previously discussed in Chapter 7.

▶ Summary

The purpose of therapeutic patient–provider and family–provider encounters is not only to obtain needed information but also to establish a relationship that serves as the context for a working alliance as these relationships unfold. Provider–patient encounters are effective to the degree to which important data can be obtained and health behaviors negotiated.

Trust is so basic to these relationships that it is often taken for granted. Trust, defined here as confidence in provider competence and perceptions that providers have one's best interests in mind, is critical to therapeutic alliances. Trust in providers helps patients deal with the fears and uncertainties surrounding their care and conditions. Patients are simply unable to do many of the things providers do, and in many ways are forced to depend on them. Patients and their families need to be able to see health professionals as both competent and caring. Providers who foster trust will seek to build their professional-clinical credibility as well as their reputations to be interpersonally trustworthy.

Patients and even families may have generalized global trust of most things and people or they may be inherently suspicious and guarded. They may also display a range of trust with specific providers and in specific contexts. Some are generally trusting individuals but have a specific mistrust of health care providers or health care delivery systems. Patients' reactions to hospitals is a case in point. This mistrust can originate from a previous negative or traumatic experience or from a lack of information. Each time a patient and family encounter a new provider and/or new health care delivery system, trust must be negotiated or renegotiated.

The ability to create trust in the patient–provider relationship is dependent on certain individual predispositions as well as specific communication strategies. Approaches that demonstrate honesty, genuineness, comfort and caring, competence, and encouragement contribute to faith and trust in providers.

Provider training in trust building is critical. Also, institutional commitment to building trust in patients and families through securing quality care is important. Providers might lament that there are too many demands on their time during this era of managed care to build trust in their relationships with patients. Very vulnerable patients in acute care settings who do not have the luxury of long, continuous processes to build sound relationships are expected to put their trust in providers as if this was an easy exercise in relinquishing control when it is not.

No matter how forced or fragile, patients and/or their families will develop expectations of beneficence, even in emergency care situations. While the building of trust does take time, it is a task that cannot be neglected even under the most challenging situations and in this era of greater demands on provider time. Thom, Hall, and Pawlson (2004) optimistically summarize the potential of trusting patient–provider relationships by explaining that lower levels of trust can be changed, and improved trust might reduce disparities, increase access to care, and improve health outcomes. Otherwise the issue is not whether we have the time to devote to trust building, rather the issue is one of we cannot afford not to take the time to build trust.

Discussion

1. Discuss the potential positive outcomes of trust on patient outcomes.
2. What is the interconnection between patient trust of providers and provider trust of patients?
3. Discuss examples of patients having global trust but lacking specific trust of health providers.
4. Identify examples of patient mistrust and the possible negative effects on the patient–provider relationship.
5. Discuss the possibility that different populations might have different levels of trust in providers and health care institutions.

References

Berry, L. L., Parish, J. T., Janakiraman, R., Ogburn-Russell, L., Couchman, G. R., Rayburn, W. L., & Grisel, J. (2008). Patients' commitment to their primary physicians and why it matters. *Annals of Family Medicine, 6*, 6–13. doi:10.1370/afm.757

Doescher, M. P., Saver, B. G., Franks, P., & Fiscella, K. (2000). Racial and ethnic disparities in perceptions of physician style and trust. *Archives of Family Medicine, 9*(10), 1156–1163. PMID:11115223

Erikson, E. (1993). *Childhood and society*. New York, NY: W.W. Norton & Company.

Giordano, G. N., & Lindström, M. (2015). Trust and health: Testing the reverse causality hypothesis. *Journal of Epidemiology and Community Health, 70*(1), 10–16. doi:10.1136/jech-2015-205822

Gopichandran, V., Wouters, E., & Chetlapalli, S. K. (2015). Development and validation of a socioculturally competent trust in physician scale for a developing country setting. *BMJ Open, 5*(4), e007305. doi:10.1136/bmjopen-2014-007305

Halbert, C. H., Armstrong, K., & Gandy, O. H. (2006). Racial differences in trust in health care providers. *Archives of Internal Medicine, 166*(8), 896–901. doi:10.1001/archinte.166.8.896

LoCurto, J., & Berg, G. M. (2016). Trust in healthcare settings: Scale development, methods, and preliminary determinants. *SAGE Open Medicine, 4*, 1–12. doi:10.1177/2050312116664224

Moreno-Peral, P., Conejo-Ceron, S., Fernandez, A., Bereguera, A., Martinez-Andres, M., Pons-Vigues, M., … Rubio-Valera, M. (2015). Primary care patients' perspectives of barriers and enablers of primary prevention and health promotion-a meta-ethnographic synthesis. *PLoS One, 10*, e0125004.

Northouse, L. L., & Northouse, P. G. (1992). *Health communication—Strategies for health professionals* (2nd ed.). East Norwalk, CT: Appleton and Lange.

O'Malley, A. S., Sheppard, V. B., Schwartz, M., & Mandelblatt, J. (2004). The role of trust in use of preventive services among low-income African-American women. *Preventive Medicine, 38*, 777–785. doi:10.1016/j.ypmed.2004.01.018

Pearson, S. D., & Raeke, L. H. (2000).Patients' trust in physicians: Many theories, few measures, little data. *Journal of General Internal Medicine, 15*, 509–513. doi:10.1046/j.1525-1497.2000.11002.x

Rogers, W. A. (2002). Is there a moral duty for doctors to trust patients? *Journal of Medical Ethics, 28*, 77–80. Retrieved from www.jmedethics.com

Shenolikar, R. A., Balkrishnan, R., & Hall, M. A. (2004). How patient-physician encounters in critical medical situations affect trust: Results of a national survey. *BMC Health Services Research, 4*, 4–24. doi:10.1186/1472-6963-4-24

Tarn, D. M., Meredith, L. S., Kagawa-Singer, M., Matsumura, S., Bito, S., Liu, H., … Wenger, N. S. (2005). Trust in one's physician: The role of ethnic match, autonomy, acculturation, and religiosity among Japanese and Japanese Americans. *Annals of Family Medicine, 3*, 339–347. doi:10.1370/afm.289

Thom, D., Hall, M., & Paulson, G. (2004). Measuring patients' trust in physicians when accessing quality of care. *Health Affairs, 23*(4), 124–132. doi:10.1377/hlthaff.23.4.124

Thom, D. H., Wong, S. T., Guzman, D., Wu, A., Penko, J., Miaskowshi, C., & Kushel, M. (2011).Physician trust in the patient: Development and validation of a new measure. *Annals of Family Medicine, 9*, 148–154. doi:10.1370/afm.1224

CHAPTER 9

The Art and Skillful Use of Questions

CHAPTER OBJECTIVES

- Identify question format choices in encounters with patients and their families.
- Differentiate between question formats in terms of response burden.
- Discuss the role of questions in establishing patient–provider relationships.
- Identify instances in which questions can be used with deleterious consequences.
- Discuss the provider's role in encouraging and supporting patients and their families to ask questions.

KEY TERMS

- Advisement purpose (of questions)
- Close-ended questions
- Direct/indirect questions
- Leading or loaded questions
- Open-ended questions
- Multiple-choice questions
- Question response burden
- Ruling out/ruling in questions
- Questions used as self-disclosure statements

▶ Introduction

Asking questions is an important skill to health providers when conducting health care assessments, diagnostic interviews, and evaluating patients' preferences. If patients are not able to answer questions, providers seek the assistance of patient representatives or family caregivers to provide the information needed to assess and care for them. Pawar (2005) maintains that perhaps the most critical skill in uncovering the needs of a patient is that of inquiring or seeking information by questioning. Asking questions, the right questions at the right time is not always easy. But asking an *answerable question* is one of the most important skills providers can master. The quality of answers received depends on what is asked and how it is asked.

Patients' answers to our questions are part of the database around which we collaboratively plan and evaluate their care. Health histories and the majority of patients' assessments are the direct result of the skillful use of questions by health care providers. Thus, a primary goal of establishing therapeutic relationships with patients and conducting patient interviews is essentially to elicit information from patients about their condition.

For this process to occur effectively, the provider must have knowledge of, as well as skill and judgment in, the art of questioning. This chapter will review basic principles behind the choice of and use of questions. Before launching this important discussion, it is important to remind the reader that questions do not happen in a vacuum; that is, they occur in the immediate context of the provider–patient encounter. Characteristics of this relationship influence which questions will be asked and how they will be worded.

Discussion or dialog between patients and providers and between families and providers is not communication between strangers even when they know little about one another.

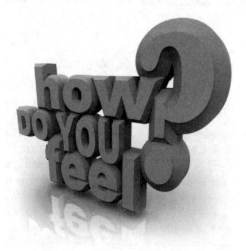

Questions are asked in a context known to both—discussing health issues in a health care setting.

In the best case scenario there is mutual trust and understanding so that these *strangers* are not strangers at all. Each patient, family member, and provider enter the encounter with their own concept about what should be discussed. What they think should be discussed is highly influenced by many factors like age, gender, race, ethnicity, role, and prior history with the health care system.

In few instances do patient and provider characteristics match. The word for the matching of patient and provider characteristics is *concordance*. There is considerable literature addressing barriers to engaging patients in medical interviews due to lack of concordance in patient–provider encounters. For example, female patients may prefer and be more open with a female provider. Patients whose primary language is not English are usually more comfortable with providers who speak their language and share or understand the basis of their cultural beliefs. Studies have reported that lack of concordance, especially along racial and ethnic lines, may account for providers' not asking as many questions as they should or patients not asking questions that they should.

Researchers have examined how ethnic and racial differences impact patient and provider question-asking behaviors. In a study by Eggly et al. (2011), differences in patients asking questions of providers were associated with racial differences. For example, African American patients asked fewer questions than Whites. It was suggested this fact could result in African Americans receiving less information from their physicians (oncologists) than White patients. Penner and colleagues (2016) concluded that implicit racial bias is a likely source of disparities in treatment among oncologists and should be addressed in oncology training and practice.

Receiving less information means lower levels of health literacy which in turn limits patients' abilities to grasp public health messages and follow medical regimens as directed. Furthermore, patients who do not ask questions may be less health literate and not know what questions to ask. These complex domino effects could explain, at least in part, health disparities. The important point is that providers need to be aware of the multiple reasons why patients might ask questions, and in turn, why certain patient populations will not ask questions of their providers.

Instead of passively receiving information and recommendations from providers, engaged patients are likely to ask more questions, seek health information, and use this information to make decisions (Gruman and colleagues, 2010). It is critical that space and opportunity be provided for patients to ask their own questions. Frequently, patients' questions reveal their informational needs and their understanding or misunderstanding of their condition and treatment. For example, patients might ask about whether a certain medication will cause high blood pressure.

This question and the way it is phrased reveals to the provider the patient's level of comprehension. Patients' questions should be asked because when answered they result in greater comprehension of treatment and treatment options (Mazor et al., 2016). Otherwise, patients who ask questions of health providers reveal what is important to them and their needs for clarification. This in turn increases their knowledge and understanding, placing them in a better position to make decisions.

Frequently, providers encourage patients to make a list of their questions prior to a visit. This enables the patient to ask relevant questions that can have significant effects on their adherence to treatment recommendations (Galliher et al., 2010). Patients' and family members' feelings of connectedness with the health care system and/or the health provider are essential, and the back and forth questioning process promotes understanding and adherence to their treatment programs.

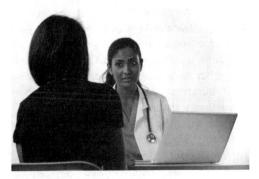

© Stuart Jenner/Shutterstock

▶ Therapeutic Use of Questions

Obviously questions are important in the initial interview and assessment of patients, but they have a significant impact as well on the therapeutic relationship that forms between the patient and provider. Patients are familiar with questions; asking and answering questions is a common mode of human communication that begins early in life and is refined over time. People are generally aware of different question formats; questions are generally formatted to begin with who, when, where, what, and why.

This approach to questioning is insufficient in therapeutic relationships where embellishment is needed and a helping relationship is the goal. The skill of inquiry (gaining information through the use of questions) is customarily the primary tool for health care providers. While patients can and are asked to fill out fact sheets in advance of visits, the most important source of information comes from the dialogue. What prompts a string of follow-up questions is frequently the provider's visual clues during a face-to-face encounter.

Providers are diagnostically driven, and are continually seeking to assess patients' conditions. In fact, the provider role is characterized by the privilege and expectation of asking questions. Patients know that when they encounter a health provider they will be asked questions and will be expected to answer these questions. The only way of avoiding this exchange is either to avoid these encounters altogether or to carefully screen and control what questions they will answer and how much they will disclose.

For the most part, providers engage the patient in an interpersonal context through the use of questions (Tongue, Epps, & Forese, 2005). Familiar openings used by providers include "What brings you here today?"; "How are you feeling?"; and "What seems to be the problem?" Tongue and colleagues suggest that providers should be careful with the use of some questions that place the patient in the awkward position of answering, "Fine." Although typical salutations are common, other ways of engaging the patient are preferable.

Questions yield data; data provide information needed to begin assessments of patients' needs and health problems. Evidence has shown that when information exchange (the process of asking questions and getting answers) is weakened, the quality of health care, including costs of care, also suffers. Incomplete information or no information can significantly inhibit the ability of providers to distinguish the best care for the patient. It can also lead to unnecessary tests and referrals. Family members, particularly family caregivers, are critical sources of information and add to the necessary knowledge base. Providers use several types of questions to obtain, clarify, and specify information about the condition of the patient. Furthermore, questions enable providers to follow, focus in-depth, and redirect patients' statements about their needs and concerns.

Collecting Information

Collecting patient information is central to the patient health history-taking process but also for the implementation and evaluation of the care planned. At any time through the process of establishing trust, it allows for patients'

stories to unfold more fully. Frequently, questions are used to begin the dialogue. From there, the provider encourages patient elaboration while becoming focused and using more specific questions. When the patient gives ambiguous or unclear responses or statements, providers are challenged to alter the question format to meet the specific circumstances of communicating with the patient, especially when there are no available family members at the time.

Questions can be likened to "an invitation." They invite patients and/or their family caregivers to collaborate in identifying problems and creating solutions. But this invitation is not always welcomed. What the provider does not want to do is make the patient or family feel inadequate and uncomfortable in struggling to answer questions asked of them. They may have trouble answering questions but also in understanding why they are asked. With the invitation to answer questions an explanation is helpful (e.g., "The reason why I'm asking you these questions is that it gives me information about your health as a whole before I ask about something specific"). Questions are lead-ins for the patient to begin talking.

Information collected from a patient may include health history data (e.g., previous diseases, surgeries, hospitalizations, and medications). Background and sociocultural data (e.g., age, income, race, ethnicity, years of education, marital status, and number of dependents) are usually collected beforehand in standard office forms. Although this information appears to be straightforward and easy to extract, this is not always the case. For example, unless patients have made a point of bringing a list of concerns, questions, and an outline of their health history, they may not know how to respond or have difficulty answering these background questions. Data about primary language (language spoken at home), educational level, gender orientation, and racial or ethnic background may be sensitive. Yet, to be seen for a health care problem, it is helpful to understand a patient's cultural background and perception of health issues.

These questions along with others—immigration status, religious affiliation, mental health, sexual history, alcohol and drug use, and even the number of pregnancies—can be sensitive topics, and not all patients or their families are convinced that responding to these kinds of questions is a good idea. Having never had to give this data to health providers before, some patients and families may be suspicious about why providers are interested and if this information will be used against them. For example, for patients whose immigration status is an issue, such questions may make them feel uncomfortable and uneasy.

Some questions are uncomfortable, and others can elicit embarrassment or even stronger feelings of fear, guilt, and shame. For this reason, the skillful use of questioning and the supportive and respectful ways inquiry occurs may make the difference in the completeness and accuracy of data collected. Giving patients choices about the amount of data disclosed (if it is not directly related to their condition) and the context in which the data are provided (privately) are always important principles to keep in mind. A helpful strategy to use is to address their fears and concerns up front before asking these questions. For example, "Patients sometimes wonder why we ask these questions and what we are looking for; let me tell you a little about that."

Clarifying and Specifying

Questions are used to clarify and specify information patients or families give. Because patients are not usually able to assemble information in ways that are meaningful to health care providers, a second function of the use of questions is to clarify the information already provided. In this case, the provider begins to focus on relevant areas as the conversation unfolds. For example, when a patient complains of abdominal pain, the clinician wants to know the location, character, and severity of the pain. This assessment requires assisting the patient to clarify and specify features of the pain experience. The following provider questions help to clarify patients' experience. "Is it a dull or sharp pain?" "A radiating pain or localized pain?" "Is it mild or very severe?" Depending upon what providers are looking for these questions will vary. These data are essential and require providers to focus their questions to elicit clarity and specificity. While open exploration can be helpful (e.g., "Tell me about your pain"), carefully worded questions that seek clarification or specificity work well, at least in gathering basic information.

When patients are having difficulty describing their experience due to emotional distress, language deficits, or some other barrier, the provider must thoughtfully sort through those phrases or words that will evoke clarification but are absent of jargon. Using the patients' own terms or phrases can be quite useful. If patients refer to their pain as "pressure," then providers can seek to clarify this "pressure." The provider uses the patients' terms to engage them further in the collaborative effort to further describe and understand their needs and problems.

In conducting a health history, performing a physical exam, or delivering some aspect of care, it is very important that the provider become specific about the data needed. For example, when changing dressings, providers need to know exactly which dressing changing movements are very painful and which are less painful. Questions that are focused help to specify the experience and reduce distress from the procedure. Carefully chosen questions direct and focus the interview or assessment in productive ways.

Ruling Out and Ruling In

Ruling out and **ruling in** is a way of gaining specificity about patients' concerns. Ruling-out questions include those that seek clarity and are generally more direct (e.g., "Does the pain extend to your left shoulder?"). They also can require the patient to observe a phenomena, compare the experience, and choose a response that fits the choices that the provider has given (e.g., "If I press here, do you feel the pain as sharply when I press there?").

Some ruling-out and ruling-in questions require patients to recall past experiences and compare them with present experience. For example, the provider might ask, "Does this medication cause you to feel nauseated if you take it before a meal?" And, "Is the nausea you feel different from what you always feel?" In this dialogue, the provider is seeking to pinpoint and rule out various possibilities and generate certain hypotheses about patients' concerns or problems.

In summary, while questions seem to have very specific information-gathering purposes in the clinical interview, they also have a more subtle secondary effect of providing support and reassurance as the provider seeks to form a therapeutic alliance with the patient and patient's family. Sometimes questions are used in a slow-moving encounter as a filler. An occasional question lets the patient know that the provider is still listening and is attentive to the patient's concerns and needs. Pawar (2005) reminds providers to "think dialogue, not monologue" by asking questions, exploring concerns, and making connections. Rather than hearing concerns and responding with an immediate solution, all dialogue with patients requires digging deeper and more fully.

▶ Nontherapeutic Use of Questions

While questions are the primary vehicle for gathering information in therapeutic communications with patients, questioning is not always therapeutic. Questions are effective when interviewing but can also be misused. Thus, questions can be used therapeutically or nontherapeutically. The following discussion highlights various ways in which questions can be inappropriately positioned in provider–patient interactions. These questions do not ask legitimate questions but they are intended to tell something to the patient.

Interpretative Purposes

Sometimes providers pose questions but these questions are not used to gather information. They are used to deliver interpretations or judgments. Interpretative questions are not used to collect data; they are used to express provider opinions. An example would be "If you choose not to let your daughter have braces, wouldn't that make you an irresponsible parent?" The point is that the provider is not asking for a yes or no answer. Neither is the provider interested in whether the parent shares this opinion. Rather, the provider appears to be more interested in the mother knowing that if she refuses having braces for her daughter, she is neglecting the health of her child. While this interaction focuses around a question, no new information is sought. Under the guise of this question, the provider delivers an opinion and an interpretation of the parent's behavior. In some sense, it is a disguised accusation without being expressed directly.

Self-Disclosure Purpose

A second type of question used to give, not request, information is the **question using self-disclosure statements**. An example would be, "Do you know that your rolling back on the bed (after I got you in position) is making it hard on me?" In this scenario, the provider wants to tell the patient not to do something; instead of being direct and clear, the provider uses a question. The question is another form of a telling response. It tells what the provider is experiencing (i.e., difficulty and hardship). The underlying message which may be missed is "Don't move after I position you." Patients might be confused by this comment; what is the provider really saying? However, they might also get the point that the provider is irritated, but the message, "Don't move," is missed. Patients feeling or thinking that providers are irritated at them may damage the trust and working alliance that may have developed thus far, either with this provider or the team of providers.

Advisement Purpose

A third type of question that tells and does not ask is one that gives advice or attempts to persuade, referred to as the **advisement purpose of questions**. Consider the following question: "Don't you think that if you take a little juice first, that pill will be easier to swallow?" Behind this question is advice—"It will be easier to take your pill if you drink some juice first." Usually when providers put advice in the form of a question, they are attempting to soften their advice and appear less authoritative. They may actually believe that they will have greater success in changing patients' behavior if this advice is **indirect** because **direct** advice can be offensive and might evoke negative, resistant behavior.

Telling questions, presented as self-disclosures, interpretations, or advisements, are used when more direct telling is seen to be too harsh or in some other way ill advised. Some providers may think that directness is disrespectful. Telling questions may be viewed as more tactful and sometimes kinder ways of making observations or giving judgmental feedback or stating opinions. The major problem is that telling questions can be confusing. It is not always wise to be more tactful with advice when it is absolutely essential that the advice be understood and followed.

The repeated use of telling questions can also be distracting and annoying to patients and families. Some patients may feel they are being manipulated and mistrust these questions which are really remarks, not legitimate questions. Because using telling questions carries a risk, a good rule of thumb is to use as few telling questions as possible. Even when using this type of question to vary the structure and pace of the dialogue, questions may be viewed negatively and therefore should be avoided. Interpretation, self-disclosure, and advice are more appropriately delivered directly if at all. These communication approaches are discussed in detail in the chapters to follow.

Defensive Use of Questions

Questions, whether telling or authentically data-gathering, can be used defensively. Using questions defensively is also inappropriate. Questions are used defensively to evade the spotlight. Beginning practitioners, when confronted with patients who ask direct and personal questions of them, might answer a question with a question. Being asked, for example, if they are married may be something the provider finds inappropriate; it might be followed with "Why do you want to know?" Furthermore, the process of being asked a number of personal and direct questions by the patient may be disconcerting because it may disrupt the process of collecting patient data. Providers may respond defensively to evade the spotlight and to avoid the discomfort at the moment.

Deleterious Use of the Direct Questions

Perhaps the most frequently misused question format is the endless use of direct questions. Examples of direct questions would include "Are you taking your medicine?", "Are you following the diet and exercise plan I gave you?", and "Did you use the ice packs every 2–4 hours?" There is no formula about how many direct questions can be asked within a particular period of time. However, asking direct questions in *machine gun-like* fashion is inappropriate and can add to patients' frustration. Repeated direct questions may have several negative effects on patient–provider relationships. In their earlier work, Gazda, Childers, and Walters (1982) identified several undesirable outcomes that occur if direct questions are misused. A number of these are described here.

The first problem these authors cite is the creation of a dependent relationship. The use of multiple direct questions can give the effect of provider "takeover"; the respondent learns to expect that important outcomes are a result of provider dominance.

A second deleterious effect, related to the first, is that direct questions can put the responsibility for problem solving on the helper. The provider, assuming the role of expert by asking many direct questions, gives the message that a solution will come as a result of the patient answering a series of questions. Provider dominance is clear. The provider's solution, however, is not always one the patient can use. Although prescriptive actions are appropriate, much more of health care and medical practice is the result of collaborative patient–provider problem solving. Responding passively to direct questions prevents patients from actively modifying solutions so that the solutions work uniquely for them.

Patients who take a less active role in formulating solutions may also be less likely to accept responsibility for their behavior. Over-reliance on experts primes the patient to hold the provider responsible for success or failure of the treatment plan. Again, use of direct questions by the provider might have the impact of lessening the willingness of patients to be active participants in planning and evaluating their care.

Another important deleterious effect of direct questions is their tendency to result in information that might not be altogether valid. Almost every direct question has within it the preferred answer (Gazda et al., 1982). Consider the following direct questions:

- "Are you ready for your bath?"
- "Would you like help getting out of your chair?"
- "Would you like to be discharged tomorrow morning?"

In every case, the patient can read between the lines; their answers should be affirmative because that is what the provider expects. Most patients want to be agreeable, approved of, and liked by providers. Conversely, they may fear that if they disagree, their care will suffer. If this is the case, they are more likely to answer as they assume the provider wants them to. The agreement elicited merely reflects the patient's obligatory response to the provider. The fact that the patient is not really ready to have a bath or wants to go home but thinks his family is not ready to care for him yet goes unexpressed. Thus, the brief response to the question, whether yes or no, may not be the true picture of the patient's preference and gives incomplete information about the patient's circumstances.

An additional critical attitudinal problem can arise from the misuse of direct questions. The overuse of direct questions by providers can lead to resentment. Sometimes questions appear to relentlessly probe for hidden motivations when patients and their families have no hidden motivations, at least that they are aware of. Additionally, relying on direct questions too much can make the provider inattentive to other aspects of the entire experience of the patient. The first problem relates to the fact that sometimes providers' questions can be asked out of curiosity rather than because the answers are needed or relevant. Many questions asked at one time can be irritating if they are not interspersed with reflective thought on the part of both provider and patient.

EXHIBIT 9-1 reveals how misplaced, probing questions can make the patient feel resentful.

This series of direct questions can be irritating and confusing to patients. It appears that the provider is interested in the patient's need to see the doctor. However, the specificity and line of questioning suggests that the provider may have other reasons for wanting to know the doctor's schedule. Had the provider explained why more exact information was important, the patient might have been less irritated and confused.

EXHIBIT 9-1 Dialogue Box Illustrating Probing Questioning

PROVIDER:	"Did you see your doctor this morning?"
PATIENT:	"Not yet."
PROVIDER:	"When did he say he'd be here?"
PATIENT:	"He really didn't say."
PROVIDER:	"When did he come yesterday?"
PATIENT:	"In the morning."
PROVIDER:	"Probably between 10:00 and 11:00 o'clock, right?"
PATIENT:	(Angry tone of voice) "Probably; why?"

Questions usually carry demands. Too many questions increase the demand aspect in the patient–provider encounter. The patient and/or family member may feel pushed and pulled in ways that are uncomfortable, especially if the line of inquiry lacks warmth, respect, and empathy. The consequence could also include replies that are hostile and superficial. Sometimes providers ask too many questions because they are feeling pressure to keep the conversation going or because they are uncomfortable with silence. Providers who have what appears to be an endless list of questions to ask are better off allowing for silence between what the patient says and what they say. This will also enable the provider to reformulate additional questions that are meaningful and to the point.

The inattentive provider is in serious jeopardy. This provider will rely on direct questions and miss the numerous cues that come from the patient's nonverbal communication. The provider may pay little attention to the person in the patient and be "out of touch" in attempts to understand how and what help is needed. In some respects, the greater the number of direct questions that result in minimal data, the less likely it is that patients will be helped in meaningful ways. This principle is important to remember both in using questions and in choosing the appropriate format for questions. The reason that many direct questions

can impose limitations on the helping process is that they severely curb the quality of listening that occurs.

Asking "**leading**" or "**loaded**" **questions** is another type of question to avoid. These questions, usually closed-ended in format, restrict or influence the patient's response because the wording suggests what the appropriate answer should be. Actual data collection is blocked due to the fact that response options are limited. An example might be, "This doesn't hurt, does it?" This type of questioning is used when the provider's needs or goals are paramount. The patient may respond out of deference to the provider and give the desired response, such as "No-o-o." Still, this answer could be invalid. Patients might deny feeling pain or pain intensity when they are feeling more than a moderate amount of pain. There is the possibility that the patient will minimize the pain by describing the experience as a "little achy," for example. In either case, patients feel the need to alter their responses out of deference or even intimidation.

A final type of question that should be avoided is the double-barreled question. This format allows only one answer when really two or more separate questions are asked. An example, "Would you like the chair lowered, a glass of water to rinse out your mouth, a magazine while you're waiting?" While this particular double-barreled question format seems acceptable, it can be annoying. More than one double-barreled question may anger the patient and family members. These questions are disrespectful because they rush the patient to compare these alternatives and give a quick response.

While using questions properly may seem simple, there are many dos and don'ts associated with the therapeutic use of questions. The next section of this text focuses on formats for therapeutic questioning and the effects of different types of question formats. Question formats allow providers options in meeting data collection objectives. Each type of question elicits a certain type of answer. Collecting information, clarifying and specifying, and ruling out/ruling in are the major purposes for using questions. Different question formats perform these functions.

▶ Types of Question Formats

When providers think of questions that they want to ask patients or their families they need to consider how to word the question in order to get the best result and this is more than just the basic purpose of the question. This includes knowing more about the patient's level of health literacy and experience with health care services. Providers usually prefer to utilize the most efficient approach to arrive at the maximum information. Patients' potential reactions to questions are important because providers are not only interested in what approach will provide the most information, but also concerned that what is asked and how it is ask will build on the therapeutic relationship they want to achieve and maintain.

In all instances, before choosing an approach, providers need to know the unique characteristics of the patient and family and think about how these characteristics might influence the choice of question format. This includes the patient's age, gender, race, ethnicity, culture, health literacy, and health status. This information will influence which formats will work best and when and how to use them. There are many options; questions can be framed in a variety of ways to elicit information and engage patients and their families in discussions. The following description outlines the several types of question formats available (**EXHIBIT 9-2**).

Closed-Ended Questions

The most common category of questions is *closed-ended*. This question format does not require significant creativity or demand expansive elaboration. **Close-ended questions** require short, one- or two-word responses. Usually the responses are simply one-word replies: yes or no. Providers frequently ask "Do you have

---

EXHIBIT 9-2 Question Formats and Usual Responses

Close-ended: These questions ask for a short answer, even one or two words. The response is usually a short answer in return. For example—Question: "Do you eat healthy?"; Response: "Yes…most of the time." This close-ended question could be followed with an open-ended question to get more data (e.g., "What do you usually eat for breakfast, lunch, and dinner?").
However, having previously said "Yes, most of the time"; the patient is likely to report the healthy foods consumed.

Open-ended: Unlike close-ended questions, open-ended questions elicit more detail without priming the question with projecting a value. For example—Question: "In an average 24-hour period, what do you eat?"; Response: "I usually eat cereal or an egg in the morning, coffee, toast or muffin, but sometimes I don't have time and just grab coffee; for lunch a subway or grilled cheese sandwich, hamburger and French fries, or soup and garlic toast; for dinner I go out with friends a lot…we have a couple of beers, nachos, then tacos or burrito." This open-ended question can be followed by a closed-ended question to get specific information, for example, "Do you have snacks or eat anything after dinner?"

Multiple choice: Multiple choice questions offer a number of potential responses, and the patient is asked to choose between them. Question: "So, if you don't go out for dinner do you skip dinner altogether, grab a snack after work, or go home and eat something at home?" Response: "I do all those things…I guess mostly grab a snack after work." This type of question fails to give a lot of detail and is usually hard for the patient to decide on which option best fits them.

any questions?" This is a commonly used question to close out a patient visit; it is not a question that seeks detail. What do you expect the answer will be 9 times out of 10? Right, the answer is no. When patients are asked closed-ended questions requiring a yes or no response (e.g., "Do you understand?") they may be embarrassed to admit they do not know (Graham & Brookey, 2008). A better approach would be to ask them to describe what they know or ask them to put what they know in their own words.

While close-ended questions may not require significant elaboration and are therefore easier for some patients and families to answer, there are clear drawbacks. Closed-ended questions have the effect of restricting patients' or family members' range of response. Because of this, patients are not encouraged to explore their experience or help to express their thoughts, concerns, or feelings. Closed-ended questions ask for specific data and provide limited possibilities for response, running the risk that information gathered is incomplete.

The following example illustrates this possibility.

Provider: "Are you having much pain?" (Closed-ended question)

Patient: "Yes."

Provider: "Is it about the same?" (Closed-ended question)

Patient: "I think it's worse."

Observe that the provider's questions call for brief responses from the patient; one to three words is the result. The patient is not encouraged to describe the pain or give details concerning the character of the pain.

Important information may be missed because the patient does not expand on the answers provided. In the example provided, the patient could have given important information about the pain experience (strength, nature, and location) and whether the patient's tolerance for the pain has changed. Because a second closed-ended question is used it does not open up the opportunity to explore the patient's experience (again, requires a yes or no response).

Consequently, providers learn little additional facts about the character of the patient's pain unless they change the question format.

Although information comparing the current pain with former pain is relevant, it does not improve an assessment of how the patient is tolerating the pain or whether and how this pain is different. Additionally, patients may also feel that there is a chance that the provider will not understand the nature and experience of pain they are having. Asking closed-ended questions when patients need to talk openly about their pain can cause them to question the provider's interest in really knowing them and the provider's competence in adequately assessing and treating their pain.

Closed-ended questions are not always inadvisable, however. Closed-ended questions can be effective in focusing the discussion. In fact, this is the major advantage of this type of question format. When closed-ended questions are asked after patients give their own account of their experience, they help focus, clarify, and specify certain essential details. In this way closed-ended questions, placed judiciously in the conversation, do not hinder communication. In summary, the actual characteristics of closed-ended questions that can hamper therapeutic communications are also those that can also be useful. When a patient is in an emergency situation and it is difficult for him or her to verbalize the experience of pain, closed-ended questions are preferable. Vital information must be collected quickly, and closed-ended questions are very useful in cases where, for example, the level and location of pain must be rapidly assessed in emergency situations.

Open-Ended Questions

Unlike closed-ended questions, **open-ended questions** require patients or their families to respond with more than a yes, no, or nod of the head. Although open-ended questions are underused, they are preferred for several reasons. Because these questions are looking for no specific answer, they encourage patients to provide a more in-depth and detailed response. This detail can reveal patients' understanding or lack of understanding of their condition and treatment, their unique cultural orientation, their expectations for the provider, and any areas where they harbor inaccurate assumptions about their condition and future treatment. These questions give providers clues about where to go next.

Because they allow for patients to answer in *free-form*, unbound by providers' specific clinical inquiry, they encourage patients to explore different experiences and provide more information. Tongue et al. (2005) explain that open-ended questions allow patients to define the conversation, both in content and direction. Robinson and Heritage (2006) recommend that patient visits begin with opened inquiry (e.g., "What can I do for you today?") emphasizing that patients value opportunities to express their concerns in their own time and terms even though they might not use the opportunity.

In contrast with closed-ended questions, open-ended questions give patients considerable more influence over the direction of the conversation to follow. Tongue advises that while it might be hard to do, providers should also wait until the patient is finished responding to the open-ended question asked; it takes 2 minutes for patients to tell their story, but providers typically interrupt the process in the first 18–23 seconds.

Open-ended questions are powerful because they invite full disclosure. For example, the questions "What barriers do you face in following your diet?"; "Taking your pills?"; "Calling for an appointment?" are questions that ask the patient to tell more. They are effectively used as lead-ins to a topic and ways to gain data on patients' perspectives of an event, issue, or condition. Certain open-ended questions have the impact of delivering an important person-centered clinical orientation. For example, the Patient Dignity Question (PDQ) "What do I need to know about you as a person to take the best care of you that I can?" used

to understand the patient as a person is one example (Johnston et al., 2015). This question has been studied for its effectiveness in delivering patient-centered care to persons facing end-of-life care but clearly is useful in a wide range of patient care situations. Open-ended questions not only invite a range of responses, they tend to elicit in-depth thinking and active participation on the part of the patient and/or patient's family.

Open-ended questions work very well at the start of an interview because they identify unrecognized needs for information. First, the patient is not only encouraged to provide information but also to establish an open, collaborative relationship with the provider. Responses to these questions also reveal what the patient does know and does not know, which may be the target of the providers' teaching plan. Generally, open-ended questions have more of a tendency to convey caring and concern when compared with the closed-ended format (**EXHIBIT 9-3**).

Notice that the nurse started the interview with a brief introduction followed by a broad lead-in. Although the lead-in was not a "what" or "how" phrase, the result was effective. It led to open exploration of how the patient viewed surgery and the prospects of functional recovery. Because the lead-in was broad, the patient was able to elaborate on some feelings and concerns that he or she had had throughout the past year. A point worth noting here is that the provider could have reflected upon and validated the patient's feelings of frustration and helplessness in order to communicate an empathetic presence, but the open-ended method of inquiry provided the patient maximum freedom to explore the issues relevant to them.

As with closed-ended questions, open-ended questions have limitations. First, because these questions are broad in scope, they result in a certain amount of unpredictability in the direction of the dialogue, and it is frequently the case that some very relevant information or facts might not be included. Open-ended

EXHIBIT 9-3 Dialogue Box Illustrating the Time and Attention Allowed with Open-Ended Questions

PROVIDER:	"Hi, Kristina."
PATIENT:	"Hi."
PROVIDER:	"I'm Dr. Landon's nurse, Julie. He wanted me to speak with you for a few moments before he comes in to talk with you. I understand this may possibly be your fifth surgery."
PATIENT:	"Yeah…yeah." (Nodding head)
PROVIDER:	"Can you tell me how you're feeling about the possibility of having a fifth surgery?" (Open lead-in)
PATIENT:	"Um, I'm getting really frustrated because when they did my leg surgery last September, they told me that was it. I could go to college, play volleyball, and do whatever I want. Now it's giving out on me (sounding exasperated). I don't feel happy at all…not that I'd feel happy about my leg giving out. But it's just that when they tell you that you should be OK, and that you'll be a normal young person again, and then you're not allowed to and they can't do anything about it, it's hard. I know I'm gonna be here again. I'm gonna probably go to surgery so they can look and see what happened. But, I mean, I can't even walk down a hill because it is so painful, and I'm favoring the weak leg and putting too much weight on my opposite leg. I had to be carried down the hill and it was really humiliating, especially when, you know, you've gone through a surgery and you expect it to be like normal again. After that surgery I had to go through a year of physical therapy. And you're supposed to be fine. And then it's not fine and hurts; you just don't know what (who) to trust anymore."
PROVIDER:	"What has the doctor told you about your problem?" (Open-ended question)
PATIENT:	"Oh, well, he…well, ya know, he reconstructed the anterior cruciate ligament which, um, I don't know what the problem is right now. Because finally I'm walking on regular land, and I'm walking uphill—it's just the downhill part. He didn't tell me what the possibilities were for the surgery. He didn't tell me if it was, uh, if it was the cartilage, or if the meniscus was torn, or what. So, I don't know. Maybe I could talk to him about that."
PROVIDER:	"Yeah, maybe you could talk to him about that so you can get a better picture for yourself…understand why another surgery might be needed. How did your last surgery go?" (Open-ended question)
PATIENT:	"It was OK. It was OK because I went in there really hopeful, ya know, because I hadn't played volleyball in 4 years and I thought I could play again. I skipped my entire high school career of volleyball. And I figured, not that I'm planning on playing in any big way when I get to college or anything…but I want to be able to go outside and play and have a good time. I haven't been able to run, or dance, or swim, or anything. The surgery was just a really big hopeful thing for me. But, now I think it didn't work."

questions then are rarely completely effective if not interspersed with other types of questions that focus patients and direct them along the lines of an in-depth exploration of a specific topic. Sometimes it is very important to limit and focus patients' responses. Patients in crisis or those unable to carry on an extended dialogue are examples of situations in which open-ended questions may not be the format of choice.

In summary, open-ended questions allow patients unlimited answers. While patients feel free to express themselves, providers can gain essential knowledge needed to build a better understanding of the care that the patient needs. Also, open-ended questions usually evoke more self-exploration by the patient, increasing the probability of further collaborative problem solving.

Effective use of open-ended questions requires careful wording of the questions to give some, but minimal, direction. The provider's conscious effort to actively listen to patients' responses and willingness and ability to introject when needed to keep the patient focused on the topic is important. Even though open-ended formats invite many possible responses, they should never be completely without structure and direction. Still, the open-ended question format (e.g., "What questions do you have?") is more productive than closed-ended formatted questions (e.g., "Do you have any questions?"). Clearly, expertise in asking open-ended questions is a skill that needs to be developed and maintained in clinical practice.

Multiple-Choice Question Format

A third question format is the multiple-choice question. Typically, this question offers a number of alternative topics or decision routes, and the patient is expected to choose among the options provided (**EXHIBIT 9-4**).

In view of the dialogue presented, the patient was clearly given a choice, was able to assess the options, and was able to select among them. This process can be extremely helpful to patients who feel as if control has been taken away from them and who feel as if they are mere objects not people. When patients are given the opportunity to choose and prioritize aspects of care, some feelings of dependency are lessened.

The multiple-choice format is helpful when the provider is attempting to sort issues and prioritize concerns but needs the patient's cooperation to fully explore these areas. For example, providers may want to know whether the patient is concerned about postsurgical recovery but also needs to discuss the type of anesthesia and the expected surgical outcomes.

EXHIBIT 9-4 Dialogue Box Illustrating the Use of Multiple-Choice Questions
Consider the following dialogue between a nurse's aide and a patient.
PROVIDER: "Good morning, Miss Wilson."
PATIENT: "Good morning."
PROVIDER: "Miss Wilson, in what order would you like me to help you with your morning care? Would you like to brush your teeth, wash up a little, or eat breakfast first?" (Multiple-choice question format)
PATIENT: "Brushing my teeth first, then eating my breakfast."
PROVIDER: "OK. Now, the doctor recommended that you walk twice a day for 15 minutes. Do you want to take a nap before you walk or take a shower?" (Multiple-choice question format)
PATIENT: "Let me take a nap because I was not able to sleep last night. Then we can walk."

The provider can decide, independently of patient input, what topics will come first or give the patient some choice.

It is not that the provider presents a menu of topics from which the patient selects; rather, the patient is informed of all the issues that need to be addressed and selects areas in sequential order based on their interest and readiness to explore the topics presented to them. The multiple-choice question format may work well with adult patients as well as with adolescents because it provides security in structure while at the same time engaging them in active participation and shared decision-making.

The major drawback of **multiple-choice questions** is that they are frequently complicated. They can be experienced in much the same way as double-barreled questions, where two or more questions are posed at the same time. If patients are not cognitively able to separate, sort, and evaluate options, the result may be frustration. Like double-barreled questions, multiple-choice questions can also cause the patient and/or family member to feel rushed and confused.

▶ Choice of Question Format and Response Burden

In considering which question format will be best, providers might use a variety of criteria. These include the purpose of the data-collection activity, details about the patient's condition, and the nature of the provider–patient relationship.

Factors about the patient that determine which question format is best includes the patient's present level of physical and emotional distress, the patient's actual and potential responses to the subject matter, cultural preferences, and the patient's knowledge and experience. All of these factors significantly affect patients' desires and abilities to communicate verbally and meet the demands of the question–answer task. These elements comprise the **question response burden**. As indicated earlier, types of question formats have certain response burdens. When using a question format, it is always important to consider not only what type of information this format elicits but also likely response burden the patient will experience.

Open-ended questions allow the patient to verbalize without restriction. They require a minimum amount of sorting and processing. Decisions about what is appropriate or inappropriate are not imposed on the patient. Patients who respond positively to open-ended questions are usually those who need to talk, like to express themselves verbally, and have the energy to engage in extended conversations. They usually have moderate levels of trust and positive attitudes toward providers.

Other patients may not be as amenable to data collection with the open-ended format. These are patients who are less comfortable verbalizing or may not have the energy or freedom from symptom distress to engage in lengthy conversations. They might also have language deficits or have fairly low literacy levels and feel inadequate in having this type of conversation. Even when offered a broad open-ended leading question (e.g., "How are you doing today?"), they are likely to be parsimonious in their response (e.g., "Not so good" or "OK"). While the response burden of open-ended questions, at first glance, seems to be negligible, there are many situations in which open-ended questions tax the patient's ability to respond.

Closed-ended question formats impose a different response burden. With closed-ended questions, responses are brief. Those patients in pain or distress usually respond better to this type of question. However, it is important to understand what is required of the patient. When a provider asks, "Do you feel pain?", several requirements are made of the patient. First, the patient must decode the provider's terms (e.g., *pain*).

Patients must discern what is meant by these terms and why the provider is asking for this information. Additionally, patients must identify their experience as pain or perhaps something else. Patients must be able to focus, decode, and encode their experience and, at the same time, be brief. While not much is required in terms of verbal response, more is required in terms of decoding and encoding communication between the provider and the patient.

Questions worded in the multiple-choice format are like closed-ended questions because they require further data-processing and decision-making capabilities on the patient's part. As indicated previously, this format is usually used to pinpoint (i.e., to rule in or rule out) different possibilities.

If the provider asks the patient, "Are you having pain here, here, how about here—and, where is the pain worse? Here or here?", certain patient skills are needed. As with closed-ended questions, the patient must be able to focus and decode the provider's language and encode his or her own. However, what is also required with this format is the ability to compare and contrast, cross-referencing different experiences of pain or pressure. For some patients under certain circumstances, this requirement is beyond their capability. They may have problems in encoding and decoding and also have problems with comparative analysis. While it would seem that the multiple-choice question format leads to efficiency in data collection, providers also run the risk of getting very little data. Language barriers, present distress, and cognitive deficits can all contribute to patients' inabilities to use this question format.

▶ Summary

As indicated in this chapter, the provider–patient relationship is characterized by the privilege and expectation of asking questions of the patient. However, this privilege and expectation also extends to the patient and the patient's family. In effective therapeutic relationships, patients and their families are encouraged to ask questions, whatever questions that will help them to understand the provider's assessment process and choice of treatment. The primary therapeutic motive for providers asking questions is to derive complete and accurate data on which to plan and deliver care to patients. Secondary to this purpose is the opportunity questions afford in building a therapeutic connection which will always include patients and/or their families asking their own questions.

Questions help open dialogue, direct discussions, command attention in a given area, and clarify. In our society, people experience questions of all types. Many questions seem irrelevant. Still, within the patient–provider relationship, questions are more deliberate

than accidental or capricious. Providers are diagnostically oriented, and this orientation is based on the thoughtful selection of the appropriate context and format for questions.

The appropriate use of questions includes gathering data, seeking clarification and qualification, and pinpointing or ruling in or out possible conditions. Question formats—closed, open, or multiple choice—are options in the provider's exploration of the patient's condition and experience. Different question formats elicit different responses, and it is important to understand the strengths and limitations of each of these formats. In truth, one format alone will not suffice. Rather, providers need to be able to draw on each format discriminately.

Questions are not always used in therapeutic ways. Clearly, they can be misused. Several examples were provided in this chapter. Questions can mask interpretations and advice. In these cases, while questions are used to soften the impact and directness of other response modes, the provider runs the risk of confusing the patient. Direct questions are particularly problematic because too many ill-placed direct questions can be confusing and cause patients to feel defensive. The consequences can defeat the essential purpose for which questions were designed. Questions should always allow reply without intimidation or defensiveness.

Questions, whether open, closed, or multiple choice in format, are a primary means of providers gathering information from patients and their families. The idea however is not that providers have questions but patients and their families do not. It should be stressed again that the goals of collaborative care planning can be met more fully when providing the opportunity and encouragement to ask questions. The art of questioning and the skill of asking an answerable question are central to conversing therapeutically. However, the provision of patient opportunities to ask questions and answer questions when asked is equally important to securing and maintaining therapeutic relationships.

Discussion

1. Explain the link between the provider asking questions and better patient outcomes.
2. Discuss the need to ask questions but also encourage patients to ask questions of providers.
3. Differentiate between therapeutic and nontherapeutic questioning.
4. Describe instances in which close-ended questions may be better than open-ended questions.
5. Explain why telling questions are not really asking questions for the purpose of gathering patient information.

References

Eggly, S., Harper, F. W. K., Penner, L. A., Gleason, M. J., Foster, T., & Albrecht, T. L. (2011). Variation in question asking during cancer clinical interactions: A potential source of disparities in access to information. *Patient Education and Counseling, 82*(1), 63–68. doi:10.1016/j.pec.2010.04.008

Galliher, J. M., Post, D. M., Weiss, B. D., Dickinson, L. M., Manning, B. K., Staton, E. W., … Wilson, W. D. (2010). Patients' question-asking behavior during primary care visits: A report from the AAFP National Research Network. *Annals of Family Medicine, 8*(2), 151–159. doi:10.1370/afm.105

Gazda, G. M., Childers, W. C., & Walters, R. P. (1982). *Interpersonal communication: A handbook for health professionals.* Gaithersburg, MD: Aspen Publishers, Inc. (Epigraph from pp. 141–142).

Graham, S., & Brookey, J. (2008). Do patients understand? *The Permanente Journal, 12*(3), 67–69. PMID:21331214

Gruman, J., Rovner, M. H., French, M. E., Jeffress, D., Sofaer, S., Shaller, D., & Prager, D. J. (2010). From patient education to patient engagement: Implications for the field of patient education. *Patient Education and Counseling, 78,* 350–356. doi:10.1016/j.pec.2010.02.002

Johnston, B., Pringle, J., Gaffney, M., Narayanasamy, M., McGuire, M., & Buchanan, D. (2015). The dignified approach to care: A pilot study using the patient dignity question as an intervention to enhance dignity and person-centred care for people with palliative care needs in the acute hospital setting. *BMC Palliative Care, 14*(1), 9. doi:10.1186/s12904-015-0013-3

Mazor, K. M., Rubin, D. L., Roblin, D. W., Williams, A. E., Han, P. K. J., Gaglio, B., … Wagner, J. L. (2016). Health literacy–listening skill and patient questions following cancer prevention and screening discussions. *Health Expectations: An International Journal of Public Participation in Health Care and Health Policy, 19*(4), 920–934. doi:10.1111/hex.12387

Pawar, M. (2005). Five tips for generating patient satisfaction and compliance. *Family Practice Management, 12*(6), 44–46. Retrieved from www.aafp.org/fpm

Penner, L. A., Dovidio, J. F., Gonzalez, R., Albrecht, T. L., Foster, T., Harper, F. W. K., … Eggly, S. (2016). The effects of oncologist implicit racial bias in racially discordant oncology interactions. *Journal of Clinical Oncology, 34*(24), 2874–2880. doi:10.1200/JCO.2015.66.3658

Robinson, J. D., & Heritage, J. (2006). Physicians' opening questions and patients' satisfaction. *Patient Education and Counseling, 60,* 279–285. doi:10.1016/j.pec.2005.11.009

Tongue, J. R., Epps, H. R., & Forese, L. L. (2005). Communication skills for patient-centered care. *The Journal of Bone and Joint Surgery, 87,* 652–658. Retrieved from JBJS.org

CHAPTER 10

Therapeutic Use of Silence and Pauses

CHAPTER OBJECTIVES

- Define silence as a therapeutic response mode.
- List several therapeutic purposes for the use of silence and pauses in patient–provider relationships.
- Analyze the meaning of silence in patients' responses and reactions.
- Describe how one might intervene with defensive silences.
- Identify potential negative effects of silence and pauses.

KEY TERMS

- Active listening
- Defensive silence
- Interpersonal space
- Interresponse time
- Interruptive response
- Overtalk
- Pauses
- Self-reflection
- Silence

▶ Introduction

People from various cultures have different perspectives and understandings of silence. Cultural views evolve from religious or spiritual beliefs, and variations are reflected by country and region. Any generalities about cultural differences and proclivities to be comfortable or uncomfortable with silence can be stereotypic but some are worthy of consideration.

In some cultures *talk* is valued, and **silence** is considered a deficit in social skills and/or a lack of knowledge. People subscribing to Western or Eastern philosophies have been shown to hold almost opposite attitudes about talk and silence. Many Western cultures are uncomfortable with more than a few seconds

201

of silence, while Eastern cultures are comfortable with minutes of silence.

"Silence is louder than words" depicts the belief that much is to be gained by observing silences. Stewart (2009) explains that silence is one of the least understood nonverbal behaviors partly because people use it and understand it in many different ways. Silence has received both positive and negative acclaim—"silence is golden" and the notion that silence is to be "overcome" are largely contradicting attitudes.

Silence can be felt as a respite and a time to collect one's thoughts. "Silence speaks louder than words" depicts the belief there is something valuable going on in silent periods. Akin to Eastern philosophy the idea that there is something going on in periods of silence subscribes to meditative periods to discover one's experience and that of others. Otherwise, during silence, insight emerges to help people understand the world within and the world outside.

Among Americans in the Western world an unwillingness to converse can be perceived as unfriendly; silence can be interpreted as impolite, unkind, or arrogant. In many instances, silence is viewed to be devoid of meaning and something *to fill*. Talkativeness exemplifies intellect and social poise and are signs of leadership capabilities. Schools and colleges teach *public speaking*.

Within geographical regions there are differences. For example, among Latin Americans and Italians, talk occupies social relationships and there is rarely times of silence; persons from these groups and others are observed to talk freely and openly and even interrupt or talk over each other. In Western cultures, reactions to silence are, in part, triggered from very early uses of silence. When children are bad, they are told to be "quiet." Adults punish one another by withholding thoughts and feelings. The reasons behind silence are not always clear; to the extent that an individual's silence is unclear or possibly punitive, these quiet periods can evoke uneasiness and increase social distance.

Silence is not considered to be negative in Eastern philosophy, and evidence of communicative patterns document comfort with silence. For example, among Chinese people, silence is positive and regarded as a sign of wisdom and as a way of gaining wisdom. People who are talkative are generally perceived as lacking an awareness of the natural order of things. Pausing in silence for a few seconds before answering a question or introducing a topic is the polite thing to do.

These mixed cultural perspectives and interpretations of silence influence how we feel about the use of therapeutic silence and whether we will use it universally and with all patients. During therapeutic encounters patients and providers may have similar or different levels of comfort with silence. For those providers whose culture values talkativeness, silence may be uncomfortable. Some providers measure the success of an interview on whether silence is kept at a minimum. For those who come from cultures that value silence, talkativeness may be uncomfortable. Thus, for the latter group, spacing remarks with silent periods or **pauses** is not difficult or uncomfortable.

Silence can be excessive and when it is it can increase both patients' and the providers' anxiety. Too much silence can be confusing and be interpreted as unwillingness to communicate or withdrawal from the relationship. Silence can also be interpreted as fear, anger, depression, disinterest, withdrawal, confusion, and inability to express one's thoughts or feelings.

In therapeutic encounters, silence on the part of the provider can be perceived as warmth and understanding or seen as withholding. Some providers intentionally use silent periods to help patients take stock of their situation and feel accepted in an understanding, supportive, and safe environment (Lane, Koetting, & Bishop, 2002). On the flip side, patients can feel threatened and confused about why providers remain silent. Lane and colleagues describing the use of silence in psychotherapy remark that if not skillfully done, this technique can be perceived as therapists' distancing, disinterest, and disengagement. Still, learning to listen in silence is a skill valued by psychotherapists.

As with all therapeutic responses, silence and pauses can be underused or overused. This chapter emphasizes the need to become comfortable with silences, to understand their meaning when it is the patient who is silent, and to draw on them in the therapeutic interview to enhance the productivity of patient–provider encounters and patients' experience of provider empathy.

▶ Definitions of Silence

Silence is the absence of audible sound or noise. In interpersonal interactions it is the absence of audible speech or verbal utterance. A distinction should be made between speech that is inaudible and incoherent speech. Speech that is incoherent or mere utterance is still speech even though it is not understood. It is inappropriate to call a patient silent when in fact they spoke but could not be understood.

Utterances or speech fragments are used not only by patients but also by providers to communicate. According to Hein (1980), silence periods are those times in the therapeutic relationship in which the provider waits, without interruption, for the patient to begin or resume speaking. Further, when used therapeutically, silence can be interspersed with utterances (e.g., "humm" or "uh-huh") which are sounds that display encouragement without interrupting the patient's elaboration of thoughts and feelings.

In actuality, there are two types of silence in the therapeutic relationship. The first is when the patient stops speaking and there is absence of speech before the provider starts speaking, or when the provider stops speaking and there is absence of speech before the patient speaks. The implicit understanding behind conversation is that patient and provider verbalize in the pattern of first one, then the other.

A second type of silence refers to the absence of speech that occurs when either patient or provider stops speaking and then the same person resumes speaking. In either case, the silent space may be long or very short, such as in a pause (see **EXHIBIT 10-1**). A *pause* is said to be a natural rest in the melody of speech, whereas silence is longer. Usually, absence of speech beyond 3–4 seconds is considered a silent period, not just a brief interruption in the course of conversation.

Another way to perceive silence is as **interpersonal space**. Silent periods can say something about psychosocial space in human encounters. The psychosocial space between two individuals, even between the same two people, continually changes.

This phenomenon is also apparent in patient–provider interactions. The space between talk and silence gives clues about patterns of interpersonal space, and this space can be expanded or reduced, depending on the patient or provider. Applying this principle to our daily experiences, it is obvious that

EXHIBIT 10-1 Basic Principles Underlying Silence as a Therapeutic Response Mode

- There is a relationship between an interviewer's and respondent's use of silence; the more silent the interviewer, the more likely the respondent will follow with silence.
- The speech–silence behavior of any given individual in the context of an interview is highly consistent, despite large individual differences in the characteristics of interviewers.
- In some cultures, silence means wisdom; in others, silence might be viewed as withholding, defensiveness, insecurity, and dullness.

increases or decreases in silent periods do occur and reflect the nature of our moods and the characteristics of our relationships with one another. Changes, even small ones, in how interpersonal space is used can make a difference in the quality of our social and professional interactions.

The following illustration demonstrates changes in the quality of interaction when the provider introduces pauses and silences, expanding or decreasing interpersonal space. The example describes the impact these changes can have on personal distancing in this physician's first visit with a new patient (**EXHIBIT 10-2**).

In this case, the introduction of silence by the provider shifted the apparent "power struggle" in the relationship. The patient was openly resisting the provider's advice. Even the idea of doing much more than getting an antibiotic was out of the question for the patient. Through the use of silence the provider moved the patient from a position of resistance to one of being receptive to advice.

Although the physician did not persuade the patient to take the blood test, agreement about increasing the patient's routine medications was established. There may be other reasons the patient refused a blood test. These reasons could reflect noncompliance with some routine medications which would be apparent with the blood test. In this case, the patient would not risk discovery. There are other less directive approaches the physician could have used. Still, the use of silence seemed to successfully reduce the patient's noticeable resistance to following the physician's orders.

EXHIBIT 10-2 Dialogue Box Illustrating the Use of Silence and Pauses

PROVIDER:	"What we should do is take a blood test, then we may need to increase your Theophylline. Also, I think we should add…"
PATIENT:	(Forcefully) "I don't want to have the blood test."
PROVIDER:	"You're not going to get significant results if your dose is not at therapeutic level." (Silence)
PATIENT:	"I go to an allergist. He told me what I need to do. I just want an antibiotic for my bronchitis. (Pause) I don't think a blood test is necessary!"
PROVIDER:	(Silence)
PATIENT:	"You think I should increase my medicine? And I should probably increase my inhaler, right?"
PROVIDER:	"Yes, that's right." (Pause) "And, if you're not feeling better in a week, come back and see me."
PATIENT:	"OK."

▶ The Characteristics of Silence

To understand silence, it is important to question what occurs during silence. There are three basic aspects of silence that are worthy of attention: (1) interresponse time, (2) the interruption response, and (3) the overtalk response.

Interresponse Time

Interresponse time refers to the number of seconds or minutes in a silence period. A typical social conversation contains many interresponse times that are less than a second long. This feature of conversation, many short silences, tends to characterize social interaction. It would be peculiar to engage in longer silences when speaking with casual acquaintances, yet it is expected in therapeutic encounters, especially in psychotherapy sessions.

As in previous discussions of silence, in some cultures shorter response times are typical. However, other cultures abide by longer response times. Longer response time and slowness of speech are common in certain regions of the United States. For example, some people from Maine, the Appalachians, and parts of the South and Southwest may speak slower and use interresponse times that are more than a second in length.

These communities can be contrasted with regions in the city of New York where fast-paced speech is common and may be experienced as crowding. Crowded speech can contain many examples of interresponse times that are much less than a second. These tendencies become even more obvious when situational or environmental situations affect speech. For example, the city dweller on a camping vacation in the mountains or on a sailing excursion may feel out of sorts but adapt to the slower pace of everyday life. In turn, those slower-speaking individuals may find it very irritating to stand in line at Kennedy Airport or hail a cab on Fifth Avenue (New York). Over time they might adapt and view it as exciting.

Patients' health conditions and illness frequently affect the speed of their speech and their tendency to use short or long durations of silence between phrases. For example, patients who are suffering pain, fatigue, or lethargy, or who are depressed, will tend to exhibit longer interresponse times. The elderly usually require added time to assemble their ideas due to physical and mental processes as do people with limited literacy or developmental delays. Patients who are anxious, excitable, agitated, or manic may exhibit more rapid speech that allows for fewer interruptions.

Interresponse times of 3 or 4 seconds or more are more than brief pauses between expressed ideas. They are frequently used as space to think about something new or to think over a previously expressed thought. These times are distinct and do not resemble pauses where little thinking is occurring.

In a fast-paced conversation, however, 2-seconds interresponse times may be enough to provide additional thinking and feeling experiences and, thus, are not merely pauses. In a helping relationship or therapeutic dialogue, silences can last up to 10 seconds, sometimes longer. Also, a change in dialogue where 1 or 2 seconds of silence are added may communicate allowance to think and feel, and assists patients to sort and regroup their thoughts or develop a new slant on the feelings they have expressed.

In an early classic study of response times in patient–provider encounters, the character of silence periods and patients' reactions were reported. Adult patients evaluated providers' use of silence. The study revealed that the use of silence (reaction-time latency) between speakers contributed to patients' satisfaction (Rowland-Morin & Carroll, 1990). Otherwise, patients were more satisfied not only when silence occurred in interviews but also when physicians utilized words that the patient used and interrupted with reflections.

Patients' views of provider interruptions cutting off patient communication and not allowing for interspersed silences were also studied in an analysis of residents' medical consultations with clinic patients. This study reported that intrusive interruptions by these providers resulted in lower patient satisfaction (Li, Zhang, Yum, Lundgren, & Pahal, 2008). Further, sicker patients were interrupted more frequently and were less satisfied with the way they were treated by the provider.

Interruptions

Just as adding a mere 2 seconds to silence can provide patients interpersonal space, taking 1 or 2 seconds from the silence pattern can create a feeling of being crowded or rushed by the provider. Consider the following dialogue and the effect of changing interresponse time in periods of silence. This is a dialogue between a nurse and a patient describing his headaches (**EXHIBIT 10-3**).

EXHIBIT 10-3 Dialogue Box Illustrating the Impact of Changes in Interresponse Time

PROVIDER:	"Did the medication help you?"
PATIENT:	"Yup—but it was hard…"
PROVIDER:	"Do you have any ideas about what you can do?" (Interruption)
PATIENT:	(Looking at the nurse) "No—I feel frustrated!"
PROVIDER:	(Silence, 4 seconds).
PATIENT:	"I really don't know what I'm going to do about this stuff the doctor gave me. If I take it, I'm worthless as far as working goes and actually everything else, and so I just get further and further behind. If I don't take it, I can't see straight and I don't get much more done. God, I feel frustrated!"
PROVIDER:	"Yes…" (Silence, 2 seconds)
PATIENT:	"Actually, I wonder what would happen if I only took half the pill? Maybe I'll run that by the doctor and see what he thinks. Or, I could call him and see if there is anything else he could give me."

Notice that in the beginning of this conversation the provider crowded the patient, even interrupted him in midthought. When the patient was provided extended interpersonal space he was able to gather his thoughts and decrease his frustration by coming up with a plan. He constructed two potential solutions to the dilemma he was facing. By altering the interresponse time between statements, the nurse was able to modify the pressure he felt generated from the frustration and create a climate for problem solving.

Interruptions have a significant impact on conversation. Interruptions or **interruptive responses** are disruptions of another individual's speech and generally have the impact of cutting short the expression of the person's ideas. Interruptions can occur in the middle of a statement or in the brief lull that occurs between expressed thoughts and feelings. The circumstance in which both parties begin speaking simultaneously is called overtalk.

Overtalk

Conversation can be filled with interruptions. This is referred to as **overtalk** and usually results in significant barriers to communication for both individuals. There are specific instances in which most people will engage in overtalk. The most familiar circumstance is when people are arguing. When either or both parties are feeling threatened, overtalk may be a defense against any distress they experience. Overtalk essentially communicates the message "cease or stop this." What might occur is the opposite, an escalation of comments, which may be accusations.

Some people habitually interrupt. This style of communicating influences the way they work with others and the way others feel about them. Frequently the behavior is interpreted as bullying, but can really represent something opposite. Patients who habitually interrupt may feel exceedingly threatened. Because they crowd out others in their communication, they may also be prone to fears of rejection.

Their interruptions can also reflect boredom, the need to dominate others, reactions to redundancy, or reactions to freshly stimulated thoughts and feelings. Providers can overtalk because the patient is not providing quickly enough the information they need. In this way, the provider is saying "Don't finish, listen to me!" Or, "I can guess what you are going to say—let me say it." Conversations with many interruptions and a good deal of overtalk can be filled with incomplete messages. If one individual does not back off for 3 or 4 seconds, overtalk fills the space, and significant interpersonal crowding sets in. There may be many incomplete messages because neither person was able to voice a complete thought or idea.

In summary, overtalk and interruptions are important aspects of interresponse boundaries when there is no silence. As previously explained, overtalk and interruptions crowd conversation. Silence allows for thoughtful reflection and the development of understanding and insight, which is the primary objective in provider–patient relationships. Hence, silence in helping relationships can extend to 10 seconds or even longer. Crowding can actually reduce the tendency for patients to disclose. With crowding, patients can experience being misunderstood, frustrated, and dissatisfied. Patients who are recipients of crowding might fear that their needs to be understood will go unmet.

A final point should be made. Providers can actually elicit interruptions and overtalk from patients by using them first. So, the idea is not only to avoid using them but avoid eliciting them. If providers do not initiate these response patterns they might mirror them back to the patient almost unconsciously, matching the pace and character of patients' overtalk or interruptions. The results are two frustrated and dissatisfied individuals. In the event that this happens, the primary corrective measure is the provider's conscious and deliberate use of silence to alter the nature of the encounter. Providers can use silence to slow down the pace and change any tendency to interrupt and overtalk.

▶ Therapeutic Purpose of Silence in the Provider–Patient Relationship

As previously noted, silences can be used therapeutically. There are several important purposes for using silence in therapeutic dialogues with patients. These include (1) providing space for reflection in order to assess and analyze the patient's condition and (2) communicating empathy and compassion. However, the primary purpose in providing interpersonal space through silence is to encourage patients to take the lead in explaining their condition and experiences more fully.

Encouraging Patients to Speak

Silence can encourage patients to speak, especially if the provider shows interest and expectation. This kind of silence invites patients to initiate the topic that they feel is most pressing or important. Further, silent interludes give patients the opportunity to collect and organize their thoughts and think through what they want to say next. Using silence can also reduce the pace of the interview, creating more interpersonal space in the dialogue. This strategy can encourage patients to delve more deeply, weigh a decision, or consider alternative actions—in essence, be more participatory in assessing their condition, planning, and evaluating their care.

These therapeutic effects of silence were illustrated in the earlier dialogue between the nurse and patient. By providing the patient with silent interludes, the nurse enabled the patient to delve more deeply into his dilemma; as a result, he thought of a new course of action. By not asking pointless questions, the provider gave the patient room to be spontaneous and to move from simple to more complex analyses of his dilemma.

Rather than remaining confused and upset about the medication he was prescribed, he decided to talk to his doctor and request a change in dosage or a new drug. While the nurse could have cut short this decision process by merely advising the patient what to do, the real value of this interchange was that the patient came to his own decision. This process acknowledged both his responsibility to communicate with his physician and his right to receive better care.

Communicating Empathy and Compassion

Silent periods have been noted for their ability to touch emotions and inspire compassion (Tornøe, Danbolt, Kvigne, & Sørlie, 2014). Emotions are experiential and complex, having origins in personal history. Sometimes words that are used to describe emotions are inadequate and simplistic. It is important to recognize what is being communicated by silence during each silent period.

Communicating empathy and compassion in a therapeutic interview is facilitated with the use of silence. Silence conveys **active listening** which is essential to both empathic and compassionate responses. To successfully achieve active listening, the provider must display interest.

Active listening during silence communicates that providers want to hear what patients have to say—to enter the world of the patient and understand it more fully. It conveys an interest in the patient's well-being beyond that demonstrated by specific gestures that "do" something. The power in silence is that it provides an unhurried atmosphere in which patients can reflect on their experiences in the presence of their provider.

While it would appear that the provider is doing nothing in these moments of silence, in actuality much is going on. During these interludes, the provider is observing what patients do, hearing what patients say and how they

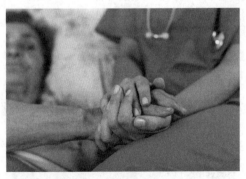

© Lighthunter/Shutterstock.

say it, feeling how patients feel, and sensing what patients have not said but may want to say. Silence often communicates caring when words are superfluous. In a summary of interviews of hospice nurses describing their experience with terminally ill patients, Tornøe and colleagues spoke of the concept of "consoling through silence." These nurses explained that sharing the silence with patients could have a powerful consoling effect. They also revealed that sharing silence with patients required a shift from "doing something for the patient" to "being with the patient."

Providers during hurried states are usually perceived as incapable or unwilling to know patients more fully. When they relinquish their distractions and focus in silence with the patient, they are conveying not only the capability to understand the patient but also the willingness to do so.

Assessment of Patient Condition

In addition to encouraging patients to describe their experiences and to convey empathetic and compassionate understanding, silent interludes are critical for focusing for the purposes of conducting in-depth and detailed assessments of patients. Finset (2016) aptly describes the value of slowing the pace of patient–provider discussions. He explained that slowing the pace and allowing for brief silences may facilitate patient disclosure of relevant concerns and thoughts. This idea goes beyond the obvious point that to obtain clinical data, providers will lapse into silent periods as they listen for chest sounds, palpate a pulse, or examine a severe overbite.

During silences, providers have opportunities to observe verbal and nonverbal behaviors. They also have opportunities to look for incongruencies in how patients feel about their condition or the prescribed plan of care. To be aware of incongruencies, providers must understand the full range of nonverbal expressions—fear, anxiety, hostility, sadness, depression, relief, happiness, and excitement.

Because silences provide open-ended opportunities to observe, providers may need to organize their points of focus—use verbal and nonverbal messages of thoughts and feelings, pick up subtle attitudes and underlying beliefs, observe patients' own reactions to their disclosures, and construct a composite picture of the patient's experience as witnessed by the clinician. This process then tends to further convey understanding on the part of clinicians as well as their ability to be helpful.

Thoughtful Self-Reflection

A final purpose of silence is the provision for thoughtful **self-reflection** on the part of the provider. This process is one of becoming aware of one's thoughts, feelings, and actions without assigning judgment. Many researchers have identified the importance of self-reflection and reflective practices in preparing competent health professionals (Amini, Bilan, & Ghasempour, 2015; Mann, Gordon, & MacLeod, 2007; Murdoch-Eaton & Sandars, 2014). Reflection is frequently addressed and for good reasons. As health professionals are functioning in more complex health care settings, the need to solve multifaceted patient and health care problems and the need for reflective practice become even more important.

The opportunity to observe oneself in therapeutic encounters is not something that is familiar to all clinicians but can be easier for seasoned professionals. The skill of reflection can draw the provider away from the immediate task at hand. When providers observe themselves in the context of their encounters with patients they learn that a great deal is happening between them and their patients, some of which they will not immediately understand. This includes becoming aware of attitudes, judgments, and feelings.

The following data can be retrieved by simply reflecting on one's own thoughts and feelings in the silent periods of a therapeutic interview.

- How am I feeling about what the patient is saying? What am I not saying?
- How am I reacting to the manner in which the patient is communicating?
- How is the context of this interview affecting me and what I do and do not say?
- What am I trying to achieve? How well is it working?
- What do I want to communicate above all else to help this patient?

Just as silence gives patients the opportunity to think through a point or to consider introducing a topic, providers are given the same opportunity to collect and reassemble their thoughts through reflective practice. In actuality, silent periods provide both providers and patients important time-outs that serve the therapeutic aims of the interview.

▶ Analysis of Silence in Patients' Responses

Sometimes patients are silent, but this silence does not seem to serve the patient therapeutically. The answer as to why the patient is silent is usually a very complex one. First, silence may be a function of their physical condition. Beyond physical reasons there is a host of other underlying reasons. Patients' silences may indicate anger, fear, depression, disinterest, withdrawal, or a whole host of feelings, including absence of emotion. Silence can be a response to cultural differences. Davidhizar and Giger (1994) suggest that a number of problems may arise when silence occurs in an interpersonal situation. Among these problems are the different meanings that silence may have from culture to culture.

Sometimes patients refuse to talk, and while these cases are not as common as lapses into silence, they are extremely important to understand. There are three reasons patients may refuse to talk: (1) defensiveness against perceived threats, (2) provocation—to get the provider to seek them out, or (3) underlying hostility and resistance. These reasons are discussed as follows.

The Basis for Defensive Silences

Patients' silences can mean many things. But, the defensive use of silence can demonstrate patients' beliefs that if they are silent and withhold thoughts and feelings, they will avoid being scrutinized or criticized. There are several potential reasons for this silence. For example, patients may have a history of repeated exposures to being insulted or shamed when they expressed themselves; their families may have shunned expressions of different thoughts or ideas; or significant mental and physical abuse could have occurred when the patient spoke up or spoke out. In any case, the patient could develop a patterned response to withdraw and/or to remain silent in situations they perceived to be threatening. Over time, they may have become unaware of this defensive reaction. Therefore, it is possible that patients will not respond to such queries as "Why are you quiet?" They may not know or not fully understand the meaning of their silence.

A second dynamic behind patients' refusal to speak might be their desire to be sought out. This silence is conveyed as provocation (e.g., treat me as special). In essence, the provider is being tested. These behaviors are manipulative and when used repetitively by patients tend to cause anger, hostility, and resentment in providers. While the original intent of the patient was to secure a helping relationship, the outcome is the opposite—the patient has provoked the provider, who, in turn, withdraws. Providers' reflections about the underlying meaning of patients' motives can reverse this process and motivate providers' to respond differently.

A third explanation for silence in interpersonal situations is harbored feelings of hostility, anger, and resentment. Patients who exhibit silence out of hostility, anger, or resentment communicate these feelings but act as if they did not. These silences are usually cold, rejecting, punishing kinds of silence. Silences of this kind are frequently used in social relationships (e.g., to communicate anger when one's partner is late or has forgotten an important occasion such as an anniversary). They are generally regarded as passive-aggressive. In fact, some individuals will use the ambiguity surrounding silence as a punishment (i.e., "You think you know why I am quiet, but I know you don't know for sure…You will have to suffer with uncertainty until I decide to tell you why I won't speak to you."). In the context of a patient–provider encounter underlying feelings of hostility and anger, patients may refuse to answer provider questions or answer the provider's question with a question.

Finally, patients' silences can reflect their health condition and both verbal and cognitive barriers to enter into open dialogue or even respond to one or two questions. Providers understand that the patient's capacities to communicate may be limited due to illness but they may not be fully prepared to understand anger and hostility in periods of silence.

Providers seem to assume that patients will not exhibit these behaviors in their interviews with them. Usually this belief does not reflect all the dimensions of what the patient–provider relationship might mean. There are many reasons why patients may communicate their hostility through silence:

- Providers are generally regarded as authority figures. Patients might have early programming that causes them to be passive-aggressive in the context of dominant-submissive relationships.
- Patients may fear reprisal if they communicate their anger directly. They may be fearful of being neglected or of receiving inferior care.
- Whatever irritation or upset they experience may be perceived as insignificant in the context of the larger picture. That is, patients may recognize their distress and deliberately minimize it because there are so many other issues of equal or greater importance to them.

Nonetheless, the result is the same. The pattern that can occur is that patients contain their feelings and lapse into silence. Still angry, they can passively communicate their anger and this becomes a barrier to patient–provider participatory decision-making and care planning.

Intervening with Defensive Silences

It is important to understand that patients' silences may mean many things. Also, the negative use of silence by patients is not easily discussed with them. In fact, one's first take should always be understanding silence at face value where silence means "I am not ready to talk about that" or just "I'm not able to talk or answer you." It is important to acknowledge this meaning and invite them to respond at their own pace (provided that this offer does not interfere with their care). When silence proves to inhibit disclosures that are necessary to deliver care, providers are likely to help them to open up; but, if this is not possible they will turn to identified patient representatives or family members.

There are important steps in dealing with negative, **defensive silence** in patients. As previously suggested initially, the provider needs to demonstrate acceptance of the patient's silence. One method is to listen beyond the silence, reflecting and attending to the patient. This behavior will demonstrate acceptance. Second, providers need to note the context of the silence and if there is a trend. Does the patient lapse into silence about certain topics, such as about embarrassing details or sensitive subjects like sexual behavior, drug and alcohol use, or abusive spousal experiences? Approach these topics with respect. If patients lapse into silences, they are generally more sensitive about these topics. If patients' silences are interrupted, they may become more defensive and be increasingly anxious. The provider runs the risk of permanently cutting short patients' self-disclosures and worse yet, force them to terminate their care prematurely by not returning for follow-up.

One rule of thumb is that when asking for verbal replies in these situations, begin with neutral themes or superficial material, or talk around the topic until the patient feels more comfortable. Providers also need to consider silences as symptomatic of something else. A gentle lead—"I'm trying to understand what's on your mind…but, I'm having difficulty knowing exactly what's bothering you," or "I am interested in helping you through this…."—is helpful. Exploring the meaning behind silences is important. But this cannot always be done directly (e.g., "Why are you silent?"). Direct questions can reduce disclosure because they come across as critical, not supportive.

Most effective is a simple suggestion that their silence is a sign that something else is bothering them and that if they share it (all or in part) they may feel different or better. Patients generally understand that sharing difficulties with others can feel supportive. They just do not know whether providers will extend the same level of support. Exploring these dynamics can enable patients to feel providers' support.

▶ Negative Effects of Using Silence

Silence is not always a helpful technique for providers to use in provider's interactions with patients and their families. Providers use of silence responses are often difficult to apply in a manner that will achieve maximum benefit and minimize the chance of sending the wrong message (e.g., aloofness, uncaring, coldness) or otherwise being counterproductive. Silence can extend beyond the point of usefulness, thoughts tend to drift, and the focus of the interview can be lost (Collins, 1977). When this occurs, the silence becomes uncomfortable and may provoke anxiety in both the provider and the patient.

Mixed messages about providers' tolerance of silence can also defeat the therapeutic effects of silence. The ambiguous message, "I accept your need to be quiet but at the same time don't like the stillness in the room," gives two conflicting messages.

The amount of silence always depends on the tolerance of both provider and patient and might vary from time to time. Providers might be needing to fill every lapse in conversation with verbiage. Remember, providers own cultural beliefs and past experiences can impact their comfort with silence. When providers have difficulty dealing with silence, they run the risk of inadvertently punishing the patient while remaining mostly silent. Punishment can be delivered by insincere or sarcastic responses or simple gestures that suggest, in subtle ways, "If you have nothing to say (ask, talk about) then I won't waste my time with you." A potential therapeutic encounter becomes unproductive when providers' needs take precedence over those of the patient and produces a negative tone.

The opposite situation in which the provider feels more comfortable with silence and the patient's natural mode is to be talkative can elicit similar outcomes. Essentially the patient will experience little direction from the provider. The patient's need for a response and feedback is thwarted, again because the provider's needs take precedence. Usually when patients don't receive the feedback they need, they will begin to repeat themselves in a second or even third attempt to get a response.

They might feel confused and wonder about how the provider feels about them. With patients who are distrustful, silence of any length can evoke more anxiety. Also, too much silence from providers tends to put pressure on patients to speak when they are not feeling well or unable to speak. Generally, an interaction

filled with too many pauses or silent periods can result in feelings that the purpose of the conversation is unclear and unfocused.

The tendency to respond in kind can also present problems in the therapeutic interview. In this case, the provider's silence can even become "a game" where the patient offers little, waits to hear from the provider, or simply plays "who can hold out the longest." Communication becomes a game and the therapeutic benefits of silence are lost.

While effective silence is useful to collect thoughts and determine what should be conveyed next, confused, uncomfortable, or resistive silences are seen as unconstructive and should be remedied. An example of confused silence is displayed in this interaction between a provider (counselor) and a patient.

PROVIDER: "Do you think your wife truly supports your decision (to return to school to get a degree)?"

PATIENT: (Says nothing for approximately 6 seconds.)

PROVIDER: "You look confused. Did you understand my question?"

PATIENT: "I don't know what decision you're talking about."

Had the provider not picked up on the fact that the patient had not answered or that the patient looked confused, clarification may not have occurred because the provider may have focused on an alternative theme or topic. One instance of confused interaction can take a toll on providers' relationships with patients as patients might interpret too long a silence as disinterest or lack of genuine caring. Reversing this outcome will emphasize the fact that the interview is purposeful, and that providers are sincere in their attempts to understand patients.

In summary then, silences can elicit significant therapeutic gains; however, they can also be detrimental in the course of patient–provider encounters. It is important to distinguish and evaluate their impact and reverse any negative effects that occur and turn into complete inability to interact effectively.

▶ Summary

The use of silence and pauses can be an effective therapeutic skill. As with any of the therapeutic response modes discussed in this text, an awareness of how to use it, what should happen, and how to reverse negative consequences is important.

Suffering in silence is a phenomenon experienced by patients in primary care settings who are suffering but avoid asking for help (Bell et al., 2011). There are many reasons why patients might remain quiet or silent. Feeling uncertain about how to bring up a topic, not wanting to distract the provider or bother them unnecessarily, the stigma of their illness, not wanting the treatment, or reluctance to discuss personal issues can all can underlie patients' silences.

It may be surprising to learn how much can be learned from patients by the use of the right question in the right question format. But we also need to be quiet and listen to what fills the space when there is silence…what comes from within us and what is revealed by patients and their families. Virtually all interpersonal relationships depend on verbal communication. In truth, in contemporary Western society, conversation is highly prized. We are often judged by how often and to what degree we engage in conversation. Being socially acceptable is, in part, related to our ability to relate verbally to others. The verbal form of communication is believed to be preferable, at least for some groups. This is not the case universally, particularly for individuals from other cultural groups where silence is regarded positively and associated with wisdom.

While the absence of verbal communication is silence, this silence does not mean that there is no communication. It may sound paradoxical, but silence is a form of communicating

where meanings are shared nonverbally. What is shared nonverbally is accessible through active listening combined with empathy and compassion. Communicating empathy and compassion in a therapeutic interview is facilitated with the use of silence.

Therapeutic silence occurs when providers deliberately use silence to facilitate patient exploration of problems. The provider conveys understanding or at least a desire to understand the experience of the patient. Silence in itself tends to encourage patients to verbalize if it is an interested, expectant silence. Silence conveys *active listening* which is essential to both empathic and compassionate responses.

The major barrier of providers' therapeutic use of silence is their assumption that nothing significant is occurring in during silence periods. They may judge that their time is being wasted, become bored, and let their attention wander. If providers are able to observe themselves and their patients in these periods of silence, they will learn that a great deal happens in these moments. Listening beyond the surface of the spoken word is facilitated by silent interludes.

Either providers or patients can modify the amount and length of silence in an interaction. But silence begets silence, meaning that responding in silence will eventually result in the giving of silence in return. Short interresponse times may lead patients to feel understood. Sudden changes from short interresponse times to very long silence periods may cause confusion either in the provider or patient, or both. If providers use too long a period of silence patients may become distracted. Silence and the length of silences in therapeutic encounters need to be thoughtfully brought into the interaction to avoid confusing the patient.

Providers can slow down crowded communication by intentionally giving a series of medium-length-silence responses. Repeated crowding in an interaction can also cause a chain reaction when crowding is reciprocated.

The chain reaction where crowding begets crowding, silence begets silence, is referred to as "response matching" and is described further in Chapter 11.

Overall, it behooves the provider to be aware of both the positive and negative effects of silence and pauses in patient–provider interactions. Effective interviewing requires a skillful application of pauses and silences, where thoughtful observation of the patient directs the pace and depth of the interaction. Otherwise, providers should be asking "Is this an appropriate use of silence, and is it achieving something that will benefit participatory care planning?"

The essence of being present with the patient is often thought of as a prime feature of silence. As described by many seasoned health professionals, providers can lessen the burden of patient suffering by "coming alongside" the patient using active listening and acknowledging expressed thoughts and nonverbal responses. The therapeutic use of silence is frequently overlooked or not thought to be a technique or intervention. In this chapter, substantial discussion was provided to describe its importance and ways in which it can be used effectively in patient–provider interactions.

Discussion

1. Discuss the differences in comfort with silence across cultures.
2. What is therapeutic about pauses and silence?
3. Describe how mutual silence can be effective as well as therapeutic for both patient and provider.
4. Describe *response matching* when used to describe patients' and providers' silence and pauses in any given interaction.
5. Distinguish between defensive and therapeutic silence, and discuss ways to modify defensive silence in patients.

References

Amini, A., Bilan, N., & Ghasempour, M. (2015). Effects of reflection on clinical learning of medical students. *International Journal of Pediatrics, 3*(2.1), 39–44. Retrieved from http://ijme.mui.ac.ir/article-1-458-en .html

Bell, R. A., Franks, P., Duberstein, P. R., Epstein, R. M., Feldman, M. D., Garcia, E. F. y., & Kravitz, R. L. (2011). Suffering in silence: Reasons for not disclosing depression in primary care. *Annals of Family Medicine, 9*(5), 439–446. doi:10.1370/afm.1277

Collins, M. (1977). *Communication in health care: Understanding and implementing effective human relationships.* St. Louis, MO: C.V. Mosby Co.

Davidhizar, R., & Giger, J. R. (1994). When your patient is silent. *Journal of Advanced Nursing, 20*(4), 703–706. PMID:7822606

Finset, A. (2016). Silence is golden. *Patient Education and Counseling, 99*(10), 1545–1546. doi:10.1016/j.pec .2016.08.025

Hein, E. C. (1980). *Communication in nursing practice* (2nd ed.). Boston, MA: Little, Brown & Co.

Lane, R. C., Koetting, M. G., & Bishop, J. (2002). Silence as communication in psychodynamic psychotherapy. *Clinical Psychology Review, 22*(7), 1091–1104. PMID: 12238247

Li, H. Z., Zhang, Z., Yum, Y., Lundgren, J., & Pahal, J. S. (2008). Interruption and patient satisfaction in resident-patient consultations. *Health Education, 108*(5), 411–427. doi:10.1108 /09654280810900026

Mann, K., Gordon, J., & MacLeod, A. (2007). Reflection and reflective practice in health professions education: A systematic review. *Advances in Health Science Education Theory and Practice, 14*, 595–621. doi:10.1007/s10459-007-9090-2

Murdoch-Eaton, D., & Sandars, J. (2014). Reflection: Moving from a mandatory ritual to meaningful professional development. *Archives of Diseases in Children, 99*(3), 279–283. doi:10.1136/archdischild -2013-303948

Rowland-Morin, P. A., & Carroll, J. G. (1990). Verbal communication skills and patient satisfaction: A study of doctor-patient interviews. *Evaluation and the Health Professions, 13*(2), 168–185. doi:10.1177/016327879001300202

Stewart, J. (Ed.). (2009). *Bridges not walls: A book about interpersonal relations.* (10th ed.). New York, NY: McGraw-Hill.

Tornøe, K. A., Danbolt, L. J., Kvigne, K., & Sørlie, V. (2014). The power of consoling presence-hospice nurses' lived experience with spiritual and existential care for the dying. *BMC Nursing, 13*, 25. doi:10.1186/1472-6955-13-25

© Excellent backgrounds/Shutterstock

CHAPTER 11

The Impact of Self-Disclosures

CHAPTER OBJECTIVES

- Define and discuss self-disclosure as a therapeutic response mode.
- Discuss how self-disclosure may be different by intent and level.
- Describe the potential nontherapeutic effects of self-disclosure.
- Identify several types of provider nontherapeutic self-disclosures.
- Discuss how to manage requests for self-disclosure from patients and when it is appropriate to do so.

KEY TERMS

- Competitive or Attention-getting disclosures
- Disclosures in service of aggression or manipulation
- Irresponsible or accidental disclosures
- Meta-disclosure
- Response matching
- Role reversal
- Self-disclosure

▶ Introduction

In any human interaction we are always disclosing aspects of ourselves whether verbally or nonverbally. In this sense self-disclosure is unavoidable. Nonetheless, deliberate self-disclosure to facilitate therapeutic aims is different. There is a therapeutic objective supporting the decision to reveal something personal.

Self-disclosure by a health care provider is a somewhat foreign idea in the history of health care. This is due, in part, to the fact that personal self-disclosure was viewed early on as a violation of the patient–provider relationship. In fact, the idea was to not disclose anything of a personal nature. In the field of psychotherapy, Freud emphasized the idea of appearing like a blank slate, mirroring back to the patient what the patient is revealing. There was no room for disclosures of a personal kind (e.g., marital status, number of children). However, from the 1960s forward, there was a shift toward a more humanistic approach that viewed provider self-disclosure as helpful in establishing therapeutic alliances with patients.

In recent years, patients have been empowered to know much more about the training and expertise of their health care providers implying that some information is expected particularly when it discloses the professional background of the provider. Still, the open disclosure of personal data beyond professional credentials is met with mixed reviews with both negative and positive evaluations.

Henretty and Levitt (2010) present a balanced review of the pros and cons of using self-disclosures in the field of psychotherapy and concluded there is support for its helpfulness. They also emphasized that there were no risk-free therapist disclosures. In a later paper, Henretty, Currier, Berman, and Levitt (2014) summarized evidence from an extensive review of the literature and highlighted the potential benefits of self-disclosure for building rapport, strengthening therapeutic alliances, and eliciting client disclosures.

Are patients entitled to know more about their providers; what are the boundaries in professional roles with patients and their families? Perceptions of the advisability of provider self-disclosure remain mixed. Although self-disclosure was once judged largely as inappropriate, some level of self-disclosure is now viewed as acceptable and, in some cases, an important adjunct to therapeutic relationship building.

While self-disclosures by providers can facilitate therapeutic aims, they can also be problematic. The issue is one of anticipating the potential impact and judiciously using self-disclosures. The amount and timing of self-disclosures become particularly critical in judging their appropriateness in the therapeutic relationship.

In an example of when the patient confronted the physician with being more interested in his golf game. "What about me 'doc'?" was the patient's attempt to redirect the conversation away from the physician's ramblings to a focus on his own concerns. This left the patient wondering about the physician's sincerity and interest. Rarely would we expect this

violation of roles, but this is a true account. Would the timing have been better if the physician's self-disclosure came at the end of the patient's visit? Maybe, but either way, it is difficult to understand what therapeutic value this disclosure had and the possible negative effect it can have.

The purpose of this chapter is to discuss the use of self-disclosures as aids to therapeutic communication with patients but also to present a balanced view of this response mode. Before addressing the deliberate use of self-disclosure in the patient–provider relationship, it is important to describe the nature of self-disclosure, present arguments for and against this response mode, and identify types of nontherapeutic as well as therapeutic self-disclosures.

▶ Definitions of Self-Disclosure

Self-disclosure in the context of providers disclosing to patients is defined broadly as any statement made to a patient that describes a provider's personal experience—usually thoughts, experiences, attitudes, and feelings. In short, provider self-disclosures entail any self-revelation of a personal nature. Such disclosures have been classified among mental health groups as unavoidable, accidental, or purposeful (Psychopathology Committee of the Group for the Advancement of Psychiatry, 2001).

In general terms, all statements beginning with the pronoun "I" could be categorized as self-disclosures. For example, "I think," "I feel," "I had the experience." "I" statements, however, are also used to introduce other intentions—advising, interpreting, and expressing opinion. For example, "I think you should get up and walk for short periods," or "I think a high-protein low-fat diet is best." In these situations, the primary impact of the message is some other purpose. These statements also proceeded by "I" disclose what the provider is thinking but the primary intent is not to share personal data about oneself but to influence patients' behaviors. These statements are examples of the *advisement response mode*.

Because "I" statements also introduce advisement, interpretation, and the expression of opinion, it is not accurate to say that all "I" statements are only self-disclosing. A distinction needs to be made between statements made with self-reference and those that are clearly self-disclosures. Self-reference statements refer to "I" or "me" but disclose little personal data about the sender.

Self-disclosure, then, is when an individual reveals nonobvious aspects of the self (e.g., thoughts, feelings, attitudes, or experiences) through a distinct and meaningful self-reference. While "I feel upset with my care in the hospital" is a self-disclosure, "I think you need to close the curtain" is not.

Conceptualizing Self-Disclosure

Self-disclosures are made by both patients and providers. They may be delivered in very intimate circumstances or to many people at one time. Self-disclosures (e.g., "I like you") made in the context of a one-to-one relationship are very different from public disclosures. Public disclosures (e.g., "I live in the Midwest" or "I have a BS degree in Biology") made to many persons at the same time are usually more superficial even though they convey personal information. Although they also reveal the nonobvious, they present much less threat of exposure than do self-disclosures of personal information in either a one-to-one or group settings.

Self-disclosures can be conceptualized in terms of the content of the disclosure. Content in disclosures may vary. In social situations, this content may be personal attitudes or the type of work one does. Other disclosures, say, about one's personality, religious beliefs, and perceived body image, are likely to be offered in more intimate situations or when a certain level of trust has been established and a desire for a relationship has been expressed.

Finally, self-disclosures can be categorized as here-and-now, present experience disclosures, or historical disclosures that refer to the past. Consider, for example, the remark, "You make me anxious." This statement refers to the sender's immediate experience. Statements such as "That reminds me of how I felt before my surgery" refer to past feelings but a present experience. This distinction is important in judging a patient's level of trust. When patients feel free to disclose a concern, fear, or impression about their current relationships with providers, it is usually indicative of moderate to high levels of trust.

Intent and Level of Self-Disclosures

There is still another way of classifying self-disclosures that addresses the intent and level of intimacy of the statements. The following types of disclosures will be described in this section: (1) **meta-disclosures**, (2) **irresponsible or accidental disclosures**, (3) **disclosures in the service of aggression or manipulation**, and (4) **competitive or attention-getting disclosures**.

The first type of disclosure is *meta-disclosure*. Typically, *meta-disclosures* are disclosures about a disclosure. For example, "I lied to you because I wanted you to think I was better than I am" is a meta-disclosure. It reveals something about a previous self-disclosing statement (namely, "I told you a lie"). Meta-disclosures are useful in helping providers refocus on the difficulties of understanding the patient. For example, "I'm having trouble understanding what you are saying about your breathing—let me ask some questions" comments on the character of the communication and creates a potential for clarifying the patient's communication. These statements are also referred to as *process disclosures* because they focus more on the process of communication rather than the content of the dialogue.

▶ Types of Problem Self-Disclosures by Providers

Several types of self-disclosures are problematic when made by providers.

Irresponsible disclosures are made without any real regard for the receiver. In the patient–provider relationship, when made by providers they are considered *boundary transgressions* and are forbidden (Beach et al., 2004). If a patient is describing, for example, his difficulty maintaining an erection, a provider's statement "Getting an erection has never been a problem for me" would be irresponsible. Sometimes such statements are also accidental, meaning that the provider really did not mean to share something, but it "slipped out."

Disclosures in the service of other feelings—aggression and anger—are common in social interactions. For example, "I don't want to hear about it, you always complain about my cooking." This type of disclosure is frequently used to punctuate negative judgments ("you complain too much").

In the context of patient–provider discussions, they tend to be disruptive to any level of empathy that was previously established. Consider the following dialogue beginning with this statement by the provider: "You're always

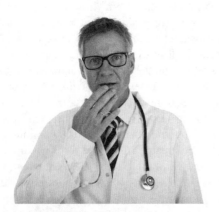
© Sebastian Gauert/Shutterstock.

cheating on your diet, so how do you think I can help you if you keep doing this? (angry tone) I have never had as much trouble with other patients." Angry disclosures of this kind express aggression and are generally received as hurtful. While the underlying intent of the provider may not be to inflict shame, disgrace, or distress this is generally what happens. Providers' frustrations are unleashed on the patient, not only in unhelpful ways but in ways that are hurtful.

Disclosures can also be made to *persuade* or *manipulate* the patient. Persuasion and manipulation are also used in instances where the patient is felt to be resistant or recalcitrant, and the provider is trying to convince the patient to make some changes. "Come on now, you can tell me whether you took your medication. I can find out anyway" is manipulative. This disclosure is used strategically to get the patient to disclose when he is hiding something from the provider. This type of disclosure not only manipulates (e.g., "I'll find out anyway if you don't tell me"), it projects a level of intimacy that is not there. "You can tell me" suggests a level of trust and intimacy that does not exist because if it did the patient would probably have disclosed his actions or lack of action without the provider's need to persuade or manipulate.

Competitive or attention-getting disclosures are also frequently used in social situations. The primary purpose is to gain special recognition. Statements like "Guess what, I'm so cool I just got asked to be the group's representative" is announcing something that sets the person ahead of the group and could evoke a competitive counter—"I've been the representative for 3 years already. They want me to be the chair because they like how I handle the budget." The aim is to take the floor from the first person, making oneself better or more important than another.

In provider–patient dialogue, competitive disclosures can occur even though they are clearly disruptive. Consider the following dialogue.

PATIENT: "I wonder when I'm going to see my doctor. Is he here yet? I think he forgot me today. He's usually here by now. I don't think I can go a whole day without talking to him."

PROVIDER: "That's nothing. I'm going a whole week without talking to my husband. He is on a business trip, and I can't reach him by phone because of the time difference. If I don't get some help with the kids—the babysitter is sick—I don't know how I'm going to work these two 12-hour shifts coming up." (Competitive self-disclosure jockeying for importance.)

Clearly, the provider's motive in self-disclosing is not patient-centered. The provider is focused more on her own problems than on the concerns of the patient. In this dialogue, there is a reverse priority: "You think you have problems reaching someone important to you, wait until you hear this!" The provider's needs seem to take precedence over those of the patient, and clearly the provider has lost an opportunity to be patient-centered.

▶ The Therapeutic Effects of Self-Disclosure

Provider self-disclosure has been alternatively considered either as a role boundary violation or a way to foster trust and rapport with patients (Beach et al., 2004). Self-disclosure on the part of the patient is, without a doubt, essential and hopefully therapeutic. Patients interact with providers to disclose a health issue or problem they want help with. Providers rely on patient disclosures to conduct accurate assessments of their condition. Patient self-disclosures can also be healing if they promote feelings of being supported and understood. Every patient has a basic need to be attended to and understood. Curran (2014) explains that few providers would argue

against the use of "small disclosures"; but when role boundaries are crossed this is an entirely different story.

Although controversial, there can be therapeutic value when providers self-disclose personal data. Thus, while in some cases provider self-disclosures can be counterproductive in other instances they can be helpful (Lussier & Richard, 2007). The most significant contributions to our understanding of the therapeutic value of self-disclosure comes from the early work of Jourard (1971), who expressed the view that self-disclosure begets self-disclosure. That is, open-disclosure statements on the part of the provider generate further disclosure on the part of the patient. Provider self-disclosures (**EXHIBIT 11-1**), however, must meet certain criteria, they:

- Must be true statements.
- Are subjectively perceived statements about the self.
- Are intentionally revealed to the patient with a therapeutic aim in mind.

First, compare this provider's self-disclosure (EXHIBIT 11-1) with the earlier example of the physician preoccupied with his golf game. Do you recognize the difference? As it would appear, this provider's string of self-disclosure statements could be of significant therapeutic value. The provider shares some intimate details about his reflections and feelings about the patient. Although the disclosures began at a superficial level, the level of intimacy increased with additional self-disclosures.

The conversation culminated with the provider and patient sharing attitudes about their relationship in the here-and-now—"we're in it together, whatever happens." The provider evokes self-disclosure from the patient by making personal disclosures. These statements encouraged the patient to express what might be her innermost thoughts and feelings affecting her outlook about future treatments. The nature of these disclosures suggests that there is a context for mutual trust building in this relationship.

EXHIBIT 11-1 Dialogue Box Illustrating Effective Use of Provider Self-Disclosures

Review this dialogue between the provider and patient:

PATIENT: "I'm worried about my tests. What if they come back 'bad?'" (Self-disclosure)

PROVIDER: "We won't really know until next week."

PATIENT: "I have problems enough without…you know, I don't think I could get through another surgery after all I've been through." (Self-disclosure)

PROVIDER: "You have been through a lot, and I can understand it isn't easy."

PATIENT: (Begins to cry)

PROVIDER: "You know, when I think back on how you have 'held your own'—gone through these last 2 years, I feel a deep respect and admiration for you." (Self-disclosure)

PATIENT: (Smiling and tearful) "I didn't know that."

PROVIDER: "Yes. I care. I'm in this for the duration." (Self-disclosure)

PATIENT: "Then I'll get the courage from somewhere—can't let you down." (Jokingly)

There is a tendency for communication to be expressed in symmetry; that is, responses of one kind are likely to evoke similar responses. This tendency for one person to open up on a subject and the other to follow suit is called response matching. **Response matching** in the patient–provider relationship means that if providers self-disclose they are likely to evoke self-disclosure in patients.

Otherwise, self-disclosure begets self-disclosure. When patients are reinforced or encouraged to continue to talk about a subject in a meaningful way, providers' self-disclosures are said to facilitate the therapeutic goals of the relationship. Thus, interpersonal penetration—increasing depth and breadth in disclosures—increases over time. In this way, provider self-disclosures are productive in that they elicit more data and engage the patient in mutual problem-solving. The principle of response matching is the primary justification for using self-disclosure in the provider–patient relationship.

There are other therapeutic effects of self-disclosure. These effects arise when patients realize that providers are human (too). Four positive effects will be elaborated upon: (1) a sense of being understood, (2) the enhancement of trust, (3) decreased loneliness, and (4) decreased role distance.

The Sense of Being Understood

One of the major tensions in the provider–patient relationship is the uncertainty about whether the patient will be understood fully enough for the provider to offer and choose the best possible intervention. When providers self-disclose pertinent personal data, patients can gain reassurance that the provider:

- Listens carefully.
- Is processing the patient's experience.
- Is empathetic.
- Can understand, at the human level, what this illness or injury and its prognosis means to the patient.

In the best of cases, patients whose providers offer brief but well-timed disclosures are more likely to feel that the provider really understands, whereas those patients whose providers never self-disclose and assume *a neutral position* are likely to view the provider as impenetrable and therefore impervious to the worrying and suffering that are important to them.

The Enhancement of Trust

Building on the previous potential benefit, when patients feel that providers more fully understand them they are likely to sense that the provider can be trusted. Trust in the patient–provider relationship has two elements: (1) the patient perceives the provider as knowledgeable and competent and (2) the patient perceives that the provider has his or her best interests in mind. An example of this kind of self-disclosure might be the following statement coming from an expert: "Together we are going to get you better." Otherwise, patients are reassured that the provider is competent and has their best interests in mind.

Decreased Loneliness

Provider self-disclosures can reduce feelings of loneliness in the patient as it alters the level of intimacy in the relationship. The provider's self-disclosure confirms that the patient is not all alone in the process of coping with and fighting his illness. The provider's self-disclosure clearly communicates presence (e.g., "I am present not only as a provider but at the human level").

To some extent, decreased loneliness occurs as patients realize that they are not so different from other people; in this case, the provider. Providers disclosures can communicate shared experience, and this works directly to alter the personal isolation that the patient encounters. Interestingly enough, the provider's disclosure may increase positive attitudes toward the provider. Clinicians have observed that self-disclosure induces "liking." Perceived as a reward, the patient feels singled out in a special way to hear the provider's usually unexpressed thoughts and feelings. One such example of this kind of self-disclosure might be: "If I were in your shoes, I would feel stressed too."

Liking and self-disclosure are positively associated. When asked to selectively disclose to several clinicians, the patient is more likely to disclose more intimate data to those for whom he or she has a greater liking. Also, at the end of a period of mutual self-disclosure, patients will indicate a greater liking for those with whom they have exchanged more intimate disclosures.

The patient who views the provider as someone with whom intimacy is possible will most often apprise the relationship as desirable, be less likely to avoid, and more likely to approach the provider. Providers' appeal (quality to be liked) is a subtle but important factor in many issues concerned with treatment, including patients' willingness to be treated by the provider, patient comfort in disclosing intimate details to the provider, and patient compliance with the treatment program prescribed. Patients' discussions with friends and family of their experiences with providers can often be bracketed with "I like" him or her. This is said as if that were the main reason they look forward to seeing the provider again.

Decreased Role Distance

A fourth and final potential therapeutic outcome in providers' use of self-disclosure is that role distance is decreased when providers self-disclose. As previously noted, decreasing role distance by using self-disclosures is controversial in the sense that these self-disclosures can violate patient and provider role boundaries. While it is not advised to blur role boundaries, decreased role distance can have positive effects. Decreasing role distance can modify patients' dependence on providers for answers and direction. In the context of building shared decision-making interactions with patients, some level of decreased role distance can maximize the likelihood that mutual, collaborative problem-solving will occur between patients and providers.

In summary, when providers use self-disclosures for the expressed purpose of achieving a therapeutic outcome (e.g., to build empathy, evoke patient self-disclosure, or communicate the human touch) certain steps will ensure success. First, the provider carefully listens to and observes the verbal and non-verbal aspects of the patient's communication. Second, the provider responds empathically.

Third, the provider might reveal a similar personal experience thereby increasing the impact of the empathetic reflection. Following the disclosure, the provider needs to evaluate the relevance of both the empathic response and self-disclosure. By using these steps, the provider increases the likelihood that the self-disclosure will serve a therapeutic purpose.

▶ Types of Nontherapeutic Self-Disclosure

Provider self-disclosures of a personal nature (beyond name, specialty, and credentials) continue to be controversial. In part there is little direct evidence that it is helpful or preferable over other steps to engage the patient. In a study by McDaniel et al. (2007), 85% of the self-disclosures were not considered useful to the patient by the research team and 11% were deemed to be disruptive. In explaining these results, the investigators stated that there was so little time in the space of the interview that the probability of the provider disclosure promoting a patient disclosure was also very limited. Provider disclosures were more distracting than helpful.

Thus, just as there are therapeutic outcomes with the use of self-disclosures, there is also the potential for these disclosures to produce no effects at all or even nontherapeutic results. Providers need to be fully aware of the following potential drawbacks. There are at least three key difficulties that can arise.

Decreasing Understanding

The provider might express thoughts and feelings but these will not be within the patient's current frame of reference. This is a common error. In an attempt to make the patient feel better, the statement actually could make the patient feel worse. For example:

PATIENT: "I've put on a lot of weight—can't seem to get it off."

PROVIDER: "I've lost 20 pounds this year myself. Couldn't feel better." (Self-disclosure)

The topic is weight gain and the difficulties of losing weight. The provider tells of her success. It is obvious that the provider has mastered the challenge (to lose weight) but the patient has not. This might be confusing and unsettling. If the provider had remained focused on the patient's concerns, distraction from the patient's needs would be avoided. In this example, the patient may feel more social distance and doubtful about whether the provider can actually focus beyond the patient's preoccupation with her own weight issues. The result is more social distance and decreased hope of being helped.

Role Reversal

A second major nontherapeutic consequence is that as the provider uses self-disclosure, the patient and provider switch roles. When **role reversal** occurs, the provider becomes the helpee and the patient, the helper. This is a violation of role boundaries. Patients may benefit at least temporarily by getting off the hook as a result of the role reversal but this is therapeutically counterproductive. They are relieved of the expectation to collaborate on their own treatment program, but this is the opposite of what providers hope to achieve. The following dialogue describes this process as the provider is trying to encourage a resistant patient to follow a low-fat diet (**EXHIBIT 11-2**).

In this scenario, role reversal occurs. The patient has distracted the provider from the purpose of exploring his own diet restrictions. He has participated in the provider talking about her own difficulties instead. He is even beginning to give her advice about her problems of coping with diet restrictions. Role reversal is evidenced by the fact that (1) the focus switched to the provider's problem; (2) the patient assumes a helping role; and (3) the provider

---

EXHIBIT 11-2 Dialogue Box Illustrating Role Reversal When Provider Self-Discloses

PROVIDER:	"There are reasons that the doctor wants you to keep your diet low in fat."
PATIENT:	"I know—but I like salami, chopped liver, fries—a meal is not a meal without bread and butter."
PROVIDER:	"I can understand that it is hard for you. I've had to eliminate nearly all fat from my diet, and it is difficult to turn my back on things I like so much." (Self-disclosure)
PATIENT:	"What foods have you turned your back on?"
PROVIDER:	"Ice cream (my favorite), butter, cheeses, bacon, and sausage…" (Self-disclosure)
PATIENT:	"It probably wouldn't hurt you to have an occasional piece of cheese or an ice cream cone."
PROVIDER:	"If I start cheating, I seem to have no control." (Self-disclosure)
PATIENT:	"Maybe what you can do is check into some of those low-fat ice creams or yogurt—my wife eats a lot of yogurt."

---

replies to the remarks in a complementary fashion, reinforcing the reversal of roles.

There is more than one possibility to explain why this occurred. First, the patient may have felt that the provider's questions were too intrusive and wanted to avoid answering them. Second, the patient might have wanted to avoid changing his eating patterns and simply wants to stop the provider from putting pressure on him. A third possibility is that the patient does want to comply and is unwilling to work with this provider on the problem.

Also, there are a number of potential reasons the provider failed to remain a helper in this encounter. First, the provider may not have anticipated the consequences of a self-disclosure with this patient. The provider may even have been unaware of the patient's desire to take the focus off himself. Second, the provider may have perceived resistance in the patient but decided that expanding on her own experience would increase the patient's trust. Finally, the provider may have some strong feelings about her own problems with compliance and was unaware of these. The patient's questions may have elicited awareness of problems that she needs to discuss with her own physician.

The surprise element for the provider—"Gee, I thought I accepted my restrictions and the realization this is not the case"—may further distract her from focusing on the patient's problem. Thus, the provider might not be fully cognizant of the role reversal because she is caught up in thoughts about her own problem.

Role reversal is itself reversible. That is, providers can regain their focus on the patient and maintain their professional roles. Ways of doing this include stopping and turning the focus back on the patient's problem, stating that "well we are talking more about me than you" and "it seems you are struggling with this yourself." In these statements the provider regains control by summarizing what the patient has said about his problem.

▶ Criteria to Judge the Benefits of Self-Disclosure

Because provider self-disclosures are both beneficial and problematic, criteria have been developed to evaluate its usefulness. One set of criteria was identified by the early work of Auvil and Silver (1984), who identified four guidelines for judging the merits of a disclosure (**EXHIBIT 11-3**).

Finally, one rule of thumb to keep in mind in employing self-disclosures therapeutically is that self-disclosure needs to be tied to a goal or aim. If the provider does not have a patient-centered objective for using a personal self-disclosure, then it probably should not be used. If providers are not patient-centered in their use of disclosures, they are probably acting on other motives, including getting their own needs met. Meeting your own needs rather than the patient's is, in most cases, nontherapeutic for the patient. In McDaniel et al. study (2007), only 29 of the encounters studied (21%) actually returned to the concerns of the patient after the provider used self-disclosure.

▸ Deflecting Patients' Requests for Self-Disclosure

There are times when providers are asked by patients to disclose personal data about themselves. Sometimes providers feel that they must answer to be courteous to the patient. Patient requests for self-disclosure are frequently felt to be uncomfortable because they distract from the task at hand and cross professional boundaries. The following discussion addresses ways to avoid self-disclosing when it is not appropriate or when the provider is uncertain of the therapeutic value. In some cases, the patient's lack of clarity about the intent of the interview will cause a shift in focus to the provider (**EXHIBIT 11-4**).

This patient might be asking for personal data from the medical student because he is unsure about the purpose of the student and not sure that the student knows what he is doing. The patient is "sizing up" the student and asks several questions to establish whether the student is competent enough to assume any part of his care.

Self-disclosures on the part of the provider can be uncomfortable. When such disclosures are requested by the patient or patient's family, they are not readily linked to a patient-centered objective—although it appears that by responding to the request, the provider is meeting the patient's need. The need for the information is obscure, and the provider does not know exactly how the information will be put to use. Additionally, there is the threat that what providers disclose may cause the patient to dismiss or reject them. While the provider may not be rejected, the mere threat or anticipation that rejection could occur can make the provider more self-conscious and hesitant. All uncomfortable self-disclosures have the impact of exposing vulnerabilities.

There are cases in which requests for self-disclosures need to be deflected. These cases are determined on the basis of certain criteria that will help the provider know how to respond. The criteria are listed and discussed as follows.

Absence of Patient-Centered Rationale

Does the provider's self-disclosure have a patient-centered rationale? Sometimes complying with the request to self-disclose will benefit the patient directly or indirectly. Benefits that occur directly as a result of provider

EXHIBIT 11-4 Dialogue Box Illustrating Requests for Self-Disclosure

Take, for example, this dialogue between a medical student and patient.

PROVIDER: "Mr. J _____, I'm here to gather some information about the symptoms you're feeling right now."

PATIENT: "Who are you?"

PROVIDER: "I'm a medical student. I work with Dr. S _____."

PATIENT: "How long have you been in school?"

PROVIDER: (Feeling somewhat uncomfortable) "Several years."

PATIENT: "Am I your first patient?"

PROVIDER: "No, I've seen many patients."

self-disclosure include those identified earlier—the patient derives a sense of being understood, trust in the provider is enhanced, the patient experiences a decrease in feelings of loneliness, and role distance (between provider and patient) is reduced.

Indirect patient-centered benefits include (1) balancing the dialogue, (2) giving the patient an opportunity to relax—a break from the intensity of the interview, and (3) communicating the humanity of the provider so the patient will feel more comfortable in disclosing around a selected topic.

If an invited self-disclosure does not seem to address one or more of these direct or indirect benefits, then chances are the request for self-disclosure needs to be deflected.

Highly Personal Information Requests

In addition to a lack of patient-centered purpose, there is still another instance in which the provider should deflect a request for self-disclosure. When a request is too personal and causes provider discomfort, the request should be denied. Examples of these requests vary, but can typically include any or all of these topics—the provider's age, religion, marital status, if they are dating, where they live, and how much money they make.

Sometimes these requests are even more personal and include questions about sexual partner preferences, health status, and other personal life events experienced by the provider and/or the provider's significant other. The questions may be innocuous or intrusive. "Are you married?" seems innocuous. "Do you and your wife fight a lot? Who wins—you or her?" is more intrusive and involves information that the provider would not even share with a stranger.

Although providers may choose to answer and answer honestly, there are other options. If the provider feels uncomfortable with a request, then a statement to the effect, "I'm not really comfortable answering those kinds of questions" is appropriate. It is not required that the provider give an explanation, but explanations such as "I don't discuss my personal life with my patients" helps clarify the provider's response. With these remarks, the provider is setting limits (relationship boundaries) on the discourse. Frequently, the patient means nothing behind the question and may have resorted to social chitchat because nothing else seemed to be important. Nonetheless, the provider needs to set limits on these requests for self-disclosure.

Guidelines in Deflecting Requests for Self-Disclosure

Auvil and Silver identified five ways to circumvent a situation where providers' self-disclosure, at the patient's request, may be problematic: (1) express benign curiosity, (2) redirect or refocus the patient, (3) interpret the patient's request, (4) clarify the meaning behind the request, and (5) offer feedback about the patient's need to ask personal questions and set limits.

Provided the provider can be sincere about it; the easiest and most nonthreatening response is benign curiosity. The patient requests personal data and the provider responds with, "I'm wondering why you are asking me this." This reply calls for further information about the patient and gives clarity to the relationship (e.g., the patient's explanation that "I asked you that because I didn't think you understood about my holding things back from my wife.").

Redirecting or refocusing the patient is a technique to bring the patient back to the original topic that came before the patient's request. This is done in a manner that indicates that the provider may not have heard the patient's request. It does not negate the fact that the patient did make a request; it simply reestablishes priorities in the therapeutic encounter. The following example illustrates how this is achieved in a relatively benign way (**EXHIBIT 11-5**).

The provider deflects the patient's request by responding as if she did not hear him. This was not done critically or judgmentally. The provider simply redirects the patient to follow her line of inquiry.

Interpreting why the patient is asking for personal data requires a great deal more knowledge and skill. It is appropriate but less frequently used, especially by inexperienced clinicians, because it calls for judgments that the provider may not be able to make.

Consider the following exchange:

PATIENT: "Are you married? Do you have kids?"

PROVIDER: "Knowing something more about me as a person makes you a little more comfortable with me, doesn't it?" (Deflected request for self-disclosure and interpretation of the patient's intention)

This type of response requires patients to examine the context of the relationship and their inability or unwillingness to engage in a dialogue about themselves. If patients are not capable of such insight, the interpretation usually loses its impact even though it may successfully deflect the patient's request.

Clarifying the patient's request is a less-presumptuous strategy. For example, "You asked me if I were married, had kids—I wonder what concerns or uncertainties you might have about me." The provider expresses acceptance and positive regard for the patient's desire to know but seeks clarity about why the information is important to the patient.

Finally, responding with feedback deflects patients' requests for self-disclosure.

EXHIBIT 11-5 Dialogue Box Illustrating Deflecting Patient Requests for Self-Disclosure

PROVIDER: "So tell me how this feels when I press here."

PATIENT: "It hurts but not as bad as it did yesterday."

PROVIDER: "How about here?"

PATIENT: "Nothing—has anyone ever told you that you have pretty eyes?"

PROVIDER: "What about here, feel anything when I press harder?" (Deflected request for self-disclosure)

PATIENT: "Yeah, that hurts."

Some patients might come across offensively. For example: "What do you like, Doc—blondes, brunettes; big ones, small ones, huh?" Some patients need concrete feedback about their manner of asking questions. The provider needs to feel that it is appropriate to instruct patients about the effect of their behavior not only on the provider but also on others. For example, "I'm not going to reply to that (patient's name), I don't think many people would."

▶ Summary

In the most general sense, all communications disclose something about the speaker. Even nonverbal gestures disclose something personal. Still, when statements are made that reveal the nonobvious—a personal fact, thought, feeling, attitude, or experience—and a distinct self-reference is made, the communication is more deliberately or accidentally self-disclosing.

All providers at some point ask themselves whether they should disclose personal aspects of their life during encounters with patients. In some instances self-disclosure can be helpful and advance the therapeutic aim; in other instances it is not and can even be counterproductive (Lussier & Richard, 2007). On the positive side, self-disclosure can promote open communication that is critical in the establishment of a therapeutic alliance with the patient. When used effectively, self-disclosure can convey empathy while promoting a deeper closeness between provider and patient. There are some very therapeutic outcomes that can occur with self-disclosure that are not a product of other response modes. Trust and the feeling of being understood can be achieved with other response modes to some extent; however, feeling less lonely and decreased role distancing are outcomes

relatively unique to this therapeutic response mode.

However, the use of self-disclosures is controversial. It may not have a therapeutic effect, there may not be time to use this approach, and the technique could result in negative outcomes. There are various reasons for self-disclosure to be problematic. First, it opens the door for patients to ask more personal questions. These self-disclosures can appear misplaced and can alienate patients because the disclosure is outside the expectation for the provider to remain professional. Interrupting the flow of patients' own disclosures can occur, shifting the attention to the provider instead of the patient. McDaniel et al. (2007) found the probability that the focus will get back to the patient's concerns seems to be lower than we think in the average work day in a primary care practice.

Self-disclosures are difficult, and it may not be the provider's first choice in encouraging the patient to tell more. Self-disclosure by the provider takes courage and exposes one's vulnerabilities. Providers are not immune to the fear of rejection or disapproval that comes from disclosure. For these reasons, deliberate use of self-disclosure is a therapeutic response mode that needs to be well thought out and practiced. If there is no patient-centered purpose for this self-disclosure, the provider cannot help the patient using this approach.

In summary, although self-disclosure is used in social relationships, its application to therapeutic relationships with patients is still another matter. Provider self-disclosure is a skill that needs to be thoughtfully executed and evaluated. In those who believe disclosure is a pathway to their patients' trust, disclosure may elicit very positive alliances. One of our most important tasks is to understand how much personal information is comfortable for us to share and for patients to witness.

Discussion

1. Discuss examples of provider self-disclosure and evaluate the potential positive and negative effects.
2. Identify and discuss potential patient responses to provider self-disclosure.
3. Discuss the process of redirecting or refocusing the patient back to their concerns rather than a focus on provider personal information.
4. It might not be fully apparent but if the provider does not have a patient-centered objective for using a personal self-disclosure, should it be used?
5. What criteria would you use to evaluate the merit of using a self-disclosing response?

References

Auvil, C. A., & Silver, B. W. (1984). Therapist self-disclosure: When is it appropriate? *Perspectives in Psychiatric Care, 22*(2), 57–61. doi:10.1111/j.1744-6163.1984.tb00205.x

Beach, M. C., Roter, D., Larson, S., Levinson, W., Ford, D. E., & Frankel, R. (2004). What do physicians tell patients about themselves?: A qualitative analysis of physician self-disclosure. *Journal of General Internal Medicine, 19*(9), 911–916. doi:10.1111/j.1525-1497.2004.30604.x

Curran, K. A. (2014). Too much information—The ethics of self-disclosure. *The New England Journal of Medicine, 371*, 8–9. doi:10.1056/NEJMp1404119

Henretty, J. R., Currier, J. M., Berman, J. S., & Levitt, H. M. (2014, March 17). The impact of counselor self-disclosure on clients: A meta-analytic review of experimental and quasi-experimental research. *Journal of Counseling Psychology*. Advance online publication. doi:10.1037/a0036189

Henretty, J. R., & Levitt, H. M. (2010). The role of therapist self-disclosure in psychotherapy: A qualitative review. *Clinical Psychology Review, 30*(2), 63–77. doi:10.1016/j.cpr.2009.09.004

Jourard, S. M. (1971). *The transparent self*. New York, NY: Van Nostrand.

Lussier, M.-T., & Richard, C. (2007). Self-disclosure during medical encounters. *Canadian Family Physician, 53*(3), 421–422. PMID:17872674

McDaniel, S. H., Beckman, H. B., Morse, D. S., Silberman, J., Seaburn, D. B., & Epstein, R. M. (2007). Physician self-disclosure in primary care visits: Enough about you, what about me? *Archives of Internal Medicine, 167*(12), 1321–1326. doi:10.1001/archinte.167.12.1321

Psychopathology Committee of the Group for the Advancement of Psychiatry. (2001). This month's highlights: Evidence-based practices. *Psychiatric Services, 52*, 1425. doi:10.1176/appi.ps.52.11.1425

CHAPTER 12

The Proper Placement of Advisement

▶ Introduction

Advice can be found in many forms of social media. Early on, advice columns (e.g., "Ann Landers" and "Dear Abby") and, to some extent, national syndicated television shows (e.g., *Geraldo*, *Oprah Winfrey*, *Montel Williams*, and, of course, *Dr. Phil*) served as model avenues of advising the public about relationships and health issues. These sources, once dominating the public media, have been expanded to include an enormous variety of public service and social media through Internet postings, websites, and chat rooms as well as professional and administrative sources for evidence-based health care information.

Most early sources served the function of helping their audiences choose the better course of action. Sometimes their advice was direct, stating the best way to solve a problem, and came from insightful considerations by the program host. An alternative approach used by live audience episodes put viewers into situational dilemmas and created a form of "groupthink" (i.e., the audience was encouraged to solve the problem together). A form of *audience opinionaire,* sometimes supplemented with invited experts' judgments, was the format.

Audiences learned from this "quick advice" even if it is not totally relevant to their life circumstances. Both the advice columns and the television shows addressed two aspects of the problem:

- How one should think when confronted with the situation.
- What conclusions one should come to at the end of the process of thinking about the problem or dilemma.

In short, what we were exposed to was public media-sponsored mass instruction in problem solving for a wide range of common and not so common problems. Along the way, we may have even learned something new about which diets have the best rate of rapid weight loss, how to reduce fine lines in aging facial features, who you should invite to your wedding, how to deal with a boyfriend/girlfriend who was cheating on you, how to improve troubled parent–child relationships, and what to do when a roommate does not pay their share of the rent.

The popularity of such media suggested that we were and are "hungry" for advice. Enter the era of public service and social media through Internet sources and postings from official sponsored websites (e.g., the National Institutes of Health, the American Cancer Society, the American Heart Association, hospital and medical center health alliance websites, interactive patient education programs, and mobile apps, just to name a few). Our choices for advice are so vast we need a system for navigating the data and resources available to us.

In society, most people both seek advice and express it. Furthermore, some groups like to challenge advice, particularly if the **advice or directive** is not something they accept or want to follow. Generally, advisement situations can generate a great deal of discussion because, by disclosing opinions, one invites open dialogue about what one should do and how it should be done. A matter of importance to health providers is that they frequently get asked to give advice in informal interactions with family and friends. Eastwood (2009) details the circumstances of these kinds of interactions and provides guidelines for responding to these kinds of requests that every provider will encounter at some point.

In this chapter, the proper placement of advisement is explored. The differences between opinion-giving and advisement are described. The misuse of advisement and opinion-giving are discussed as they potentially interfere with mutual problem-solving in patient–provider relationships. Finally, principles behind the therapeutic use of advisement are identified and specific guidelines presented. An indirect, open style of advice-giving generally prepares patients to be less resistant and skeptical of the provider. It also increases the chances for patients' thoughtful exploration of their own needs and concerns.

Advice-giving in the provider–patient and provider–family member relationship has made significant shifts. Formally, the major role of the provider was to give advice and evaluate the extent to which patients followed this advice. However, the shift in health counseling toward motivational interviewing infers that simple advice given is inadequate in, for example, motivating patients to change unhealthy behaviors. Young (2014) explains the need "to make the healthy choice the easy choice." This principle of behavior change is core in helping people to substitute unhealthy behaviors with those that are healthy. The role of the provider is not only one of advice giving but one of removing barriers that individuals face when trying to make changes.

Another reason for providers' hesitancy to give advice is a function of how the health care system works today. Increasingly, patients are seeing a number of different providers and specialists to manage their care over time. It is unusual for a provider to have enough information about a person and health condition to be able to give advice that may in fact be changed down the road.

Providers are sometimes reluctant to give advice when they are uncertain about what other providers and specialists will tell or have told the patient. Otherwise, providers do not want to work at cross-purposes. In the case when there is no clear demarcation of who is in charge, providers may also assume that advice-giving is down the line when the patient sees the expert. Other reasons for provider hesitancy can include providers' views that the patient will not follow the advice (so why give it) or their advice may contradict that of other members of the health care team. Current health care system factors (e.g., the varying length of time providers have to see the patient) can influence the extent to which providers feel comfortable in their assessment of the patient and their appraisal of the patient's motivation and readiness to change.

▶ Definitions of Advisement

Advisement is one of the least-studied therapeutic response modes. This is surprising when one considers the pervasiveness of advice-giving in our society and the probability health care providers will use advice-giving frequently in the course of their relationship with every patient and their families. In broad terms, **advisement** is the act of disclosing what one thinks or feels about another's experience, namely, what one thinks they should or should not feel, think, or do. It is unilateral in that most of the data and assessment of facts come from the provider and goes to the patient or the patient's family.

In specific terms, advisement is the provider's use of suggestions, directives, instructions, or commands. Its aim is to effect change in the patient's behavior, attitude, and/or emotional response. Advice is given at all stages of the health–illness continuum—prevention, treatment, and evaluation of care.

Advice-giving is characterized in descriptions of providers' roles but also relevant in organizing an entire health care service to meet patient needs. The integrative behavior change model outlined by Kaiser Permanente, titled "Idealized Behavior Change Navigation," is an excellent example of a total health care system's approach to supporting patients in the change process (2013). Advise is one element under the concept of "guide me" in which advice, support, coach, and help me develop a shared plan (of care) is fundamental to the mission of the entire institution.

Intensity of Advisement

Intensity of Advisement can be characterized by level of intensity. Low-intensity advisement is the process of giving information, opinions, and recommendations, but the patient has maximum control over the ultimate course of action. This form of advisement is nondirective. For example, telling patients that "if they continue to smoke their health will suffer" illustrates that low-intensity advisement is advisory but not prescriptive.

High-intensity advisement, on the other hand, is a powerful suggestion, frequently worded as a command. Patients essentially abdicate some control over their behavior. Providers might state it as a prescription: "I want you to stop smoking gradually so that you reduce smoking to one pack a day. I will see you back here in 2 weeks and we will see if you are ready to move on from there."

Providers get more directive in their advice-giving with patients who have already developed a health problem related to the problem behavior or the behavior worsens a chronic illness, such as the case with smoking and lung cancer, cardiovascular disease, and emphysema. This latter type of advisement is taken up again in Chapter 14 where the judicious use of commands, directives, and orders are discussed.

Advisement differs from the act of giving information and expressing opinions. Essentially, giving information and expressing opinions are preferable because they are more likely to result in mutual problem-solving and shared decision-making. In a study of general practitioners' discussions with patients about stopping smoking (Coleman, Cheater, & Murphy, 2004), more than three-quarters of these physicians used approaches that would elicit collaboration rather than those that would be confrontational. Advisement, especially high-intensity advisement, can be more forceful and may not be given in a way that is respectful of patients' thoughts and preferences. Stewart (2009, p. 385) goes as far to say advice can be *hurtful* because it asserts power over others. This can occur if patients are led to feel belittled, inadequate, or incapable. Expressing opinions and offering information, on the other hand, tend to communicate respect for patients' views and are intended to persuade patients to participate in the decision-making process.

Patient Responses to Advisement

Patients' responses to advice often depend on whether the advice was sought. Early on, Bertakis, Roter, and Putnam (1991) found that patients were less satisfied in health care encounters when providers (physicians) dominated the interview by excessive talking, such as giving too much advice, or when the emotional tone was provider (in this case, physician) dominated. Usually, when patients ask for advice, they are open to hearing and modifying the information to fit their individual circumstances. Accepting advice may also be a function of cultural orientation. In some cultures, individualism is stressed and individual rights are valued above all else. Individuals with this orientation may be less inclined to accept advice than are those individuals whose culture stresses conformity.

Advisement, and to a lesser extent, opinion-giving can be misused. Essentially, when providers are telling patients what they *should* think, how they *should* feel, or how they *should* behave, they are implying that they (the providers) know best. This position tends to prevent patients from struggling with and thinking through their own problems. Providers do not use advice solely to assist patients. Advisement can be used for ulterior motives such as to avoid uncomfortable patient–provider situations or lapse into a comfortable approach during encounters. Some patient's health care decisions are difficult, and sometimes providers use advisement to avoid uncomfortable silence. Resorting to advice-giving can serve to avoid focusing on difficult or painful thoughts and feelings that patients' situations evoke.

Perhaps the most common misuse of advisement is to solve a problem *quickly*. In this case, the provider may be given too much credit for the resolution of the problem. Using advice in this way tends to discount explanations as to why some suggestions will not work. It is as much the provider's task to assess why something may not work as it is to offer medically sound advice.

Providers' responses to patients' needs for and reactions to advice are critical. Patients seek provider advice. Patients who openly ask for advice, but are denied, may feel cheated and unhappy with the provider or the service. In the study by Williams, Beeken, and Wardle (2013), cancer survivors wanted more advice about lifestyle issues (e.g., weight management and physical exercise). Unlike what providers thought, namely to give advice would be *insensitive*, study participants favored this advice and said they would not receive the advice as *insensitive*.

Sometimes patients are given advice but they do not understand the advice, and providers have little time to elaborate. Reactions (e.g., "She said I should...but, I don't know why she said that...and it happened so fast I didn't think to ask her") can occur on a somewhat frequent basis. Providers need to be aware that for every piece of advice given, room needs to be made for assessing whether patients have

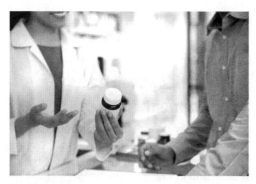

© Atstock Productions/Shutterstock.

understood. Checking patients' understanding can be done in a variety of ways, such as teach-back, where patients put in their own words what they heard providers say.

Patients and providers alike may be uncertain about the course of action. Any ambiguity that exists can be uncomfortable and disconcerting. This ambiguity contributes to patients' inability to grasp the advice given and to feel confident that they can successfully do what providers advise them to do. Additionally, providers will find it necessary to be accepting of patients who did not answer or who do not follow advice given. Providers' reactions to a patients' accepting or rejecting their advice should not be received solely as a reflection of their competence. Many factors account for patients and their family members adhering to medical advice; more importantly it is helpful to identify and understand patient and family reasons for not adhering to provider advice.

▶ The Misuse of Advisement and Opinion-Giving

Studies seem to suggest that advisement, while common in provider–patient relationships, is frequently problematic. Within the landmark work of Carl Rogers and description of the client-centered framework (Rogers, 1951), advice was discouraged for four reasons:

- It is comparatively poor in generating rapport and unconditional positive regard.
- It can produce more guarded responses in patients who are resisting the advice.
- It may encourage dependency and diminish learning which is contrary to developing a collaborative relationship.
- It tends to increase resistance in the patient, particularly if the advice is given in an authoritative way.

The following discussion and examples illustrate some of Roger's reasons and the ways advisement and opinion-giving is misused.

Taking Control from the Patient

Taking control from the patient limits opportunities to establish a collaborative relationship. Consider the following dialogue between a provider and a young adult patient who is being seen in the clinic for an injury to her arm (**EXHIBIT 12-1**).

EXHIBIT 12-1 Dialogue Box Illustrating Advisement that Could Interfere with Patients Making Changes

PROVIDER:	"So how did you hurt your arm?"
PATIENT:	"I fell while I was snowboarding. It didn't hurt too much at first, but about an hour later it started to swell and throb."
PROVIDER:	(Silence) "Well, my children are not allowed to snowboard for that very reason. I have three rules: no snowboarding, no skateboarding, and no rollerblading. The same goes for you." (Advisement—indirect)
PATIENT:	(Silence) "Oh…well, I've been snowboarding for 3 years and snow skiing for 10 years, and this is the first time I've gotten hurt."
PROVIDER:	"Well, you have just been very lucky, young lady!"

The physician in this scenario approached the patient parentally, suggesting that she was a "bad" girl and "look what happened." His advice—"follow my rules"—was posed indirectly through a self-disclosure. The effect on the patient was problematic because she judged the self-disclosure irrelevant but also got the point that she should obey the provider by following the advice given.

The patient already felt bad, and the physician's comments might have made her feel worse. His parental tone was annoying to the patient evidenced by her later statements inferring she has her own parents and they allow her to participate in these sports. Further, the physician's comment, "You've been very lucky!" was taken as indirect advice (i.e., "No more snowboarding, young lady!"). Resistance was evoked, though not verbalized. No doubt, the patient felt that her snowboarding was her decision. She came to have her arm X-rayed and set, that's all!

Advising this patient not to participate in the sports she enjoyed was counterproductive. Not too surprising, this patient's experience caused her to request a change in the provider before her next visit for follow-up care. Hypothetically, she saw little benefit in continuing with this physician because she did not feel supported or free to express her feelings without being judged. She experienced an absence of unconditional positive regard, did not learn anything new (diminished learning), and felt no desire to follow up with this provider (increased resistance and lack of cooperation). Had the physician listened and kept his advice "low key" and tried to make the patient feel better, the outcome might have been different.

By giving directive advice, even disguised, providers can take away from patients the responsibility that is rightfully theirs. As per Roger's warnings, this typically puts patients in a state of dependence on the judgment and guidance of the provider. By giving the patient information such as about the incidence of such injuries—offering low-intensity advice— the provider is supplying patients with data

and support for formulating their own decisions and choice of future actions.

Altering Negative Effects of Advisement

Consider how the previous dialogue could be altered to achieve a therapeutic aim. Assume that the physician deeply cares about the health and well-being of his patient. What could he have done? First, he could have explained that he has treated many of these injuries and that this was like the others he has treated. He could also ask his patient to describe how it happened, expressing interest in the trauma aspect of the accident.

Actively listening to the patient describe how the event was a shock and what put her at risk would make two points: (1) even though we are pretty certain that you will not be injured, it does happen; (2) reliving the movements she did or did not take that resulted in the injury would have provided her with information about how to prevent future injuries of this type. Data from the provider, such as "There is 1 chance out of 25 that this injury could occur" would encourage the patient to consider the odds that it will happen again. The overall purpose of advisement is to alter behavior. Subtle and indirect advice can be more effective than straight-on directives. Phrased as it was in the previous dialogue with a self-disclosure masking the advice might have been indirect but not very subtle.

Unlike advisement, expressing opinions establishes equal opportunity and mutual respect between patients and providers and families and providers. Expressing opinions is assertively interactional. That is, provider opinions are offered as additional information for the patient's decision-making process. Consider, for example, the feelings that these statements evoke: "It's my opinion..." and "Based on what I've read (heard, seen), I would say that this course of action is better." Expressing opinions is not making the decision for the patient, it is simply giving the patient the benefit of the provider's knowledge to make their own decision.

In contrast, giving advice is the *one-sided* process of solving problems or making decisions for the patient. Salter, Holland, Harvey, and Henwood (2007) concluded from their study of pharmacists giving advice to older patients about medication use, that pharmacists' advice-giving role seemed to undermine and threaten patients' assumed competence, integrity, and self-governance. These findings complemented what was known about giving advice during health care communications in general and across the board in health care encounters of providers and patients.

▶ Principles Behind the Therapeutic Use of Advisement

In some ways, providing patients and/or their families with information about their condition is the provider's duty, and neglecting to do so would be very poor practice. The balance that must be achieved is to provide information and opinions without negating patients' rights to express their own opinions and to ask for further data to come to what they believe is their best course of action.

Differentiating When to Give Advice and When It Is Not a Good Idea

Giving advice means telling the patient what to do. Giving patients information when they need it is an act of providing facts and a perspective which enable patients to make decisions on their own or with guidance of health providers. A major challenge is understanding when to give advice.

Consider the following life issues that patients might want to discuss with health providers and whether advice-giving is appropriate in which the patient wants advice about:

1. Delaying a surgical procedure indefinitely
2. Being discharged from the hospital a day early
3. Whether to continue an extramarital affair
4. Whether to purchase long-term health care insurance
5. Stopping a prescription medication

This list contains topics that may benefit from advice from others but not advice from a health care provider. An underlying principle should help a person decide: *Is this request within the scope of practice of the health care provider or is it best answered by someone else* (e.g., a clergy member, psychologist, marriage family counselor, or financial advisor)?

Using Less Direct Advice

A basic principle in using advisement is that for many patients and their families, the less direct the advice, the less likely it is that resistance will occur. To hold to this principle, providers must have an open style—a willingness to have their advice rejected. Advice that must be followed is not an offer of advice but rather a command or directive. It is advice or direction that needs to be followed as directed and providers must clearly say so.

Many patients and their families are sensitive to advice, even though they have come to providers for help or a consultation. At its worst, advice communicates that the patient is incapable of self-direction, which can be humiliating and belittling. Sometimes patients do receive advice that was not helpful or received directives in an unhelpful manner. Just the words *"You should…"* may be the first and only thing the patient hears before tuning out and turning off. Some people have been subjected to critical parental figures, and are

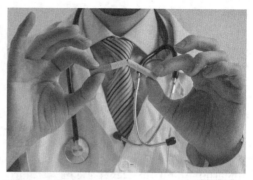

© Vchal/Shutterstock.

not able to set their reactions aside when providers begin to advise with parental inflections. These patients may have more than the average resistance to advice from anyone because authority figures have not proven to be trustworthy.

A useful way to present advice to persons who are suspicious of advice-giving is to present the advice in ways that do not resemble advice. Suggesting an "alternative" or "a possibility" lessens the emphatic tone behind the message. Presenting ideas as hypothetical is also a way to soften the harshness of advice (**EXHIBIT 12-2**). The following phrases juxtaposed on an idea can soften the impact of direct advice.

Providing a Rationale

Another method for giving advice indirectly is to credit it to experience, another source, or another authority. This is called providing a rationale. In actuality, providers formulate rationale based upon advice from one or more of the following sources—observations from treating similar patients, opinions of other providers about the direction for care, and standards of practice that are published on authoritative sources, or publications in professional journal articles.

For example, providers may preface their statements with "Patients that I have treated who followed this treatment for 2 years experienced better results" (observations from treating similar patients), or "According to research on the effects of the long-term use of sleeping medication..." (the use of published evidence-based practice). These approaches provide rationale to support patients' decisions about their care. In these cases, providers can appear to be unbiased while at the same time offer the best evidence to help patients with the dilemmas they may be experiencing. Together, patients, their families, and providers come to a joint agreed-upon decision, although in actuality, it was the provider who swayed the patient and/or family to select a specific course of action.

Decreasing Confusion

Other response modes used with advice-giving create confusion. One example illustrated in the dialogue between the physician and his patient who suffered a snowboarding injury was self-disclosure used with advice-giving. Was it effective? Most likely not. The addition of the physician's self-disclosure about rules in his family did not add to the therapeutic aim. Another confusing use of persuasion when giving advice is the following example. Imagine this same patient being asked, "Don't you think that if you continue to snowboard you will suffer an even more serious injury?" This leading question clearly is not one to be answered simply "yes" or "no." The implication is that patients in their right mind would understand this fact (i.e., "What's wrong with you that you don't see this?"). Advisement can inhibit the exploration of a problem by causing a defensive counter-response.

Recognizing Problematic Patient Responses

Blocked patient exploration can take many forms. In earlier scenarios between provider and patient, the advice given was ignored and the patient responded, at least initially, with silence. Some typical patient responses to advisement include (1) placating, (2) changing the subject, (3) ignoring the advice, (4) reacting with silence, and (5) passively agreeing with the advice. If providers study the reactions of patients to their advice-giving, these problematic responses might be recognized.

Placating is a response that is frequently given by patients. The classic exchange, "You should…" and "Yes, I will…" establishes that the patient has heard the advice and intends to follow it. But is this really the case, or did the patient not want to explore the idea and really had little intention of taking the advice? This placating response is used to make the provider "back off."

Patients might also change the subject or transition to the next topic as if the advice is "a done deal." The underlying message is, "Let's go on to something else because I really don't want to discuss your recommendation." (**EXHIBIT 12-3**).

The patient probably did not have enough time to seriously answer the question asked of her. Additionally, the advice was worded as a "warning," potentially making the expectant mother feel guilty and ashamed. The patient never really got a chance to explain how well she was caring for herself because the nurse practitioner answered the questions herself. Had the nurse's nonverbal behavior displayed interest and if the questions were open and

---

EXHIBIT 12-3 Dialogue Box Illustrating Problematic Advice-Giving Approach

Consider the following comments of a patient who is receiving prenatal care from a nurse practitioner in a community clinic.

PROVIDER: "You have been taking care of yourself, right?"

PATIENT: "Yes."

PROVIDER: "I hope so. You need to control using alcohol and eat well, because if you don't it can cause great harm to your baby." (Advisement)

PATIENT: (Silence. Feeling somewhat guilty and humiliated.) "When do I have to come back again?" (Change of subject)

---

accepting, the patient might have taken more time to discuss these lifestyle issues. Just the mere gesture of sitting down to talk gives the message of authenticity that was previously missing. This patient may have concluded "There was no talking to her—might as well change the subject." By transitioning to the next subject or changing the topic, the patient avoids a discussion of her concerns and the advice she was given.

Ignoring providers' advice with open defiance is yet another potential negative patient response. Sometimes patients can argue just as convincingly against advice as the provider can argue in support of the advice. *A battle of wits* over who is more right than the other may ensue. The provider offers advice and can be puzzled or maybe even angered by the fact that the patient does not reassure the provider she will follow it. The natural unvoiced counter would be, "Why do you even ask my advice if you're not going to take it?" The provider verbally and/or nonverbally expresses frustration and might or might not pursue the topic further during this visit or the following visits.

Silence and unelaborated-upon passive agreements are still other responses patients may give to direct advice. Silence occurs when the provider suggests a course of action (i.e., "You should…") and gets no answer. Unelaborated passive agreement occurs in circumstances where the provider suggests a course of action (i.e., "You should…") and gets a curt response ("Uh-huh").

No response or nonverbally nodding and then looking away from the provider in silence is an indication of passive agreement.

Guidelines That Enhance Patient Acceptance of Advice

Whether expressing opinions or giving advice, there are specific guidelines that are more likely to ensure acceptance. An important practice is to ask the patient (or the patient's family) if they want to hear your ideas or points of view with statements such as, "I have cared for other patients with this illness and have read a great deal on the subject. I could provide a summary if you would like to hear it."

If the patient's nonverbal response is avoidance or if the patient argues with these views, it is best to drop the discussion and reestablish trust and harmony before continuing again using a less-direct approach. Remember, you have not changed your mind; you will just wait for another opportunity to discuss the problem. The following approaches— giving tentative advice and assessing patient readiness—are established ways of giving advice (**EXHIBIT 12-4**).

Advice That Is Tentative

Advice that is tentative is more likely to be accepted. Providers who avoid being dogmatic and make allowances for the uniqueness of the individual patient, the advice will be more palatable. Questions such as, "What do you think about the suggestions I've given you?" also discourage being too

EXHIBIT 12-4 Guidelines in Offering Advice

- Advice should be offered tentatively; advice that is tentative is offered as a request to consider something and is more likely to be accepted.
  - "What do you think about the suggestions I've given you?"
- Avoid being dogmatic; leave room for the patient to accept or reject any aspect of the advice.
  - "You may find some of this advice easy to accept, but is there anything that you have trouble accepting?"
- Assess the patient's readiness to accept the advice; if needed, offer parts or aspects of the advice step-by-step.
  - "Would you like to discuss what I would suggest, or is there something special that you need to know first?"

presumptuous about patients' readiness to accept direct advice.

It is always good practice to adapt your advice to both the situation and the patient and/or family. If the patient is someone who rarely appreciates advice it may be better to cushion the advice with a story, a self-disclosure, a link with another source, or all of these approaches.

Additionally, it is important to stay close to the patient's own language, cultural viewpoint, or age-related jargon (e.g., by using patients' own language as you initially talk about patients' problems). This approach triggers familiarity and decreases the personal distance between patient and provider. In the case of young adults or adolescents, it is particularly useful to frame advice in terms that are important to them, because this group may be particularly sensitive to criticism and orders from adults and authority figures. If patients' dilemmas were simple, then solutions could be straightforward. By helping patients save face, providers minimize threats to patients'

EXHIBIT 12-5   Readiness to Change: Five Sequential Stages

At **stage 1** (uncertainty and confusion), the patient has not yet realized the problem or the magnitude of its effects. Facts and feelings about the situation may be diffuse but still upsetting. Shocked, in denial, or otherwise overwhelmed, patients are not ready to explore either the problem or potential solutions. Attempting to give patients advice at this stage would be useless.

However, in **stage 2** awareness, patients are more prone to identify a problem and examine the effects that the problem has on their lives. Advice-giving at this stage might also be futile. Patients may still be attempting to sort through the various thoughts and feelings that have been evoked by the problem. It is appropriate to discuss how the problem came about and what the potential consequences are. While the need for intervention can be discussed, providers need refrain from discussing specific solutions.

In **stage 3**, patients are increasingly developing a realization and an understanding of the problem. At this point, patients are ready to receive information about solutions. This information can be communicated in a variety of forms—as information (written form) or as professional opinions.

In **stage 4**, patients are ready to select a course of action. This stage is met with constructive interventions and can be supplemented by evaluating actions taken thus far. Patients' knowledge increases significantly in depth as well as in breadth.

In **stage 5**, a discussion of rationale is important. Discussing the rationale behind the advice given establishes a guide for patients to judge the wisdom of the advice. Again, it turns the final decision back to the patient. Sometimes, in stage 5, patients will learn more from providers' discussion of the rationale than they could ever learn with simple statements of advice. And it is this discussion that might carry more weight in convincing patients to make these changes.

When all is said and done, however, providers must be ready to be wrong about their advice or experience rejection of advice. Also, their opinions may not always agree with patients' readiness to change at the time.

---

self-esteem and increase the likelihood that they will accept the advice or opinions offered.

Assessing Patient Readiness

Considerable attention has been given of the need to know where patients are in the process of making behavioral changes. Many of these theories provide descriptions of stages of change that can be used to identify patient readiness for accepting and making changes. An in-depth description of the Transtheoretical Model of Change (Prochaska & Velicer, 1997) is presented in Chapter 24.

According to this model, the stages of change are precontemplation, contemplation, preparation, action, and maintenance. Before offering advice, information, or rendering opinions, the provider will need to assess the readiness of the patient. Carkhuff and

Rordan (1987) describe a model for determining patient readiness. Essentially, the patient may be at any one of the following five sequential stages—uncertainty and confusion, awareness, understanding, constructive action, or learning (**EXHIBIT 12-5**).

▶ Summary

In offering advice or opinions, providers must be aware that depending on how it is delivered, advice-giving might diminish a patient's responsibility for decision-making. This responsibility is rightfully theirs, and keeping patients in a state of dependence on the judgment and guidance of providers minimizes patients' abilities to formulate their own course of action. Sometimes the process of advice-giving does not afford patients the opportunities to sort through their own thoughts and arrive at their own decisions.

Providers may find it difficult to let patients make their own choices. They may be especially inclined to put their expertise to work. Remembering that each patient requires a unique solution to their problem enables providers to forestall the enthusiasm for a "quick fix."

With regard to very tough decisions and courses of action, providers must remember that lack of advice is just as bad as poorly communicated advice. Uncertainty and indecision are uncomfortable for patients, and patients have difficulty with prolonged uncertainty. In the primary care setting or specialty clinics, patients have generally come for a consultation; they want to know more about what providers' think about their condition or health status and are asking for advice or expert opinion.

Getting caught up in the reasons to avoid advice-giving is counter-productive. Rather, it is important to understand this response mode, practice giving advice, and study the effect of advice-giving on patients and their families. Accompanying patients (and patients' families) in the journey to arrive at the best possible course of action requires that providers not be timid about their professional opinions and not make assumptions about patients' need for information. There is generally a great deal of diversity in patients' acceptance and understanding of providers' advice requiring providers to be aware of unique aspects of patients' acceptance and understanding of advice. The challenge is to create a patient-centered collaborative relationship to explore, together, what is best, and this will include patient's active participation along with provider advice-giving about patient care needs and concerns.

Discussion

1. Describe the role of advisement in patient–provider relationships.
2. Identify and discuss reasons why advice-giving may_not achieve the aims for patient behavioral change.
3. Differentiate between patients' valid requests for advice and the superficial need to engage the provider when no real change is contemplated.
4. Discuss the Carkhuff stages of readiness to change.
5. Some patients and patients' families express the need to get more advice from providers. For example, the study by Williams and colleagues reported that cancer survivors and members of their social network expressed the need for lifestyle advice, which would prevent other chronic illnesses (e.g., about physical activity, diet, and weight management). What other patient groups might want more advice, not less advice-giving?

References

Bertakis, K. D., Roter, D., & Putnam, S. M. (1991). The relationship of physician medical interview style to patient satisfaction. *Journal of Family Practice, 32*(2), 175–181. PMID:1990046

Carkhuff, R., & Rordan, J. W. (1987). *The art of helping.* Philadelphia, PA: W. B. Saunders Company.

Coleman, T., Cheater, F., & Murphy, E. (2004). Qualitative study investigating the process of giving anti-smoking advice in general practice. *Patient Education and Counseling, 52,* 159–163. PMID:15132520

Eastwood, G. L. (2009). When relatives and friends ask physicians for medical advice: Ethical, legal, and practical considerations. *Journal of General Internal Medicine, 24*(12), 1333–1335. doi:10.1007/s11606-009-1127-1

Kaiser Permanente. (2013). *Idealized behavior change navigation in forum for healthy behavior change-connecting health care to healthy choices.* Retrieved from https://www.kpihp.org/wp-content/uploads/2013/10/hbc_report/

Prochaska, J. O., & Velicer, W. F. (1997). The transtheoretical model of health behavior change. *American Journal of Health Promotion, 12,* 38–48. doi:10.4278/0890-1171-12.1.38

Rogers, C. (1951). *Client-centered therapy*. Boston, MA: Houghton-Mifflin Co.

Salter, C., Holland, R., Harvey, I., & Henwood, K. (2007). "I haven't even phoned my doctor yet." The advice giving role of the pharmacist during consultations for medication review with patients aged 80 or more: Qualitative discourse analysis. *British Medical Journal, 334*, 1101. doi:10.1136/bmj.39171.577106.55

Stewart, J. S. (2009). *Bridges not walls* (9th ed.). San Francisco, CA: McGraw-Hill.

Williams, K., Beeken, R. J., & Wardle, J. (2013). Health behavior advice to cancer patients: The perspectives of social network members. *British Journal of Cancer, 108*, 831–835. doi:10.1038/bjc.2013.38

Young, S. (2014). Healthy behavior change in practical settings. *The Permanente Journal, 18*(4), 89–92. doi:10.7812/TPP/14-018

CHAPTER 13

Reflections and Interpretations

CHAPTER OBJECTIVES

- Discuss how reflections can be used therapeutically in provider communications with patients.
- Analyze how reflections differ by content, intensity, and length.
- Differentiate between reflections and interpretations.
- Differentiate reflections and interpretations from other therapeutic response modes.
- Analyze guidelines in using reflections and interpretations.

KEY TERMS

- Interpretations
- Paraphrasing
- Reflections
- Restatement

▶ Introduction

An important aspect of therapeutic relationships with patients, whether it is helping them cope with significant health conditions or make lifestyle changes, is the process of promoting insight. When patients exhibit poor recognition or acknowledgement of their circumstances they are said to have *poor insight*. Poor insight sometimes co-occurs with poor judgment. Poor judgment refers to the inability to make appropriate decisions. Limited insight with or without poor judgment is critical to patients' self-management competencies and for this reason are the targets of many counseling efforts and health care provider–patient education efforts. This chapter discusses several ways to convey to patients an understanding of their behaviors which has been or is outside their immediate awareness. There are several therapeutic response modes that offer patients insight into factors that impact their behavior and behavior change.

The use of **reflections** and interpretations are designed to increase patient insight. These response modes can assist patients in making significant behavior changes. Because they reveal an idea behind an idea or feeling, underneath a feeling they tend to provide new insight. Much like looking in a mirror they show the patient a new angle, a different side to what was said. Like all other modalities, there are both therapeutic and nontherapeutic uses of these techniques. The practice of these modalities requires in-depth knowledge of one's own interpretation bias and self-reflection skills. With abilities to reflect on one's self (thought, feelings, and behaviors), the chances of staying within the range of therapeutic exchanges that will positively impact patients is greater.

Certain response modes are known to make a difference in the kind and quality of patient insight. For example, reflections, or mirroring back to patients what they say or might feel, are likely to promote increased self-awareness. However, this same reaction might or might not be an outcome with the use of interpretations. By exploring and comparing the different effects of reflection and interpretation, we illustrate the principle that provider responses make a substantial contribution in shaping patients' level of insight and the quality of their self-disclosure in patient–provider interactions.

This chapter describes each response mode—reflection and interpretation—in detail. Comparisons are drawn between these two therapeutic responses. The strengths and limitations of each are also identified, and guidelines for their use are provided.

self-disclosure. With reflection, the attention is on the patient and providers withhold their personal thoughts, feelings, and experiences. With self-disclosure, varying amounts of personal information about the provider are shared with the patient. Both therapeutic response modes have the potential for promoting patient exploration of their own thoughts, feelings, and experiences.

What is the character of reflection? Reflection can simply be a restatement or paraphrasing of what the patient has communicated; in the classical sense, though, reflection is more than this. While reflection includes repeating or restating patients' statements, it frequently contains references to stated or implied feelings. Early on, the rationale for using reflection in psychotherapy was that patients' suppressed feelings needed to be connected with patients' verbal descriptions or expressions.

Reflections can include many clues to feelings (e.g., that observed in patients' physical positioning, nonverbal expressions, and tone of voice).

Reflections can stem from patients' current or previous statements or reference to the context of the interaction between the patient and provider. They can also include the provider's observations when knowing the patient. Reflections may be phrased tentatively or as affirmative statements. Quite frequently they are stated as observations (e.g., "As you are talking about your surgery, I hear some uncertainty in your voice" or "So you are saying that you are worried about recovering from surgery without help at home; I can tell this is troublesome for you"). Note that reflections return a

▶ Definition of Reflection

The technique of reflection was first endorsed in the detailed landmark work of Sigmund Freud (1995). Essentially, Freud believed that if the therapist presented a human mirror to the patient, there would be growth and healing through increased awareness. Reflection in a sense is the opposite of provider

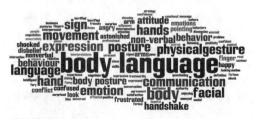

© Boris15/Shutterstock.

synopsis of the patient's feelings, and let the patient make sense of what was said.

Reflections, then, are responses by providers that redirect patients' ideas, feelings, and/or content of their message but, at the same time, bring new ideas to the table. Reflections are always followed by pauses or short silences to leave patients the opportunity to respond.

While reflections include paraphrases and restatements they usually display more depth. Paraphrases and restatements do let patients know you are listening by reiterating what they have said. It is paraphrasing or restating patients' actual words such as "You are talking about your surgery…" and "So, you are saying you are worried about recovering…" that tell patients you are listening and following what they say. **Paraphrasing** what the patient said is simply choosing parts of the patient's verbal message and stating these ideas again ("Surgery is worrying you"). **Restatement**, unlike paraphrasing, involves reiterating almost word-for-word what the patient has said. Reflection adds more depth to paraphrases and restatements by adding observations of how the topic is impacting the patient.

Consider the following example. The patient is describing a concern about having general anesthesia that will be used in surgery (**EXHIBIT 13-1**).

This series of statements by the provider illustrates the use of restatement, paraphrasing, and finally, reflection. Notice that the reflective remark makes reference to a stated or implied feeling—fear—while both the restatement and paraphrasing did not. Also notice that the reflective response elicited an in-depth discussion, while paraphrasing and restatement allowed the patient to stay with the theme but on a more superficial level.

Reflections, then, are not only statements by providers that summarize what the patient has said, they explore what are saying. Providers may reflect the early, middle, or later parts of what the patient said or some part of all three patient disclosures. Reflections focus on in-depth understanding and at the same time communicate providers' empathy.

Reflections demonstrate provider understanding; restatement, while similar to reflection, focuses more exclusively on the underlying meaning of the content and words the patient uses, particularly patients' feelings about the topic. Carl Rogers' (1951) description of *reflective listening* techniques was initially misunderstood. Rogers used the

---

EXHIBIT 13-1 Dialogue Box Illustrating Restatements, Paraphrasing, and Reflection Response Modes

PATIENT:	"I still don't know. What if I get real sick from it? They don't really know if they'll use a general anesthesia."
PROVIDER:	"They don't know if they'll use a general." (Restatement)
PATIENT:	"That's what they said."
PROVIDER:	"So, let me see; you don't know yourself what they'll use or whether they will use a general?" (Paraphrasing)
PATIENT:	"Yeah—it makes me nervous. My mother never could have a general."
PROVIDER:	"So as I'm listening to you—I sense that this is very much on your mind—what anesthesia they'll use—and I hear that you are afraid you'll get sick if they do give you a general anesthesia." (Reflection)
PATIENT:	"Yeah—maybe I worry too much, but I want to know ahead of time. I don't want a general because I'm afraid of having the same problems with it that my Mom did. Maybe I won't, but it still scares me."
PROVIDER:	"Yes, I understand why you are worried."

term to teach providers to listen and reflect in order to make sure patients' thoughts and feelings are understood. Otherwise, the purpose is not just to demonstrate that providers are listening but also to check whether they are understanding the subjective experience of the patient.

While it would seem that reflection is an easy response mode to use and has relevance to a broad range of situations, this is not the case. Reflection is a specialized response mode unfamiliar in the context of everyday conversation. Could you imagine yourself at a party and someone says to you, "I'm feeling kind of sick." And, you answer back with a reflection such as, "I can hear you say you're feeling sick, you must feel disappointed that you have to leave the party." Reflective listening is unfamiliar in the context of the give-and-take of social discourse. In fact, for this reason, providers may feel somewhat artificial and clumsy when first learning to use this response mode. Successful use of reflection can be more difficult to master than, for example, the therapeutic use of questions and silence because it is a less-familiar response.

▶ Therapeutic Uses of Reflection

While reflection is an unfamiliar response in social conversations, its use in therapeutic discourse has a substantial history, particularly in psychotherapy. As previously noted in the work of Freud, the term *reflection of feelings* became a well-known facet of the counselor's approach to people in distress.

Additionally, since the advent of Rogerian client-centered therapy, reflection has slowly infiltrated the American, European, and Asian professional cultures. Reflective techniques are now used by a wide variety of providers to demonstrate an understanding of their client's feelings and experience.

Reflection is understood to heighten empathy. The reflective response is excellent in capturing the emotional meaning of the discloser's expressed message and is often used to show the patient that the provider is not only listening but also understands his or her feelings. The desired impact then is to give the patient the experience of being known. Today, reflection is viewed as a pathway to building empathy, encouraging patients to synthesize their experience, and reassuring patients that providers are listening and understanding what patients are feeling, thinking, and doing. Slowing down the interaction by inserting a reflective statement allows patients more time, sometimes doubling the time, to think about what they mean to say.

Reflective listening is an important response mode in motivational interviewing (MI) (Miller & Rollnick, 2013). MI is not a single technique but a complex approach to supporting patient behavior change; it is more a clinical or communication method (Miller & Rollnick, 2009). Reflective listening as used in MI is just one approach to strengthen patients' own motivation and commitment to change. Miller and Rollnick explained that patients are more likely to be persuaded to change by what they hear themselves say (2013, p. 13). Thus, reflection can assist in motivating patients to change because it mirrors back to them their own thoughts and feelings about changing as well as their perceptions of barriers to changing.

From the beginning work of Rogers and others the benefits of using reflection have been enumerated. They include reducing isolation and loneliness and promoting positive self-worth, and these benefits are clearly important in patients' coping with illness and injury. Patients receive reflective remarks as a request to elaborate (Lussier & Richard, 2007). Reflections acknowledge the patient's right to have opinions, to make decisions, and to think for themselves. With reflections, patients are doing most of the thinking and feeling (**EXHIBIT 13-2**).

EXHIBIT 13-2 Potential Therapeutic Outcomes of the Use of Reflection

- Reduces sense of isolation.
- Reduces sense of loneliness.
- Promotes patients' positive self-worth.

Reducing Isolation and Loneliness

In the face of dealing with an injury or illness, patients sometime experience acute feelings of being alone with their problem. Reflective statements, when communicated empathetically, can give patients the experience of being with others that are interested and concerned. As Rogers (1951) so aptly explained, accurate reflections serve as a companion as the client (patient) explores (sometimes) frightening feelings.

It is believed that with sustained experiences of being known by providers, patients feel safe, courageous, and to have company. Reducing the experience of isolation and loneliness is something that providers can do with skillfully placed reflections. The following dialogue is between a student nurse and a patient diagnosed with leukemia. Chemotherapy has caused the patient's white blood cell count to drop, necessitating the patient's transfer to protective isolation (**EXHIBIT 13-3**).

The student nurse stayed with this patient for a few minutes talking about ways in which she could feel less isolated. Subsequently, the patient called her husband to talk about how she could feel more connected with her family at home.

In this interaction, the student nurse listened empathetically to the patient, observing that the half-hearted smiles could be clues to some underlying distress. Not knowing exactly what was bothering the patient, the

---

EXHIBIT 13-3 Dialogue Box Illustrating the Therapeutic Use of Reflection

PROVIDER:	"O.K., Mrs. R ____, it is time to move to the other room. Are you ready?"
PATIENT:	"Yes, I am." (Not smiling, looks worried.)
PROVIDER:	"You seem quiet right now." (Reflection) "Are you feeling OK?"
PATIENT:	"It is just that Mrs. Y (her Korean-speaking roommate) thinks that I am moving to another room because I don't want to be around her. I've tried to explain, but she doesn't understand."
PROVIDER:	"Would you like me to get an interpreter to explain it to her? One of the nurses speaks Korean."
PATIENT:	"Yes, I would appreciate that so much!" (Smiling, then quiet and looking worried again while fighting back tears.)
PROVIDER:	"It seems like you are unhappy or sad about something else." (Reflection)
PATIENT:	"I just don't want to go to isolation again. It is so quiet in a room by yourself. Well, at least I can play my music louder." (Smiling, half-heartedly, then looking away.)
PROVIDER:	"It seems to me that you are afraid of being lonely in isolation." (Reflection)
PATIENT:	"Yes, I was so lonely last time. The day just drags on and on. I feel cut off from the world."
PROVIDER:	"Going to isolation must make you feel even more alone since your family is so far away." (Reflection)
PATIENT:	"Yes. Until now, it has been OK that my husband and kids couldn't visit me because I could go in and out of my room as I pleased."
PROVIDER:	"You sound very sad." (Reflection)
PATIENT:	"Yes, that is exactly it." (She begins to cry)

student nurse used reflections to help both herself and the patient identify the problem and explore the patient's feelings. The patient's self-disclosures seemed to decrease her sense of isolation and feelings of loneliness and motivate her to explore ways of staying in close contact with her family.

Promoting Positive Self-Worth

When providers use reflections with patients they are imparting powerful messages about the value and worth of the patient. Reflections also encourage communication to continue beyond the point where it might have been stopped. Because reflections highlight feelings as well as content, they increase patients' awareness of feelings through a greater sensitivity to what and how thoughts are communicated. Bernstein and Bernstein (1985) suggest that by re-presenting the patient's message, reflections provide patients with new insight. Reflections mirror back to the patient important thoughts and feelings that are made more apparent because of the added attention they receive.

Reflections, used to affirm or clarify, have become such an integral part of the helping process that the issue is not whether they are useful, but rather how best to learn and teach reflection. A reflection used mechanically in the absence of empathy, however, loses its impact.

The superficial introjection of providers' observations becomes mechanical and distancing, the exact opposite of what is intended.

▸ Kinds of Reflections

As with most other response modes, reflections differ qualitatively—in content, intensity, and length and depth.

Content

Reflections differ is in the content that the provider chooses to paraphrase. From a wide range of content the provider will select and paraphrase what the patient has communicated. This content may not only include words but nonverbal clues about how the patient is feeling. Because providers will condense what patients have said, exactly what providers use in their reflections can vary across providers and even in the same provider at different times or with different topics. In some instances, providers may focus on the feeling aspect of patients' communication; in other cases, the content in the message. With repeated exposure to what and how patients think, providers are more likely to link content with feelings. Otherwise, not knowing the patient very well may cause providers to hesitate in making inferences about the patient's feelings that are associated with the content or words used.

Intensity

Another way reflections differ is by level of intensity or depth. Reflections can be graded as light, medium, or heavy according to their intensity and the insight expected from the provider. *Heavy reflections* come with high demands for provider skill and knowledge. Like interpretations, heavy reflections might be misunderstood and resisted by patients. Essentially, the provider is asking the patient *to take a leap* from what they know and what it means at a profound level. Generally, the difficulty is that providers are reflecting (mirroring back) what is obvious to them but may be outside the patient's awareness. Providers might, for example, label the distress that they hear in the patient's tone of voice and refer to rather strong labels (e.g., anger or rage).

These labels may be too threatening to the patient, especially if the feelings labeled are not familiar and have never been acceptable (e.g., anger or rage). Essentially, patients will not identify with the providers' labels. The patient's predictable response in this situation is to quickly deny or challenge the validity of the reflection. Other patient reactions may include blocking exploration, ignoring the provider's statements, or attempting to clarify the provider's observations (e.g., "Why? Do I really sound angry?"). If the provider recognizes what occurred, an alternative would be to reword the observation using less-threatening labels (e.g., "upset" instead of "angry" and "uncertain" instead of "anxious"). Backing off allows patients to relax, lower their resistance, and explore more comfortably the feeling dimension behind their statements.

It would follow that medium-level reflections are less offensive than heavy reflections. Still, patients may not understand why the provider's summary includes the labels used. Patients might not openly resist medium-level reflections and might be interested in hearing more about the provider's insight. With a little explanation or a passage of time, the patient might become open to the connections that are presented (**EXHIBIT 13-4**).

Consider, for example, the following dialogue.

The reflection accomplished two things: (1) it acknowledged the patient's request, and (2) it identified the experience the patient had (shock and disbelief about having discovered the tumor).

The reflection re-presents the patient's experience without much addition or subtraction from the verbal and nonverbal aspects of the communication. Feelings were addressed without adding too much new data. The provider was able to demonstrate empathy. While the patient did not initially address the shock that the patient felt, this aspect of the diagnosis was something the patient addressed after surgery. All in all, the patient seemed reassured by the provider that what was said made sense and was understood at a deeper level.

Light reflections are rarely resisted by patients. Essentially, they are comments that patients may have made themselves. They frequently come across as "mind-reading" comments. Essentially, the provider puts things together for the patient, sometimes just before the patient is about to reflect these same thoughts. An example might be—"It hurts like crazy" (patient) and "The pain is hard to deal with" (provider). The key to light reflections is that they rarely interrupt the flow of the interaction, and the patient almost always responds in ways that validate the content of the reflection. Otherwise, the patient is saying that the provider's statement accurately reflects what they said and meant. The patient might reply, "Yeah" or "That's right," and then embellish on their experience.

Short and Long Reflections

In addition to the specific content of a reflection and the level of intensity, reflections also differ in how much is re-presented to the patient. Shorter reflections (e.g., a few words)

EXHIBIT 13-4 Dialogue Box Illustrating Medium-Level Reflections

PATIENT: "If you want to know the truth, I'd rather you take it (tumor) out right here. It's got to be done. Take this thing out."

PROVIDER: "You want me to take it out here—now? We'll do it. Finding the lump must have been a real shock to you." (Reflection)

PATIENT: "Good." (Falls into silence expecting the procedure to be carried out, makes no reference to feeling shocked.)

At a return visit to the surgeon's office, the patient offers:

PATIENT: "This was the shock of my life—I couldn't believe it when I found it. I just wanted to get it out of my body."

PROVIDER: "Yes…." (Empathizing with the patient) "You caught it pretty early."

are generally considered better than those that express several thoughts simultaneously. If the provider has been listening carefully, summarizing the patient's communication in a few words is not difficult.

The problem arises when the provider fails to respond and allows the patient to roam aimlessly from thought to thought and topic to topic. At this point, providers have probably lost the essence of the discussion and will need to prioritize, using their own frame of reference. However, using the provider's frame of reference instead of the patient's frame of reference nullifies the value of the reflection. To the extent that this frame of reference does not re-present the patient's, the provider's reflection will fail to stimulate awareness and communicate empathy. Capturing the patient's remarks in a few words also presents less demand on the patient. As a receiver, many thoughts and ideas are confusing, need sorting, and are sometimes difficult to decode, so short reflections tend to preserve the steady flow of patient problem solving.

As noted earlier, the therapeutic purpose of reflection is clear. Reflections help patients examine their plight, feelings, and attitudes toward their health problems. They invite the patient to explore, in a gentle nondirective manner, their experience. Communicated with warmth and openness, they provide empathy.

Sometimes reflections act to reinforce or reward patient responses. In other words, as the provider selects from the patient's statements, the attention paid tends to reinforce what is restated and increases the potential for exploration in this area. Reflection has also been observed to promote relaxation, which may come from patients' realization that they have been heard. Uncertainty about being heard and understood can be lessened through well-placed and well-worded reflective statements. Finally, reflections can be used to clarify patients' experience so that providers have a better idea of what is important to them.

▶ Reflections and Interpretations

Reflections Differ from Interpretations

To fully understand reflections, it is important to differentiate them from interpretations. These response modes are similar in some ways, and the differences between them are not always clear and distinguishable.

When patients communicate something to the provider, the provider can use either a reflection or an interpretation to better understand the patient's communication. If the provider fits the message into some language that fairly accurately portrays what the patient said, the provider is using a reflection. However, if the provider associates or links what the patient has said with some theory or data about the patient's past experience or life events, then the provider is using interpretation.

Otherwise, when providers give their understanding of the patient's remarks using the patient's point of view, they are more likely using reflective therapeutic responses than interpretations. If, however, the provider's attempt to understand the patient's remarks through a theory or through the provider's experience, the provider is more likely using interpretative therapeutic responses. The intent of the reflection is to give the patient the experience of being

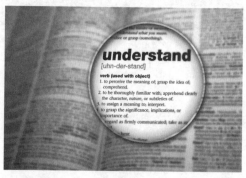

© Castleski/Shutterstock.

understood from their point of view or frame of reference. The intention of interpretations is to convey an understanding of the patient greater than the patient's own understanding of him or herself.

In very simple terms, reflections are simply to let the person disclosing know that he or she has been heard. Reflective listening enables providers to examine the accuracy of their assumptions. Reflections can be given frequently throughout a single interaction with a patient or family member. In contrast, interpretations are offered less frequently and only after a great deal of informative has been gathered (e.g., at the end of an interview and well into the patient–provider relationship).

For example, the provider might say, "When first I saw you, you were having difficulty even considering your diagnosis. Now you're saying, 'Why did this have to happen to me now?' I know this is all very upsetting. This distress will pass—what you're going through is the process of adapting to a serious illness; most patients go through this in situations like you are facing. At some time in the future your distress will lessen and you'll come to some level of acceptance" (interpretation).

This interpretative response accomplishes two goals. First, it links the patient's past and present experiences in some meaningful way (that disbelief and current distress are related to one another and both are part of the patient's lived experience of the illness). Second, it reports on a theory of adaptation to illness, where responses occur in predictable sequences. Reflections, however, are not intended to link past and present or give patients a window into a theoretical explanation of their experience.

While reflections do not provide the level of insight that interpretations do, they may still provide new information. Reflections allow patients to concentrate, a second time, on material they have shared. Reflection promotes exploration that generally does not occur in the absence of a helping person. Reflections can

provide new data because it is impossible to re-present material exactly as it was presented. Even minor or subtle changes can stimulate new thoughts on the part of patients.

Definitions of Interpretation

A good interpretation, or one placed at the right moment, can significantly increase both patients' faith in the provider and patients' insights into their own experiences. Essentially, the purpose is to facilitate patients to see beyond the surface of their thoughts, feelings, and behavior. **Interpretations** are the explicit statements of providers that give meaning to a segment of patients' feelings or behavior. There are essentially two types of interpretation—one links past and present events and the other links theoretical significance with a patient's experience.

In either case, these interpretations are speculations. The linking of past and present events (e.g., about a childhood experience and a current event) assumes that there is some cause and effect relationship that justifies the association between these two points in time. Both past and current experience need to have been discussed in the patient–provider relationship at some point in time, but not necessarily during the same visit. Assumptions about a likely connection are speculative and not easily verified. Such interpretations are made on shaky grounds because much of the speculation is out of the patients' awareness.

The second type of interpretation, introjecting a theoretical premise, requires both a reformulation of the statements of the patient and the application of a concept or principle. For example, a young mother who is describing a problem with her infant would be assisted by understanding the theoretical explanation for the reasons behind her infant's behavior and her response. This particular theory of growth and development may not be familiar to the young mother. For the theoretical interpretation to be of value providers assess what this mother already knows about stages of infant development and early mother–child interaction and build upon what the mother already knows.

The major way interpretations depart from either restatements or reflections is the depth of understanding evoked. Interpretations take patients further along the continuum of understanding than do either restatements or reflections. Interpretations actually offer explanations (reasons behind patients' experiences); reflections simply mirror back words and implied feelings. While reflection can be applied early in the helping relationship, interpretations require the collection and analysis of a good deal of patient data. Interpretations are offered much later in the relationship. In fact, if interpretations are given too early, it appears that the provider is jumping to conclusions, stereotyping the patient, or simply projecting a personal bias. Interpretations are more successful when they are preceded by one or more restatements to assist patients to follow the connections providers are making.

Reflections and Interpretations Differ from Other Response Modes

Therapeutic response modes—the use of silence, questions, and self-disclosure—differ from each other in terms of the direction they lead the patient and in the amount of work that the patient will be required to do. That is, the person who does most of the talking, thinking, and feeling may be different depending on the response mode used and the stage of the relationship. When providers are interested in helping patients explore their problems, reflections are recommended.

Providers who are exploring patients' problems from the provider vantage point might use more questions and fewer reflections. Directive statements and closed-ended questions asking for yes or no responses tend

to be followed by less reference to the meanings or feelings behind (e.g., symptoms or problems). It is believed that reflections generate less resistance from patients than do direct questions and interpretations. In either case, as suggested many times in this text, the use of these response modes must consider the characteristics of the patient (age, gender, ethnicity, education, cultural and religious beliefs). Some groups might learn from these discussions, but others may resist especially if they strongly feel that there is little the provider can really know about their values and beliefs.

Providers' use of reflections is not intended to understand patients better than patients understand themselves. Unlike interpretations, reflections do not fit patients' experience into some theory or explanation of cause and effect. Reflections are also less likely than advisement to communicate provider values. Less direct than questions, reflections tend to let the patient chart the direction that learning and insight will take.

▶ Guidelines in the Use of Reflections

If there is one single principle that applies to using all therapeutic response modes, it is that of moderation. Moving too quickly and too rigorously is not advisable. Likewise, delving too deeply into patients' experience when they are not ready or not willing is ill-advised. Ill-spaced, ill-timed reflections and interpretations can undermine providers' attempts to better understand patients and establish a collaborative helping relationship. How to phrase reflections and how and when to use interpretations are important issues.

Goals for Using Reflections

When providers use reflections the goal is to convey empathy and, at the same time, promote exploration of the needs and concerns of patients. To achieve this balance, several guides are useful. One way to approach reflection is to shift attention from the content of the patient's message to the feelings the patient seems to have, then silently reflect on how the feeling is associated with the content. Having evaluated whether this is a useful connection to share with the patient, providers can then reflect back as to what seems to be the essential thoughts and feelings of the patient. Rogers (1951) points out that the provider's tone of voice is critical.

Reflections without empathy appear as declarations that have a somewhat judgmental tone. Reflections need to be kept light. These are reflections that simply let patients know the provider has heard and is following their line of thinking. They are also intended to confirm with the patient that the provider is correctly understanding what the patient said. Interrupting the patient in order to offer a reflection should be avoided, but pauses can occur that allow some space between the last remarks of the patient and the reflection of the provider. In choosing a paraphrase, the provider should stay within the patient's frame of reference, inserting little, if any, new material and using the patient's own words. Keep the reflections centered on the here and now of what is communicated.

Forming a Reflection

Providers are not always confident about their reflective remarks. Beginners frequently worry about sounding "phony." However, skill at forming appropriate reflections can be taught and in time, and with practice, providers can become more confident. It is true that providers who concentrate too much on a few key words might miss the gist or essence of the patient's message altogether.

Inflection at the end of a speculation communicates providers' uncertainty about the importance of what has been said and/or the understanding of patients' remarks. Reflections that are worded as statements (e.g., as observations) communicate confidence and

generally encourage patients to focus on their own experience rather than on providers' struggle to come up with appropriate words and terms. Dutiful reflections—offering a reflection because providers feel it is time to or because they should—are rarely effective. What can be absent is the empathetic character needed to communicate the presence of a sensitive provider.

Countering the Awkward Aspects of Making Reflections

Reflections are not always easy to make even when one has learned to make them and feels comfortable. There are several difficulties in giving effective reflections. Self-consciousness, awkwardness, inability to capture the patient's words in vivid remarks, and confusion about what aspect of a long message should be reflected are difficulties most providers experience.

These difficulties can be managed with actions that enhance reflections. Long interresponse times before reflecting allow the provider to sort and carefully examine patients' remarks. Silently reflecting on what the patient has said and using one's imagination to tap into the patient's experience is also useful. Repeating key words or using metaphors can capture patients' experience, as will introjecting a disclosure before a reflection when patients' words seem confusing. An example might be, "Let me see, I'm not sure I understand what you mean by 'sticking to my diet isn't worth it.'"

A common beginner's problem is a tendency to add too much or to omit important content when re-presenting patients' experience. Sometimes this results in distortion or exaggeration that just does not fit the patient. For example, "So you are saying that it is impossible to follow your diet." The patient might reply, "No, I mean that it is difficult but because I don't seem to lose the weight I need to…is it really worth dieting in the first place?"

While the provider was bordering on the concerns of the patient, it was not that the diet itself was impossible to follow; rather, the diet is not getting the results desired. These are related but also two separate issues. Asking questions to clarify what the patient meant before reflecting on the patient's experience could have avoided this faulty reflection. It is also important not to sound too mechanical. If this happens, reflections are presented stiffly and sound strained. In learning to use reflections it is helpful to practice both one's tone of voice and to try out 50 or more reflections to feel authentic when using this response mode.

In the beginning, providers can feel like they are merely echoing what the patient is saying. This happens when providers have not thought through how to word a paraphrase or reflection. Silence response modes or pauses, however, can promote associations and enhance providers' abilities to use metaphors. Statements like, "You feel you're on slippery ice" (fear) or "You must feel like you're in a corner and can't get out" (helplessness) are vivid images that help capture the essence of the patient's story. When choosing which images to use, providers need to be aware that certain statements might not be commonly used by the patient; images that correspond with the patient's age, gender, culture, and educational level are likely to be more meaningful and acceptable.

When the patient talks too quickly or too long without giving providers an opportunity to introject a comment, reflection is difficult. Sometimes the patient has presented confusing or even contradictory messages, and precise interpretations are not always possible. Reflecting the most useful parts of a complex disclosure is a skill that develops over time. One strategy is to reflect silently, assess the most important aspect of the message, and reflect it back verbally to the patient.

A second option is to use self-disclosures to enlist patients' help to clarify what they have said. If the patient communicates contradictory or confusing material, it is advisable to reflect the contradiction. For example, "I've heard you express good and bad things about this change; on the one hand…but…" If the confusion is complicated, the provider may offer, "It's hard to really know how you're feeling about this change." Remember, the patient may not be confused at all; it may be that the provider's ability to track and comprehend all that the patient has said is limited. In this case, it is better to disclose one's inability to comprehend what the patient has said while taking accountability for not being able to understand—"It might be because I didn't hear all of what you said, are you saying…?" or "I might have misheard you, can you help me understand it one more time?"

Avoiding Overuse of Reflections

Reflections can be used too frequently or indiscriminately. When this occurs, providers may appear disinterested. Hemphill-Pearson (2008, p. 25) suggests that in using reflections the temptation may be to "parrot" what the patient said, and parroting can anger patients and make them question the provider's competence as well as sincerity.

Sometimes when too many reflections have been used providers begin to appear that they are mimicking patients' expressions. This can make reflections and other nondirective techniques seem ludicrous. Consider the following dialogue between a person in pain and a medical student.

PATIENT: "I have pain in my shoulder."
PROVIDER: (Scanning patient chart) "You have pain?" (Restatement)
PATIENT: "Yes, right here—my left side—it hurts a lot."
PROVIDER: "Your left side is really painful—it concerns you?" (still thumbing through chart) (Reflection)
PATIENT: "I told you twice—my shoulder hurts. Aren't you going to look at it?"

Understandably, the patient is getting agitated with the provider. The overuse of the reflective response mode might actually worsen feelings of not being attended to properly. Notice that one therapeutic benefit of reflection is establishing empathic understanding; yet this use of restatement and reflection, which is ill-spaced, actually communicates the opposite, no real empathy is offered.

▶ Interpretations Used in Social and Therapeutic Contexts

Interpretations go beyond patients' surface messages and into the less apparent territory of the meanings and motivations behind remarks. Because they deal with less obvious material, they are subject to error.

In Social Contexts

In social situations or social relationships, interpretations are frequently received negatively. There is seems to be no justifiable reason to support interpretations in these interactions. Frequently, they make the receiver feel vulnerable and the sender feel superior. All providers who are trained in interpreting patients' or family members' remarks need to be careful to avoid slipping into this mode outside the therapeutic relationship.

In some instances providers may get into very complicated situations and come across as arrogant. Consider, for example, the provider who meets an eligible dating partner, and after learning something about the young lady, offers this explanation about her hesitancy in accepting a date. "From what you've told me, you've been burned badly. Many girls I know carry around excess baggage. You probably struggle with problems of intimacy coming from your early childhood years." These interpretative remarks are interesting and might even be accurate. However, the balance in this social relationship has shifted. The young

woman is led to believe that she has major problems—some she did not even know about. Her reaction may be to hesitate even more to get to know her prospective date—why would she consider getting to know someone who makes such giant leaps with just a little bit of knowledge about her?

Because interpretations violate the norms of social relationships, they may not be comfortably used in therapeutic relationships as well. Ways that interpretations are misused in social relationships can color providers' attitudes about using them in patient–provider relationships. In addition, providers may hesitate to use therapeutic interpretations because they are concerned about response matching by patients. An example might be, "You need to know what to do with…" (provider); "It's clear to me that *you* need to know what to do with…." (patient). That is, providers' interpretations may be matched with patients' interpretations of the provider. In reality, this type of "turnabout is fair play" rarely occurs, although providers do worry about the possibility.

Therapeutic Uses of Interpretation

Interpretations are, however, therapeutic response modes that can provide comfort to patients. Interpretations can be experienced both as providing new information and providing new order to old information. A sound interpretation by the provider can increase the faith and confidence of the patient in the provider. Thus, interpretations have the potential to decrease patient distress and increase feelings of security if they reflect patients' experience.

Consider the following dialogue between provider and patient. The patient is distressed over the physician's refusal to discharge him from the hospital. The nurse caring for this patient has observed and read the patient's chart describing past history and multiple hospitalizations.

PROVIDER: "It seems you're upset you can't go home earlier—I understand that."

PATIENT: "Yes, they said that I would...I can't take this much longer."

PROVIDER: "I think you're also reacting to the long struggle you've had with repeated hospitalizations."

PATIENT: "It seems this is going on and on and nobody can help me like they should."

PROVIDER: "You may be more angry with your illness than with any of us.... We are safe targets for this frustration. It happens a lot with our patients...."

Note here how the past is drawn into the present and how the nurse suggests that the health care team, not the patient's illness, is the target for the patient's stored-up frustration and feelings of futility. The patient can learn that these reactions are not random and disconnected but form a continuity that reveals a problem over time and, in this case, might be related to acceptance of and adaptation to chronic not only ones's illness and the treatment that is required.

In this way, interpretations can translate a set of apparently unrelated or surface-related events into a coherent whole. This process in turn gives patients a more meaningful understanding and deepens their awareness of what is happening to them. Said differently, the need for receiving interpretations is a need for creating new meaning from a series of events that evokes feelings of helplessness. Even minor interpretations can be perceived as helpful by someone who is struggling to make sense of frustrating or unmanageable situations.

The use of interpretative remarks in helping relationships has not always been judged helpful or advisable. In fact, there are some psychotherapeutic schools of thought that view interpretations as irrelevant and possibly dangerous. Some cognitive behavioral therapists, for example, generally regard theoretical interpretations as, at best, chancy, and interpretations linking past and present as unimportant in supporting patient growth. These therapists

and practitioners, in keeping with cognitive behavioral therapy techniques, emphasize the present and education to deal with patient problems in a time-limited structured format. What is important is what is manifested here and now.

Therapists subscribing to the psychodynamic motivational approach use reflective listening in their model describing change cycles; reflective listening is recognized as a counseling task in both the stage of precontemplation and the stage of contemplation when patients are first thinking about making behavioral changes (Douaihy, Kelly, & Gold, 2014; Duffy, 2011). During these stages, patients are beginning to examine decisions to change versus reasons to stay the same. The reasons that the past relates to the present are not critical to achieving behavioral changes. Some clinicians view provider interpretations as mere projections of the provider's own conflicts or dilemmas. If interpretation is putting on the patient what is truly only relevant to oneself, then providers could be making gross errors in their assessment and treatment of patients.

A more moderate view suggests that interpretations can be therapeutic, and because no single therapeutic response will do in all situations, it is better to have more options. Thus, interpretations are suitable options if utilized properly. Most providers caution that interpretations should be offered only when patients have established a connection and are about to expand their insight in a particular area.

Research indicates that interpretations that are much more removed from patients' awareness are more likely to be resisted. Dr. Maggie Turp (2017) addressing the potency of interpretations stated that providers need to understand that interpretations will challenge a patient's way of seeing things because providers are bringing "previously unavailable awareness and insight to our client's self-understanding..."

Denial, blocking, and inattention on the part of the patient are important clues that patients' readiness to hear and deal with the implications of the interpretation is not what it needs to be. The patient should be able to listen to, ponder, and ultimately understand the interpretation if it is to be successful. Patients' readiness to receive an interpretation is felt by some to be more important than the accuracy of the interpretation, because patients can always correct interpretations if they are ready to engage in explanations of their experience at the level of interpretation-making.

It is possible to plot reflection and interpretation on the same continuum with the expectation that as the provider moves from simple reflections to restating material not immediately within the patient's awareness, the depth of interpretive responses increases. That is, reflection begins with a restatement of remarks. When comments are made to link previously unrelated statements, the provider is moving into the realm of making interpretations.

▶ Guidelines for the Therapeutic Use of Interpretations

Patients' exploration of situations, dilemmas, or problems must be nurtured and developed. Principles for the effective use of interpretative remarks stem from this idea. The basic outcome—to enhance patients' sense of control over the situation and to allow them to grow in knowledge—directs the choice and placement of interpretations (**EXHIBIT 13-5**).

EXHIBIT 13-5 Guidelines for the Therapeutic Use of Interpretations

- Place interpretations after reflections
- Validate any interpretation offered
- Use interpretations sparingly

Placing Interpretations After Reflections

Interpretations placed after reflections tend to make problem exploration go smoothly. Also, interpretations that start out simple and build on increased awareness of the situation are likely to be less obtrusive.

Validating Interpretations

Interpretations need to be evaluated and validated. Validation can include comments such as, "Can you see the connection I described?" or "How does this idea fit with your thinking about this situation?" Delivering a few interpretative remarks with adequate evaluative follow-up generally permits more self-exploration than does direct unsubstantiated interpretations. Interpretation, though, can lead to the abandonment of self-exploration with the result of silence, denial, or blocking.

Usually, interpretations made tentatively are less likely to confuse and therefore preserve the flow of patient self-disclosure. While an interpretation may be true, there may be several other interpretations that are also true. Providers' interpretations then may be true but not salient. For this reason, evaluative comments are needed to help both provider and patient put interpretative remarks in perspective. Providers should leave time to discuss interpretations and to ask patients if they have any questions about these interpretations.

A common problem when making interpretations is the juxtaposing of one theory with every instance. Using one principle to explain all behaviors within and across groups of individuals is a faulty application of interpretations. No theory exists that adequately and accurately explains a single behavior across all groups of individuals. Interpretations using theory, then, are always tentative.

To summarize, effective interpretations can be made by even the beginning practitioner. However, adequate observations of the patient and a theoretical basis on which to draw one's conclusions are essential. The delivery of an interpretation will meet with more success if it is communicated as a tentative suggestion, inviting the patient to collaborate in validating the idea. Sometimes self-disclosure (e.g., "I'm wondering how your frustration about your (hospital) discharge is related to the total experience of your illness") presents the interpretation in a mild, nonobtrusive fashion, or a question in the service of interpretation can be delivered more palatably (e.g., "Do you see a connection between your frustration with (your hospital) discharge and your experience with your illness as a whole?")

Using Interpretations Sparingly

Interpretations need to be used sparingly. Because accurate interpretations require thoughtful reflection by the provider, the ability to deliver several interpretations in a single encounter is not the point. In fact, patients who are encouraged to stay on this intellectual plane, kept at the thinking level, may miss the feelings associated with the several interpretations offered at the same time.

▶ Summary

Reflections and interpretations are two additional therapeutic response modes. While they are similar to some degree, they are also very different. Interpretations move the patient to a deeper level of exploration of experiences because they mirror the patient's behaviors and feelings that may not be within the patient's immediate awareness. Because of this, they are also more open to error if the provider misses some relevant and critical information about the patient. If reflections are tied closely to patients' current experience and providers correctly paraphrase words and feelings that are reflected in patients' stories,

there is less chance for error. When empathically expressed, reflections tell patients that the provider is present, listening, and respectful of patients' needs to make sure they are heard and understood correctly.

Providers need to pave the way so that patients are ready and can understand the purpose of restatements and interpretations. Patients receive reflective remarks as a request to elaborate, and reflections acknowledge the patient's right to have opinions, make decisions, and think for themselves. With reflections, patients are doing most of the thinking and feeling.

Reflective listening is the most valuable skill for giving the patient or patient's family members the assurance that their concerns are truly being heard. Interpretations can elicit deeper understanding and even reduce anxiety by explaining, for example, why they feel confused or out of control. The major drawback of interpretations over reflections is that interpretations can be more provider-driven and therefore, less patient-centered. In the case of interpretations, providers are doing most of the thinking, and there is the chance they will introject their own subjective experience rather than actually reflect the experience of the patient. Both reflections and interpretations also give the patient the opportunity to make sense of what they are saying.

Guidelines in using both response modes include forming reflections and interpretations so that they can be understood, phrasing them accurately, using them sparingly, and presenting them in ways that are least offensive to the patient. It is counterproductive to provide too many interpretations in a single patient–provider encounter. Timing is important, particularly with interpretations, so that the revelation is accepted or, at the very least, provides useful material for further discussion.

Using interpretations prematurely and before empathy and trust has had time to form is ill-advised. Interpretations should never be presented as accusations or moral judgments but rather as supportive remarks offered as tentative explanations. Finally, while reflections can be made early in the provider–patient relationship, interpretations are best reserved for a period when provider–patient rapport has been secured over time. If not, the patient is likely to react negatively and missed readings of patients' thoughts and concerns occur.

While reflections express patients' experience from the patient's frame of reference, interpretations tend to express patients' experience from the provider's frame of reference. Basic patient–provider communications training is helpful, but specific in-depth training in these modalities is essential. Deficits in knowing how to employ these modalities are not confined to the new provider; the guidelines for their use may be forgotten or become "rusty." It behooves us all to evaluate our use of these response modes over time and make corrections as needed.

Discussion

1. Describe ways in which reflections can be used therapeutically in interactions with patients.
2. How do reflections differ by content and intensity?
3. What are the key differences between reflections and interpretations?
4. How do the use of reflections and interpretations differ from other therapeutic response modes?
5. What are some important guidelines when using interpretations and reflections?

References

Bernstein, L. S., & Bernstein, R. S. (1985). *Interviewing: A guide for health professionals.* New York, NY: Appleton-Century-Crofts.

Douaihy, A., Kelly, T. M., & Gold, M. A. (Eds.). (2014). *Motivational interviewing: A guide for medical trainees.* Oxford: Oxford University Press.

Duffy, F. D. (2011). Counseling and Advising for behavior changes. In L. Goldman (Ed.), *Goldman's cecil medicine* (Part 3, Chapter 13, 24th ed.). New York, NY: Elsevier.

Freud, S. (1995). *The basic writings of Sigmund Freud.* In A. A. Brill (Trans.). New York, NY: Random House.

Hemphill-Pearson, B. J. (Ed.). (2008). *Assessments in occupational therapy mental health: An integrative approach* (2nd ed.). Thorofare, NJ: SLACK Inc.

Lussier, M. T., & Richard, C. (2007). Feeling understood: Expression of empathy during medical consultations. *Canadian Family Physician, 53*(4), 640–641. PMID:17872713

Miller, S., & Rollnick, S. (2009). Ten things motivational interviewing is not. *Behavioural and Cognitive Psychotherapy, 37,* 129–140. doi:10.1017/S1352465809005128

Miller, S., & Rollnick, S. (2013). *Motivational interviewing: Helping people change.* New York, NY: The Guilford Press.

Rogers, C. (1951). Client-centered therapy. Boston, MA: Houghton-Mifflin Co.

Turp, M. (2017). *Proceedings from Brighton Therapy Partnership: Perspectives on interpretation in psychoanalytic counseling.* Brighton Therapy Partnership: Training and CPD for therapists. Retrieved from www.brightontherapypartnership.org.uk/btp-interview-with-maggie-turp/

CHAPTER 14

The Judicious Use of Confrontations, Orders, and Commands

CHAPTER OBJECTIVES

- Define confrontation and differentiate between levels of confrontation.
- Describe how the intensity of confrontations can be modified.
- Differentiate between commands, orders, and confrontations.
- Identify ways of assessing compliance to commands, orders, and directives.
- Describe ways to ease the impact of confrontational discussions with patients.

KEY TERMS

- Caring confrontation
- Commands
- Confrontations
- Directives
- Experiential confrontation
- Factual confrontation
- Orders

▶ Introduction

Up to this point, the therapeutic response modes presented have been largely supportive and facilitative. Providers respond to patients and their families with unconditional positive regard; they do not judge or scrutinize them or their health care decisions. Rather, providers try to facilitate an atmosphere in which patients feel comfortable and will share their concerns and worries about their health or disease and its treatment. Essentially, the idea is to show empathy, confirm the value and worth of the patient, and establish trust. Questions, advisement, reflections, and interpretations can be rather gently used to prompt patients' collaborative problem-solving. These approaches respect patients' readiness to change and work to motivate them to change lifestyle behaviors.

The question is, is it more appropriate in selected instances to express judgment and urgency? In the profession of medicine, doctors give orders to control the administration of medical care. In hospitals, nurses and medical assistants receive these orders and are bound by law and ethics to follow them. When discharged, patients receive doctors' orders (e.g., prescriptions for medications, instructions in wound care, directions for introducing physical activity). These orders or directives are now the responsibility of the patient and patient caregivers.

In fact, doctors and medical providers have a term that is ascribed to a patient who does not follow these orders; the patient is noncompliant or nonadherent. If the patient resists following an order (such as taking a medication or limiting physical exercise), a notation is usually placed in the patient's medical record and describes the patient's behavior as resistant or noncompliant.

From here forward, patients may be treated as a "problem patient," not necessarily as a patient with problem behavior. Herein is the process of labeling patients. In some instances, patients are right to refuse a medical order; participatory and shared decision-making stress the idea that patients are integral in ensuring that care is both effective and safe. Any medical order that causes harm or serious side effects should be stopped immediately. But there is a difference between patients who stop following orders on their own and do not communicate this to their health provider, and those who want to stop or have temporarily stopped and have communicated with their health provider. The first type of patient will, no doubt, be labeled noncompliant, while the second type would not.

In health care settings, not only are orders routinely used, so are **confrontations** and to a limited extent, **commands**. These response modes involve critically evaluating what the patient is or is not doing and communicating judgment and advice. In this chapter, the judicious use of confrontation, orders, and commands is discussed. It is through the use of supportive communications—empathy and unconditional acceptance and positive regard—that providers establish their therapeutic connection with the patient.

Confrontations, orders, and commands involve being judgmental and evaluative. The contribution of these types of modalities (confrontation, orders, and commands) is that they make sure that directions to patients are clear and concise and, in some instances, express the seriousness of moving ahead quickly to protect the patient's life and welfare. However, providers are cautioned to remember that an empathic and supportive style is the appropriate context for providing effective confrontations (White & Miller, 2007).

Confrontations are usually employed to ensure action—to cause a response so necessary that the avoidance of action has serious consequences. These response modes are not considered useful in long-term behavioral change situations. In fact, confrontation, for example, is considered counterproductive in cases with patients needing to reverse a pattern of behavior that has been or is very difficult to relinquish (e.g., smoking, alcohol, or drug use).

In these instances, the closest example of something like confrontation is the approach to "present contrast," where the provider confronts patients with the difference between what they say they are doing or want to do and what they are actually doing. The feedback is direct and clear. The purpose of this technique is to build awareness in patients, which should reinforce motivation to change. In the counseling literature, this approach is sometimes referred to as *therapeutic confrontation* or **caring confrontation** (Clark, 2012; McGuire-Bouwman, 2006).

Confrontations: Definitions, Levels, and Types

Definitions of Confrontation

Confrontation or *acts of confronting* in therapeutic encounters is the deliberate use of statements or questions with patients to point out certain discrepancies. As previously indicated, behavioral change theories suggest presenting discrepancies as a means to motivate patients, and sometimes their families, to change what they are doing or not doing. These discrepancies may be (1) differences between what patients say they do and what they actually do, (2) differences in statements or behaviors observed over time, and (3) differences between what patients should do and what they are actually doing.

The value of confrontation is that it offers both providers' and patients' alternative views about what is really going on. Assuming that patients are truly interested in providers' viewpoints, feedback about discrepant behavior can be informative and can actually contribute to patient knowledge, insight, and understanding.

When this feedback comes from a health care provider, it is generally presumed that the observations are valid and have some bearing on the patient's well-being. In some cases, providers' observations may be more complete and accurate than those of the patient. Confrontations that increase patients' knowledge or self-awareness stem from providers' extensive experience and high level of expertise in learning and working with patients. The point is to share this knowledge in a way that the patient will understand and probably follow.

Levels of Confrontation

Like other therapeutic response modes, confrontations may be more or less intense, and, like interpretations, they may be more or less threatening. Low-level confrontations are less intense and consequently arouse lower levels of emotional response. Consider this dialogue between patient and provider; the provider is speaking to the patient about the necessity of a low-fat diet:

PROVIDER: "OK, Janice, now I know you like fast foods, but, if I catch you at a fast-food restaurant I'm going to get upset." (Smiling)

This confrontation delivers a message; despite an urge and desire for fast foods, the patient must avoid them. This confrontation is low level because it is offered in a friendly manner. It is also delivered in a jovial, somewhat ambiguous fashion. Is the provider really that serious or not? Just as it might evoke a friendly response from the patient: "then I'll have to go there very late at night" (frowns and smiles), it might also arouse negative feelings.

After all, is the provider confessing to going to fast-food restaurants, and how is the provider really going to catch the patient at a fast-food restaurant? While the patient might make use of this feedback, the informality may dilute the impact of this teaching moment. The depth and intensity of this confrontation and feedback seems to be too weak.

Confrontations that are moderately intense but are not so direct as to damage collaboration are middle-level confrontations. Consider the following dialogue between the patient just described and provider.

PROVIDER: "Janice, I know you like fast foods, but, if you continue to over-indulge, you will gain more weight and your ability to control your diabetes will get harder and harder with this high-fat and high-calorie diet. I have had lots of patients in your situation and have seen this happen time and time again. Did you read the information I gave you?"

There is nothing ambiguous about this confrontation. This confrontation is more intense and the need to comply is clearly articulated. The provider, without a doubt, warns the patient about the seriousness of the situation and uses emphasis in choice of words and tone of voice. The provider wants to "arm" the patient with important information and expects that the patient will hear it loud and clear.

There are also instances in which confrontations might be too strong. Typically, these high-level confrontations arouse intense feelings and can be perceived as very threatening. They are not likely to encourage change and more likely to be upsetting to patients. Consider this third version of the same patient–provider encounter.

PROVIDER: "Janice, I know you enjoy fast foods, but you've got to cut them out of your diet. I can't continue to treat you if you self-indulge like this."

This confrontation reprimands the patient. The patient may feel inadequate, "bad," embarrassed, and ashamed. It does not elicit constructive problem-solving nor does it show patient support which would empower the patient to correct unhealthy eating patterns. The purpose of the confrontation is lost in the idea that the provider may decide to release the patient and not treat him or her in the future. As such, the threat is actually the loss of provider, not the loss of health which is where it should be. This confrontation is very threatening and is likely to arouse very strong negative emotions.

Gazda, Childers, and Walters (1982, p. 143) addressed the problems with strong confrontations. They stated that if confrontations are too strong, five undesirable patient outcomes may occur (**EXHIBIT 14-1**).

Any one of these undesirable responses reduces the probability that further communication between provider and patient will be constructive and collaborative.

If the confrontation is too weak, however, the outcomes can be equally undesirable.

> **EXHIBIT 14-1** Undesirable Effects of Confrontations That Are Too Strong
>
> - Patients may respond defensively, giving explanations and reasons, and building a wall against the provider's influence.
> - Some patients may be driven away altogether.
> - Patients could become angry and go on the attack.
> - Patients can pretend to accept the advice but actually ignore it.
> - Patients feel helpless and become inappropriately dependent on the provider.

There are three undesirable outcomes as a result of confrontations that are too weak. Patients might:

- Lose respect for the provider. Otherwise, patients may assume that providers do not really believe in what they are talking about or that they lack the courage to be forceful about their judgments.
- Neither notice nor pay attention to the providers' statements.
- Receive the confrontation as reinforcing. The impression given to the patient is that the discrepant behavior is really okay (i.e., "You shouldn't eat fast foods—but, it's OK if you do").

In the example of the provider who confronts the patient about unhealthy eating patterns, the first example (low intensity) resulted in the patient's feeling confused about the convictions of the provider. The high-intensity confrontation, however, runs the risk of causing a defensive response that ranges from withdrawal to dependency.

In summary, the intensity of any confrontation needs to be strong enough to elicit positive actions but not so strong that it immobilizes the patient. To achieve this aim, it is important to regulate the intensity of the confrontation. In accordance with patients' reactions, confrontations can begin as gentle statements with feedback and progress in intensity if patients demonstrate confusion or fail to grasp the seriousness of the situation.

Types of Confrontation: Experiential or Factual Confrontations

Confrontations can also be described as either **experiential** or **factual**. That is, providers can speak from their firsthand experience of patients' behavior or they can present data of a factual nature that will provide patients and/or their families with information and feedback. For example, if providers state that the patient is trying to avoid fast foods but is not able to, the confrontation is experiential. Otherwise, the provider learned this through direct experience with the patient. Two observations communicate discrepancy: the patient's attempt to avoid fast foods but apparent inability to be successful. If the provider, however, states, "Janice, if you continue to eat fast foods the way you are, your blood sugar levels will fluctuate significantly," then the provider presents clinical judgments that are substantiated by factual data about the disease and its management.

Confrontations, as has been explained, present discrepancies. They may be more or less intense and more or less threatening. They may reflect providers' direct observations of the patient and/or draw from providers' expertise and knowledge in the field, or both. For any confrontation to play a positive role in change it should be coupled with trust and empathy. High levels of trust and empathetic responsiveness in the patient–provider relationship are prerequisite to effective confrontations.

Easing into Confrontations and Regulating Intensity

Easing into confrontations and regulating intensity have been described in the literature in some detail. The following six steps seem

---

EXHIBIT 14-2 Steps to Complete Before Using Confrontations

- Establish a relationship built on trust and caring.
- Use empathy, positive regard, respect, warmth, active listening, and genuineness in building this relationship.
- Lay a foundation for the purpose for addressing the patient's unique concerns and problems.
- Avoid appearing overly judgmental and critical in instances in which there are no emergent threats to the patient.
- Identify any discrepancies that were obvious and plan an approach to communicate them.
- Define the provider's role and level of commitment to the partnership.

---

to follow logically and ensure that confrontations occur when the patient–provider relationship itself is substantially strong enough to permit the provider to confront the patient (**EXHIBIT 14-2**). In this case, the provider has done the following.

Returning then to our scenario of the provider and the patient who is overindulging in fast foods, and therefore placing her health at risk, the following process exemplifies how to prepare the patient to receive the confrontation. The provider first acknowledges how difficult it is to resist fast foods and recognizes the patient for having made some attempts in this direction.

To communicate further respect and appreciation, providers can ask patients how they see the problem and what solutions they would propose. Before zeroing in on this patient's difficulty, the provider can speak generally about other patients' difficulties and/or what the provider has learned through professional experience and research. At this point, expressions of tolerance, if not previously expressed, may be given: "I know, it's tough," or "The most difficult thing is to resist those

'Golden Arches.'" Finally, the provider states clearly and succinctly, "Eating fast foods is going to prevent you from staying well. You're going to need to change this pattern—I don't expect you to do it without help. But we are definitely going to get very serious about this."

In most cases, this process is sufficient to both gain patients' attention and increase their interest in making changes. If the provider determines that what is really called for is a great deal more forcefulness, there are five specific ways in which this confrontation could be strengthened (**EXHIBIT 14-3**).

Considering that providers can either strengthen or weaken confrontations, and that they can even do both within a single encounter, it is important to consider general instances in which confrontations are appropriately intense.

Most patients will respond to simple first-level confrontations; however, there are instances that require more direct approaches. When patients are asked to make changes, these changes are not always easy to implement. Some changes involve altering rather deep-seated repetitive behaviors and/or culturally or religiously supported patterns. Patients may not be easily convinced that the change is worth it. In this instance, providers' will need to decide whether there is time to use one or more motivational interviewing approaches.

In the following dialogue, the nurse practitioner is trying to persuade an elderly patient to adhere to a low-fat diet. The patient is recovering from hepatitis that was incurred as a result of a blood transfusion at the time he was hospitalized for hip surgery. The patient was hospitalized but has been discharged and is receiving follow-up care and instruction because his liver damage was significant and recovery has been slow (**EXHIBIT 14-4**).

In this scenario, the patient expressed how difficult it was to follow the dietary restrictions. Chances are, he was cheating on his diet but not enough to feel the effects. At first, low-level confrontation strategies were used. Then the nurse practitioner intensified his or her confrontations in several ways: the provider presented factual information that had specific meaning to the patient, raised discrepancies, and used a confrontation backed by expert knowledge.

By not giving in but repeating and more emphatically stating the need to remain on the

---

EXHIBIT 14-3 Ways to Strengthen Confrontations

- The more personal the reference is, the more direct the confrontation. By making it clear that it is the patient's behavior, and nothing else, that is the issue and the confrontation becomes decidedly more direct.
- The more concrete the examples are, the more difficult it is to challenge the accuracy of a confrontation. For example, providers could remind patients that they are becoming more resistant than they were 6 months ago.
- The more recent the events are, the more powerful the examples. Behaviors that occurred in the past are less threatening even if they reflected poor judgment on the patient's part. The provider could remark, "In the last month you've shown me you cannot go a week without going off your diet."
- The more behaviors, not just words, are dealt with the more pressure can be applied because behaviors are not easily dismissed or invalidated. Thus, the provider's reference to specific examples of patients going off their diet cannot be argued.
- The more using what patients have said or done earlier to contradict what they are saying or doing now the stronger the confrontation. The provider may comment, "The last time you were in the office you said you would stay on your diet, yet you tell me you didn't."

EXHIBIT 14-4 Dialogue Box Illustrating Low- to Higher-Intensive Confrontations

PROVIDER:	"Mr. O_____, I've looked at your test results, it looks like you're going to have to stay on your low-fat diet for a while more."
PATIENT:	"But I love chopped liver, poor-boy sandwiches, pizza…."
PROVIDER:	"I know it's hard being on a restricted diet; have you ever been on a restricted diet before?"
PATIENT:	"A low-salt diet…."
PROVIDER:	"And did you stick to it?"
PATIENT:	"Mostly…yes. I had a stroke."
PROVIDER:	"So you stuck with it because you were afraid something bad would happen to you?"
PATIENT:	"Uh-huh."
PROVIDER:	"Do you know why you are being kept on a restricted diet?"
PATIENT:	"No, not really, no."
PROVIDER:	"The liver and gall bladder are involved in digesting fat. Your liver was traumatized because of your hepatitis. It cannot work as well as it should. So, we need you to keep fat out of your diet so we can give your liver a chance to heal. Right now, your liver needs a rest."
PATIENT:	"But I've been on it (the diet) a long time; how long will it last?"
PROVIDER:	"The liver needs time to heal, especially when you are older."
PATIENT:	"But I love corned beef and cabbage, a beer before dinner, and…."
PROVIDER:	"I know, but, for now, you really need to stick with your diet. I'll get you a copy of the revised food list. Later we can be a little more lenient; but for now the thing you need to do is stick to it."
PATIENT:	"So, you think I'm better off, uh, if I give this another try?"
PROVIDER:	"Yes, I can't really release you from the restrictions until your tests are better."
PATIENT:	"Sure I can't have just a little pizza and beer?"
PROVIDER:	"No, I'm afraid not. It's not going to be this bad forever. Try to think ahead to when your liver is healthy. Going back over the information I gave you, what would happen if you ate lots of fatty foods?"

diet, the nurse practitioner gave the patient very clear messages. Also, by applying authoritative leverage, suggesting to the patient that he was *under orders*, the nurse practitioner gave the patient very clear information that for his own welfare under no circumstances was this order to be changed, at least not at this time. Finally, by asking the patient to look at the discrepancy between what the nurse practitioner wanted to do and what would happen if he did, discrepancies are raised again.

Health care providers are particularly committed to promoting and maintaining health. If they observe that patients are doing things that run counter to these values, they are likely to become more concerned and even express judgment. Patients who resist necessary health-promotion or disease-management recommendations generally require skilled confrontational and motivational interviewing approaches as in the use of confrontations by presenting discrepancies near the end of the dialogue.

▶ Orders and Commands as Explicit Directives

Confrontations are frequently associated with two additional therapeutic response modes: orders and commands. Orders do not refer exclusively to written orders that are typically found in the patient's chart. Rather, what are meant by *orders* (and commands) are providers' actions to elicit change by insistence.

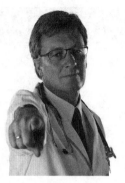

© CRoger Jegg - Fotodesign-Jegg.de/Shutterstock.

When a patient must adhere to a course of action and this course of action is related to an emergent life-and-death situation, providers need to issue an order if it is within their authority to do so. Orders and commands are used to increase the probability that a certain action will occur immediately. They are delivered with authority and require immediate response. In many respects, giving orders or commands is simply directing patients about what the provider wants them to do under serious circumstances.

For example, if the provider advises an elderly patient to stop driving his motor vehicle, this is an order or command to be taken very seriously. Not only is the patient's health and welfare at risk, so are the lives of friends and family passengers and other drivers on the road when the patient no longer has the capacity to drive safely.

There is yet another important element—the demand aspect of the directive—that separates commands from simple **directives**. In the scenario between the nurse practitioner and the patient with hepatitis and liver damage, the provider gave directives (e.g., "For now, you really need to stick with your diet," and "I can't really release you from the restrictions until your tests are better"). These directives were clear and firm. They were, in fact, statements of the medical order stating that the patient must stick to his diet expressed a demand. Phrased differently, it would have

been a directive but not a command. For example, the nurse practitioner's statement, "I've looked at your test results, and it looks like you're going to have to stay on your low-fat diet for a while more," comes across as a directive and the tone is less insistent. While it is clearly a directive, it is not expressed as a strong command.

Differentiating Orders and Commands from Confrontation and Advice

Orders and commands in health care differ from confrontations and advice-giving. Also, orders differ from commands—both need to be followed—but *commands* denote critical and immediate necessity for the action or change.

It is providers' responsibility to see that every order is understood. Thus, in our scenario, the nurse practitioner spent time giving the patient information about liver damage and the healing process as well as feedback about his specific condition—his liver-function tests did not warrant the relaxing of restrictions.

To avoid confusing the issue, the nurse practitioner was clear and succinct in presenting facts and imperatives. This is a requirement of issuing orders: procedures or steps to be taken need to be worded simply. When orders are very complicated, requiring many steps, and/or when patients' memory and concentration are impaired, orders need to be followed with written instructions and shared with family caregivers. In most cases this is true under any circumstance even if the patient or patient's caregiver is taking notes.

Pharmacists and nutritionists are particularly aware of the need to specify orders in writing. Usually there are so many important details that these orders need to be written. Consider what would seem to be a very simple instruction about a patient's medication (**EXHIBIT 14-5**).

EXHIBIT 14-5 Dialogue Box Illustrating Complexity of Orders About Medications

- "The doctor wants you to take these medications two times a day."
- "Take two capsules of this medicine and one pill each time."
- "Take these medications after your meals—in the morning after breakfast, at night after dinner."
- "This medication should be taken within an hour after eating."
- "Continue taking these medications until they are gone—7 days for this medication, 14 days for the second medication."
- "While you are on this medication, you should drink ample amounts of water— eight glasses a day is advised."
- "Also, you should avoid alcohol while taking these medications."
- "If you have excessive nausea or drowsiness while taking these medications within the first day or so, you should call and speak to your physician."

It is obvious that this information is more than good advice. Embedded in these instructions are orders.

As with advisement, an order is always more acceptable to a patient when the provider has established a relationship and uses the language and knowledge of the patient. This is an important principle with all patients but particularly so with patients who have low literacy levels. Providers need to accompany orders with ample explanation and time for the patient and family caregiver to respond and ask questions. Providers can even ask that the patient or patient caregiver to reiterate what they were told. When possible, orders need to be linked with the patient's own goals (e.g., to be able to eat certain foods again).

In the scenario between the nurse practitioner and the patient, the nurse practitioner was not certain if the patient knew enough about his condition or treatment to understand the

medical orders that were part of his plan of care. And, the patient responded as if he were confused or puzzled. It was important for the nurse practitioner to notice the patient's verbal and nonverbal responses, because both gave clues about the patient's readiness to hear, accept, and implement the directions and orders.

While head-nodding or the patient's reiteration of the directive are good signs, blank stares, confused expressions, and repeated questioning about the necessity of the order are not. Such signs suggest that the patient will have difficulty following the orders. The provider must ascertain both the patient's intentions to comply and the reasons for being reluctant. In some cases, orders can be revised to incorporate the specific preferences of patients. However, in most cases, orders are to be followed precisely as they are given. Even though the provider may want to relax the order, as in the scenario between the nurse practitioner and patient, orders generally cannot be altered.

Responsibility for Assessing Adherence

Once an order is issued, members of the health care team must evaluate the patient's level of adherence. Nonadherence to treatment plans, especially medication regimens, is a common problem, particularly among patients with asymptomatic stages of chronic illnesses such as diabetes and hypertension. However, these patients are not the focus in this discussion. The patients important to this discussion are those facing urgent health issues. When a patient is found to be nonadherent under these circumstances, what the provider does is critical. Still, some principles applying to chronic conditions that are not immediately life-threatening do have applicability here. In each instance, the provider's response is important in further modifying the patient's behavior.

In our scenario, the nurse practitioner did not assess the patient's level of adherence but assumed it was less than what it should be. It is also possible that the nurse practitioner did not want to stir up the patient's defensiveness by suggesting that the patient was lax in following the medical regimen. Assessing nonadherence, however, is extremely important for several reasons. When nonadherence or incomplete adherence occurs, some medications do not reach therapeutic levels and thus do not work the way they should. The original order may need to be changed or extended.

Special adherence education and support might be required for patients and their caregivers. Frequently, patients' responses to one aspect of treatment will raise issues of adherence to other aspects of treatment including physical activity. The reasons for poor adherence are usually multiple, including fears, suspicions, lack of knowledge, cultural beliefs, past experiences with health care providers, mistrust in the provider and the treatment, treatment side effects, and demands of the particular treatment or medication regimen. Providers are encouraged to review sections of this text that address health literacy (Chapter 15) and patient adherence to treatment (Chapter 18).

Generally, it is advisable to accept some part of the blame for patient's nonadherence if it is appropriate. In truth, patients' behavior is only one factor impacting nonadherence. In the case of the hepatitis patient and nurse practitioner, part of the problem might be that the patient and family were not provided support and education early on. Instead of blaming the patient, the nurse practitioner offered to get the patient a copy of the revised diet outline.

If the nurse practitioner had discussed this with the patient sooner, the patient might have been more knowledgeable and receptive. In taking this step, the provider does not ignore the patient's role in nonadherence but conveys the collaborative nature of the two working together to achieve treatment goals. Although the seriousness and immediacy of the problem should be made the focus of the discussion, there is still opportunity to explore and problem-solve with the patient how he could be more adherent (see **EXHIBIT 14-6**).

Commands Differ from Orders and Directives

Commands fit into the category of needing to be heeded immediately. These directives, like

EXHIBIT 14-6 General Guidelines for Assessing Patient Adherence and Nonadherence to Treatment

- "What do you remember about (specific action or change directive)?" (Open-ended question to explore)
- "How are you doing with (specific action or behavior change)?" (Open-ended question)
- "There are probably things that keep you from (specific action or behavior change)." "What are yours?" (Normalizes and encourages exploration of barriers)
- "Looking back at it, what do you think helped you do it or kept you from doing it?" (Open-ended question, still exploring barriers and facilitators)
- "What did you think you should do instead?" (Open-ended question, encouraging problem-solving)
- "What happened when you did it?" "What happened when you didn't, or did it only partially?" (Open-ended questions, exploring evaluation of attempts to change)
- "Given the same situation again, what would you do?" (Open-ended question, problem-solving)

orders, are phrased as necessities, but the seriousness of the context is usually more apparent. Directives that command not only convey that a behavior is mandatory, they imply immediacy.

"Take this medication now" is a command. The behavior is mandatory and the immediacy of the action is clear. While some providers may be uncomfortable with commands, the skill of issuing both orders and commands is a necessary addition to their less-directive response modes.

In issuing orders or commands, which should be communicated clearly and simply, it is extremely important that patients and family caregivers not only understand the action to take but also that these orders or commands are not mistaken for advice or extraneous information. Unlike advice, orders and commands must be followed. Because there is much at stake in noncompliance, verbal orders are best complemented by written instructions. In cases of orders and commands, the inference that patients have a choice to not comply or comply only partially must be avoided. Also, patients must understand that noncompliance or partial compliance cannot be ignored or excused.

If, for example, the patient will die if a directive is not followed, the expected action must be clear and the importance must also be clear. Orders and commands must always be received as critical advice. Discussing difficulties that patients may have to endure (such as social losses due to changes in behavior) fail in comparison to the necessity of immediate changes. Orders can, but should not, be perceived as a choice. In the earlier scenario, the patient wanted to negotiate relaxation of the diet restrictions—"sure I can't have just a little pizza and beer?" The responsibility lies with health care providers to reaffirm the seriousness of these directives.

Summarizing Directives for Patients

Closing discussions with patients when confrontations, orders, and commands have been used is sometimes complicated. Essentially, providers must assess not only what has and has not been understood but also how it was interpreted. Usually, to assess patients' response, providers will summarize important points of the discussion, including any directives given.

Some providers will prompt patients with a gentle command using the "teach-back" approach (e.g., "Tell me what you heard me say." And then, "What do you plan to do?"). Asking patients and/or family caregivers to assemble the points they remember is a good way to assess the level of shared meaning as well as any misconceptions they may have about what the provider said. If directives have been successfully used, the patient will be able to give feedback reflecting the discussion, including awareness of any adverse consequences if the directive is ignored.

As in any interview or consultation encounter with patients and/or their family caregivers, patients need to be told that the session is ending. This awareness can prompt patients to ask questions or clarify points that were not clear to them before the provider leaves the room. They should understand that if they are unsure about a directive or are feeling that they cannot comply, they have limited time to address their concerns but can always contact the provider immediately if necessary. It is very important for patients to understand how to get further information because the likelihood is that other questions or concerns will occur to them as they leave or when they talk to other friends and family members. In all cases, it is important to summarize the exchange in a positive manner.

Providers need to focus on the shared understanding, consensus, and plans that have come from the discussion with patients. Additionally, they may take particular notice of gains or progress made in previous attempts to patients following directives. Acknowledgement of this kind can raise patient self-confidence and self-efficacy about managing their critical health problem.

▶ Summary

Assisting patients to cope with illness and manage disease requires more direct strategies as well as the more supportive approaches (empathy, trust, respect, and warmth). While many times providers will opt for behavioral change theories that respect patients' stage of readiness and strive to avoid confrontation, there are specific instances in which it is appropriate to make more deliberate and assertive efforts to convince patients to change or take on a new behavioral approach to their problems and do this quickly. Providers are acting on their best clinical judgment and evidence-based practice. Providers generally agree that the seriousness of the situation dictates, in part, what strategy they will use. If their patient is in immediate threat for death or disability, they are likely to think more active and assertive strategies are appropriate if not essential.

It is widely understood that the action potential of confrontations, orders, and commands are best delivered when providers have earned the right to use these techniques. Confrontations can be more or less harsh, but they are important, action-oriented therapeutic responses. Confrontations deal openly with patients' displayed discrepant behaviors or with discrepancies between what patients should do and what they are actually doing.

The most threatening type of confrontation is one that deals with the present and is accusatory. Patients usually respond defensively to these high-level/high-intensive confrontations, so it is important to assess the need and wisdom of using confrontations of this type. In actuality, a provider has many options in any given encounter beginning with a mild, low-level confrontation and proceeding with more direct, intense confrontations if needed.

Although orders and commands are frequently used along with confrontation, they are actually separate strategies to promote change.

Both orders and commands are directives; however, commands are usually issued more forcefully and require immediate response. Situations requiring rapid response are best treated with commands.

Confrontations, orders, and commands are frequently preferred over advice and opinions. Advice can lack strength and influence while confrontations, orders, and commands, even mildly phrased, do not. Patients who are at risk for ignoring advice and instructions require strongly stated imperatives. For example, if the patient is going to die in a year if he continues to do what he is doing, you are going to use confrontation about health consequences related to ignoring medical advice. It is the provider's duty to share this factual information. Will you wait for his readiness to change before explaining this to him? Not likely. You will do it immediately.

While confrontations, orders, and commands increase self-awareness and help promote change, their distinct contribution is that they stress the seriousness of the situation, punctuating the necessity to listen and comply with providers' directives. Just as providers cannot rely completely on this approach, neither can providers abdicate their responsibility to use these responses in appropriate contexts. Because these modalities are frequently used in a context of punctuation with affective involvement by the provider, it is necessary that providers be aware of their own emotional responses.

Historically, the use of confrontations, orders, and commands involved the sequential escalation of provider influence and power. Power and authority resided with providers with minimal recognition that patients were active participants in their own care. Sometimes providers decide they need these more direct approaches to clearly state the seriousness of the situation and get the responses they are looking for in the short run. Confrontations are more indirect. Orders clearly state one or more recommendations, and commands demand a specific response (avoidance of which would involve critical consequences). Quite often these responses are used together. That is, orders or commands are often given in an encounter where confrontation has occurred.

In summary, despite the fact that our orientation to behavior change in this text discourages the use of high-intensity confrontation approaches, there are times when this therapeutic response mode is appropriate. Not all patients are willing or able to participate collaboratively in their care. But, clearly they need this care. So, while providers may limit "ordering" the patient, they are not likely to eliminate orders from their repertoire of skills.

Discussion

1. What are the basic similarities and differences between confrontations, directives, and orders?
2. Explain the difference between offering an experientially based confrontation and a confrontation based upon providers' professional expertise and evidence-based practice.
3. Identify ways the intensity of confrontations might be increased or decreased.
4. Give details about what is communicated in any directive where the consequence of not complying is a threat to patients' health and well-being.
5. Discuss the following idea: confrontation without a strong therapeutic relationship based upon empathy and respect is rarely effective.

References

Clark, F. (2012). *Caring confrontation with involuntary chemical dependency clients.* Master of Social Work Clinical Research Papers. Paper 13. Retrieved from http://sophia.stkate.edu/msw_papers/13

Gazda, G. M., Childers, W. C., & Walters, R. P. (1982). *Interpersonal communication: A handbook for health professionals.* Gaithersburg, MD: Aspen Publishers, Inc. (Epigraph from pp. 141–142).

McGuire-Bouwman, K. (2006). *Caring confrontation in experiential psychotherapy.* Retrieved from http://www.cefocusing.com/pdf/2F2cCaringConfrontationin ExperientialTherapy.pdf

White, W., & Miller, W. (2007). The use of confrontation in addiction treatment: History, science and time for change. *Counselor, 8*(4), 12–30.

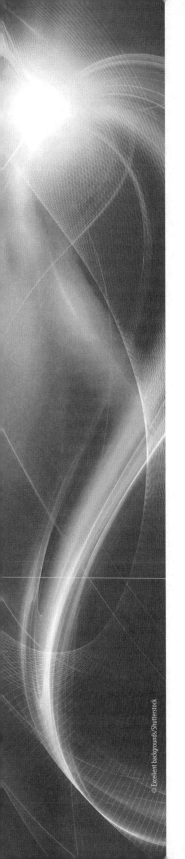

PART IV

Communications to Ensure Comprehensive and Continuous Patient-Centered Care Under Challenging Circumstances

Most people would agree that communication can be difficult, and providers would add that communicating with patients and families are often difficult. Under the best of circumstances, a provider can get poor results. Providers or patients and their families can fail to send messages in ways that they can be understood. What is said is not always perceived and processed in the manner that was intended. By definition, human communication can be both awe-inspiring and, at times, problematic.

What if one "upped the ante," so to speak, and tried to communicate under already difficult interpersonal circumstances? Would providers need to quadruple their skills and knowledge? Most likely, because to communicate effectively in these instances one would have to know a considerable amount about the specific so-called difficulty. In health care, providers are confronted time and time again with challenging circumstances that are intense and emotional and have a high risk for not turning out well, circumstances in which patients successfully resist our good judgment and care.

Part IV of this text introduces issues surrounding communicating therapeutically with select populations that pose a variety of challenges: those with limited low literacy, those patients facing the long-term stress of coping and managing chronic illness, patients who are facing a life crisis either due to illness or other situational event, and those patients displaying significant negative or resistant coping responses. In actuality, there are populations of patients that experience these challenges simultaneously making effective communications even more challenging.

In this section of the text, specific attention is drawn to communicating with patients and families under challenging circumstances. But, what is difficult for one provider may be elementary to another, so the situations chosen for discussion in this section may or may not be challenging to some providers, but at least for the beginning clinician, they are likely to be. Barriers to communication in these situations have been described in the literature.

In Chapter 15, "Communicating with Patients with Low Health Literacy," the challenges of communicating effectively with patients who by virtue of education, language, minority status, culture, and previous experience or lack of experience with health issues are described. These individuals and their families may have difficulty in understanding and navigating the health care delivery system to receive the best care possible. Specific steps in assessing levels of literacy in general, and specifically health literacy, are described along with recommendations for shaping communications to meet the needs of these groups and communities.

In Chapter 16, "Communicating with Patients with Chronic and/or Life-Threatening Illness," the concepts and principles of communicating with patients take on particular specificity. Knowing what patients and their families may be experiencing at a certain phase of illness and treatment is important in understanding how to respond therapeutically. Knowing how to address patient noncompliance in disease self-management is yet another dimension of communicating with these groups and their families.

In Chapter 17, "Communicating with Patients and Families in Crisis," the deficits in communication that individuals in crisis typically exhibit are detailed. Patients' subsequent reactions to the stimulus and crisis events are also presented. Finally, guidelines for communicating effectively with individuals in crisis are presented and discussed.

Providers who are engaged in the management of chronic disease and life-threatening illness must know a great deal about patients' actual and potential responses to illness. Managing care includes managing responses to illness (and treatment). Providers are to be both healers of disease and healers of maladaptive coping responses. Communicating with patients who display emotion, specifically when the display is negative, can be moderately to extremely difficult for most providers. In the final chapter of this section, Chapter 18, "Communicating Effectively with Patients Displaying Significant Negative or Resistive Coping Responses," emotions underlying patients' situations and choosing the best among several response options can be challenging.

If a thousand health care providers were asked which specific patient behaviors have been difficult to handle or contributed to negative affects there may be some level of agreement. Difficult patient behaviors discussed in Chapter 18 have also been addressed elsewhere in the literature. Patients' accusatory, complaining, demanding, aggressive, and self-pitying presentations usually arouse emotions in providers. These emotions are frequently followed by defensive reactions from providers—reactions that unfortunately can aggravate a preexisting challenging situation. Understanding these patient behaviors, their underlying causes, and what providers can do to avoid interpersonal traps are essential to communicating effectively with these patients.

In summary, Part IV of this text addresses communication skills at a somewhat higher, advanced level. This is not to say that the basic generic therapeutic response skills are not useful. Rather, generic skills must be added too. Experiences with actual patients in the context of health and illness provide depth and wisdom for communicating effectively as health professionals.

CHAPTER 15

Communicating with Patients with Low Health Literacy

CHAPTER OBJECTIVES

- Discuss the problem of low literacy in the United States, and identify populations and communities at risk for poor literacy.
- Differentiate between general literacy skills and health literacy.
- Identify at least four barriers to health literacy.
- Discuss the potential relationship of low health literacy and poor health outcomes.
- Describe ways to assess and enhance health literacy in patients.

KEY TERMS

- Functional health literacy
- General literacy

- Health literacy
- Matematical literacy

▶ Introduction

Speak slowly and with as few words as possible and always use the language of the person might be the single best advice for communicating with patients and families, but particularly so when they experience challenges due to poor literacy skills. This advice is probably what is meant by "communicating in plain language." It is particularly important in health care because all aspects of care center around understanding patients and discussing approaches to assess and manage their health issues.

Knowing the degree to which patients or patients' families understand what you communicated and its significance is challenging when communicating with persons with low literacy. On the flip side is the question of *to what degree* you *understand* them. How often would you admit, "I think I understood, but really can't be sure."?

Although seldom disclosed, the reality that neither you nor your patient nor the patient's family understood completely what was communicated can be rather high. Providers' mode of communicating with low literacy patients is critical in determining desired treatment outcomes.

`Low literacy has been associated with poor knowledge of disease, poor adherence to treatment regimens, and problems in disease self-management. Descriptive as well as randomized controlled research studies have reported the link between low literacy and these outcomes.

This chapter addresses the concepts and strategies for communicating with persons of low health literacy and strategies to assess literacy levels and plan accordingly. Strategies in this chapter include using the smallest amount of information at a visit, reinforcing information with visual handouts, repetition, teach-back, using the words of the patient, and using storytelling.

▶ The Problem of Literacy in the United States

According to a study conducted in late April 2013 by the U.S. Department of Education and the National Institute of Literacy and reported in several sources, 32 million adults or 14% of the population in the United States cannot read (U.S. Department of Education, National Institute of Literacy, OECD, 2016). Furthermore, 21% of adults in the United States read below a fifth grade level, and 19% of high school graduates cannot read. In the United States, data on reading levels differed by populations: 41% of Hispanic adults read below a basic level, compared to 24% Black, and 9% White. It was suggested that the illiteracy rate had not changed in 10 years.

While the United States competes favorably with other technology-rich countries on measures of literacy in general (defined as average score not significantly different from the international average), scores were significantly lower on other measures of literacy (Rampey et al., 2016). For example, the United States was significantly lower on numeracy and problem-solving skills. Numeracy (sometimes called **mathematical literacy**) refers to the ability to reason and comprehend fundamental arithmetic (addition, subtraction, multiplication, and division), while problem-solving skills refer to the ability to work through details of a problem to reach a solution.

The reason why level of literacy (in all its dimensions) is important to health care and health care providers is that it is intimately linked with health literacy or individuals' abilities to obtain, process, and understand health information and services needed to make appropriate health decisions (Berkman et al., 2011). Low health literacy, like low levels of basic literacy, is a significant problem in the

United States. The Agency for Healthcare Research and Quality (AHQR) stated that in 2003 approximately 80 million adults in the United States had limited health literacy, and this varied across groups with higher rates of limited literacy among the elderly, minorities, individuals who did not complete high school, adults whose primary language was not English (before starting school), and people living in poverty. Furthermore, AHQR stated that in a 2004 systematic review of the literature found that low health literacy (reading skills) was associated with poor health outcomes. These outcomes included health-related knowledge and comprehension, hospitalization rates, global health measures, and some chronic diseases.

To fully understand the problem of health literacy, providers need to have a working knowledge of the problem of low literacy (the ability to read and write and calculate basic math) and the extent to which it affects patients' abilities to understand aspects of their illness and to follow the treatment that is planned for them.

Taken as a whole, significant numbers of the U.S. population may have difficulty communicating with health care providers, navigating the health care system, and understanding the important meaning and instructions. These patients and their families present a special challenge in that they may not easily understand materials and instructions presented even at the sixth-grade level. Frequently, they feel reluctant to reveal their illiteracy and may not try to engage in dialogue with providers in fear of risking exposure of their poor understanding. If this happens, both provider and patient will be handicapped in ensuring the best care possible.

▶ Functional Health Literacy

Results of the various agencies reporting on low literacy and poor health literacy raise

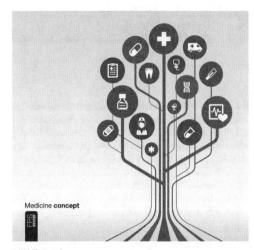

Medicine **concept**

© Hilch/Shutterstock.

considerable concern about patients and their families to function adequately in a health care setting. While *literacy* speaks generally about the ability about read and write, **functional health literacy** refers more specifically to the skills and knowledge necessary to understand illness and treatment but also the ability to navigate the health care system.

These skills include understanding how to read and interpret medication prescriptions, appointment slips, and referrals, and understanding the concept of need for follow-up of illness through additional medical appointments (**EXHIBIT 15-1**).

An underlying purpose of providers' communications is not only to communicate at a level that the patient can understand but also includes improving patients' health literacy. Maximizing patient encounters to improve patient health literacy is complicated by a variety of personal, patient–provider, and system factors that are not always under providers' control. Nonetheless, the goal is to advance the patient's understanding of illness and treatment through singular or sequential contacts communicating with patients and/or their family members.

In a report by the AHQR (2004), it was concluded that low literacy is not only associated with poor understanding of medical

EXHIBIT 15-1 Reasons Health Professionals Value Functional Health Literacy

1. Health literacy can empower patients to form an active alliance with their providers, enhanced primarily by the patient's ability to understand basic medical terminology and procedures.
2. Informed patients are more likely to initiate and sustain adequate self-management behaviors that will also result in

health-promoting behaviors and improved health outcomes.
3. Patients who do not understand health providers' instructions are less likely to receive quality care. This is particularly a problem with the elderly who bear the greatest burden of disease but are known to have low levels of health literacy (Safeer & Keenan, 2005).

advice but with adverse patient outcomes and even negative effects on health. Taken as a whole, low health literacy can lead to substandard care. It was noted that patients with low literacy had not only poorer health outcomes (intermediate disease markers, measures of morbidity, and general health status) but also poorer use of health services.

The research is marred by a number of methodological issues (reliance on cross-sectional designs, inconsistency in the type of health literacy measure used, and problems with generalization due to small and selective sample sizes). Furthermore, most studies measured short-term knowledge gain and immediate health outcomes without building in the measurement of long-term effects. An issue of importance is whether these relationships would hold up over time and what exactly is the nature of this relationship. For example, it has been shown that literacy also correlates with economic and insurance status, which is linked with use of health care and preventive health services. The impact of health literacy on health service use could be confounded by many other related factors.

Nonetheless, the literature supports a positive and significant relationship between level of health literacy and patient outcomes in a wide array of studies through time of patients with chronic conditions (e.g., HIV [Miller, Brownlee, McCoy, & Pignone, 2007], diabetes [Schillinger, Barton, Karter, Wang, & Adler, 2006], and the use of health services [Miller et al., 2007]).

Early on the U.S. Department of Health and Human Services, in its report *Healthy People 2010*, included improved health literacy as an objective (Objective 11-2), stressing the need for equity in health care. In this document, health literacy is defined as "The degree to which individuals have the capacity to obtain, process, and understand basic health information and services needed to make appropriate health decisions."

According to this document, health literacy includes the ability to understand: (1) instructions on prescription drug bottles, (2) appointment slips, (3) medical education brochures, (4) medical directions and consent forms, plus (5) the ability to navigate complex health care systems. Health literacy is not simply the ability to read materials. "It requires a complex group of reading, listening, analytical, and decision-making skills, and the ability to apply these skills to health situations." It is the same document listed above: Healthy People 2010.

In health care situations, health literacy includes both verbal and written comprehension and numeracy skills. Understanding cholesterol levels, calculating how many medications to take and when, and reading labels all require math skills, and, while most of it is simple math, still the probability that any one patient with low literacy skills may not understand what to do is significant enough to address. In addition to basic literacy skills, health literacy includes background information about how the body works, what infection and injury mean, how the body recovers with medical intervention, and the relationship of lifestyle patterns and illness (e.g., nutrition and obesity).

Unlike basic literacy skills, health literacy is not necessarily related to years of education. A person who has attained a graduate degree may not function well in a health care setting nor understand the importance of preventive care. A person who is well educated but was educated more than 20 years ago may no longer have an accurate understanding of many chronic illnesses. Other reasons accounting for poor health literacy include the individual's previous exposure to chronic illness and health care environments. On the contrary, someone who has not graduated from high school may be particularly knowledgeable about how to navigate the system and the meaning of chronic illness due to their own history of a chronic disease or the treatment of a close family member.

Due to the complex nature of health care forms and regulations, not even persons with very high levels of **general literacy** may easily interpret their lab tests, and not even a physician could help a patient complete insurance forms or use the best insurance coverage plan. All things considered, it is important to conduct an individualized assessment of the patient's knowledge and ability to function in the health care setting. This should be the standard of practice but attention to populations at significantly higher risk—the elderly, those whose familiarity with the English language is weak; minorities, those who have not completed high school; and those living in poverty—is critical.

▶ Barriers to Health Literacy

Barriers to adequate **health literacy** for everyone are multiple and vary depending on cultural and educational differences. All potential barriers need to be assessed in each encounter with patients and their families. As previously noted, health care providers have a role in improving the health literacy of the patients and families they see, not only for those who lack basic skills to successfully navigate the health care system but for everyone encountered. In fact, patients and their families at the close of an encounter should be saying, "I didn't know that," "Ok, I understand," or "Well…that was pretty interesting."

As agents for change, providers must first be able to identify low health literacy and understand the barriers to achieving higher levels of health literacy. Approaches to solving the health literacy problem would be enhanced if those factors that influence health literacy were understood. The state of the science in studying health literacy is preliminary with many studies focusing on the assessment of literacy and others on the connection of literacy with health-seeking behaviors, with a minor concentration on the factors that influence health literacy. This is, in part, due to the absence of a conceptual framework from which to view the problem in a broader context. The following discussion places health literacy in a context affected by multiple barriers, some of which are mutable (within providers' control) and others which are not.

Barriers to patients achieving health literacy are multiple and occur at many levels: individual-level barriers (demographic, health status, complexity of illness/treatment, illness experience, and health care system exposure), patient–provider relationship barriers, and system-related barriers (number, length, and quality of encounters, patient-centered care delivery). **FIGURE 15-1** is a diagram of these factors and illustrates how they may interact with each other to affect level of health care literacy.

Individual-Level Patient Barriers

As previously described, certain populations are vulnerable to low levels of health literacy. Age, culture, language, education, and income

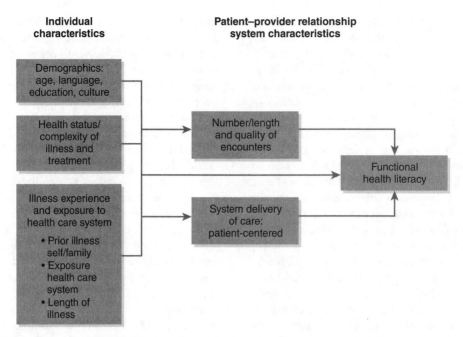

FIGURE 15-1 Multiple Interacting Factors Affecting Functional Health Literacy.

all play an independent and collective role in affecting individuals' level of health literacy. The following populations are at particular risk for low health literacy: youth, the elderly, those with low socioeconomic status with no health insurance, minority and marginal or vulnerable populations, the medically or cognitively impaired, and the medically underserved.

A population previously under-appreciated are groups of patients and families that have defined disabilities. By disability, it is meant those having sensory or communication deficits; functional limitations; or physical, mental, and/or emotional injuries or illnesses that impair their ability to acquire health literacy skills placing them at higher risk for health disparities.

In a recent report from the National Academies of Sciences, Engineering, and Medicine examining health equity, health disparities, and health literacy among people living with disabilities (2017) Havercamp and others explain that it is not that people with disabilities are destined for a life of poor health status,

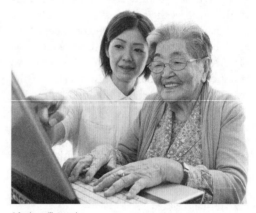

© Sunabesyou/Shutterstock.

rather, the lack of institutional support for this underserved population contributes to poor health outcomes.

Vulnerable populations have been shown to be at risk for disparities in health care and health. For the 14th year in a row, the AHRQ, as mandated by Congress, reported on disparities in health care quality received. The report continues to raise awareness of disparities as a function of race, ethnicity, and socioeconomic status, but also reports on age and potential literacy differences resulting in disparities in health care quality received in the U.S.

A number of studies have examined the association of low literacy and age. Most of the studies investigate the problem for the elderly with fewer studies on youth and adolescents. In a comprehensive and noteworthy study of the relationship of literacy and mortality in the elderly (Sudore et al., 2006) found that limited literacy (using the Rapid Estimate of Adult Literacy in Medicine [REALM]) was independently associated with a nearly twofold increase in mortality among 2,500 Black and White, community-dwelling elders without functional difficulties or dementia. This was the case even after adjusting for a number of confounding factors (demographics, socioeconomic status, comorbidities, self-rated health, health-related behaviors, access to health care, and psychosocial status). While limited literacy is prevalent in the elderly, no prospective study to date was conducted to link literacy with mortality in this population.

The aging of the population and the prevalence of chronic disease in the elderly raises the question of how literacy does and will play a role in both comorbidity and mortality in this population. It is possible that low literacy is implicated in health screening and continued use of appropriate health care. Because of the impact of low health literacy on hospital visits, health care expenditures, and poor health outcomes, much attention has been placed on adults and the elderly. For youth, the issues are different; but the problem of the use of health services and following preventive practices could, in part, be similar to that of adults and the elderly.

The relationship of low health literacy and adolescents' willingness to follow disease prevention messages and health promotion practices has been studied. Brown, Teufel, and Birch (2007) reported that in addition to age, difficulty understanding health information

and belief that kids can do little to affect their future health decreased their interest in and desire to follow what they were taught about health.

The investigators concluded that more attention should be placed on increasing student interest in health issues and feelings that they could control health outcomes. Culture and ethnicity have also been studied for their influence on health literacy. Language and education affect health literacy in that not all health promotion and disease prevention literature is comprehensible, and this might affect patients' repertoire of information about disease and treatment.

Given that multiple problems in these areas increase the risk that their health care literacy will be very low, these individuals may have difficulty finding or accessing health providers, completing health care forms, making decisions when offered alternatives, describing their history of health care problems and the course of treatment, understanding the role of preventive health care, understanding the relationship of risky behaviors and health promotion and disease prevention, self-managing chronic or acute health conditions, understanding directions on health information sheets, and making decisions about their care. Recognizing individuals with these deficits is important early on, and, as suggested, sufficient time and attention needs to be given to bringing these individuals to a place of even basic understanding (**EXHIBIT 15-2**).

An example of this kind of misconception would be the following. A 34-year-old Hispanic male with HIV and Hepatitis C expresses the opinion that he thought that he could not transmit Hepatitis C to someone else *unless his liver touched the liver of this other person*. What is lost in the translation here is knowledge of how disease is transmitted and the effect of the disease on body systems. Another example is the patient who interprets the directions on his or her medication bottle reading *take twice a day* to mean

---

EXHIBIT 15-2 Deficits in Patients' Understanding Health Conditions

- Patients do not recognize what they do not know. Many patients do not know what they do not know. These groups frequently include the elderly, those with impaired judgment, and those with limited exposure to disease and health care delivery systems.
- Patients think they know but do not know. Many patients harbor misconceptions about disease and treatment. They may have no reason to doubt their understanding so rarely ask questions to clarify what they believe.

---

take two pills at once. In each of these examples, there were apparent barriers to effective communication including the patients' low levels of health literacy, language problems, and misunderstanding of disease (how disease and treatment work).

The identification of the barriers just listed focuses almost exclusively on what the patient brings to the encounter. In addition to these factors, several other factors affect patients' health literacy and our ability to educate them and communicate effectively. Patient–provider encounters, health and treatment complexity, and system issues affect patient–family–provider communications and providers' capacities to improve patient health literacy.

Provider–Patient–Family Relationship Barriers

While one hopes that provider–patient–family encounters promote health literacy, this is not always the case. In fact, training in the health care professions has been studied for its ability to favorably affect professionals' abilities to identify and reach patients with low literacy,

and this occurs across disciplinary boundaries and health professions. Improvements are needed.

A good deal of the health literature has been directed at improving the written word to communicate more effectively with patients and their families. The expectation is that if the materials are sufficiently user-friendly, the problem of low literacy has been addressed. The problem with this assumption is that the impact of the relationship between providers and patients is not taken into account. In this case, it is not only the quality of the printed matter but the provider's interpersonal approach to the patient. Several theorists have attempted to describe the essence of the patient–provider relationship that will successfully affect patients in positive ways. Several of the interventions described in Part III (listening, pausing, and judicious use of silence) are included in explanations of what makes for therapeutic communications with persons of low literacy.

It has also been suggested that the patient and his or her family may or may not understand the provider and, if confused, may not ask for clarification. The presence of an interpreter is not always the answer because what might occur is that the focus of the relationship shifts from patient and provider to interpreter and provider. Although necessary and welcomed at times, the use of an interpreter might be problematic if the therapeutic alliance with the patient is disturbed. The appropriate use of interpreters has been addressed in several publications.

System-Level Barriers

System-level factors that may act as barriers are perhaps the least explored category. They include the mission of the institution, the organization of services, the proportion of providers to patients, and time and schedule of care activities. If the mission of the institution is to serve primarily low-income populations at risk for disease and illness who have not perhaps received adequate screening and preventive care, then the institutional philosophy may be to focus on methods to enhance receptive approaches to gain the trust and confidence of the population they serve.

However, if the system of care is such that the ratio of providers to patients is inadequate and the time provided for medical visits is limited, then organizationally, any opportunity to improve health literacy may be compromised. Studies of provider–patient ratios and health outcomes, including patient and family satisfaction with communication received, indicate the importance of a system that *talks the talk and walks the walk*.

Paasche-Orlow, Schillinger, Greene, and Wagner (2006), in a careful account of the system-level barriers suggest that changes need to occur at the level of organization and delivery of health care systems to improve the overall quality of U.S. health care and produce a more health-literate society. They advocate that *comprehension* should be a standard in clinical care to the extent that it is a basic universal precaution.

To effectively do this, providers will need system-level supports, including time, education about assessing and addressing health literacy deficits, and built-in incentives, to encourage this facet of their roles. Above all, these structures and incentives, including reinforcements, should be targeted for vulnerable populations. It is in these populations, in particular, that a variety of biophysical, economic, environmental, and cultural factors influence the health and health care to those with limited literacy.

Summarizing the nature of the link between the system and outcomes for those that have literacy deficits, Paasche-Orlow, Schillinger, Greene, and Wagner (2006) propose three distinctive organizing principles:

1. Promote productive interactions between providers and patients to improve communications, exercising universal precautions to assure comprehension, improving

providers' communication capacities, and developing communication technology platforms.

2. Address the organization of health care, making patient-centered care a system property and streamlining, simplifying, and targeting vulnerable populations.

3. Embrace a community-level ecological perspective, using intervention models that acknowledge the multilevel nature of population vulnerability and advocate and develop an independent and trusted public health voice.

▶ Communication Interventions to Improve Health Literacy

Health providers have an important role in assessing, planning for, implementing, and evaluating health literacy and problems directed at enhancing health literacy. It has been estimated that up to 80% of patients forget what their provider (doctor) has said as soon as they leave and nearly 50% of what they do remember is inaccurate.

By assessing and addressing health literacy, providers can improve communication with their patients and increase the probability that patients will understand what they say, ultimately leading to better treatment adherence and ultimately, better health outcomes. Health care systems can enable and support providers to play significant roles in addressing literacy issues. **EXHIBIT 15-3** describes the elements of health care systems promoting health literacy.

The first thing health providers need to know is how to identify individuals with low levels of health literacy. Because patients with low health literacy often feel shame and a sense

EXHIBIT 15-3 Elements of a Health Care System Promoting Health Literacy

- Time to construct reading materials using plain language and illustrations.
- Opportunity to test and evaluate all written materials and medical instruction information sheets.
- Provider–patient time to communicate to exceed 6–10 minutes.
- Advocacy for health literacy in the organization and recognition of the value of assessing health literacy.
- Providers knowledgeable and skilled in concepts of and assessment of limited literacy.
- Opportunity to conduct feedback loop (patients are asked what they do or do not understand as well as time for the provider to clarify the patient's communication).
- Development of population-based health literacy best practices.

of inadequacy they may hesitate to ask the provider to repeat instructions or explain treatment or other important relevant information (Safeer & Keenan, 2005).

▶ Assessing Health Literacy

Reviewing the literature on physician assessment of health literacy, Safeer and Keenan (2005) bring attention to the fact that health providers do poorly in assessing literacy. The usual approach is to identify the patient's potential understanding by obtaining the patient's level of education. Safeer and Keenan also indicate that the grade level of the patient may underestimate the level of illiteracy and, as the age of the patient increases, declining cognitive skills, decreased sensory abilities, and increased time since formal education place people at greater risk for poor health literacy.

There are a number of health literacy assessments that have been used for research purposes and some are useful to providers. The Test of Functional Health Literacy in Adults (TOFHLA) is a short-measure S-TOFHLA in English or Spanish to measure language proficiency. The REALM, or more recently, the REALM-R, is an eight-item measure to rapidly screen for health literacy problems.

The REALM is easy to administer and is quick, whereas the TOFHLA provides a formal overview of patients' abilities to comprehend material but is generally more time-consuming and less practical in the everyday clinic setting. Thus, the short form of the TOFHLA was designed. Another instrument, developed to be used exclusively with Spanish-speaking patients, is called the Short Assessment of Health Literacy for Spanish-Speaking Adults (SAHLSA-50) (Lee, Bender, Ruiz, & Cho, 2006) and is based on the REALM. This instrument contains 50 items and could be used in the clinical setting to screen Spanish-speaking patients for low literacy.

The shorter versions of the S-TOFHLA (in Spanish or English) or REALM-R may be useful in the community clinic setting; however, the provider interviewer approach is key in assessing health literacy. The S-TOFHLA is useful in measuring written comprehension but does not capture language competency. Recently, the BEST (Basic English Skills Test) has been tested for its use as an oral interview that can be used in the emergency department (Downey & Zun, 2007).

Basic medical language is usually graded on a continuum, as in the REALM. There are terms that are easy to understand (at the third grade level or below), moderately difficult (at a fourth to sixth grade level), slightly more difficult (seventh and eighth grade levels), and most difficult to comprehend (high school level).

Asking patients if they have heard any of the words in the *moderate* (fatigue, prescription, depression, nutrition) category may give providers some idea about whether patients are at the very low end of health literacy or may be health care-experienced and knowl-edgeable to the point that they have a high level of health literacy. As suggested in the REALM, providers might ask patients whether they have heard the term and what they think the term means. In this way, providers capture information about both patient recognition and comprehension which are needed to tailor patient instruction and teaching.

There is still another assessment tool that has been developed, and it can be used as a quick screening tool in primary care settings (Weiss et al., 2005). The Newest Vital Sign (NVS) uses a nutrition label (the ice cream nutrition label) and six questions to ascertain patients' compre-hension. It takes approximately 3 minutes to complete. Fewer than four correct answers indi-cate a patient may have limited health literacy.

The English version has been shown to have good reliability. However, the reliability of the Spanish version was not as good and was explained as a function of so many subgroups of Latino subjects tested. The investigators rec-ommend further testing of the NVS. This tool is available online only at http://www.annfammed .org/cgi/content/full/3/6/514/DC1 (Weiss et al., 2005, p. 516).

Because little has been done in the assess-ment of health literacy in adolescents, Chisolm and Buchanan (2007) validated a tool specifi-cally to examine the TOFHLA in adolescents. They found that the reading comprehension component of the TOFHLA was valid for ado-lescents. While most literacy tools have been used and validated with adults, there is an over-pressing need to have adolescents make health care choices, and this requires them to be knowledgeable about health promotion and disease prevention.

One of the most practical and conven-tional assessment tool which does not require administering a survey is the *teach-back* method, also referred to as the "feedback loop" or "closing the loop." The idea behind this assessment and intervention is that in order to fully understand patients' comprehension of the information given to them, it is important

to assess their grasp of the content that was communicated. Patients are asked to restate the information in their own words, not simply repeat what the provider said, to better ensure that the information is both understood and remembered. Thus, this strategy is used to assess the comprehension of medical informa-tion and aid in the patient's remembering what it is that the provider taught them.

When patients' understanding is inac-curate or incomplete, providers repeat the process until they are confident that patients understand the information needed to be com-pliant to the treatment regimen or recommen-dations for health promotion. Patients can also be asked to act upon the information given as if they were, in real life, performing the action. For example, they would read the prescription bottle and demonstrate the number of pills they would take of this and other medications twice a day. They could also demonstrate their knowledge of how many pills they will take in a single day as well as morning and evening intervals and what secondary conditions are needed (e.g., before meals/after meals, avoid-ing use of alcohol, and reporting significant side effects).

In the use of the teach-back or closing the loop techniques, it is important and possible to avoid a "test-like" atmosphere. Rather, the provider is testing how well the patient was taught, not how well the patient performs. By putting the responsibility on the provider, it is possible to avoid provoking feelings of embar-rassment, shame, and anxiety that may result from patients' feeling they failed and disap-pointed the provider. Review the following dialogue and formulate your opinions about the success of this approach (**EXHIBIT 15-4**).

Each time providers use teach-back they can learn how the patient has processed instruc-tions and what directions need clarification or enforcement. While the example of instructing about medication was used, this same tech-nique could be used in teaching patients about other parts of their treatment or in their under-standing of their illness and symptoms.

EXHIBIT 15-4 Dialogue Demonstrating the Teach-Back Approach

PROVIDER:	"So what the instructions mean is that you will need to take this medication in the morning before you have a meal. You are free to eat after 1 hour from the time you take this pill. But, if you forget to take it before 2:00 in the afternoon you need to wait until the next day."
PROVIDER:	"Now, I want to see how well I did in explaining everything you need to know in order to take your medication. What's important about taking this medicine in the morning?"
PATIENT:	"I have to take it before 2."
PROVIDER:	"Ok, you got one part. The other important thing to remember is that you need to take it before you eat and wait an hour before you have something to eat."

EXHIBIT 15-5 Potential Indicators of Poor Comprehension and Low Health Literacy

- Ambivalence about asking staff for help. (Tends to avoid being an imposition)
- Reserve questions until after leaving the interview or exam room. (May ask another staff member in passing what something means)
- Ask a question and then withdraws it as if they understand but do not.
- Miss appointments and do not call to reschedule. (May give no reason)
- Nonadherent to a treatment plan and medication regimen. (May simply reply, "I forgot")
- Quiet and unassuming in the treatment room.
- Come with adult companions who can offer advice or reword what provider says.
- Delay making decisions about treatment options, and ask for things to be put in writing.

If patients are unable to repeat what they were told, providers will need to assess what the problem is and how the provider can reframe the teaching approach. If providers choose to repeat the information, it is advisable to restate the material without using the same words. For example, try to simplify perhaps using fewer words and observe patients' attention span. Another approach is to repeat the material several times throughout the course of the discussion to assess whether the patient is getting more comfortable with the words and terms that are used. This method is also used to determine whether patients have the capacity and skill to handle management of their disease whether it is giving themselves insulin injections or simply how they are going to organize their medications in their weekly medication tray.

An insightful description of clues to understanding patients' comprehension of details and level of health literacy is helpful (Baker et al., 1996). **EXHIBIT 15-5** lists several indicators that will help build providers' skills in assessing patients.

▶ Documenting Health Literacy Problems

Patients' medical records contain a wealth of information about their health condition and the plan of care. What is often missing is information about patients' comprehension of their illness and treatment. A simple approach to documenting patient comprehension is to draft a flow sheet with the essentials of what is required for the patient to adequately self-manage their care, in essence a skill checklist. For example, for a diabetic patient on insulin such a chart might include monitoring skills (e.g., checking blood glucose levels and complications resulting from poor control of sugar levels, the beginning signs of insulin shock, how to inject insulin, and what diet and exercise plan needs to be followed).

One column of the flow sheet would list the skill, the second column would indicate the date and time the patient had received instruction, and the third column would contain information about the patient's skill level (e.g., on a scale of 1 to 5 with 1 indicating low level of comprehension and 5, high level of comprehension). Added to this flow sheet may be directions to other providers about what information needs to be reinforced or supplemented. The documentation of health literacy problems is critical because of its associated links to patient adherence to treatment regimens.

▶ Health Promotion Messages and Media to Improve Health Literacy

A multitude of agencies have concerns about the health literacy deficits in the United States. For disease prevention awareness programs to be effective they need to address communities at their level. Many groups and communities cannot understand messages that are broadcasted or communicated in narrow circles or over social media.

Public media are instrumental in communicating disease-prevention and health-promotion messages. Viewing these messages will inform providers about what works and with whom. Notice that messages are brief, and persons who are or are not yet affected by the disease speak (they are persons like those at risk). The context of the message is important, and usually the audience can identify with the context (the importance of the family or needs to be there for grandchildren).

An example, a young Hispanic couple and their children are pictured in the context of a loving family unit. The words are: "Protect YOUR family!" (from HIV/AIDS). What is known about this population is that the family (*familia*) is a high priority, and the man in the family is strong and powerful. Thus, the concept of *machismo* is intrinsically addressed in the message to take positive action. As is, this message has significant impact on those who read it. Although the message is very brief, the context makes it powerful. Few who read this message are likely to forget the content.

The literature on improving health literacy through good communications with patients and their families is extensive. A list of references is provided at the end of this chapter. **EXHIBIT 15-6** provides a composite list of approaches that are recommended and/or have been used in communicating to patients with limited health literacy.

In summary, health literacy levels should be assessed and specific steps need to be taken to enhance the effectiveness of encounters to enhance patients' health literacy. At the very least, providers need to make sure that patients advocate for themselves on a regular basis at patient–provider contacts. They should ask:

1. What is my problem?
2. What are you going to do?
3. What am I supposed to do?
4. Why is it important for me to do this (take medication, follow a particular diet and exercise program, monitor my blood glucose levels)?

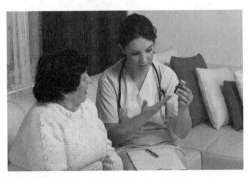

© Blaj Gabriel/Shutterstock.

EXHIBIT 15-6 Communications to Improve Patient Health Literacy

- Take a moment to develop a *gestalt* of the patient and situation (demographics [age, gender, ethnicity, educational level], culture, cultural similarities and differences, presenting problem and history, previous treatment plan), including first response.
- Assess the patient's health literacy (not educational level).
- Assess in a manner that avoids suggesting that this is a test and that it is shameful to not know.
- Be aware that the patient's level of comprehension may be at even fourth grade or lower. Use small, brief, and simply worded messages.
- Communicate messages at a pace the patient can follow.
- Place these messages in some context known to and valued by the patient.
- Repeat material at selected intervals, being careful to use similar but not the same words.
- When possible, supplement information with visuals: cartoons, videos, pictures.
- Choose visuals that the patient can identify and associate with, such as common fears, values, or goals.
- Initially use the patient's words, then carefully move to the known medical terms for the condition or treatment (presuming the patient will never comprehend a medical term may be as humiliating to the patient as shaming him or her for not knowing).
- Draw pictures if there are no pictures or diagrams to use.
- Tell stories about other hypothetical cases (while protecting the confidentiality of case materials) that would pique the interest of the patient.
- Use the teach-back or return demonstration technique to judge how much the patient has understood and retained.
- Using the patient's level of understanding, carefully fill in any gaps or clarify any misconceptions (patients will rarely understand the first exposure).

In the context of these questions and answers, patients should become more familiar with how the body/mind works, how the disease/illness/injury affects the body, how other conditions might result from this primary condition, how long it will be before they notice improvement, and what alternatives exist to treat the condition. All this should happen in the context that the patient may have very limited accurate and complete information and that in-depth learning will require repetition of facts and discussions.

▶ Improving Health Literacy in Patients with Chronic Illness

Patients with a chronic health condition may appear to know a great deal about their health status and medical treatment. Over time, their exposure to the health care system, different medication regimens, different providers, and information they have gleaned from printed materials or the Internet have given them some foundation to self-manage their care.

What they might not know are the particular patterns of disease self-management that may affect their health behaviors. They may not understand that as their treatment is prolonged they are likely to tire of the routine and even experiment with altering their care plan, even without discussing this decision with a health care provider. They may also become nonadherent due to the long-term demands (costs and life-style limitations) put upon them by their illness. If they do not have a good alliance with their provider, where there is open communication and an environment that is shameless, they may not disclose to the provider steps they have taken to give themselves "a break."

Among those at particular risk for literacy-associated self-management problems are those with not only chronic illness for reasons that the majority are elderly and have chronic diseases but also more comorbid conditions due to their prolonged condition or new chronic illnesses. These patients have more problems managing their care, greater rates of hospital and health service utilization, and poorer health outcomes (**EXHIBIT 15-7**).

EXHIBIT 15-7 Case Study Medication Taking in Elders

Consider an 88-year-old elderly woman living alone in a one-bedroom apartment. She is taking medications for diabetes, high blood pressure, osteoarthritis, and depression. She is also taking several over-the-counter vitamins and minor pain suppressants with the notation "prn" (Latin phrase, pro re nata or only as needed). She understands that she must take medications on a regular basis but several times a week finds that she is just not able to read the prescription on the bottle or remember if she already took her medications.

She has several prescription aids to help her (e.g., weekly pill box and refrigerator magnets). She knows she has several pills to take and cannot read the writing on the pill bottle, so she just takes one, the one she thinks she needs to take. Then an hour later, returns to take a second pill. This time she remembers the doctor told her to take two pills twice a day so she takes four (2 × 2 = 4) thinking she is doing the right thing. Occasionally, her daughter calls and asks, "Are you taking your medication, Mom?" She is not sure that she is, but she does not want to bother her daughter, so she replies: "Yes…I know how important my pills are." The discussion ends there and because her daughter is an hour away, there is no real investigation as to the reality or truth behind the reply.

Although this example seems exaggerated, this event occurs more often than one would think. Unless patients' dosage errors are discovered their medication-taking behaviors can go unnoticed for some time.

▶ Importance of Using "Plain Language"

Earlier in this chapter the use of plain language was alluded to. It is a tool in the briefcase of the provider. But for health providers, it is not as simple to do as it would seem. Health providers are trained and educated to know and use medical terminology in their relationships with other providers. To some degree, this language is abbreviated and is specific to the setting in which health care is provided.

Think of all the shorthand versions providers use to communicate with one another. For example, those referring to certain health conditions might be AMI (acute myocardial infarction or heart attack), IBS (irritable bowel syndrome), PE (pulmonary embolism), and TSH (thyroid stimulating hormone). Those referring to treatment choices are BID (twice a day), PRN (only when necessary), and NPO (nothing by mouth). Sometimes medical terminology is abbreviated purposively to allow providers to talk about medical conditions in front of patients and family without their fully understanding what is being said and its significance.

Using plain language requires a paradigm shift for most providers. They need to be consciously aware that they speak a different language and this is not the language of the patient and patient's family. They need to shift to communication that is plain language if they are to be heard and understood effectively by patients and their family caregivers. Plain language is such that the very first time a patient reads or hears a message they can understand what is communicated. Even when providers think they are communicating in plain language it may not be may plain enough.

The U.S. Department of Health and Human Services, in its *Quick Guide to Health Literacy*, lists the various elements of plain language: (1) presenting important points first, (2) organizing complex thoughts and ideas into understandable parts, (3) using simple terminology and language and defining technical terms whenever used, and (4) using the active voice instead of passive voice in making statements to the patient. Active and passive voice is clearly different. The following is an example of the use of active or passive voice using the same message.

ACTIVE VOICE: "The clinical specialist will contact you by telephone to set up an appointment for you to come back next week."

PASSIVE VOICE: "To provide you a new appointment for next week, you will be contacted by telephone by the clinical specialist."

These messages virtually contain the same information but as they are read the message in the active voice is easier to follow and to understand and, controlling for all other factors (e.g., stress at the time), is more likely to be retained in the patient's memory. Using plain language is just one step in ensuring messages will be received as intended. But because groups differ in how and what they understand, not all messages will be received similarly across groups. A case in point is patients whose primary language is not English and whose culture is other than the dominant culture. Clearly, there is a definite need for cultural and linguistic competence in sending and receiving messages to many patients and their families. Consider the following dialogue carefully identifying the problem areas in the discussion with the patient (**EXHIBIT 15-8**).

Analysis of the communication in this clinic visit of a patient being diagnosed with type 2 diabetes pinpoints many potential

---

EXHIBIT 15-8 Example of Failing to Completely Accommodate Explanations to Meet the Needs of Patients

PROVIDER: "Many people have diabetes. You have what is called type 2 diabetes. Diabetes occurs when the pancreas doesn't produce enough insulin or the body can't effectively use the insulin that the body does produce. Type 2 diabetes occurs later on in life but many younger people are being diagnosed with this condition now."

(Pause)

PATIENT: "Diabetes…the 'sugar disease'?"

PROVIDER: "Actually, diabetes can be controlled with proper diet and exercise. However, if your diabetes cannot be controlled, there are medications you will need to take, and you will have to monitor your blood glucose level on a regular basis. This is how we will know whether the medication is working for you at the dose we prescribe. It is very important that we treat this condition because serious consequences can occur if it is not. You may have heard about retinopathy, impotence, kidney disease, or even heart disease associated with diabetes that have not been effectively treated."

(Pause—no response by the patient)

PROVIDER: "Do you know what the signs and symptoms of diabetes are?"

PATIENT: "No…what are signs and symptoms?"

PROVIDER: "Signs and symptoms are what is going on that are typical with diabetes. Some of them are unusual thirst, frequent urination, weight changes (either gain or lose weight), blurred vision, extreme fatigue, cuts that are slow to heal, tingling in your hands or feet, problems in getting or maintaining an erection. As you can see, diabetes affects many bodily functions. So today I want to give you a list of directions to follow. I want to see if we can control your diabetes with exercise and healthy eating. To get you in to check your blood glucose level, we will have the nurse practitioner set up an appointment for you today."

problems. Clearly, to effectively educate the patient the dialogue needs to change to accommodate a patient with low health literacy (at least about the patient's illness and treatment).

First of all, the information shared with the patient must be accurate and comprehensive. The information should include a description of what the patient's condition is, what this means in terms of the body's functioning, what the provider will do, what the patient may need to do, and why it is important for the patient to follow the medical regimen planned.

What is problematic, however, is how this information was presented and the level of discourse between the patient and provider. All else considered, although the provider expected to see compliance with this plan, the patient is not prepared sufficiently to effectively participate in self-managing diabetes. A large part of the problem was instructions that did not reflect the patient's actual level of understanding and comprehension.

In analyzing this interaction, note whether the messages were in "plain language." Remember that plain language would mean something different to different groups. The following words could be misunderstood by many with low literacy:

Pancreas: Many people do not know what a pancreas is, where it is, or even that it is a part of the human body. It is not something visible, and people rarely talk about their pancreas.

Signs and symptoms: The average layperson does not talk in terms of signs and symptoms. They may not understand that things that occur are considered in clusters. They are more likely to understand them as single isolated events.

Concept that the body produces insulin: Again, some people may not have heard the word or know what insulin is and where in the body it is located. They may not know that it is the function of the

pancreas to make insulin because they did not know about the pancreas either.

Age and diabetes: The data about the late onset of type 2 diabetes raise the issue of what is type 1 diabetes and if there is a type 3 diabetes. Patients might wonder if they were supposed to know they were going to get diabetes when they were younger. The issue of risk factors for diabetes was indirectly touched upon in a short discussion of diet and exercise. Patients are not likely to understand this issue or why the provider raised the issue.

Diabetes and control: Providers cannot be certain that the patient knows what it means to "control" diabetes. Control may mean getting things to slow down. But how does this jive with making the body effectively use insulin?

Blood glucose level: The person with low literacy may not know what glucose is and what it is doing in the blood. Monitoring blood glucose means what? Does that mean something is attached to the blood vessel and that sends messages to the doctor when the blood gets too much glucose? What does "regular basis" really mean?

Consequences: Retinopathy, impotence, kidney disease, and heart disease. The majority of these concepts are likely to be unfamiliar to the patient, or if familiar, the patient may not understand whether these consequences all occur at the same time.

Exercise and healthy living: Exactly what does this mean? Does it mean joining a gym, eating only fruit and vegetables, cooking without wine and oil? The concept of exercise means something different to people as does the concept of "healthy living" which may include native foods that would be contraindicated in a diabetic diet.

On first appraisal, the provider is not only accurate but is communicating what generally should be explained to patients about their condition. However, in the conversation the provider uses several not easy to understand words and concepts.

What is equally concerning is the manner in which the provider conducted the discussion. Despite pausing, examine the fact that the provider asked only one question about what the patient understood ("Do you know what the signs and symptoms of diabetes are?"). It should be noted that this opportunity for the patient to share personal knowledge comes late. And, while the provider tries to explain signs and symptoms, the patient is inundated with new and unfamiliar terms by now. The patient did not make good use of the pauses, perhaps thinking that any personal questions would be answered later. What occurs over the entire discussion is an overload of cascading new and foreign-sounding ideas. As a result, the patient might feel overwhelmed

and retreats into silence, possibly thinking that the only way to understand what the provider said is to go home and talk about it to friends and family.

The provider had a final opportunity to complete the feedback loop by having the patient discuss in his own words what the provider said but fails to take this opportunity to do so. To add to the difficulty of the discourse, the provider, while well intended, uses too many words and slides for teaching points without asking if the patient understands what was said. Also, using messages in the passive voice are more difficult to understand than those in the active voice.

For the purposes of learning from this example, consider this same discussion using some of the principles of communicating with patients that have limited health literacy (**EXHIBIT 15-9**).

EXHIBIT 15-9   Alternative Approach to Accommodate Patient's Level of Understanding

PROVIDER: "You have a condition called diabetes. Have you heard about diabetes before?"

PATIENT: "I think it is the sugar disease. My father had it and lost a toe."

PROVIDER: "Sometimes people talk about diabetes as 'the sugar disease.' What it really means is a problem with your pancreas, an organ in your body that makes insulin. Insulin is a hormone that helps your body turn blood sugar into energy. It is necessary for everyone, and everyone has a pancreas. (Pause) So when someone has diabetes, their pancreas is not making enough insulin or their body is not using it the way it needs to. This might be hard to understand at first. Do you understand what I said?"

PATIENT: "Well…I have a pancreas…everybody does…it's not working, so I have diabetes. But how do you know I have diabetes; you didn't look at my pancreas?"

PROVIDER: "Right, I didn't. But we take blood tests and we can tell if you have too much glucose, or blood sugar. The blood test helps us know if you don't have enough insulin to do the work it needs to do. (Pause) …also, when you came in you said you were 'tired' and don't have enough energy to do the regular things you usually do. You also said you were always thirsty, peed a lot, and had gained weight. From the results of your blood test and the information that you gave us, we call these signs and symptoms,…we think you have diabetes."

PATIENT: "Well, what are you going to do?"

PROVIDER: "You and I will be partners. I need your help, too. We will talk to you about physical activity and what you eat and how you cook your food."

PATIENT: "I don't know…my wife does the cooking."

PROVIDER: "So it is going to be important that she also understands what diabetes is, what the plan is, and what can be expected if you follow the plan. We would like to have your wife come in next time we see you. The nurse will schedule a visit for you."

The dialogue is exemplar in the use of some principles of communicating with persons with limited health literacy. Notice that the information was cut into sections (breaking complex information into smaller chunks). Notice also that the pace was much slower than in the previous dialogue (slow down the pace of information giving). Also in this example, the provider tried to use simple language, avoiding technical terms when possible.

When technical jargon was used it was done sparsely, and the provider took care to define terms (use simple language and define technical terms). Finally, the active, not passive, voice was used, simplifying the messages considerably (use the active voice). The differences in communication between the first and second dialogue point to several important issues. The second dialogue reflects care practices that recognize and value knowing the patient's health literacy level. Time is provided to implement health literacy best practices. The health care setting is one that seeks and trains providers in the concepts and principles of enhancing health literacy. Finally, the health care setting encourages patients and their families to be active participants in their care and treatment decision making.

▶ Summary

The United States fairs favorably when the nation's level of literacy is compared to other technology-rich countries. However, among those groups within the United States that score low in numeracy and problem-solving skills the United States scores significantly lower than other technology-rich countries. The level of health literacy across the United States shows considerable differences among high-risk groups: the elderly, poor, minority, those who have not completed high school, and those whose primary language is not English, have lower levels of health literacy or the capacity to obtain, communicate, process,

and understand basic health information and services to make appropriate health decisions. These groups are also at risk for poor health care and poor health.

Health literacy has a direct impact on the quality and quantity of communication between providers and patients and community caregivers. Furthermore, health literacy has found to be associated with health outcomes, disease management, and use of health services. The exact mechanism by which health literacy affects health outcomes and disease management is not completely known. However, it has been suggested that health literacy has a direct impact on quality of disease self-management, which, in turn, affects health outcomes. Sentell and Halpin (2006), in a secondary analysis of the data from the 1992 National Adult Literacy Survey, concluded that literacy inequities may be a significant factor in health disparities having powerful effects on work-impairing conditions as well as long-term illness.

The relationship of education and self-management is also not completely clear. Schillinger et al. (2006) suggest that it may be that literacy mediates the relationship of education and self-management, however, more research needs to support this premise. The idea here is that health literacy not educational level explains disease self-management and control. Some highly educated persons have low levels of health literacy. This idea explains why some people who are very well educated may not understand self-management tasks while those with little to no schooling might be very health literate. The reason for this is that there are several factors responsible for higher levels of health literacy: age, exposure to illness and health care systems in the past, and the system of care that fosters health literacy.

Evaluating a patient's level of comprehension and capacity to participate in shared decision-making (health literacy) has been recommended to be *a universal precaution* because of the relationship between health literacy and patient self-management, and patient safety. This chapter provided an overview of the concept of health literacy and its relationship to health outcomes. Barriers to health literacy and some general concepts, principles, and interventions that are effective in communicating with low literacy populations were discussed.

The assumption is that health literacy is modifiable and every health care professional has a role in improving health literacy in a wide range of patient populations somewhere on the continuum of low to high health literacy. How providers go about this is contingent upon the particular setting whether delivering inpatient or outpatient care, coaching patients in disease self-management, or addressing disease prevention and health promotion services and campaigns.

Discussion

1. Describe the differences between general literacy level and health literacy.
2. Identify and discuss a tool to measure a patient's level of health literacy.
3. Identify and discuss key guidelines in communicating with patients who have low levels of health literacy.
4. Discuss the statement "Patients may be very educated but have low levels of health literacy."
5. Identify patient, patient–provider relationship, and system-level barriers to patient health literacy.

References

2016 National Healthcare Quality and Disparities Report. Agency for Healthcare Research and Quality, Rockville, MD. Reviewed January 2018, from http://www.ahrq.gov/research/findings/nhqrdr/nhqdr16/index.html

Baker, D. W., Parker, R. M., Williams, M. V., Pitkin, K., Parikh, N. S., Coates, W., & Imara, M. (1996). The health experience of patients with low literacy. *Archives of Family Medicine, 5*(6), 329–334. PMID: 8640322

Berkman, N. D., Sheridan, S. L., Donahue, K. E., Halpern, D. J., Viera, A., Crotty, K., … Viswanathan, M. (2011, March). *Health literacy interventions and outcomes: An updated systematic review.* (Evidence Report/Technology Assessment No. 199. (Prepared by RTI International—University of North Carolina Evidence-based Practice Center Under Contract No. 290-2007-10056-I.) AHRQ Publication No. 11-E006). Rockville, MD. Agency for Healthcare Research and Quality. Retrieved from http://www.ahrq.gov/clinic/tp/lituptp.htm

Brown, S. L., Teufel, J. A., & Birch, D. A. (2007). Early adolescents' perceptions of health and health literacy. *Journal of School Health, 77*(1), 7–15. doi:10.1016/j.jadohealth.2007.04.015

Chisolm, D. J., & Buchanan, L. (2007). Measuring adolescent functional health literacy: A validation of the test of functional health literacy in adults. *Journal of Adolescent Health, 41*(3), 312–314. doi:10.1016/j.jadohealth.2007.04.015

Downey, L. A., & Zun, L. (2007). Testing of a verbal assessment tool of English proficiency for use in the healthcare setting. *The Journal of the National Medical Association, 99*(7), 795–798. PMID 16775913

Lee, S. Y., Bender, D. E., Ruiz, R. E., & Cho, Y. I. (2006). Development of an easy-to-use Spanish health literacytest. *Health Services Research, 41*(4, Part 1), 1392–1412. doi:10.1111/j.1475-6773.2006.00532.x

Miller, D., Brownlee, C. D., McCoy, T. P., & Pignone, M. P. (2007). The effect of health literacy on knowledge and receipt of colorectal cancer screening: A survey study. *BioMed Central Family Practice, 8,* 16. doi:10.1186/1471-2296-8-16

OECD. (2016). *Skills matter: Further results from the Survey of Adult Skills,* OECD Skills Studies. Paris: OECD Publishing. doi:10.1787/9789264258051-en

Paasche-Orlow, M. K., Schillinger, D., Greene, S. M., & Wagner, E. H. (2006). How healthcare systems can begin to address the challenge of limited literacy. *Journal of General Internal Medicine, 21,* 884–887. doi:10.1111/j.1525-1497.2006.00544.x

Rampey, B. D., Finnegan, R., Goodman, M., Mohadjer, L., Krenzke, T., Hogan, J., & Provasnik, S. (2016). *Skills of U.S. unemployed, young, and older adults in sharper focus: Results From the Program for the International Assessment of Adult Competencies (PIAAC) 2012/2014: First Look* (NCES 2016-039rev). U.S. Department of Education. Washington, DC: National Center for

Education Statistics. Retrieved from http://nces.ed.gov/pubsearch.

Safeer, R., & Keenan, J. (2005). Health literacy: The gap between physicians and patients. *American Family Physician, 72*(3), 463–468. PMID:16100861

Schillinger, D., Barton, L. R., Karter, A. J., Wang, F., & Adler, N. (2006). Does literacy mediate the relationship between education and health outcomes: A study of a low-income population with diabetes. *Public Health Reports, 121*, 245–254. doi:10.1177/003335490612100305

Sentell, T. L., & Halpin, H. A. (2006). The importance of adult literacy in understanding health disparities. *Journal of General Internal Medicine, 21*, 862–866. doi:10.1111/j.1525-1497.2006.00538.x

Sudore, R. L., Yaffe, K., Satterfield, S., Harris, T. B., Mehta, K. M., Simonsick, E. M., … Schillinger, D. (2006). Limited literacy and mortality in the elderly: The health, aging, and body comparison study. *Journal of General Internal, 21*, 806–812. doi:10.1111/j.1525-1497.2006.00539.x

The National Academies of Sciences, Engineering, and Medicine. (Prepublication 2017). *People living with disabilities: Health equity, health disparities, and health literacy: Proceedings of a workshop.* Washington, DC: The National Academies Press. Retrieved from www.nap.edu

U.S. Department of Health and Human Services, Office of Disease Prevention and Health Promotion. Healthy People 2010. Retrieved from www.healthypeople.gov/Document/HTML/Volume1/11HealthCom.htm

U.S. Department of Health and Human Services, Office of Disease Prevention and Health Promotion. Quick guide to health literacy. Retrieved from http://www.health.gov/communication/literacy/quickguide/healthinfo.htm

Weiss, B. D., Mays, M. Z., Martz, W., Castro, K. M., DeWalt, D. A., Pignone, M. P., … Hale, F. A. (2005). Quick assessment of literacy in primary care: The newest vital sign. *Annals of Family Medicine, 3*(6), 514–522. doi:10.1370/afm.405

CHAPTER 16

Communicating with Patients Who Have Chronic and/or Life-Threatening Illness

CHAPTER OBJECTIVES

- Identify the several sequential phases in the adaptation to illness process.
- Describe potential losses that patients and their families may experience when coping with chronic illness and/or injury.
- Discuss the impact of patients' potential responses to chronic illness (e.g., powerlessness, helplessness, and hopelessness) on their ability to cope effectively.
- Providers working with these patients and their families may also experience high levels of stress. Describe several coping skills that providers might use to fend off the effects of the professional stress syndrome.
- Discuss several barriers to and facilitators of patient and family and provider communications in end-of-life care.

KEY TERMS

- Adaptation to illness
- Behavior control
- Cognitive appraisal
- Cognitive control
- Denial (first, second, and third order)
- Emotion-focused coping
- Maladaptive coping
- Problem-focused coping

▶ Introduction

There is something "special" about patients and their families who live with the stresses of chronic and, in some cases, life-threatening illness. Their remarkable resilience and persistence show us the strength and beauty of human existence and teaches us to be humble in their presence. Humble but not overwhelmed. Our knowledge and experience to a certain extent insolate us and prepare us to come along with patients and their families in the journey of coping, managing, and surviving under extreme odds.

These observations do not negate the unique demands placed on patients and their families with respect to their specific disease and stage of illness. For example, experiences of persons with lung cancer differ from those who are disabled by painful arthritis. These diseases are different and usher in very different treatment trajectories with different prognoses. In this chapter, patients are discussed with reference to the stressors of their particular condition (e.g., cancer, diabetes, cardiovascular disease). They are also discussed according to stage of adaptation to their health illness: beginning, intermediate, and late stages of adaptation to the demands of their illness.

Why are patients grouped together and categorized? Providers do so because there are particular things to look for with patients who have certain chronic or life-threatening conditions. Knowing from the start that we will be communicating with a patient and family facing a serious life-threatening illness prepares us in advance to anticipate what is important in order to design a specific care plan.

There are communications that might be unique to these patients that do not apply to patients experiencing time-limited illness and injury. Our assumption is that patients with chronic debilitating diseases (e.g., arthritis and emphysema) and terminal illnesses (e.g., advanced heart disease and some cancers) are significantly different from those with an injury that will heal within a predictable time period (e.g., ankle fracture or torn ligament), an acute illness (e.g., a bout of the flu or pneumonia), or mild, albeit persistent, chronic disorders (e.g., asthma or sinusitis).

In some instances, patients with chronic disease may also experience life-threatening illness simultaneously. What was once considered a life-threatening condition (e.g., advanced cancer and HIV/AIDS) may now be treated as a chronic ailment. Patients with both debilitating chronic disorders and those with life-threatening conditions are discussed together in this chapter. Both similarities and differences in approaches are described. Do patients who are experiencing the debilitating effects of osteoarthritis differ from those who are dealing with end-stage cancer? One is a chronic debilitating illness and the other, a life-threatening one. Both patients might experience similar problems: depression, lack of energy, worry about their future, and experience pain and limited functioning. Although many issues are common to both, most providers would agree that the differences between these patients support their use of different approaches that are unique depending upon the diagnosis and prognosis.

In this chapter, the similarities in communicating with these two categories of patients are discussed in depth. Issues of coping and adaptation are described along with the psychological responses of helplessness, powerlessness, and hopelessness. Interventions and communications that address these patients' psychological responses are discussed. Additionally, principles of communicating with terminal patients about their prognosis and end-of-life care are explored.

The stages of **adaptation to illness** and injury affect both patients and their families. The patient's emotional state and the character of their communications with providers as well as with friends and family may differ depending upon the stage of adaptation to their illness or injury. One needs to keep in mind that these patients are coping with stressors, not all of which are shared between them, but do have a significant impact upon their communication needs with health care providers. Chronic debilitating diseases significantly alter patients' quality of life but infrequently cause death. In contrast, life-threatening conditions (e.g., advanced lung cancer and heart disease) not only limit a patient's quality of life but also significantly impact patients' lives.

▶ The Process of Dealing with Chronic Illness

Chronic illnesses are now the number one threat to the health of Americans and for that matter those in other developed countries. The rise in chronic illnesses is due to not only American lifestyle behaviors increasing the odds of chronic conditions but also technological advances that have elevated once-considered terminal illnesses to treatable chronic illnesses.

Chronic illnesses appear in children and adults of all ages and in persons of all races, genders, ethnicities, and socioeconomic groups. Their treatment can require complex medical interventions along with lifestyle behavior changes. Because chronic illnesses are so prevalent, many of our patients and their families face challenges not only in self-management tasks but also in adapting to the chronicity of these disease, from diagnosis on.

Many beginning health care professionals do not immediately grasp the importance of understanding how patients adapt or respond to illness and injury. Some providers consider this area of patients' life out of the realm of their practice, and others have little awareness that adaptation to illness impacts all phases of planned treatment: participatory planning, self-management and treatment adherence, and evaluation of the effects of their treatment. Regardless of the reasons, these providers' limited awareness needs to be replaced with a fuller understanding of every aspect of patients' adjustment to chronic illness. In our roles as health care providers, in order to adequately care for and communicate

with patients, providers need to understand something about how they experience and adapt to their illness and injury. Patients communicate with providers in the context of their response to their illness or injury. Providers at any point in time can be seen as caring or insensitive based on their patients' or patients' family perceptions of how aware they are of the challenges of the patient's illness.

The Meaning of Chronic and Life-Threatening Illness

Patients and their families respond to illness and injury in ways that are similar to coping with any stressful life events. In short, patients may have long histories of adapting to stressful life events, and this history influences how they will respond to their current illness. They have developed their own unique lifestyles and ways of dealing with unwanted, unpleasant, and painful situations, including illnesses and injuries. However, coping with an injury like a sprained foot has really little to do with what chronic illness has in store for patients and their families, for chronic illness has no end. Although there may be good times and not so good times, chronic illnesses are always in shadows to shape patients' lives, hence, some patients reflecting on the past remark, "My life was never the same."

The role of health providers in easing the process of adaptation to illness has been addressed in the literature and is an interdisciplinary concern. In most health professions, the process of adaption is studied and approaches designed and tested. In an overview on how social workers can help patients better cope with the grief associated with a chronic illness or injury, Jackson (2014, p. 18) paints a vivid picture of the experience: "Imagine a person with a chronic illness as forever walking down a dividing line between the past and the future. Looking backward, he can see everything illness has taken from him or has forced him to relinquish. Looking forward, he can't see anything quite clearly. There's no going back to the past, and the future is uncertain." Recovery from many illnesses can be unpredictable and uncontrollable leaving pockets of high anxiety and fears sprinkled throughout the course of the illness and its treatment.

In summary, for patients and their families, the experience can be overwhelming especially with numerous changes and accommodations required of them. Health providers are in key roles to help patients cope with the many changes and losses they experience in an ever-running narrative about the way these changes were handled and adaptation eased. Factors which impact patients' capacities to cope adaptively are many: their experience and knowledge from prior illnesses, cultural beliefs about illness in general and the current diagnosis in particular, the level of support they have from friends and family, and the strength of the alliance with the health care team. Providers need to know what to expect as patients go through the process of adapting to a chronic illness. The next section of this chapter describes the stages of adaptation but it is important to be cognizant of the fact that the presentation of these stages in patients will take unique shapes depending on their individual differences.

Stages of Adaptation to Illness and Injury

While each patient has a unique pattern of responding to illness or injury, there seems to be certain stages they go through that they have in common. When providers think about how patients deal with chronic illness they may have a rather narrow focus. According to Schwartz (2009), patients often perceive providers as having no concept of what they are going through both emotionally and physically even though they can be experts in diagnosing and treating diseases. What comes to mind is how patients cope with the diagnosis of a chronic illness when the process is actually much more involved. The process of dealing with chronic illness is that of adapting to not only the diagnosis but also every stage of the illness trajectory from diagnosis onward. People go through stages in learning how to cope with and manage their chronic illness. This is true not only for adults but also for children. It is also true for not only the patient but also parents or family of the patient.

Adaptation to illness has been described and studied extensively in the health care literature. Essentially, each stage of illness corresponds to events which are paired with adaptation stages and responses. The adaptation process is characterized by a position on the timeline of first learning one's diagnosis to death if applicable. **TABLE 16-1** describes an example of how the illness trajectory is linked to psychological adaptation and includes the phase or stage of illness and the corresponding illness event timeline and adaptation stage.

For example, the awareness or discovery of disease occurring during diagnosis of illness carries with it emotional reactions of denial

TABLE 16-1 Illness Trajectory and Psychosocial Adaptation to Illness			
I. Phase or stage of illness:	Discovery	Acute and chronic	Terminal
II. Event timeline:	Diagnosis (with or without symptoms)	Symptomatic (depending on exacerbations and remissions)	Significant physical decline
III. Adaptation stage:	Denial and disbelief	Anger, depression, beginning resolution	Ultimate resolution and acceptance

and disbelief. Emotional reactions to acute illness and/or chronic conditions, wherein repeated exacerbations occur, might manifest as anger and depression intermixed with beginning resolution. In terminal stages of illness, resolution and acceptance are commonly observed but the experience of the stage is uniquely tied to the provider's responses and communication skills.

Models for understanding the process of adaptation come from a number of different authors, most notable being Elisabeth Kübler-Ross, MD (1926–2004). Kübler-Ross was a Swiss psychiatrist and was the first to introduce her model in her 1969 classic book, *On Death and Dying*. The model presented in this book described five stages of grief experienced by persons confronting death or the loss of someone who was dying. Stages identified by Kübler-Ross included denial, anger, bargaining, depression, and finally acceptance. The Kübler-Ross model of stages of grief has been widely accepted by the general public and used in training health professionals. Although very popular, there is limited validity for this model in the research literature (Newman, 2004).

Kübler-Ross authored 20 books and became more specialized on topics of illness and death experience (e.g., the care of dying children, HIV-infected patients, and prisoners with AIDs). Following her first book, the model was used to describe the common experiences of reaction to losses associated with other stressful or traumatizing events including adaptation to chronic illness. It became clear that the same emotions that occur in death and dying, grief and grieving might also occur in the psychological adaptation to illness.

The model was originally pictured as linear, progressing from denial in the event of discovery to acceptance in the events near death. However, Kübler-Ross did not intend the model to be interpreted so literally in lock-step fashion. She explained that the five common experiences could occur in any phase of the adaptation process (Kübler-Ross, 1969). Many factors contribute both to how a patient progresses and to the intensity of any one response. Kübler-Ross compassionately observed and documented these reactions from statements made in interviews with patients. These observations also included patients' affective reactions to an awareness of their illness at different points in time.

Other conceptual frameworks are similar to this classic description. Today, there are many frameworks from which to choose. For example, one framework poses a model of adaptation to chronic illness that specifies stages built on the grieving process. The model includes shock or disbelief, developing awareness, restitution, resolution of the loss, and idealization. Others have used similar concepts: disbelief, developing awareness, reorganization of relationships with others, resolution of the loss, and identity change. Many theories differ only in the terms used or in the number of stages or substages observed in patients. A recent review of the lived experience of healthy behaviors in people with debilitating illness (Haynes & Watt, 2008) explained that spirituality and focus/adaptation were keys in helping patients cope with resolution of the implications of living with their chronic illness.

Providers engaged in assisting patients and their families to manage the course of their disease (e.g., caring for patients with chronic illnesses) have conceptualized the adaptation process for these patients in a similar manner. Identifying the emotional reactions of patients who are facing rehabilitation, the following four categories have been used to describe specific stages: (1) fear and anxiety, (2) anger and hostility, (3) depression, and (4) resolution and acceptance.

Any categorization is largely a question of semantics or generalization about a set of behaviors. Health care providers should observe and report their own observations of patients' emotional reactions and the particular sequential arrangement of stages. The most important principles to guide our observations are that (1) patients do have emotional reactions to their illnesses or injuries, (2) these reactions change over time, and (3) the process is not as linear as once suspected.

Since this early research, a number of studies have addressed the process of adaptation and have suggested further guidelines for understanding patients' responses. First, it has been documented that some patients seem to harbor certain reactions longer than others; this includes the observation that some patients never demonstrate certain reactions (e.g., anger) while other patients remain in one stage (e.g., denial) throughout their illness. Second, unlike the original notions about sequential stages, the process of evolving emotional reactions appears to be more complex. For example, in the case of many chronic and terminal illnesses, there are a series of events that can potentially trigger additional cycles. The initial diagnosis of a terminal illness may trigger one sequence but the reappearance of symptoms or the advent of new symptoms can trigger additional cycles.

In studies of patients with life-threatening illness (e.g., cancer, advanced heart failure, or HIV), there are a series of events that herald new emotional responses. The initial diagnosis can trigger a strong emotional reaction. During the course of the disease, the appearance of new symptoms may trigger additional trauma. For persons living with HIV, the advent of new opportunistic infections or decline in CD4 count or percentage can trigger additional responses such as fear, anxiety, anger, and depression.

Fear, Anxiety, and Disorganization

Psychosocial adaptation to illness involves many emotional reactions that can significantly affect patients' communication and behaviors. Fear and anxiety (mild or intense) are generated by an awareness of illness and injury. Adaptation to life-threatening disease calls up not only the threat of the initial diagnosis but the fear of the effects of treatment that will

follow. For example, cancer patients experience the crisis of initial diagnosis and when treated with a bone marrow transplantation can be observed to go through stages of adaptation but also substages within these stages.

The process starts with the initial awareness of the disease and continues with a reaction to this awareness. This is an important place to begin in order to lessen the stress of the diagnosis and can be reapplied in a subsequent stage when patients reflect on the success or lack of success of their treatment.

Logically, it would be presumed that minor illnesses or injuries would evoke mild fear, and anxiety and major illnesses or injuries would cause severe anxiety and fear. However, remember that patients respond uniquely and while some patients may respond with (even panic) others might not. Also, studies have shown that objective appraisals of illness and injury events do not always match patients' subjective evaluations. In some patients, minor illness would evoke mild levels of fear and anxiety; and major illness, high levels of fear and anxiety. But there are some patients, for whatever reasons, that may respond to major illness the same way they respond to minor illness. Or a minor illness may create severe distress and a major illness, mild distress. There are two principles to keep in mind: (1) patients experience levels of stress differently and (2) patients' fears and anxiety might not match objective appraisal of the level of threat.

Appropriate interventions would be to assess patients' knowledge of their diagnosis and their appraisal of the level of threat they are facing. Patients' expressed fears reflect their appraisal of the severity of their illness. They may not verbalize their fears but they behave fearfully such as watching every move the provider makes and listening carefully to remarks made to other members of the treatment team. It is as if they were waiting to confirm what they perceived. Will the provider reveal the real seriousness of the diagnosis to the team member who is in the same room? Will the team member show concern that is not readily apparent from the physician's demeanor? Patients monitor providers' communications to determine what they think they do not know, but fear.

Patients are frequently not able to put their fears and anxieties into words or terms that providers can understand especially when they are experiencing the disorganization of thoughts and behavior. Anxiety by definition is apprehension about some unknown; it could be centered around the meaning patients' illness has for them, their treatment, or their prognosis. While anxiety is uncomfortable and sometimes overwhelming it tends to lack definition and the cause may be unknown. If you ask patients about the cause of their anxiety they may not be able to tell you.

Fear, on the other hand, is also uncomfortable but is induced by perceptions of a clear and present threat or danger. Fear serves a critical role because it protects us from danger and harm by triggering a flight–fight response telling us to react defensively. Fears have more specificity, and if you ask patients what they are afraid of they probably will be able to tell you specifically (e.g., "I'm afraid the doctor is not telling me everything," "I'm afraid my incision will get infected," "I'm afraid my medication will affect my sexual performance," and "I'm afraid of the pain").

Unlike anxiety which is often "free floating" and difficult to describe; fears have specificity and can be described in some detail with simple prompting. It should be stated that fear and anxiety might occur at the same time; patients could be afraid of surgery (a clear and present danger in their minds) and have anxiety about whether they will survive. Also, it is possible that fear can trigger anxious feelings as described in this example. Anxiety can also cause fear if anxious feelings are experienced as a present threat (e.g., the fear of having a heart attack while feeling rapid shallow breathing due to anxiety).

While providers rarely question the appropriateness of patients' experiences of fear or anxiety, these reactions may be under-discussed. One reason for this is that these reactions are considered "normal" in adapting to chronic illness and can be taken for granted. The assumption is that in time these emotions will lessen on their own. But avoidance of discussing patients' anxieties or fears and, similarly, any additional emotional reactions (e.g., anger and depression) is nontherapeutic. Clearly, patients are in pain sometimes just as powerful as any physical pain. Emotional pain can accentuate the experience of physical pain and vice versa. In fact, the experience of fear and anxiety can lead to disorganizing thoughts and behaviors.

It is a standing recommendation that providers openly discuss patients' emotional reactions to their illness and treatment regardless of how appropriate or commonplace these reactions are. These and other reactions can influence patient self-care practices (Capehorn et al., 2017) and cancer survivors' fears of reoccurrence and progression (Hall, Lennes, Pirl, Friedman, & Park, 2017; Ozga et al., 2015). If they exist, they are to be discussed and patients need to receive assistance and support.

Anger and Hostility

Anger in the context of stages of adaptation is both a reaction to stress and a statement of protest. When patients experience their diagnosis as something tangible the natural response is to object. Questions such as "Why me?" may be quickly replaced with the denial "Not me." Patients who react with anger to their diagnosis can register the underlying meaning of their diagnosis to be a shortened life span (in the case of a terminal illness) or an impaired quality of life with the onset of chronic and debilitating symptoms.

When stressors are less significant, the natural reaction is usually a milder form of "anger" (e.g., irritation). In the case of either chronic or terminal illness the reaction is not irritation; the feeling is more likely much stronger. It is inconceivable to think that patients diagnosed with a chronic asthmatic condition or cancer would be irritated. Whether chronic or terminal, these conditions are "earthshaking" or "lifeshaking." One can understand the impact of these diagnoses when focusing on the primary and secondary implications of these conditions.

Depending on several factors (e.g., the patient's outlook, culture, religion, and previous history with stressful life events), these responses may be severe or modulated. Sometimes expressions of anger are present but communicated in ways that they go unnoticed or misunderstood. Feelings of anger can be directed at health providers or the health care setting. For example, patients learning for the first time they have cancer and feeling dependent and confined due to surgery and recovery might misdirect anger or overreact with health care providers.

A partial analysis in the example given might lead us to conclude that the patient pulled out her nasal gastric tubing for any of the following reasons: the patient did not like being fed this way, the tube was irritating the patient's nasal passages, or the patient did not understand the necessity of tube feeding. While these factors may have something to do with the patient's behavior, this limited explanation is very shortsighted. The trauma the patient experienced as a result of recently learning her diagnosis was terminal and subsequent physical decline may explain in greater depth her reactions and unstated communication. Being angry at everything and everybody is a potential reaction and a real experience for many patients, and even for their families.

Providers and family members who are targets of this kind of misdirected anger should understand that there is seldom anything personal in the patient's response. Patients have limited outlets for their frustration, stress, and misery. It is understandable that the objects of their anger may be the very people they need and rely on the most. Providers can understand that patients are actually communicating frustration surrounding the indignities of their illnesses. Witnessing this protest may be far better than observing the patient passively acquiesce and become "victim" to their condition. This is why depression, the next reaction or stage, is sometimes more difficult.

Depression

Most patients, sometime during the course of their illness, will experience and report being depressed. The diagnosis of any potentially chronic illness has significant ramifications for patients' lives and it has been observed that many patients early on in the course of their illness experience depression. Depression can occur later in treatment when patients tire of the many symptoms they have endured or the constant worry about recurrence of a life-threatening disease. Depression can be more intense if there is an insufficient outlet for angry feelings, limited support, and intense feelings of powerlessness and hopelessness.

Patients who exhibit depression along with hopelessness are prime candidates for suicide attempts and must be watched very carefully. Becoming more common are patients who are seriously depressed and consider suicide, especially those with chronic pain (Cheatle, 2011). Suicide can be seen as an easier way out, the only real option, or an escape from the physical and emotional pain patients experience.

In cases of chronic illness, the routines of treatment allow little flexibility and a release

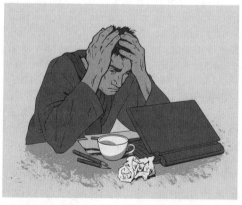

of anger can occur. In cases of terminal illness, patients' appraisal of their powerlessness over the disease can cause more anger than they are capable of releasing appropriately. Intense suppressed anger is often associated with depression. Patients who suppress anger may also hide feelings of depression. Real feelings are masked by with comments like "I'm ok," "fine," or "pretty good." Patients may even smile and attempt to be cheerful while feeling anxious and depressed. This veil of well-being is thin and will soon become obvious to the astute provider.

If encouraged, patients will explore their feelings with providers. What they say and how they say it is important. They may complain of the lack of energy and feeling tired. They also may report outbursts of crying or an overwhelming sadness, and a sense of isolation from other people. These disclosures are clues about the depth and intensity of depression, and coupled with behavioral responses (e.g., prematurely composing a will), they expose the significance of these reactions and the need to evaluate the patient's capacity to resist depressing thoughts and feelings while coping with the realities of their condition and treatment.

Resolution and Acceptance

The acute, demanding phases of illness may not prevail but over time, symptoms of disease and side effects of treatment can keep patients on edge. In some cases, physical and functional decline will lessen as if the illness experience was plateauing. The original crisis does not remain a crisis. One patient experiences a new infection and gets better from it. Another patient becomes more dependent, maybe requires life support, but eventually the power of the event recedes. Up to this stage in time many patients will have shown extraordinary resilience. Resilience is the capacity to respond to adverse situations that pose a risk to one's health or well-being (Cal, de Sa, Glustak, & Santiago, 2015).

Resolution and acceptance can occur early on but is most talked about when patients are facing the end of life. Patients' stress lessens and the patient prepares for the next major health event. For most patients, the end of health-related stress means recovery or rehabilitation. Even if the outcome is less than what was hoped for or expected, or the prognosis remains grim, a sense of relief occurs.

Having a chronic or life-threatening illness may cause patients to reflect on their life events and accomplishments. Thoughts of having "too little time" cross the minds of the chronically ill because years of healthy life will be reduced. A thought of "too little time left" concerns a terminally ill patient because the temporary nature of human existence is acutely apparent. Patients might reflect on themes (e.g., "It could have been a lot worse," "I learned so much about myself," and "I feel so lucky to have had my doctor/providers/family").

Maintaining a feeling of being in control and sustaining hope despite an uncertain or downward course are extremely important to patients. Feelings of being in control have several dimensions. Having **behavior control** and **cognitive control** are very important. Patients who feel in control of physical capacities, decisions, thoughts, and relationships have the protective layer of sensing no matter what happens they are "still myself."

Chronically ill patients may find that the intrusions into their lives by the health care system threaten their personal privacy and integrity. The ability to control this environmental intrusion and maintain privacy can preserve patients' sense of dignity and sense of self. Additionally, communicating to patients what is happening to them and engaging them in decisions about their care and treatment gives to patients the regulatory ability that preserves their rights to self-determination regardless of their compromised functional abilities.

As chronic health problems become more severe and limit even further the patient's ability to function, feelings of hopefulness will bolster the patient. Hope enables patients to avoid overwhelming despair. Despair may occur as a result of the roller-coaster effects of the illness when remissions and flare-ups are multiple or as a result of the decline that becomes more permanent than transient. Assisting patients to identify realistic and immediately relevant goals helps them cope with feelings of despair. Not only does this augment and confirm the patient's value, but it also provides a necessary distraction.

Chronic and/or life-threatening illnesses create a number of condition-related stresses, particularly losses. These have been described in research studies and include fear of pain, disfigurement or body-image change, fear of dying, and loss of work and family roles. When accompanied by actual experiences of pain, fatigue, loss of energy and appetite, self-regulatory functioning, and restricted mobility, patients' adaptive capabilities are taxed at very high levels.

Collectively, these changes present significant challenges for both patients and their significant others (see **EXHIBIT 16-1**). The resilience and resourcefulness of most patients is remarkable. They employ a high level of coping potential in dealing with their disease. Some patients dredge up coping capabilities that they, themselves, did not realize they had. Otherwise fragile individuals may demonstrate a remarkable degree of coping once they are faced with the reality of their health status. If, however, patients cannot cope with the demands of their illnesses or have difficulty accepting the realities of their decline they may remain anxious, angry, or depressed. Consultation on cases is warranted.

In summary, all patients do not proceed through stages of adaptation to illness in the same manner. The process is not linear: one, two, and then three. The process is circular. Thus, it is always important to understand the limits of applicability in using conceptual frameworks. The advantage of such models is that they provide a point of departure. The major disadvantage is that the model inadequately describes a particular patient's unique experience. Telford, Kralik, and Koch (2006) explained that blanket acceptance of the stage model of adjustment as a way of understanding patients' responses to illness has its limitations.

EXHIBIT 16-1 Potential Losses Associated with Chronic and Life-Threatening Illness

Alteration in Physical Well-Being

- Energy and appetite
- Physical strength, endurance, and vitality
- Cognitive capacities
- Mobility and balance
- Organ functioning (e.g., bowel and bladder control)
- Visual and auditory skills
- Speech and sense of taste and touch
- Inability to control pain
- Loss of sexual functioning
- Pain

Loss of Body Parts and Appearance

- Organ function
- Hair and skin
- Height and weight

Changes in Social Roles

- Loss or alteration in occupational/professional role
- Disruption of partner/family role functioning
- Loss of social and community network
- Inability to enjoy social gatherings and entertainment venues
- Loss or disruption in finances supporting self and others

Changes in Self-Esteem, Self-Concept

- Sense of self-control
- Identity
- Self-respect
- Esteem in the eyes of others
- Loss of autonomy and independence

These authors encourage providers to listen instead to patients' stories and that this is the basis of developing a truly patient-centered approach and takes into consideration the social context of patients' lives.

Recurring Responses: Helplessness, Powerlessness, and Hopelessness

Managing the care of patients with chronic and/or life-threatening illnesses requires the provider to be intimately and knowledgeably connected with patients' feelings of being out of control. It is not always easy or comfortable to connect with patients at this level but important if providers are going to comfort patients experiencing devastating chronic or life-threatening conditions. Compassionate caring requires providers to connect at the feeling level. There are three important and recurrent feeling states to understand. They are feelings of helplessness, powerlessness, and hopelessness.

Researchers have shown that extended exposure to threat and/or harm can produce a state of helplessness. When threats are outside an individual's control, are global (affecting many aspects of the person's life), and are also unpredictable, feelings of helplessness can be more intense. *Helplessness*, then, is a condition that is both perceived by and induced in patients who are experiencing illness. Learned helplessness occurs when patients realize that despite all they do nothing will help their situation. Thus, repeated exposures may reduce an individual's overall coping capability and elicit an apathetic response. Patients have learned that there are no real options and give up trying to find one. This is where providers can make a difference: (1) by changing patients' perception of their illness to something they can successfully cope with and (2) by supporting patients' efforts to continue trying.

What happens when patients encounter helplessness over time? Patients encountering prolonged, sustained helplessness will develop perceptions of powerlessness. *Powerlessness* is patients' recognition that they have no control to affect a specific outcome. Otherwise,

patients have power but have lost power when it comes to a particular circumstance (i.e., loss of function resulting from a chronic illness). Powerlessness is the perceived inability and hopelessness in controlling illness. Patients' sense of power or powerlessness is directly related to their actual control over their illness. A sense of powerlessness has been attributed to individual personality predispositions, and theorists will also argue that this emotional reaction is also situationally defined.

Feelings of sustained helplessness can result not only in feelings of powerlessness but eventually hopelessness as well. *Hopelessness* is sometimes seen as synonymous with helplessness. Helplessness is the belief that one is unable to help oneself or to act without help, while hopelessness is being without hope. In fact, if powerlessness persists, a state of hopelessness will occur. Hopelessness is also associated with depression and suicidality, and although it may be temporary, it may, nonetheless, result in a deteriorated physical and mental status.

That which alleviates helplessness will alter feelings of powerlessness and hopelessness. The primary approach to nullifying this triad of difficult perceptions is to anticipate, evaluate, and intervene in supportive ways with patients. For example, giving patients explanations about what to expect, what can be done, and involving them in the shared decision-making process in which they have control over treatment decisions (when possible) can minimize hopelessness and reminding patients of the power they do have and that they are not as helpless as they believe they are.

▶ Therapeutic Responses to Chronically Ill Patients

Certain patients whose conditions cannot be reversed can make health care providers anxious and this is one category that tends to do so. Patients whose circumstances are perceived to be fragile certainly create concern and even anxiety. To some extent, providers are not immune to the same triad of difficult emotions that patients experience: the helplessness, powerlessness, and hopelessness that their patients experience.

A common retort of providers who choose not to work with these patients but to work with patients who are going to improve and will do so fairly rapidly is, "I could never work with them. Isn't it just too depressing?" Fortunately, there are providers who become very committed to the care of these patients. Some providers who initially regard these patients as "depressing" learn to appreciate the rewards and satisfaction that come from caring for them.

Coping and Support

Providers have an important role in helping patients cope with the stressors of their chronic illness and treatment. However, patients' families and loved ones play a critical role as well.

There are two types of coping functions: (1) those that manage or alter the problem or the source of stress (**problem-focused coping**) and (2) those that regulate the stressful emotions that are brought on by the stress (**emotion-focused coping**). These functions work together, otherwise, if the stress was caused by the diagnosis of a serious illness and

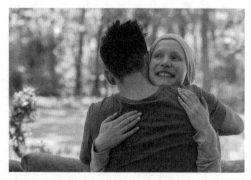

© Photographee.eu/Shutterstock.

coping was getting the help needed to treat the illness, problem-focused coping is operating. If the stress of a chronic illness includes experiences of shock and disbelief, getting help for these intense feelings would be emotion-focused coping.

The classic work of Lazarus and Folkman (1984) details how these coping processes work. They explain that individuals who face stressful events or situations use both forms of coping. As previously stated, patients use coping mechanisms to deal with the problem (their symptoms of pain and fatigue) and to alter the emotional distress they feel as a result of their symptoms (pain and fatigue). Promoting adaptive behaviors in patients necessitates recognizing not only the symptoms (the problem) but also patients' evaluation of the symptoms that are causing the distress.

Guides for assessing a patient's coping status are outlined in **EXHIBITS 16-2** and **16-3**. Exhibit 16-2 outlines specific interview questions that are useful for gathering information from patients about their coping abilities. Exhibit 16-3 identifies avenues of investigation that will help providers formulate an overall appraisal of patients' coping behaviors and their risks for maladaptive responses.

Patients who experience chronic and/or life-threatening illness will cope better if they are aware of and understand how their personal ways of dealing with their illnesses are important to their health and how they may prevent unnecessary hospitalizations. Most patients are not aware of how their illness creates stress and how their lifestyles and beliefs about self, others, and health affect them. This lack of awareness is more likely in patients who (1) lack knowledge of the stressful events and chronic strains that contribute to their health problems, (2) believe that looking at how they cope is only necessary when a crisis has occurred, and (3) believe that changing the ways they deal with stress and their illness is not necessary once they feel better. Some patients believe that learning new ways of coping will cost lots of money, and if they

EXHIBIT 16-2 Chronic Disease Management: Assessment of Coping Status—Patient Interview Probes

- "What concerns do you have about your illness?"
- "What do you expect from your treatment?"
- "What helps you to reduce stress?" (Former stress-busting measures might be employed in the current adaptation to illness)
- "In dealing with your illness right now, what works best? What doesn't seem to work well?"
- "Is there a support system for you? Do you feel it is adequate?" (When people are ill, they call on friends or family to support them; however, this system may not provide the support the patient needs)
- "What barriers keep you from getting the support you need or want?" (How optimistic are you about getting the care and support you need?)
- "Considering the difficulties you are having right now—how well are you dealing with them?" (Address each difficulty or symptom one at a time)
- "Overall, how much does your health limit you? How would you rate the quality of your life?"

EXHIBIT 16-3 Provider Guide to Formulate an Appraisal of Patients' Coping Capabilities

- What is the patient's current condition? Health status, prognosis?
- What is the patient's current knowledge of his or her illness and awareness of the significance of their diagnosis?
- What is the patient's present mood, affect, feelings of control, and level of self-confidence about dealing with his or her illness?
- What is the patient's primary coping responses at this time (denial, anger, etc.)?
- To what extent is denial used and what level of denial is manifested (first order, denial of facts; second order, denial of implications of facts; third order, denial of illness outcome)?
- What and how adequate is the patient's support network?
- How available are self-help and/or home health care resources to the patient?
- What are the patient's spiritual/religious needs?
- What stressors, secondary to health status, are particularly significant: financial, loss of family/social support, stigma and/or social alienation, loss of independence?

change an aspect of their lifestyle, this may cause other problems for them and for other people around them.

Patients' coping efforts are influenced by many factors (e.g., personal factors and available coping resources). One important factor is how patients view their stressors. The cognitive mediating process that is important in determining an individual's perceptions of threat is referred to as **cognitive appraisal**. Patients' perceptions of and processing of health-related problems will determine their emotional reactions. If patients do not see a health-related condition as a problem, the patient perceives no threat, and patients will not call into action any additional resources to handle the problem.

To understand why patients who are exposed to the same event react differently, one must draw on the principles of cognitive appraisal and the impact of cultural and religious beliefs. Through the cognitive appraisal process, or patients' way of processing information, patients evaluate the significance of current stressful health-related events. In primary appraisal, patients evaluate the extent to which an event is relevant or irrelevant, benign or threatening.

Threatening events are deemed either immediately harmful or capable of harm, otherwise, patients evaluate both the immediate and potential threat of events. In secondary appraisal, patients evaluate the magnitude of the problem by assessing the extent something can be done to alter the circumstances. When the patient's reaction is one of hopelessness, patients see they have no available options or resources available to address the threatening life event. Still, the patient's religious and cultural beliefs might buffer their perception of threat and fear of harm. Faith in a higher being or perception and attitudes about universal lifetime struggles can bring them closer to their families and communities who will provide them support. Whether patients perceive an event as threatening, the particular coping responses they use are determined by their available resources, otherwise, the tangible and material resources available to individuals clearly affect coping abilities.

It is important to understand the impact of coping on health, mortality, and morbidity. Research has shown that the effects are significant. Coping, for example, has been shown to influence the duration, frequency, intensity, and patterning of neurochemical stress reactions. Inadequate coping can affect health negatively by increasing patient's risk for morbidity and mortality. Research on **maladaptive coping** responses, for example, catastrophizing, may adversely affect health outcomes (Drossman et al., 2000) and perception of symptoms. Maladaptive coping responses are any behaviors that avoid the presenting problem and its emotional impact even though they may bring temporary relief. Examples include patients who cope with stress with illicit drugs and alcohol abuse. Engaging in any high-risk behaviors in order to cope with stressful life events exposes the patient to higher risks for morbidity and/or mortality.

Yet another very important way in which coping responses influence morbidity and mortality is the appropriateness of the response in light of the threat. For example, many patients who suspect that they have a health problem delay seeking medical screening or treatment. Medical attention then can be significantly delayed when patients fail to evaluate the situation as threatening or use a response that does not directly address the significance of the signs or symptoms that they are experiencing.

Many times, maladaptive coping is used in the service of denial. For example, substance abuse can numb awareness of the seriousness of the disease. Recall that in the discussion of stages of psychological adaptation earlier in this chapter denial was the first stage in the adaptation process. If denial continued indefinitely the process of coping would be maladaptive. Understanding the use of denial to cope with health-related threats is important. In still another classic conceptual framework, Weisman (1972) describes three levels of denial pertaining to the diagnosis of life-threatening illnesses; these include **first-order, second-order, and third-order denial**.

First-order denial is simply a denial of facts. Signs of recurrent illness may be explained away as insignificant. New breast changes in a patient with a history of breast cancer may be explained away as too minor to be upset about.

Second-order denial is denial of the implications of the facts. Thus, patients may acknowledge the facts—breast changes—but deny the significance or meaning of these changes. In denying the significance of these changes, patients minimize the importance of their primary diagnosis. Many patients go through phases in the course of their prolonged illness wherein they "will their illness away." They are tired of being hypervigilant; they may want to ignore the restrictions that their illness imposes. Most patients will be brought back into awareness with minimal confrontation; others may need additional support and counseling. Sometimes patients do not deny their illness altogether but "fractionate" their illness, rendering it significantly less threatening. Fractionating means that patients have cognitively broken their illness into smaller, manageable parts; while this process can be adaptive, an undesirable result is that symptoms may be evaluated as considerably less important than they really are. Or, the patient may focus on some small part of the illness (e.g., weight loss), thus minimizing the secondary implications of the serious illness (cancer).

Third-order denial is denial of the ultimate outcome of the illness or prognosis. For persons with life-threatening illness, it is a denial of impending death. For persons with chronic, debilitating illness that is not life-threatening, it is denial of the ultimate immobility and loss of function that may occur over time. In this case, patients acknowledge the reality of their illness (diagnosis), and even recognize the immediate consequences of their condition (e.g., pain, fatigue, and weight loss). They do not, however, accept their ultimate prognosis. The issue of death is avoided. Patients may believe and talk as if they will experience little functional decline. They may even plan future events as if their state of health will remain the same.

Denial is a powerful coping response in which certain perceptions are not processed in usual ways. Patients and their families use this response to control the anxiety and distress that they experience as a result of their illness and the changes they encounter throughout the course of their illness and treatment. Assisting patients to cope requires providers to intervene effectively with the presenting health problems. This means employing interventions to control symptoms and the disease process. It also includes having open discussions with patients about the meaning of their symptoms and illness. These discussions should be anticipated in advance and tailored to patients' unique ways of coping and their readiness to confront aspects of their disease.

Intervening with presenting health problems is a partial picture of how providers must interact with patients and their families. As previously indicated, treating patients' reactions to their health problems is imperative for effective disease management and successful self-management support. This means that providers will communicate to patients about the responses they are likely to have, how these responses change over time, and what they can do to manage any distress they experience as a result of their health-related changes. It also means providing resources and instruction to patients such as how they can monitor and manage their symptoms and conditions.

There are certain patient attitudes and beliefs that are indicative of low-level awareness about stress and chronic illness. But how do providers know when patients need instruction about stress and coping? The following list of principles of stress and coping with illness are basic but discussions with patients can be individualized to cover these basic concepts in teaching points that can assist patients and families to cope more effectively with the impact of their illness. These principles need to be translated in terms patients can understand and should be parceled out in accordance to the patient's interest and capacity to appreciate them (**EXHIBIT 16-4**).

Approaches to Truth Telling and Patients' Capacities to Receive Information

Health providers provide both *good* and *bad* news to their patients and their families. This includes minor test results as well as major facts about their diagnosis and prognosis. They need to be mindful of the patient's emotional state and their capacity to receive this news. In a section of the text to follow (Part VI, Chapter 22), a good deal of discussion focuses on the ethical practice of truth telling

EXHIBIT 16-4 Principles Helpful in Counseling Patients about Stress and Coping with Illness

- Patients who can cope effectively with problems can feel more self-confident. Realization that they are important members of the health care enterprise reinforces their commitment to their treatment and self-confidence.
- Patients' responses and coping capabilities are important in their recovery. Patients may get some satisfaction that their efforts are important in their recovery process.
- Stress can interfere with patients' ability to cope effectively and their awareness of their strengths and capabilities. Patients can plan ahead by talking with providers about how to handle illness-related stressors.
- Patients' attitudes, religious beliefs, and cultural backgrounds influence how they deal with problems. An important area to explore is ways these factors may contribute positively to coping effectively.
- There are more than a few ways to cope. Coping means different things to different people; thus, there are things to try that patients may not have explored that could help them cope effectively.
- Stressful life events (e.g., chronic illnesses) affect patients' coping abilities but chronic strain (e.g., dealing with chronic pain) also significantly affects their coping ability. Therefore, it is important that they not underestimate symptoms that cause chronic strain.
- Active coping (e.g., through diet, exercise and physical activity, rest and relaxation, social activities, and stress management techniques) as well as asking for support from providers, friends, and family are effective coping responses.
- Generally, when patients stifle their feelings, refuse to think about their problems, or dwell on them for long periods of time, this may not be helpful. How can they set aside time to think about their feelings, and when and with whom would they feel comfortable in discussing their feelings?
- Friends and family can either help patients cope more effectively or cause them to cope less effectively. How are their family and friends helpful, and what do they need to know to be more helpful?
- Learning problem-solving skills can help patients cope more effectively with each phase of illness and illness demands. How do they approach solving problems and how is it working?
- It is possible for patients to cope effectively with some problems and at the same time, ineffectively with others. This principle of adaptation refers to the fact that some problems are more "emotionally loaded" and more support is needed in these instances.
- Feeling hopeless or helpless about patients' problems needs to be checked or monitored so that they will feel better about their condition, treatment, and ability to manage their circumstances. Feeling hopeless or helpless can be reversed with the input of health providers and supportive family and friends. They should be monitored if they create distress and depression.

in communicating essential information to patients and their families.

Preliminary to this discussion it is important that providers understand that they may play a significant role in balancing patients' awareness of their illness and the emotional distress evoked by this awareness. It might not be their responsibility to convey certain medical information but they will interact with patients and their families at various times before and after news is shared with them. Denial is a preliminary stage in adaptation. Although providers may feel uncomfortable with patients who are denying what they have been told, it is critical that they understand and respect this process. It is generally understood that all patients need to maintain some level of denial in order to remain hopeful. The provider–patient–family relationship is based on mutual respect and trust.

If providers, particularly physicians, withhold essential facts from patients and/or their families they are violating the ethical basis of the relationship.

Providers are concerned about the emotional reactions of their patients and the consequences of adding stress to an already physically and emotionally stressful situation. Some believe that to evade the facts is a better course of action, particularly when the prognosis is poor. However, studies have shown that the majority of patients feel they should be fully informed. Research reveals that among those patients who were informed, the majority were glad that they were told but it is a matter of when and by whom. Among those undergoing diagnostic testing, the majority want to be told the truth.

A primary concern behind providers' hesitancy to inform patients about a poor prognosis is the fear that the patients' awareness will result in high levels of fear and stress. Providers anticipate strong negative reactions sometimes including unnecessary dependency, excessive worry, and even clinical anxiety and depression. They are concerned that these reactions will further alter patients' quality of life and that of their family. In contrast to these negative consequences it is also observed that patients who are told not only prefer to know but experience positive changes. The information may initially create imbalance but patients may then regain composure. Families may exhibit similar experiences.

Underlying the issue of truth telling is the fact that many patients actually know a great deal more than they are told. Many patients understand their condition even without providers' input. This is possible because of available information resources beyond the patient's health care team. Patients and families search the Internet and they ask friends and community advisors about what they know. Patients and their families can figure it out without facts from providers. Staff frequently fails to realize that patients

come to conclusions that they choose not to disclose to providers. Providers who believe that patients only know what they have told them are underestimating patients and their families. Additionally, patients learn "to read providers" through provider nonverbal responses. Silences, efforts at evading topics, false reassurances, and pessimistic attitudes are frequently picked up and interpreted by patients and their families.

Patients at some level also do their own self-assessments. They are able to understand their own bodies and establish for themselves that they are weaker, less alert, and irreversibly dependent on others. Patients may remain silent about what they know because they assume that provider and family silences mean that they do not want to talk about the inevitable. The problem is that all untested assumptions and conclusions may be incorrect, and providers, for this reason, need to find ways to lift the veil over these taboo subjects. One approach to use would be the following: "Patients often think that providers have given up; this is far from the truth. Providers are fighting for you every day and in many different ways."

The phenomena of each party not disclosing to the other what both know or assume but fail to discuss is called *mutual denial*. It can appear that patients and/or their families have joined a conspiracy of silence to protect those involved from feeling uncomfortable. Because patients generally know more than what they are told, providers run the serious risk of losing patients' trust and confidence by withholding aspects of their condition. Providers must be aware of their own reactions to patients' conditions and give careful consideration to how these feelings are affecting their communications with their patients.

When providers approach the issues of negative prognosis or terminal state, the actual discussion should be thoughtfully planned in advance. These conversations should not be initiated without providing patients the opportunities to clarify and react to the information. Abrupt announcements or short-lived explanations are ill-advised. Some providers will ease into a conversation by first asking questions (e.g., "Well, I suppose you've been wondering just what's going on.") or by leading with a disclosure (e.g., "This news is difficult for me to tell you," or "I wish I could give you better news.").

By easing into the subject, providers can assess patients' readiness and capability to pursue the subject. Because the provider has offered an opening, space is made for a less restricting discussion. Patients who feel sufficiently secure are likely to reveal what they have concluded and their views of the facts given them. In addition to offering the opportunity to discuss the facts, providers need to recognize that once the subject is raised there may be a continuing dialogue where many other concerns will surface and will need to be handled patiently, repeatedly, and with empathy.

The uncertainty surrounding a terminal status is difficult for most patients and significant others to deal with. Patients and significant others frequently ask for exact estimates of survival time (e.g., "How much time do I have?"). Usually, providers render an estimate very cautiously because predictions about survival time not always match actual survival time. Sometimes providers will err toward optimistic estimates. Such estimates, however, are not always helpful. Although they may sustain hope, this hope is unrealistic.

Concerns About Communicating with Patients and Family Around End-of-Life Care

For those families who need to coordinate the many aspects of dealing with the loved one's actual demise (e.g., gathering family members from long distances), over-optimistic predictions are a disservice to the patient and the family. In Part VIII, Chapter 29, a lengthy discussion of communications with patients and families during end-of-life care is provided.

There is considerable concern about whether communication is adequate around end-of-life care. These concerns have been presented in a number of professional journals, all raising the issue: "how can communications be improved?"

An editorial in the *American Journal of Respiratory Critical Care Medicine* (Azoulay, 2005) stressed that exercising compassion was not enough. Providers must sharpen their communication skills, continuously evaluate their practices, identify their mistakes and inadequacies, and correct for them. Providing information and support to families and patients is the primary goal; however, this is inconsistently achieved in many settings including critical care units. Tulsky (2005) explains that while patients have desires for information and providers cannot always predict what they want to know, health providers do not sufficiently discuss the treatment options or quality of life or respond to emotional cues from patients and their families.

Knauft, Nielsen, Engelberg, Patrick, and Curtis (2005) reported in their study of chronic obstructive pulmonary disease (COPD) patient care that when end-of-life discussions did occur, patients rated them as relatively high in quality. These authors concluded that the real issue may be addressing the barriers to these discussions because once they happened, patients were highly satisfied with them. These researchers identified two barriers that were endorsed by more than half of the patients observed: (1) patients' desire to focus on staying alive rather than talk about death and (2) not being sure which physician would be taking care of them when the time came. Providers can use empathy while acknowledging that it is difficult to talk about this important, but difficult, task.

Providers can learn to communicate better through intensive course offerings. Today, a number of communication skill training programs have been developed to specifically address end-of-life care. As previously explained, more information about end-of-life care is provided in Chapter 23.

▶ Summary

There is a growing need for advanced expertise in chronic and life-threatening disease management as conditions continue to significantly grow in numbers and proportions. In the case of the care of the chronically ill and those patients with life-threatening illnesses, the assault of these conditions on the lives of patients and their significant others is significant.

Managing the care of these patients requires not only knowledge of the specific disease processes but also basic principles related to patients' process of adapting and coping. Providers must be aware of the cognitive and affective changes these patients experience so that they can communicate effectively with them. They must be able to conduct an evaluation of coping responses over time. The majority of these patients will receive their care almost exclusively in ambulatory care settings and in the home. Because of this, providers will be expected to comprehend patients' needs in a rich and diverse cultural, ethnic, social, and economic context.

A good deal of the care to these patients will consist of effectively communicating in order to identify risk factors and detect early signs of decline. Care to these patients involves managing symptoms collaboratively with patients and those in supportive roles around them.

The issues of chronic debilitating and/or life-threatening illness must be understood if providers are to effectively help patients and their families cope. Patients, themselves, need to understand how coping responses influence their current health and the progression of their disease. In cases of terminal illness, the communication capabilities of providers are extremely important. Providers must understand their own responses to patients' conditions, individual patients' desires for information, and how these factors influence the content of their discussions and what information they share or withhold from patients. While there are general guidelines about truth telling, each situation should be treated uniquely. Providers will generally lean toward truth-telling for many reasons including ethical imperatives and patients' preferences to be told.

It is erroneous to believe that patients know only what providers have explicitly told them. Under most circumstances, open, truthful disclosures best prepare patients and families to cope with the inevitabilities surrounding their illness whether it is chronic and disabling or terminal. An estimated 50 million people die each year in the United States, many without access to sound palliative care (Paice, Ferrell, Coyle, Coyne, & Calloway, 2008). End-of-life care communications call for the removal of barriers because most patients value these discussions if they are encouraged to have them.

Discussion

1. Identify and describe the stages of psychological adaptation to chronic and life-threatening illnesses.
2. Discuss the concept that coping with chronic illness is about overcoming powerlessness.
3. Define and give examples of adaptive and maladaptive coping.
4. Discuss examples of how maladaptive coping can result in worse patient outcomes.
5. Identify and discuss principles of coping to chronic illness that patients and their families should know.

References

Azoulay, E. (2005). Editorial: The end-of-life family conference: Communication empowers. *American Journal of Respiratory Critical Care Medicine, 171,* 803–805. doi:10.1164/rccm.2501004

Cal, S. F., de Sa, L. R., Glustak, M. E., & Santiago, M. B. (2015). Resilience in chronic diseases: A systematic review. *Cogent Psychology, 2*(1), 1024928. doi:10.1080/23311908.2015.1024928

Capehorn, M., Polonsky, W. H., Edelman, S., Belton, A., Down, S., Gamerman, V., … Alzaid, A. (2017). Challenges faced by physicians when discussing the Type 2 diabetes diagnosis with patients: Insights from a cross-national study (IntroDiaR). *Diabetes Medicine, 34*(8), 1100–1107. doi:10.1111/dme.3357.Epub2017 May 21

Cheatle, M. D. (2011). Depression, chronic pain, and suicide by overdose: On the edge. Pain Medicine, *12*(Suppl_2, 1), S43–S48. doi:10.1111/j.1526-4637.2011.01131.x

Drossman, D. A., Leserman, J., Li, Z., Keefe, F., Hu, Y. J. B., & Moomey, T. C. (2000). Effects of coping on health outcome among women with gastrointestinal disorders. *Psychosomatic Medicine, 62,* 309–317. PMID:10845344

Hall, D. L., Lennes, I. T., Pirl, W. F., Friedman, E. R., & Park, E. R. (2017). Fear of recurrence or progression as a link between somatic symptoms and perceived stress among cancer survivors. *Supportive Care in Cancer: Official Journal of the Multinational Association of Supportive Care in Cancer, 25*(5), 1401–1407. doi:10.1007/s00520-016-3533-3

Haynes, D. F., & Watt, P. (2008). The lived experience of health behaviors in people with debilitating illness. *Holistic Nursing Practice, 22*(1), 44–53. doi:10.1097/01.HNP.0000306328.34085.57

Jackson, K. (2014). Grieving chronic illness and injury— Infinite losses. *Social Work Today, 14*(4), 18.

Knauft, M. E., Nielsen, E. L., Engelberg, R. A., Patrick, D. L., & Curtis, J. R. (2005). Barriers and facilitators to end-of-life care communication for patients with COPD. *Chest, 127,* 2188–2196. doi:10.1378/chest.127.6.2188

Kübler-Ross, E. (1969). *On death and dying.* New York, NY: Macmillan. doi:10.1136/bmj.329.7466.627

Lazarus, R., & Folkman, S. (1984). *Stress, appraisal and coping.* New York, NY: Springer Publishing.

Newman, L. (2004). Elisabeth Kübler-Ross. *BMJ : British Medical Journal, 329*(7466), 627.

Ozga, M., Aghajanian, C., Myers-Virtue, S., McDonnell, G., Jhanwar, S., Hichenberg, S., & Sulimanoff, I. (2015). A systematic review of ovarian cancer and fear of recurrence. *Palliative & Supportive Care, 13*(6), 1771–1780. doi:10.1017/S1478951515000127

Paice, J. A., Ferrell, B. R., Coyle, N., Coyne, P., & Callaway, M. (2008). Global efforts to improve palliative care: The international end-of-life nursing education consortium training programme. *Journal of Advanced Nursing, 61*(2), 173–180. doi:10.1111/j.1365-2648.2007.04475.x

Schwartz, J. C. (2009). Psychological adaptation to illness: A personal Odyssey and suggestions for physicians. *Proceedings (Baylor University Medical Center), 22*(3), 242–245.

Telford, K., Kralik, D., & Koch, T. (2006). Acceptance and denial: Implications for people adapting to chronic illness: Literature review. *Journal of Advanced Nursing, 55,* 457–464. doi:10.1111/j.1365-2648.2006.03942.x

Tulsky, J. A. (2005). Beyond advance directives: Importance of communication skills at the end of life. *JAMA, 294,* 359–365. doi:10.1001/jama.294.3.359

Weisman, A. D. (1972). *On dying and denying: A psychiatric study of terminality.* New York, NY: Behavioral Publications.

CHAPTER 17

Communicating with Patients and Families in Crisis

CHAPTER OBJECTIVES

- Differentiate between situational and developmental crises.
- Describe the crisis response and stages of crisis resolution.
- Identify typical dysfunctional aspects of communication in times of crisis.
- Discuss stressors, coping resources, and stress-resistance resources.
- Identify interventions that are useful for managing highly anxious and agitated patients.

KEY TERMS

- Adaptive coping responses
- Anxiety
- Crisis
- Crisis-Prone
- Maladaptive coping responses

▶ Introduction

Health providers in both acute care and primary care settings encounter patients and families in crisis. People in crisis can be found in any health care setting, during primary care visits, as well as at urgent care or hospital emergency departments. First encounters with a health care professional may vary. A patient's first contact with a health care provider may be at the site of a natural disaster or emergency. The first contact may also be during a telephone call (Kavan, Guck, & Barone, 2006). Individuals' problems can range from minor setbacks to major highly stressful events, including psychiatric and substance abuse crisis situations. In the context of health care, crisis is often linked to the diagnosis of an illness or injury and the realization of its life-threatening consequences. But it need not always be.

Providers will be called upon to identify and support patients and their families in times of crisis. Some crisis events produce severe states of stress which can even result in patients' disorganization and inability to function. Although frequently a temporary state, times of crisis can be painful and require provider recognition and sometimes rapid response. In this chapter, the patient crisis experiences are explored in depth.

The stages of crisis are discussed as well as interventions to help patients and their families overcome the potential dysfunctional responses. Crisis as a response to suffering a significant illness can occur at any point in time: at diagnosis but also when patients are discharged from the hospital and inevitability face self-care tasks without the one-to-one support of providers. Crisis can also recur for patients and families when disease takes a turn for the worse. Some of these patients could be experiencing a medical crisis as well as a developmental or psychological crisis. For example, a person who has just learned of a serious diagnosis but has also just lost a job or is going to divorce. Proper assessment and interventions are needed to assist them in minimizing dysfunctional responses to crisis and to return them to coping effectively without functional disorganization that is typical when crisis occurs. It is important to point out that the effects of crisis are usually temporary and can even be a source of strength when providers assist in crisis resolution.

How will providers know when and if patients are facing a crisis? By definition, a crisis is a time of intense stress or difficulty. What comes to mind is an emergency, disaster, or catastrophic event. This would include responses to floods, hurricanes, or tornados. It can also be observed when a difficult decision must be made, such as when patients' families are faced with the troubling decision of what to do in advance care planning for the patient. Any turning point in patient care that is marked by an important change, either recovery or death, can elicit a crisis response.

People are experienced to some degree with crisis. Most adults may have encountered one or more of the following: loss of job, divorce or marital separation, personal injury, or financial distress. Adolescents may have experience with a breakup of a significant relationship, loss of a sibling or parent, and dealing with a split in the family due to divorce or separation. These experiences can cause emotional overload or feelings of helplessness and powerlessness. Some persons experience severe disturbances in perception, in processing, and in their ability to express thoughts and feelings. From a system's perspective, stimuli input and the demands for output can exceed the capacity to respond. This can be a sign of a pending crisis. Observing adult and adolescent communication in a time of crisis shows not only the stress of the emergent situation but also their inherent abilities or inabilities to cope with the challenges they face. Patients in crisis need special consideration because their abilities to receive, process, and respond will be altered by their crisis state.

In summary, crisis occurs when the patient is presented with a critical incident or stressful event that is perceived as overwhelming and outside the individual's abilities to cope. Crisis impact relies heavily on the perception of the event (Kavan et al., 2006). Patients' abilities to cope under usual circumstances seem not to be useful enough at times of crisis.

What is the straw that broke the camel's back? As previously noted, in every crisis situation there is a precipitant (sometimes referred to as a stressor) that acts to offset whatever level of equilibrium exists for patients. Precipitating or stressful events are change-producing events of unusual significance. They may be defined as unanticipated accidental or situational, occurring without warning or in the course of ongoing events that are more or less anticipated.

Individuals are vulnerable to a variety of both expected and unexpected events depending, in part, on their evaluation of these events, the cultural perspectives, and their level of support from family and health providers. Illness and injury can fall into the category of causing imbalance and needing the strong support of health care providers.

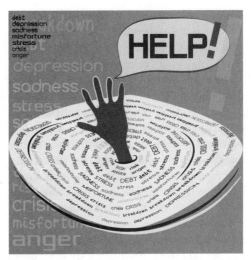

© White art/Shutterstock.

▶ Definitions of Crisis

Crisis occurs when more change or adjustment is required of individuals than they are capable of at the time. *The first major false assumption about people in crisis is that they are always incapacitated.* When one thinks of people whose tolerance has been exceeded and who become "paralyzed" in times of crisis, it is not about a simple stress response, it is about central nervous system overload. Crisis situations that produce less severe responses are more common. These situations are characterized by their more temporary nature and by their tendency to leave individuals less physically and mentally incapacitated.

A second major false assumption about people in crisis is that people experience crisis alone. Crisis is not usually a singular experience. Even in times of catastrophic events, others are also suffering and there are witnesses who suffer in different ways. Therefore, groups as well as individuals experience crises together. The most obvious examples of group crises are situational events that lie outside the normal range of expectancy. These include situations like war or significant threat of harm (e.g., bombings, shootings, or explosions), natural disasters (e.g., floods, hurricanes, or tornados), and witnessed violence (e.g., physical or emotional abuse).

Not only can individuals experience crisis along with others they are also affected by observing others who are sharing the same catastrophic experience. Viewing others in disorganizing crisis can create similar disorganizing responses. An example would be crowds dispersing after a mass shooting. On the contrary, other observers might see the crisis event as a challenge, have some experience dealing with similar crisis events, and respond

in very effective ways to protect those in crisis as well as themselves.

The phenomenon of feeling stress during a crisis and responding in kind has been studied. It is known, for example, that mood states, such as fear, anxiety, and depression can be transmitted to others. Psychologists have explained that the process of "catching the mood of someone" is like catching germs from another person. The term is *emotional contagion.* Emotional contagion can occur between people over time or more immediately in groups. It is a three-step process where one person's feelings transfer to another person.

Essentially, the stimulus for an emotion arises from one person, is acted upon or perceived by one or more persons, and causes corresponding or complementary emotions in all individuals (Hatfield, Bensman, Thorton, & Rapson, 2014). In crisis situations, emotional contagion may be responsible in part for why those who witness others in crisis might *feel* the crisis similarly.

It is also known that the interactions of individuals in crisis may worsen or improve a particular individual's responses to the event. That is, parties to the same disaster may worsen each other's responses. For example, individuals running from a scene of violence will excite others causing them to run as well. This is like a response for self-presentation. Family members can react to the patient's diagnosis as a crisis. They might calm or even accelerate the excitement and fear of the patient. Providers, then, need to be cognizant of group response to crisis because treating one patient might occur in the context of caring for a group of survivors, including whole families. Patients and families are seldom, but may need to be, sheltered from one another to limit cross-exposure to alarm, fear, and high anxiety or panic that comes with a crisis situation.

A third common misconception about crisis is that it leads to a long lasting psychological breakdown. Psychological breakdown in patients and their families during crisis is generally worrisome to providers for various reasons. Providers might worry about gaining patients' cooperation in crisis situations because they think they are incapable of good judgment. The idea that people in crisis are helpless is also erroneous. While it is possible that some patients feel helpless, have poor judgment, and cognitive distortions, many patients do not. Any temporary cognitive deficit that occurs is usually corrected in a short period of time, at least in the majority of instances. Providers learn to recognize patients' weaknesses and strengths in coping with a crisis situation. The critical issue is to assess how and to what degree their functioning is limited or impaired by the crisis and their reaction to the crisis.

Finally, a fourth common misconception is that crisis is the same as the stressor or stimulus-provoking response. While stressors or stressful stimuli are associated with crisis situations, these stimuli may not always cause a crisis. These stimuli may not result in a crisis experience. As previously indicated, the stimulus or catastrophic event may not even elicit a crisis at the level expected. In fact, there is a great deal of variability in individuals' responses to stress stimuli. This variation occurs within the same individual, over time, and across individuals when exposed to the same stimuli. What, then, explains

dysfunctional responses when individuals are exposed to stressful or noxious stimuli?

Dysfunctional Aspects of Communication in Crisis Situations

People in crisis are affected on several levels. They often experience disorganization of thoughts and behavior which has ramifications for their capacity to function. A major factor in the imbalance and disorganization that accompanies crisis is the presence of anxiety. Anxiety is characterized as a distressed state accompanied by diffuse feelings of uncertainty, apprehension, and sometimes fear of imminent danger. Anxiety, erratic behavior, and inadequate decision-making may occur as well as a set of physical signs and symptoms that parallel these responses and can be profound. Physical signs and symptoms include restlessness, shortness of breath, trembling, or shaking. Anxiety itself appears in varying amounts and with unpredictable frequency. Fluctuations can appear as if patients are getting some respite in the face of very stressful moments.

People in crisis also exhibit several forms of struggling with communication. They generally have difficulty perceiving accurately; their abilities to process information may be significantly impaired; and their ability to express ideas, thoughts, and emotions may be limited. They may or may not be able to speak, hear you, and, if they do hear you, move in response to your direction. However, these forms of communication are taxed and may not be consistently available in patients. Self-awareness of their functional limitations and declined capacities may further intensify their feelings of fear and anxiety as they perceive their state of disorganization. It is possible that persons in crisis may become even more dysfunctional as they begin to comprehend what has happened to them and observe their responses to stressful events. If they could reply they might respond, "What happened, what is happening to me…I hear somebody telling me something but I can't focus or hear what they're saying."

Dysfunctional or disorganized family units characterized by deficient and inappropriate relationships and role enactment frequently exhibit crisis states because family coping resources are severely limited even in the precrisis stage. Marginally functional families are able to maintain minimal levels of functionality when no excessive stress is present but can suffer significant disruption when demands on the family seriously exceed their resources.

Disturbances in perception: Disturbances in perception frequently occur as a direct result of overstimulation. *Overstimulation* includes a rapid or excessive barrage of stimuli that exceeds one's particular tolerance. Persons who are raped or tortured are known to endure multiple stimuli, and inherent in these situations is the fact that the stimuli exceed the tolerance level of the individual (and would do so for most people). It is adaptive in these situations to block out or selectively attend to threats around them.

Although crisis is frequently associated with overload, there are circumstances where under-stimulation or stimulation with inappropriate noxious information also creates crisis. Is the prisoner who is in isolation experiencing crisis? When sensory deprivation is involuntary, the situation may exceed individuals' capacity to act and therefore presents a crisis to the individual.

Disturbance in processing stimuli: Persons in crisis also experience the inability to process stimuli. The most common example is when recognition and memory fail which is usually at the point of peak crisis stimuli. Memory fails for several reasons. First, there may be sensory overload. Flooding a person's awareness with stimuli can create problems in properly sorting and prioritizing data. A second way in which memories fail in times of crisis is when information is constructed

or reconstructed in faulty ways because one was not expecting or have no way of dealing with the new and different signals received. Decision-making capabilities can be affected by either sensory overload or memory impairment, usually both.

Disturbance in expression: Crises also affect individuals' expressive communication capabilities. Crises frequently impair our ability to sleep and concentrate as well as our ability to remember and process information appropriately. Disturbances in perception and the processing of stimuli will also affect individuals' capacities to express thoughts, ideas, and feelings in a complete and coherent manner. When ideas are incomplete and incoherent, they fail to express themselves in ways they can be helped. Providers sometimes react to these circumstances by empathizing with patients and families as if they "read their minds." By doing this they believe they lessen the demands on patients to express themselves.

In **TABLE 17-1**, levels of anxiety are described along with their potential consequences for communications. Patients' abilities to observe, focus, and learn in crisis situations are mitigated by their level of anxiety at the time. Their abilities can fluctuate so it is not only important to identify their current deficits but their pattern of deficits and capabilities over time.

A crisis that affects groups reflects these problems many times over. Groups in crisis may behave like mobs or highly disorganized, chaotic gatherings. Additionally, groups in crisis will frequently exhibit a variety of internal changes. In response to crisis, they may change in size or composition, in reciprocity or mutuality of relationships, in symbolic or explicit goals and values, in the pattern in which information and messages flow between members and among the group, and even in how the group communicates with the external environment. For example, when observing crowds in crisis it can be seen that as they respond they scatter or run from the stimuli and even form different clusters. These clusters

TABLE 17-1 Level of Anxiety and Patients' Abilities to Observe, Process, and Learn	
Level of Anxiety (Intensity)	**Effects on Patients' Communication Skills**
Mild (+)	Sensory perception and ability to focus are intact. The ability to observe oneself and what is going on is enhanced. Connections between events are made and verbalized. At this level, learning can take place. Individuals with this level of anxiety are likely to be alert and able to function in emergencies.
Moderate (+ +)	Sensory perception is somewhat narrowed but alertness continues to the extent that individuals are able to concentrate on a delineated focus. With some effort, concentration on relevant data is possible, and appropriate connections are made as long as the individual is able to shut out irrelevant data.
Severe (+ + +)	Sensory perception is greatly reduced. Individuals focus on a small detail of an experience and are unable to make connections among scattered details. Individuals are unable to get a total picture of an experience. Learning fails to occur.
Panic (+ + + +)	There is major dissociation of experience, and individuals fail to notice or remember major experiences. Details may become enlarged and distorted. They are not able to be understood by others and some level of personality disorganization may be apparent. Individuals may experience being in a state of "terror." At this level of anxiety learning does not happen. The immediate goal is to get relief.

Reprinted with permission from Smith M. C. (1984). The client who is anxious. In S. Lego (Ed.), *The American handbook of psychiatric nursing* (p. 389). Philadelphia, PA: J. B. Lippincott Company.

could reflect the specific solution they have for escaping the crisis situation. For example, they may cluster as the group that chooses to jump the fence or to hide behind protective shields to escape injury or death.

Groups, including families in crisis, can be dysfunctional, though not all the time. Some groups that are experiencing crisis events operate at high levels of sophistication previously thought to be impossible. Catastrophic situations have shown that major threats to groups can actually improve group communication and functioning. For example, a group in crisis can problem solve the situation and assign various persons to lead or organize the rest of the group.

▶ Stress Theories and Understanding Crisis

Theories of stress and stress management provide us with a better understanding of crisis and responses to crisis. Crisis is considered to be an acute variation of stress that is so severe that disorganization occurs and functioning is impaired. It is a temporary state and can produce increased insight and feelings of strength.

Stress and Adaptation

Most noteworthy in the literature on stress and adaptation are the writings of Lazarus and

Folkman. They define *stress* as the demands placed on us from either internal or external sources that are perceived as taxing or as exceeding the resources of the individual (1984, p. 3). Researchers have operationalized stress not only as responses to stressful life events (discrete, episodic life events) but also as ongoing stressful conditions or chronic strain. As in the theory of Lazarus and Folkman, whenever stress is discussed coping with stress is also addressed. In fact, a large part of what is known about stress and stressors comes from studies of coping and adaptation. Over the past 2 decades, in particular, considerable evidence has accumulated to suggest that there is a link between levels of stress and maladaptive outcomes.

A large part of the research on stress, borrowing from the classic work of Holmes and Rahe (1967), has focused on stress that results from change of many kinds. It is hypothesized that any change—large or small—that requires readjustment in a person's life causes stress. Even seemingly benign changes such as starting a better job and forming a new friendship were believed to lead to stress and to its negative consequences. The extent of the change or change demand was viewed as important, and it was found that many people experienced elevated risks from many emotional and physical problems when they experienced either numerous life changes or several high-demand changes within a short time period.

According to the original classic work of Holmes and Rahe (1967), a clustering of life events or a high level of change demand precedes such health problems as depression, psychosomatic conditions, and suicide attempts. Additionally, it was found that the demand impact of events accumulates over time.

The number of events that occur over a 6-month or 1-year period of time may significantly increase a person's risk for physical illness. One major criticism of this early research is that too much attention was given to events that were typical of middle-class people to the neglect of things that happened to poor or marginalized people. And although life events were viewed as important, once an analysis of these events was conducted it was determined that the originally identified events had value but so did a number of other minor occurrences. Thus, being able to adjust to sporadic change was also seen as important. That is, the necessity of adjusting to unchanging (or slowly changing) conditions that must be endured daily are important sources of stress. This principle is important because it encourages providers to consider not only major events (e.g., life-threatening or debilitating chronic illness) but also less severe acute or chronic illnesses (e.g., sinusitis or thyroid disease) as legitimate stressors. Thus, a wide range of conditions are stressful from the standpoint of the strain, difficulties, and vulnerability associated with them.

Coping is a concept that is associated with the ways in which people deal with, adapt to, or adjust to stress. It is a concept that may be familiar to some patients and families; but, many may not know what coping means and why it is important to them. Coping has also been used to describe day-to-day problem solving as well as the strength of personality. Because coping is a general concept a broad range of domains are considered relevant. These include behavioral, affective, and even physiologic response modes. What has been shown repeatedly is that coping has both immediate and long-range implications. That is, people try to cope with the immediate implications of a current situation, and at the same time try to find meaning in the situation to integrate the event in their life experience. Additionally, the process of coping appears to be multiphasic; individuals seem to go through stages or phases in which they attempt to "digest" and manage the stress and the secondary implications of the stressful event. In Chapter 16, the process of patients' adaptation to a chronic illness and implications of their condition were discussed in depth.

Maladaptive and Adaptive Coping Responses

Traditionally, the literature on stress and coping tended to focus on coping strategies. The purpose of this research was to identify and evaluate strategies that individuals used to deal with certain stressors. The focus was twofold: (1) identify individual variance in strategies across situations and (2) identify strategies used across individuals facing the same types of stressful conditions.

Earlier notions of stress and coping also implied that coping responses varied and were either **adaptive coping responses** or **maladaptive coping responses**. This basic premise predominates in current analyses as providers' attempts to get patients to seek more adaptive coping strategies. Lazarus and Folkman (1984), for example, suggest that maladaptive responses are emotionally based while adaptive responses are problem-solving based. The fate of any coping response is highly contingent on its ability to address stressful events and their symptoms.

When people are asked about the ways in which they cope with stress (and if they are honest) they may identify one predominant method or a specific series of actions. Some methods are used infrequently, others almost all the time. The following are responses that people identify when they describe the way they cope with stress:

- Seek comfort/help from my friends or family.
- Try to put my stress out of my mind.
- Try to get information that will make me less worried or less afraid.
- Tell myself things (self-talk) to help me feel better.
- Turn to my religious beliefs.
- Seek to be alone, withdraw, or sleep.
- Cry, feel sad, and depressed.
- Search for a solution to my problems.
- Drink alcohol, smoke, use drugs, or eat more.
- Take out my tensions/anger on other people.
- Hope that things will get better.
- Seek out professional counseling.
- Use meditation, yoga, biofeedback, or other stress-management programs.
- Exercise.
- Take more frequent breaks or vacations.

Before advancing this discussion of stress and crisis it is important to explore the notion that some individuals are more **crisis-prone** than others. Typically, the so-called crisis-prone individual is someone who fails to use certain coping resources. These individuals, for example, lack the ability to use problem-solving and social support that helps people deal effectively with crisis. They may also be individuals also who are alienated or lack meaningful, continuous relationships. The characteristics listed in **EXHIBIT 17-1** depict ideas about crisis-prone individuals.

Providers must be careful, however, in presuming that these deficits are solely a reflection of individual culpability because several of these factors depict certain socioeconomic conditions that place people at risk through no particular fault of their own. Studies of women in crisis, for example, have shown that low-income women with young children are at higher risk and should not be seen as crisis-prone. Studies of the coping experiences of low-income women suggest that chronic and unpredictable stressors, limited options for coping, and unreliable outcomes of coping efforts significantly affect the health and well-being of these women.

It is suggested that any of these factors (alone or in some combination) can considerably erode an individual's beliefs that one's world is consistent and can be effectively controlled. It is a sad commentary that individuals whose place in society puts them at continued risk for crisis are criticized. It is important here to take a departure from this line of thinking and consider what psychologists deem as crisis-prone individuals. These patients may or

EXHIBIT 17-1 Collective Ideas about Crisis-Prone Persons

- Difficulty in learning from previous experience.
- History of multiple crises that were ineffectively resolved.
- History of mental disorder or emotional disturbance or developmental delay that makes the individual particularly vulnerable.
- Low self-esteem which may be masked by aggressive or provocative behavior.
- A tendency toward impulsive "acting out" (doing without thinking).
- Marginal income and employment, generally low socioeconomic status.
- Lack of meaningful, continuous social and/or family support.
- Alcohol or other substance abuse.
- History of numerous accidents and/or injuries, particularly within short periods of time.
- Frequent encounters with law enforcement agencies, either as a victim or suspect.
- Multiple changes in address, including homelessness.

may not experience a series of real crisis events but they act as if they have or are vulnerable to crisis. These persons are said to be of one or more personality disorders that favors living with high drama.

Stressors, Coping, and Stress-Resistance Resources

Coping methods are significantly affected by persons' actual and perceived coping resources such as the availability of social support. It has been shown, however, that the number of resources available is not always the critical factor in stress and crisis. In actuality, people that have very extensive social support networks may actually experience those resources as deficient. Similarly, persons with small support systems—just one good friend—can evaluate their network as more than adequate despite the fact that there are fewer persons to turn to.

Factors that mediate emotional distress due to crisis are stress-resistance resources (e.g., social support and a tendency toward optimism and hopefulness). *Stress-resistance resources* refer to both the internal and the external elements that a person employs to deal with and resolve the problems that are creating stress (Rice, 2012). If coping fails to provide a solution to the problem, stress continues. It may even be heightened by the

awareness of a failed capacity to handle the problem(s) or taken as perceived lack of control over an undesirable event such as in the case of incurable disease.

Most individuals use some form of social support as a means to cope effectively with stress. In many instances, social support can lessen stress, and the mere perception that adequate support is available can serve to buffer situational stress as much as the actual support itself. Still, studies have shown that social support can be variable and may have a mixed influence in assisting the person with stress and crisis.

Hope or hopefulness has also been addressed as an emotional prerequisite to overcoming major stressful events, especially those events outside the realm of expectancy. The idea is that feeling hopeful is a positive spirit that contributes to patients' quality of life and survival. But there are mixed opinions about the potential for hope and a positive spirit and outcomes for illnesses such as cancer survival. A fighting spirit is deeply rooted in some cultures and passive acceptance in others. Nonetheless, mobilizing and supporting hope is important to the patient's and family's overall outlook and active participation in managing their care.

While hopefulness generally refers to expectations that elicit a positive effect, hopelessness refers to low expectancies of success and, therefore, a negative effect. Some authors have speculated that when people find hope, meaning, purpose, and value in their existence, they are more effective and more capable of combating illness. These patients were said to demonstrate a desire to live (a positive outlook). This same perspective can be applied to those who give up hope and find meaning and purpose in surviving the last several months of their lives.

Stress and crisis events may be more or less painful for individuals. Research evidence supports the need to evaluate specific features of the events in order to understand the individual variability in responses. Why do some people view getting a new job as very stressful and others meet this challenge with ease? The early research of Holmes and Rahe (1967) suggested that all life events, positive or negative, could be assigned stress units. When these stress units are added the magnitude of change required can be known.

These researchers believed that all those events that an individual experienced within either a 6-month duration or over a year could be identified and from their total unit score, a negative health outcome, injury, or accident could be predicted with some accuracy. Judge panels were asked to assign unit values to events. The idea was that greater numbers of events, and the more events requiring moderate to high levels of adaptation (with moderate to high unit values), placed the individual at greater risk.

More recent research suggests that negatively viewed events are more likely to predict stress. Therefore, it is important not only for providers to know about patients' recent life events but they need to understand whether the patient perceives the event as positive or negative. If positive or negative, what positive or negative valence (weak, moderate, or strong) do the patients assign to these events?

Researchers who have studied the quality of stressors have described more specifically the link between events and stress.

Those events, for example, that are perceived to be outside the individual's control, to be global (i.e., affecting many aspects of a person's life), and to be enduring (not likely to change), are viewed as more threatening and are more likely to produce high levels of stress. Consider, for example, a patient who has been told he or she will never walk again. This realization is likely to create, at least initially, a state of extreme distress. Never being able to walk again will affect many aspects of this individual's life.

The ability to ambulate or move about is now outside this patient's control and the problem will endure. Because the patient's condition is perceived as enduring, uncontrollable, and global, the patient is at risk for high-level stress. The anxiety, fear, and depression that results reflect the patient's level of crisis. Usually, individuals are able to nullify the effects of crisis, at least over time. Three to six months after the stressful event is considered a benchmark separating those who have learned to adapt and those who have not. In truth, many deviations from this range and sometimes only partial adaptation can be observed where one or more areas of personal and interpersonal functioning are affected. For example, in the case of grieving, the actual relief from distress can occur much later than a year from the event and can return several years later.

▶ Types of Crisis

As previously stated, **crisis** has been defined in several ways. The essential element in all definitions is the idea that individuals are overwhelmed. The reasons they feel overwhelmed are a function of the event they face. In the literature on crisis, types of crises have been identified and include: (1) developmental crises and (2) situational crises. In psychological literature, a third type is addressed: existential crises.

Existential crisis refers to the point in life where one is reviewing and questioning their purpose in life: its meaning, purpose, and value. Middle-aged and older adults might experience an existential crisis resulting in dread and even depression. All types of crises cause stress, and the level of stress and strain experienced is variable. The primary role of health providers is a supportive function but also includes identifying the severity of stress and modifying the response to stress as needed. It is important to understand these types of crises since providers' support to patients may vary depending upon their type.

Developmental Crisis

Developmental crisis happens as a result of normal developmental changes (e.g., school age, marriage, graduation) (MacDonald, 2016). Basic individual development requires that we pass successfully through certain psychosocial task developments which correspond to our physical potential. Erikson's (1963) 6–8 stages of psychosocial development include: (1) trust versus mistrust, (2) autonomy versus shame and doubt, (3) initiative versus guilt, (4) industry versus inferiority, (5) identity versus role confusion, (6) intimacy and solidarity vs. Isolation, (7) generativity vs. self-absorption or stagnation, and (8) integrity vs. despair. The idea is that everyone passes through these stages during their lifetime with each stage building on the successful completion of earlier stages. Developmental tasks were addressed in a previous chapter highlighting Erik Erikson's theory of psychosocial development and the foundation for trust building capacities.

If mastery of these stages is not achieved, problems can occur. If the passage from one stage to the next is problematic the challenges of these stages are expected to reappear in future experiences. For example, a simplistic view of this idea is that if early development of trust fails, problems of mistrust are likely to recur in the future. In the context of health provider–patient relationships, this could result in patients' mistrusting the goodwill of providers caring for them.

To understand developmental tasks as crisis points, one must first accept the idea that

each developmental task has a potential for crisis. Erikson described the crisis as failure to master negotiating biological and sociocultural forces; each stage poses different challenges. For example, if infants (0–2 years old) pass through the stage of trust versus mistrust but the outcome is more mistrust versus trust, a future crisis may occur. Theorists did not adequately explain this phenomenon but the idea is that mastery of these stages is not automatic or a given. Just how successful one is in mastering these tasks depend not only on one's physical and mental capabilities but the nature of psychosocial environment at the time. If a satisfactory outcome is not achieved, one is set up for future problems because, in passing through developmental stages, previous mastery affects future abilities to adapt. Criticisms of this theory include questions of whether stages only occur within the age ranges suggested.

Situational Crisis

A situational crisis is most frequently mentioned by patients when being asked questions about how they are. Patients who are asked these questions can often identify situations that have impacted them in either negative or positive ways. These situations could include a new job, a lost job, a motor vehicle accident, a fall, or extreme weather conditions. These crises may also include any assaults (e.g., physical or emotional abuse). These examples are not readily raised in the first few minutes of greeting the patient. Natural disasters (e.g., floods, fires, earthquakes, and hurricanes) are situational crises affecting not one, but many persons as in an entire family.

Developmental and situational crises have similarities. They both challenge patients and are often experienced as overwhelming. Stories of patients usually describe precipitating events, initial responses, attempts to cope, and perceptions of unmet challenges. Those that are extreme require change beyond patients' capability, are temporary or more prolonged and result in a disturbance of patient equilibrium, are of concern to providers. Just how well patients are coping and whether they are able to function should be the first thing on providers' minds. Based upon how severe the crisis, a planned team approach to help the patient will be needed; and this would include a multidisciplinary approach with medical and psychosocial professionals and even spiritual or religious support services.

Phases of Crisis Resolution

The initial and most obvious sign that a patient presents in acute crisis is **anxiety**. This anxiety can be accompanied by physical signs of distress: restlessness, fidgeting, muscle tension, trembling, sweating, dizziness, headaches, and racing heart palpitations. Sometimes this anxiety is reflective of a more severe state of disorganization. Patients may fear that they are having a heart attack or going crazy. Anxiety can also be accompanied by some level of physical exhaustion due to sleep deprivation. The thoughts, fears, and concerns of someone with a high level of anxiety are not repressed, however. Patients are hypervigilant and seek optimum awareness to ward off any perceived or actual threats.

Some clinicians view the course of response to crisis in a hierarchical manner whereby acute anxiety leads to withdrawal or other deviations in behavior that place the patient in danger. Responses to crisis (e.g., exhaustion, sleep deprivation, and possibly nutritional disturbances) when uninterrupted signify a decline in individuals' abilities to protect and care for themselves. A variety of protective and injury-preventive interventions are needed to safeguard patients, their families, and others around them. At this stage, responses to crisis may have escalated to the level that patients are a clear threat to themselves (e.g., refuses to eat, active to exhaustion, or prone to injury). Some patients may be a threat to others through physical assault. The escalation process of crisis is complex. It usually includes a precrisis state and also a precipitating event.

While past experiences of patients may sensitize them to the situational stimuli, there is always a trigger that is found in the immediate situation.

Acute anxiety attacks are not uncommon outcomes with a crisis. Patients who have been assaulted may not be able to tolerate the amount or magnitude of the stimuli. Initial hypervigilance is exhausting and can further lower individuals' tolerance and a state of disorganization may occur. Studies of persons who have experienced natural catastrophic events (e.g., bombing, floods, and earthquakes) have provided a great deal of information about human responses to crisis. With high-level anxiety, people may become silent and tense. They may begin to sweat, feel weak, feel tightness in the chest, and hyperventilate. They may also feel like they are losing bowel or bladder control. If they perceive danger to be imminent, they may shake or tremble, become pale, repeat themselves over and over again, or fail to put the most elementary messages into words.

The physical paralysis that is first observed may quickly change to a state of excitation or defensive striking out. The urge to do something—the fright, fight, and flight response—can overpower them; they may run, release their temper on objects around them, or attack others. First responders in instances of natural catastrophic situations will see similarity but also differences in how crowds behave. Witnesses may respond in more- or less-helpful ways depending upon their judgments about whether the event was caused by those who are suffering; people are more likely to help innocent victims than those who are blamed for the crisis (Zagefka, Noor, Brown, De Moura, & Hopthrow, 2011).

The goals of treating persons in crisis are largely protective: shelter patients from associated consequences of a disaster, evaluate patients in an atmosphere that is supportive and empathetic, and treat both physical and emotional signs of trauma. The long-range goal is to return patients as quickly as possible to the precrisis state and preferably to a much higher level of functioning in order for them to deal with any after-effects of the crisis.

With preventive measures during the crisis experience, restoration can usually occur without severe levels of disorganization. However, when the crisis experience is prolonged and adequate intervention is not available, patients' perception of imminent threat is also prolonged and can result in a more severe state of disorganization. Full recovery is still possible but the recovery process may take longer.

▶ Managing Crisis Behaviors

Early intervention in crisis situations has been effective in not only reducing the disorganization that individuals experience but also in fortifying individuals' abilities to cope effectively with the residual aspects of the initial crisis or subsequent crises. It is now known that crisis intervention programs lead to both short-term and long-term positive outcomes: reduce fears and distress, help solve problems, coach them to avoid maladaptive coping including self-harm strengthen, and strengthen their problem-solving skills.

Clarify the patient's problems and needs: An important pervasive idea in counseling patients in crisis is that they will inevitably draw from the strength of the provider. Connecting emotionally with patients in crisis will enable providers to better assess their problems and needs. It can help providers identify patients' potential subsequent reactions and encourage patients to take direction. In some cases, this is direction that may save the patient's life. Providers' own organization and problem-solving approaches in the presence of patients' disorganization may restore patients' ability to trust their ability to overcome their current trauma.

Foster supportive interpersonal encounters: Supportive interpersonal encounters can occur between patients and friends and family but most importantly with health providers and the health provider team. A supportive relationship with the provider during crisis has been likened to a symbiotic relationship that increases dependency on the stronger, reliable problem solver. Many times, this initial dependency is necessary. The ability to connect in this way may help the patient repress or suppress the disconcerting or traumatizing perceptions and thoughts brought on by the crisis. Additionally, the partnership that the provider establishes with the patient tends to minimize perceptions of an impending threat. The patient now has someone else who knows about the trauma and the threatening aspects of the crisis and is professionally trained to help the patient. In short, patients feel like they have a capable ally. While the patient's fear may remain, generally, the experience of acute anxiety and alarm subsides.

Patients do, however, also register the level of alarm that providers experience. When they see that the providers are not particularly threatened by the event, feelings of panic may lessen. At this point, fright, fight, and flight tendencies can also be relaxed. Once patients have spent time with the provider, under the protective wing of professional involvement, they are able to begin to compare actual occurrences with anticipated feared occurrences. It is the provider's role to activate and encourage this comparison.

Encourage patients to seek additional support: When patients seem to be recovering strength it is important to support their use of additional persons in their social network. Inevitably, when patients complete their initial care they will be discharged and patient experience a void in the process of working through their crisis. Not all persons in patients' networks would be appropriate. It is advisable to explore with patients the one or two persons that they could turn to for support and understanding. In many cases, referrals to psychological supportive therapy and crisis management specialists in health care fields are important. Groups whose membership characteristics are similar to those of the patient can be helpful but judgment is needed in determining whether the patient will feel comfortable, especially when disclosing details of their crisis in a group setting.

Refer patients to therapists that can address and monitor coping mechanisms: An important, pervasive idea in counseling patients in crisis is that they will inevitably draw from the strength of the provider or other professional counselors. Connecting emotionally with patients in crisis will enable the provider to better predict patients' subsequent reactions and encourage patients to take directions that, in many cases, may save the patient's life. When initial providers cannot offer the amount of ongoing counseling a patient and their family require it is important to turn to other resources for patients. For example, mental health professionals can support and monitor patients in their choice of effective coping strategies. In the context of these kinds of sessions, providers can also monitor for inappropriate beliefs or thoughts surrounding their crisis event and their recovery.

In order to fully understand the connection between stress and coping it is helpful to refer to classic theories about the process. Crisis, in this text, is regarded as a variant of stress that is so severe that it leads an individual or group to a state of disorganization in which one's ability to function is significantly affected. All providers need to be aware of how various levels of stress can impact individuals. Stress makes demands on individuals that are physiological, social, and psychological, and these occur singularly or in combination. It should be noted that stress and anxiety are similar. They are driven by the same biochemical reactions and are both normal responses when faced with threatening situations. But there are differences. Stress is a response to a perceived threat (whether actual or imagined). Anxiety is a reaction to the stress one experiences.

In the mid-1950s, Hans Selye, a Hungarian endocrinologist, described his understanding of the stress response based on physiology and psychobiology. His theory explaining the general adaptation syndrome (GAS) included three stages of response: alarm, resistance, and exhaustion (Selye, 1976). In this model, the various stages of the stress response are paralleled with a corresponding level and type of disorganization. For example, the initial stage of alarm can be met with mobilization of adaptive behaviors which help individuals cope with stress they experience. Increased awareness of a potential threat could result in taking steps to prepare for or avoid these threats. However, when stress is very high, rather than facilitating preparing for or avoiding stressors, individuals experience exhaustion of adaptive capacities leaving them more vulnerable to these stressors. A paradigm for viewing the elements of stress and coping is provided in **FIGURE 17-1**.

General guidelines are useful in helping with patients regardless of the type of crisis. These interventions can also be practiced by crisis workers who are not professional providers. Several basic principles are summarized in the following list of guidelines:

1. Crisis victims should not be revictimized in the process of being helped.
2. An emotional or psychological connection with the patient is critical.
3. Crises are responses to real or imagined threats—the validity of the crisis stimuli should not be challenged or underestimated in judging its potential to lead to disorganization in the individuals.
4. Crisis is not merely a single event. The residual effects of crisis can continue indefinitely.

Providers must remember that patients in crisis exhibit a number of disturbances in perception, processing, and expression.

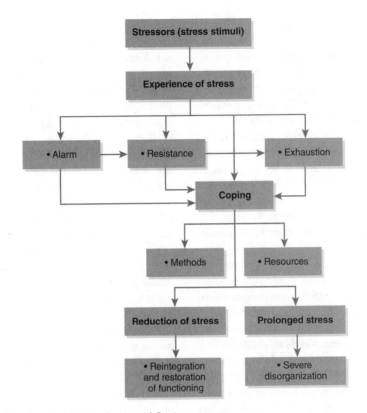

FIGURE 17-1 A Paradigm for Viewing Stress and Coping.

Therapeutic response modes as those described in Part III of this text are obviously important when communicating with people in crisis.

First, and foremost, however, providers must practice good active-listening skills. They must listen for the content in patients' messages as well as for the affective states the patient is experiencing. What does the patient say happened? What is the patient afraid of? What does the patient anticipate? What feelings are associated with what the patient says (e.g., fear, pain, generalized anxiety, depression, anger, rage)?

Second, a direct, straightforward attempt to elicit information about the situation causing the trauma is important. Rather than exploring past events, the focus needs to be on the immediate present. Due to patients' deficits in processing information they will probably respond well to directives or commands. Explorations of why, including rationale and motives, are irrelevant and can even be injurious if communicated without compassion. The provider needs to realize that this beginning exploration helps patients begin to master their experience by organizing thoughts and feelings.

Sometimes patients and/or families will express attitudes, feelings, or thoughts that are difficult for providers to accept. These ideas or observations may conflict with their personal or professional values and standards. One family's statement that their son "deserved" to be injured—he was headed for trouble... it was just a matter of time" may be difficult for providers to hear. Their immediate response may be to challenge, judge, or even criticize the family for such remarks. It should be remembered that these remarks by family members are taken out of context and rarely are families exceedingly harsh. Family members are attempting to deal with the traumatic event. To argue with a parent at this point would deny the context of the parent's experience and their own personal trauma.

Because patients in crisis are not focused or are not always clear in their verbalizations, they need to know that they are being heard and understood. Validating their experience, the pain and distress they must have, and expressing understanding about the impact of the event is extremely important in communicating compassion.

In every instance, for the patient and family in crisis, the provider needs to connect emotionally. However, connecting emotionally does not mean becoming overinvolved to the point that providers lose their professional objectivity. The reader needs to recall the differences between sympathy and the therapeutic response mode, empathy. Avoiding feeling too much but at the same time clearly communicating support and caring with an understanding of the impact of the trauma is critical in managing the patient through the crisis experience and immediately thereafter.

Communicating with Agitated and/or Confused Patients

A separate but important issue related to communicating adequately with people in acute crisis states is the appropriate responses to use when patients are agitated and confused. These disturbances can range from simple intellectual impairment to loss of conscious awareness. *Agitation and confusion* commonly occur with patients in crisis. This condition includes disturbances in orientation as well as intellectual impairment. In rare cases, delirium, a state of confusion significantly more serious, can occur and is usually accompanied by a severe state of restlessness.

There are several causes of lapses in consciousness. Brain disease, cerebral vascular accidents, brain injuries, alcohol and drug abuse, brain tumors or lesions, infectious diseases, toxins, and metabolic disturbances all contribute to altered consciousness. These conditions may be temporary and reversible or they may reflect progressive and irreversible disturbances. In addition to discovering the medical causes the depth of disturbance must be assessed because this will influence not only the patient's ability to cooperate and communicate but will also affect the level of appropriate response from the provider.

At one end of the continuum is simple reversible cognitive impairment. This condition may consist of minor disturbances in memory and poor judgment but orientation and reality remains intact and hallucinations and delusions are absent. When intellectual impairment is coupled with personality changes the condition is regarded as more severe. Ideas of reference, mood swings, and even delusions may be present. In these instances, providers must compensate for minor cognitive impairment and provide frequent reality checks for the patient.

Fluctuating levels of consciousness can be seen in patients under severe anxiety. However, rarely will providers see patients in stupor states. Although these states are rare, they can occur and providers must always be alert for the possibility because patients in prolonged states of fear and anxiety who have become significantly confused sometimes present with stupor. Examples include emergency situations in which patients wander aimlessly, sometimes in mute states, bordering on drowsiness or potential lapse in consciousness. Paramedics and frequently law enforcement officers can encounter these patients and would most often take them to emergency rooms for further evaluation. These special circumstances will alter considerably what communication occurs between patients and providers.

▶ Summary

In summary, prolonged and severe stress and crisis are becoming so predominant in our society that everywhere one turns these events and their impact can be witnessed. Stress, and even crisis, is inevitable in our society, and social changes and problems can create new events or fear of impending crisis. With this recognition, there should be no reason to question the wisdom of teaching stress resistance and coping with crisis in our major institutions—schools, churches, and health and welfare programs. In contemporary society, although there are many sources of stress that predispose people to ill health, institutions pay relatively little attention to teaching crisis–stress coping skills.

Crisis theory suggests that crises are one of two types: situational (external) or developmental (maturational). Situational crises, including being party to a natural disaster, are usually highly unpredictable, affect many aspects of peoples' lives, and often affect more than one person at a time. Developmental crises, on the other-hand, are usually predictable because they have a basis in the demands placed on individuals as they pass through sequential stages of growth and development. Erikson explained their role in psychosocial development and suggested that how well one masters these stages will influence how one responds to developmental changes down the line.

Patients arrive in settings with some degree of mastering developmental crises but have also encountered one or more situational crises. They may not always present in full-blown crisis but often have both physiological and behavioral signs and symptoms of stress from crisis. They may be acutely distressed, very worried, or experiencing chronic stressors. Providers help patients and their families weather many situations and life transitions. Just how effective providers are influences the strength of their patients to adapt to crisis situations. It will also affect their ability to help patients deal with crisis residuals and any future crisis or stressful life events they will encounter.

Individual differences in response to stress have long been recognized. More recent research suggests that individual variability in response to stress is affected by many factors such as patients' cultural and religious beliefs, their attitudes and perceptions of the stressors, perceptions of risk and danger due to these stressors, and their perceived self-efficacy. Ongoing life strains and daily hassles are now being recognized for their potential to be disruptive.

Previously, the burden of proof rested with how many stressful life events patients and/or their families have experienced within a particular time span. Now it is understood that any change, large or small, can contribute to patients' response burden. Providers' communications should be supportive but will vary, depending on patients' responses to stressful life events and whether a crisis is either medical, situational, or developmental. Empathy, assessment of the severity of the crisis response, ensuring patient safety, stabilizing patients' emotional responses, drawing on patients' cognitive strengths, and following up on crisis situations with post-crisis assessment are all important facets of the role of health providers.

Discussion

1. Discuss how crisis impacts patients and families seeking health care.
2. Describe the process of emotional contagion.
3. Discuss the difference between maturational and environmental stress.
4. Discuss and give examples of principles applying to communicating effectively with patients and families in crisis.
5. Identify interventions to manage and communicate with highly anxious patients.

References

Erikson, E. H. (1963). *Childhood and society.* New York, NY: Norton, Inc.

Hatfield, E., Bensman, L., Thornton, P. D., & Rapson, R. L. (2014). New perspectives on emotional contagion: A review of classic and recent research on facial mimicry and contagion. *International Journal on Personal Relationships, 8*(2), 159–179. doi:10.5964/ijpr.v8i2.162

Holmes, T. H., & Rahe, R. H. (1967). The social readjustment rating scale. *Journal of Psychosomatic Research, 11*(2), 213–218. PMID 6059863

Kavan, M. G., Guck, T. P., & Barone, E. J. (2006). A practical guide to crisis management. *American Family Physician, 74*(7), 1159–1164. PMID:17039753

Lazarus, R., &. Folkman, S. (1984). *Stress, appraisal and coping.* New York, NY: Springer Publishing.

MacDonald, D. K. (2016), *Crisis theory and types of crisis.* Retrieved from http://dustinkmacdonald.com/crisis-theory-types-crisis/

Rice, V. H. (2012). *Handbook of stress, coping, and health: Implications for nursing research.* Thousand Oaks, CA: Sage Publications Inc.

Selye, H. (1976). *The stress of life.* New York, NY: McGraw-Hill.

Smith, M. C. (1984). The client who is anxious. In S. Lego (Ed.), *The American handbook of psychiatric nursing* (p. 389). Philadelphia, PA: J. B. Lippincott Company.

Zagefka, H., Noor, M., Brown, R., de Moura, G. R., & Hopthrow, T. (2011). Donating to disaster victims: Responses to natural and humanly caused events. *European Journal of Social Psychology, 41*(3), 353–363. doi:10.1002/ejsp.781

CHAPTER 18

Communicating Effectively with Patients Displaying Significant Negative or Resistive Coping Responses

CHAPTER OBJECTIVES

- Describe how health care provider and patient encounters can be impacted in many ways (e.g., difficult patients, difficult tasks, and difficult care contexts).
- Discuss types of difficult patient behaviors and the underlying meaning of their communications.
- Discuss ways in which providers can assess difficult patient behaviors, apply specific management guidelines, and monitor patient responses.
- Analyze several types of patient encounters that would be difficult and identify corresponding therapeutic communication responses.
- Discuss the statement: Patients are looking for help with a medical problem and providers are motivated to help them.

KEY TERMS

- Complaining and demanding patient behaviors
- Manipulative-dependent patient behaviors
- Nonadherent patient behaviors
- Difficult patient behaviors

▶ Introduction

What is expected to be routine in health care encounters between patients and providers is not routine. Providers in all disciplines and across the full health care delivery system are confronted with difficult patient and family member behaviors. This observation runs counter to the notion that these encounters are always positive and rewarding: patients and families are looking for help with a medical problem, and providers are motivated to help them (Chepenik, 2015). However, there are instances in which this arrangement does *not* work as well as we might expect. There are conflicts, disagreements, and difficult interactions.

It has been estimated that at least 50% of the provider's time with patients is spent in communicating. These verbal encounters include taking a history, teaching, answering questions, counseling, ensuring compliance, and achieving satisfaction with care. Health providers engage patients in discussions on a variety of subjects that are organized around major categories of dialogue but there are other times when contacts are less structured. In truth, the provider is heavily influenced by patients' presenting their health condition and any psychosocial stresses surrounding their condition.

Every provider will come in contact with difficult encounters—either with patients or their family members. Patterns of health care provider dialogue with patients vary and thus there are differences in what providers will accept, how much irrelevant information they will permit, and how they will respond to patients they regard as "difficult."

The prevalence of difficult patient encounters in health care settings today is unknown but Hinchey and Jackson (2011) and Hull and Broquet (2007) estimated that up to 15% of clinical encounters are experienced as difficult by clinicians. Still others have predicted a percent as high as 30% (Hahn, 2001). "Staying grounded" in these exchanges depends a great deal on providers' understanding of not only behavioral and social science analyses but also their ability to observe and monitor their own responses in these exchanges. As stressed by the Institute of Medicine's (2004) report, *Improving Medical Education: Enhancing the Behavioral and Social Science Content of Medical School Curriculum*, it is through this knowledge that providers will be able to strengthen their therapeutic alliance with patients and increase the likelihood that patients will follow their advice.

▶ The Impact of Difficult Patient Encounters on Quality Care Outcomes

Difficult encounters with patients and families have been studied along with their impact on quality care and provider job stress. An et al. (2013) measured the link among difficult patients, health provider burnout, medical errors, and quality care in primary care settings. Difficult encounters in primary care were defined as medical practices with higher rates of underinsured, minority, and non-English-speaking patients.

The study showed that physicians with higher frequencies of difficult encounters had higher rates of dissatisfaction and burnout. However, there were no significant associations between rates of difficult encounters and either quality of patient care or errors in care management. The researchers explained that more studies were needed and that patient satisfaction should be examined for its link to difficult patient–physician encounters. Additionally, the length of exposure to any one difficult encounter and specific patient–provider interactions need further study.

In a study by Hinchey and Jackson (2011), difficult patient encounters in a walk-in primary care clinic were examined. According to this study, "difficult" patients were less likely to fully trust or be fully satisfied with their clinician and were more likely to have worsening of symptoms at 2 weeks. Patients involved in "difficult encounters" had more than five symptoms, reported having recent stress, and had depression or anxiety. Physicians involved in difficult encounters were less experienced (years of practice) and were less psychosocially oriented. These researchers concluded that direct observations of patient and provider behaviors during difficult encounters were needed.

While the chances for difficult encounters to be resolved are unknown, it is thought that most of what is deemed "difficult" will, at least in part, be resolved. In situations with "difficult patients," some aspect of the patient's physical or mental health, personality conflicts and control struggles, or a critical transition in care may be influencing encounters with health care providers. Krebs, Garrett, and Konrad (2006) explain that providers differ in their judgments of patient behaviors. In fact, there is a great deal of variability in the percentage of primary care patients perceived to be frustrating. These researchers found that highly frustrated physicians were younger, more likely to practice subspecialty internal medicine, and more likely to have high stress. Other researchers have found that providers who are less experienced and less psychosocially oriented are more likely to have difficult encounters. This may be that less-experienced providers do not have sufficient insight and ability to be receptive and compassionate.

Lorenzetti, Jacques, Donovan, Cottrell, and Buck (2013) explain that difficult provider–patient encounters may be attributable to multiple factors; those associated with the physician, patient, situation, or a combination. Common physician factors include negative bias toward specific health conditions but also poor communication skills, and situational stressors in the workplace. They explain that patient factors may include personality disorders, multiple and poorly defined symptoms, nonadherence to medical advice, and self-destructive behaviors. Situational factors include time pressures during visits, patient and staff conflicts, or complex social issues (Lorenzetti et al., p. 419). Stacey, Henderson, MacArthur, and Dohan (2009) emphasized the need to shift the focus away from the demanding patients to demanding encounters. They claimed that this shift promotes the idea that patient-provider conflict occurs in a broader sociocultural context where both patient and provider are experiencing constraints in clinical settings. Frequently, systems of care delivery will affect both the origin and resolution of encounter difficulties. Because these situations are frequently anxiety ridden for patients and providers, and even patient families, they are worthy of in-depth focus.

▶ Difficult Patients, Tasks, and Care Contexts

The first and most important principle in an analysis of difficult patient encounters is that these difficult encounters are a function of many factors including patients' health status, patient stress and anxiety, providers' responses, and any contextual situations that put pressure on both providers and patients and their families. In using this definition of difficult patient encounters, it can be argued that all encounters

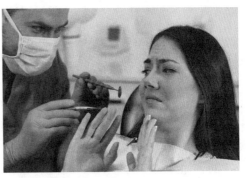

© Antonio Guillem/Shutterstock.

add significantly to the challenges providers face on a day-to-day basis.

When the label of difficult patient is used by providers, it can mean many different things. Most often it is a term used for patients whose behaviors evoke distress in the provider that exceeds what is either expected or accepted.

As previously suggested, the term *difficult patient* should be expanded to consider difficult tasks and difficult care contexts. For example, some instances of difficult patient encounters should be viewed in the context of the relationship (difficulties in the patient–provider interactions) while others should be viewed as difficult encounters due to their tasks and context of care (e.g., advance care planning in a crowded waiting room that does not offer sufficient patient and family privacy). The following scenario illustrates that provider encounters can be front-loaded to set up difficult encounters with patients.

Example: Front Loaded Patient–Provider Encounter

Before providers begin their day, they generally review a list of patients they will see. In this case, as the provider reviews the charts of these patients, certain descriptions draw attention. One patient is described as "disagreeable," one is getting end-of-life care, two want to change to another medication, one wants to be discharged early, and another patient is not getting better despite several changes and improvements in care management. The unit clerk gives this provider a message from a disgruntled family member and the charge nurse reminds the provider that the quality improvement meeting is in 5 minutes and the provider will have to chair the meeting this month.

Many providers might comment that this is a pretty typical workday. They usually do face a number of challenges. These situations set the stage for interpersonal and communication challenges to follow. The purpose of this

chapter is not to discuss the average day-to-day occurrences. Rather, the aim is to describe and discuss more-challenging encounters, those that can potentially affect care outcomes and provider stress. The examples in this chapter include clusters of behaviors shown to be difficult to handle.

In this chapter, a substantial proportion of the discussion focuses on how certain so-called difficult behaviors may be appropriately addressed. Sufficient discussion of the underlying meaning of difficult behaviors is provided so that the rationale behind recommended responses is clear. Some of these behaviors are less often experienced by providers (e.g., aggressive and condescending behaviors). Still others (e.g., **manipulative-dependent** or **complaining and demanding patient behaviors**) are more common but still difficult. In this chapter, the concept of the "difficult" patient is differentiated from difficult care context and difficult tasks.

For example, one difficult context is discussing end-of-life care with patients and their families. This is difficult because the process is usually stressful and uncomfortable for all involved. It is also difficult when providers lack an understanding of the cultural and religious beliefs that impact patient and family responses to these tasks. Generally, feelings of sadness and loss are expected but there may also be fear and anxiety. Any mixture of these responses can be difficult. Sometimes tasks are very difficult. Such is the case, for example, of a young burn patient who cries and screams during the debridement of dead tissue. The patient's behavior may be difficult; however, the task of witnessing the debridement of the wound may be equally or more distressful to the provider.

At other times, the context or task does not arouse uncomfortable feelings but the patient's behavior does. This would be the case if the provider encountered a patient who had come for an appointment or to get a prescription and complained profusely about the service received. Otherwise, the context of the encounter (a follow-up appointment believed to be uneventful) is not worrisome but the patient's communications and behaviors are. Complaining and dissatisfied patients are often seen as uncooperative and noncompliant even though their behavior may be motivated by fear and insecurity. Some patients and/or families present in ways that irritate or cause providers to be defensive. This does happen and seldom are providers fully prepared for this to occur, something that can aggravate them further.

Good communication with all patients and families—regardless of whether they are difficult or not—is important. Increasingly, the patient or family consumer is being heard and heeded, and providers will have to learn how to communicate more successfully with a broader range of patient behaviors, particularly those that elicit uncomfortable and irritating thoughts and feelings. The discussion that follows addresses five difficult patient behavior types: (1) nonadherent, (2) manipulative-dependent, (3) aggressive, (4) complaining and demanding, and (5) patient in denial. Along with a discussion of these behaviors, the underlying meaning of the behavior and selected therapeutic responses are addressed. Further attention is given to patients who are anxious and/or depressed.

▶ Types of Difficult Behaviors and Their Underlying Meanings

The following discussions cover a range of **difficult patient behaviors**. Some of them will be encountered infrequently, others happen regularly. Patients are labeled difficult usually because they evoke anger, frustration, anxiety, or similar uncomfortable reactions (Dudzinski & Timberlake, 2014). This being said, it is important to realize that labels can be assigned without examination of what the

patient is really saying or trying to achieve. Labels can apply to a wide range of patients and their behaviors. However, labeling patient behaviors is rarely useful and helpful to improving communications.

Providers' concerns about patients who are labeled in some way "difficult" usually reflect some fear that these patients will transgress a professional or personal boundary. They may lack the skill and wisdom to feel empathy and worry that they might react in anger. It is critical that providers recognize these patient behaviors and explore their underlying meaning to communicate more effectively.

Nonadherent Patient Behaviors and Communication Barriers

Adequate adherence to treatment regimens has been proven to be effective in a wide range of patient clinical conditions and populations. Adequate adherence to medications, one aspect of adherence to treatment, has been proven to be both efficacious; yet suboptimal adherence is highly prevalent across all clinical conditions and populations (Osterberg & Blaschke, 2005). In fact, Marcum, Sevick, and Handler (2013) labeled medical nonadherence as a diagnosable and treatable medical condition in and of itself.

If there was a vote tomorrow about what kind of patient elicits the most distress in providers, many would answer "patients who

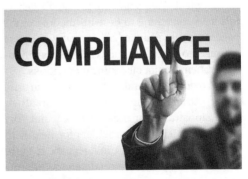

© Gustavo Frazao/Shutterstock.

don't follow their treatment program the way you instructed them to" (i.e., the patient that is nonadherent). In fact, one of the most challenging aspects of provider–patient relationships is learning how to deal with patients' **nonadherent patient behaviors** to treatment.

Patients can passively or actively refuse to follow health provider recommendations. This phenomenon can be observed across the board with all disciplines (medicine, nursing, physical therapy, pharmacy, dentistry, etc.). This is also true of patients refusing medication use or not taking their medications correctly. In medicine and nursing, patients' answers to why they did not follow instructions might be that they did not think it (medication) would work, did not have the time (too many competing demands), or did not have money to pay for the medications.

In the field of dentistry, it is patients who fail to comply with oral hygiene instructions, and in the field of pharmacy, it may be patients who do not read cautionary statements on prescription labels, do not ask questions, and proceed to combine drugs that may have serious interactive effects. (Drug interaction effects can make another medication less effective, causes unexpected and dangerous side effects, or even increase the action potential of other drugs patients are taking.)

It is mandatory that providers assess for lack of understanding, identify reasons for lack of adherence, and establish a plan to improve patients' comprehension of their condition and its treatment. Frequently, these patient behaviors have something to do with the role of the patient's family. Families' beliefs and subsequent messages to patients are powerful and can influence patients to not take some medications.

Providers generally react with surprise and frustration when patients ignore their professional recommendations. Is it not true that patients come to providers for help with a medical problem and providers are there to help them? By being nonadherent, patients break the implicit agreement and can cause providers to feel disconfirmed. Additionally, providers might feel that they know little about what the patient is really doing. Providers face a twofold blowback or setback that places the patient at risk as well as devalues the expertise of the provider. Much would be understood if providers inquired about the patient's beliefs and concerns and those of their family.

At a personal level, these patient behaviors can trigger more deep-seated issues for providers and this can cause them to make additional mistakes (e.g., unleashing their frustration on the patient, inducing guilt, withdrawing or moralizing, and preaching to the patient). Recognizing that these are less than desired responses, providers can experience even more frustration because they said the wrong thing. Breaking down barriers to treatment including dealing effectively with patient resistance is as germane as establishing a medication dose and schedule that will successfully treat infection. Nonetheless, providers are not always prepared to deal with patients who are, themselves, barriers to better care.

There are many reasons for nonadherence and a list is provided in **EXHIBIT 18-1**. They can be grouped in categories: patient, treatment and disease, and patient–provider relationship, and system barriers. At the patient level, beliefs, lack of knowledge and understanding, and language barriers are frequently affecting patients' inability to follow recommendations. Patients may not fully understand a medical order or they may not fully comprehend the consequences of refusing to follow the order. Pharmacists elicit from patients their signature when they pick up medications; otherwise, in writing is whether the patient receives or refuses consultation about their prescription drugs. These signatures attest to the fact that the patient received or refused to receive counseling. Why should such detail be documented? Obviously, these providers want some record, if things go wrong, that instruction either took place or was refused. Providers need to assess both the level of adherence and the reasons for the lack of adherence.

EXHIBIT 18-1 Assessment of Reasons for Nonadherent Patient Behaviors

Patient-Level Barriers: Characteristics of Any Patient Population Can Impact Adherence

- Patient and family beliefs and perceptions of treatment (e.g., being unconvinced of the need for treatment).
- Cultural and religious beliefs surrounding disease and treatment (i.e., patients' fate is in the hands of God, not medicine).
- Language barriers that affect patients' understanding and acceptance of medical approaches.
- Perceptions that interventions are too costly in terms of both time and/or resources.
- Low literacy and inherent cognitive deficits that impair abilities to manage their illness.

Treatment and Disease-Level Barriers: Certain Aspects of Disease and Treatment Can Lead to Patient Nonadherence Behaviors

- Serious side effects of treatment/medication use causing patients to resist treatment.
- Complicated and burdensome medication regimens resulting in patients tiring of treatment.
- Functional deficits related to disease causing them to have impaired self-care capabilities.

Patient–Provider Relationship and System Barriers: The Quality of the Patient–Provider Relationship and Barriers Created by the Delivery System Can Cause Nonadherence

- Lack of trust and satisfaction in the patient–provider relationship.
- Lack of satisfaction with the way patient care is being organized and delivered (including providers not having enough time to spend with patients and their families).
- Poor continuity of care exacerbating the problem of forming an effective therapeutic alliance and necessary follow-up.

In addition to not fully understanding health care recommendations, patients and/or their families may fear or mistrust the provider and the treatment. If they fear it, for whatever reason, they are more likely to question or challenge the provider's advice. Still another cause for nonadherence is a unique pattern of reasoning that results in patients judging the steps to be unreasonable, impractical, too costly, or in competition with another important need or goal. Time and time again the literature documents that patients may not address these issues with providers because of not wanting to bother their provider, risk provider disapproval, or just take up the time of the busy provider.

Recent research in persuading people to practice safe sex, stop smoking, or adopt healthy behaviors indicate that if the behavior changes result in the loss of a perceived positive experience (in the case of sex, loss of enjoyment; in the case of smoking, relaxation; and in the case of drugs, an altered emotional state), the behavior is not likely to be adopted. This is true even if the risk of continuing the risky behavior is known. Risky behaviors have also been associated with group conformity—peers influence both substance abuse and risky sexual practices among adolescents and adults. Despite the fact that noncompliance or lack of adherence has been an issue since the advent of medicine and health care, providers frequently lack the skill to address this problem. The motivational interviewing and other similar approaches give providers structured programs to follow that seem to result in greater commitment on the part of patients to change risky behaviors.

Manipulative-Dependent Patient and/or Family Behaviors and Communication Barriers

The term manipulative-dependent patient evokes considerable trepidation in providers. Provider teams may use this term in pejorative ways to describe their frustration when working with these patients. Patients and/or families who are *manipulative* frequently display behaviors testing the interest of others, sometimes invoking guilt.

They may make communications more difficult when threatening providers with angry outbursts or even legal action. Manipulative patients are frequently viewed as "dependent" patients, inclined to get things the way they want which usually result in more attention or more care. Examples of manipulative patients can include: "I am so glad I have an appointment with you and not the one I had last time." "You believe me when I tell you none of my pain medications have ever worked." "Can you get me another blanket?" "Some water with ice?" "I'm kind of hungry, are there any snacks today?"

Some patients may appear as "frequent fliers," signs of which are the thickness of their medical or health record. These patients may be lonely or fearful. They may have perfectly rational questions or may engage providers just for the sake of getting attention. Some providers argue that with the exception of the noncompliant patient behaviors, manipulative-dependent patient behaviors are the most frustrating of all.

While these types of patients and/or families are frequently thought to be of certain genders and socioeconomic status the fact is that manipulative behaviors can be found in patients of all ages, genders, ethnicities, and socioeconomic classes. Unlike patients who

are exhibiting dependent behaviors consistent with their disease stage and level of impairment, patients with dependent personalities exhibit this behavior in routine situations and in most of their human interactions and personal relationships. What is occurring dynamically is that these patients attempt to establish control of the provider–patient relationship usually by playing the role of a helpless, powerless patient. Their weak and passive presentation usually suggests a lack of power.

The main goal of the patient and/or the family is to control, and they may be passive-aggressive in their attempts to execute control. It is clear that through their passive role they are exercising a great deal of control, and when the provider responds in a complimentary fashion to this helplessness, the patients have actually succeeded in getting the additional needed attention. In some cases, patients' families will confide in the provider that they deal with this behavior all the time and are frustrated by it. The patient's behavior is marked by the distinct conclusion that no intervention seems to work completely. The provider has two choices: (1) to admit defeat or (2) to keep trying to find ways to meet these patients' needs.

Manipulative-dependent patients often reinforce the authority–subordinate aspects of provider–patient relationships. Some providers liken this to a parent–child relationship. When providers recognize that they are caught

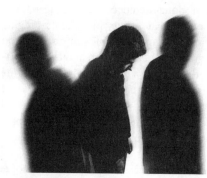

© Sjstudio6/Shutterstock.

in a parent–child relationship, they feel used and become angry. One reason for this is that these patients usually assume no real responsibility for maintaining their health and managing their illness. Patients who have negotiated this role with providers are often experts in their ploy. To behave in this manner with providers is almost second nature to them.

Providers who need patients to participate actively in their treatment (e.g., to follow nutritional guidelines, resume physical activity cautiously, or evaluate their own responses to medications) are understandably distressed by this type of patient. Characteristically, when something goes wrong these patients are likely to make it appear that it was due to some deficit in the delivery of care. Patients who abdicate their responsibility for their health and health care are typically more difficult for providers who value patient engagement and shared decision-making (**EXHIBIT 18-2**).

In keeping with the behavior of many dependent-manipulative patients, this patient asks the provider to go "beyond the call of duty," which comes as second nature to these patients who seem not to question the appropriateness of their request. While the physician seems to agree to her request, clearly, the physician agrees out of duress. The request is not appropriate, is something providers do not customarily do for patients, and puts the provider in an awkward position with the patient's employer.

Providers may anticipate a scenario where they are asked questions that they cannot rightfully answer. Manipulative-dependent patients frequently ask favors and demand more than other patients. They may threaten that they will leave if not granted their way. Although requesting that the physician call her employer is novel and it would seem that responding affirmatively would be okay (at least once), this is usually not the case. The fact that it is *novel* is a red flag that it might not be ethical. Frequently, this behavioral pattern is a learned response, reflecting former ways of coping with basic needs for attention, love, and affection.

Dependent patient behaviors in those who are suffering an acute or chronic illness present a particular challenge to providers. Continued reliance on medical care is needed; however, self-care and individual patient responsibility for symptom management is also essential. This case is complex because providers struggle with the "right" amount of dependence. Patients such as those with

---

EXHIBIT 18-2 Dialogue Presenting a Provider–Patient Encounter

Consider the following dialogue between a physician and a 56-year-old female who has been hospitalized in the early symptomatic phase of infectious hepatitis.

PROVIDER: "You know you're going to have to be on bedrest for some time until your clinical symptoms have subsided. You'll need to notify your work."

PATIENT: "Yes…doctor will you call them? I know they'll listen to you."

PROVIDER: "This is something you're going to have to do; if they want a letter—and you permit it—I'll write one."

PATIENT: "But what if they ask me questions I can't answer. Oh, my back hurts (grimacing, shifting positions)."

PROVIDER: "What could they ask?"

PATIENT: "I don't know…anything. Could you, please? It would be better if you called. I don't think I'm up to it, anyway."

PROVIDER: "I'm sorry, I don't have the time."

PATIENT: "Well, if I tell them to call you, then you don't have to call them. OK?"

PROVIDER: "All right." (Leaves the room somewhat frustrated by the conversation)

asthma, hypertension, arthritis, pulmonary disease, congestive heart failure, and many major mental illnesses require a high level of compliance to keep the disease under control.

Those patients with chronic, life-threatening diseases (e.g., advanced cancer and heart disease) are a subset of patients where medical treatment is critical to patients' quality of life and life span. Many times providers can feel that they are in a double bind where they want to avoid infantilizing patients but these patients on their own may not be able to follow even the simplest directions. Providers—nurses, physicians, pharmacists, and many paraprofessionals—are not equipped to take care of patients around the clock. Many patients, particularly the elderly and the socially disenfranchised, may not have family support or help from others. Under these conditions, the question of whether the patient's dependency on providers is appropriate is indeed difficult to answer.

Frequently, a critical deciding factor is whether the problem or need of the patient is judged to be authentic or fabricated. Some patients seek out providers because they need human contact and attention, not because they have legitimate medical issues. These patients have been known to fake complaints, call at unusual hours, or call frequently with "important" or "urgent" messages. These patients can react negatively to providers who are too busy to respond and become upset by providers who take holidays. They also tend to worship their providers and expect the same level of commitment in return. They act as if the provider has no other competing commitments but to care for them.

Providers need to recognize that passive-dependent behavior is sometimes indicative of patients with defined clinical syndromes. In the *Diagnostic Statistical Manual of Mental Disorders* (DSM-5, 2013) of the American Psychiatric Association Dependent Personality Disorder, pervasive passive-dependent behavior is diagnosed as a legitimate medical condition requiring

professional counseling. Persons who are considered to have dependent personalities will exhibit behaviors that show an excessive and pervasive need to be taken care of, submissive, clinging, and needy behavior due to fear of abandonment. These patients may have an unrealistic preoccupation with being left alone and unable to care for themselves and require others to assume responsibility for things that are their responsibility. A full list of distinguishing criteria for this diagnosis can be found in the DSM-5.

If providers have such patients, special precautions are necessary to avoid entanglements with the patient and/or family. Above all else, providers must be aware of their own feelings and reactions and try to understand why the patient is making demands which are unreasonable. Improvement in the patient's medical condition may be highly contingent upon the dynamics of patient–provider encounters. A cycle of ineffective contacts is worrisome. The provision of unending advice, opportunities for ventilation, "parental" guidance, and "free" counseling and education often fatigue the provider. The following steps are helpful in responding to these patients and advise providers about what to avoid (**EXHIBIT 18-3**).

Providers who are able to analyze their personal responses to dependent-manipulative patient behaviors and check nontherapeutic replies are more likely to succeed in managing these patients and families appropriately. Major feelings of tension, frustration, or anxiety are clues to the provider. These feelings may be followed by feelings of dread or resistance in seeing the patient again. Frequently, providers make derogatory remarks to other members of the team before, after, or even during an encounter with the patient. These discussions, while they help diffuse the tension that has accumulated, will not solve the problem.

Providers may view these situations as hopeless and consequently respond in a passive-aggressive manner. Their responses can include limiting the length or numbers of

---

EXHIBIT 18-3 Helpful Steps and Those to Avoid

Helpful Steps

1. Conduct a thorough assessment of the character and appropriateness of dependent behaviors.
2. Talk to other team members to gain insight and understanding of these behaviors.
3. Recognize and differentiate between inappropriate and appropriate dependency.
4. In some cases, it is appropriate to set limits on the demands and requests of the patient. It is important that the provider learn to say, in so many words, "no."
5. In assertive ways, providers need to establish the goals of treatment and communicate these clearly to the patient.

What to Avoid

- Socializing with the patient.
- Honoring special privileges.
- Accepting patients' exaggerations of their conditions and symptoms.
- Allowing the patient to bargain with providers for special treatment.
- Accepting flattery or positive reinforcement.
- Allowing the patient to manipulate time, frequency, and duration of contacts.

---

contacts or simply ignoring what the patient or family says or asks. Another response that is very common is for the provider to go along with the requests or demands thinking that the requests will not be that much trouble or will cease. Finally, the provider may overreact with hostility and passive or overt aggression. Expressions of anger can be overt, such as losing one's temper, or more covert, including allowing the patient to experience some uncertainty. These nontherapeutic responses do not address the problem and therefore contribute to rising tensions. The only viable solution at this point is to remove oneself from the situation in order to evaluate one's responses and regain a therapeutic perspective on these interactions.

Aggressive Patient and Family Behaviors and Communication Barriers

Although less common than either nonadherent or manipulative-dependent behaviors, *aggression* expressed by the patient and/or patient's family toward a provider or the health care team is troublesome. Caring for angry patients in intense encounters can be threatening for all health care professionals especially when the patient is threatening physical harm. In a classic study of the reactions of physicians and nurses, Smith and Hart (1994) reported that nurses reacted differently depending upon the degree of perceived threat. When the perceived threat was high, nurses managed the patient's anger by disconnecting from the patient. Low or controllable threats were generally managed by connecting empathically with the angry patient.

The attitude communicated by the aggressor is one of hostility. Behaviors that are demonstrated are usually ones of condescending, blaming, attacking, or criticizing. Sometimes these behaviors take the form of insults and sarcasm. Less often, patients may exhibit aggression through physical attacks, including hitting, pinching, biting, spitting, and pushing.

Perhaps it seems strange that patients would respond in these ways; still, these reactions do occur. Although they are abusive, they may not intend to be. Most of the time these behaviors occur because patients have unabated frustration. Either patients have not assessed the consequences or they anticipated counter-aggression which will justify their rage. It is important to recognize that aggression is a sign of unhealthy coping. Sometimes in unfamiliar, frightening, and threatening circumstances, patients' usual ways of coping may not suffice. Patients who react aggressively indicate that they may feel inferior and overwhelmed; thus, anger and aggression are secondary responses resulting from feelings of being overwhelmed or out of control.

There are times when aggression is rooted in patients' experience of their illness and disease. Anger, for example, is cited as one phase of the grief response. Once denial has been diminished, other primary feelings surface, and before patients reach a level of acceptance of their disease and its consequences, a state of "Not me!" occurs. This stage of adaptation is in essence a protest against the illness. Patients who fall victim to life-threatening illnesses or injuries often experience a reduced ability to cope and therefore sometimes project their anger and rage (surrounding their illnesses or injuries) onto their health care providers. Ironically, those individuals most capable of helping and understanding the patient become targets of the patient's anger. In these cases, even minor problems or unexpected events can trigger the patient to "let go" a barrage of feelings and accusations.

Witnessing these behaviors can be like observing a volcanic eruption: a powerful, forceful barrage of words—perhaps accompanied by movements and gestures—gush to the top, displaying intensity far beyond anything anticipated. Usually patients' or families' angry, aggressive outbursts do not last long. While providers may fear that the patient will harm someone or damage objects in the immediate environment, this rarely happens. When patients become agitated and potentially assaultive, avoiding direct confrontation is important.

Providers can learn to recognize signs of escalated agitation, can practice presenting oneself as a calm, caring professional, and maintain control even when facing a potentially violent patient. Efforts should be made to provide opportunities for patients to be in control of their own behavior. Physically apprehending the patient should be used as a last resort only when there is a clear danger of immediate physical harm. Effective use of therapeutic communication encourages patients to express their feelings and concerns. While these guidelines apply particularly to hospitalized patients with a psychiatric diagnosis, they have relevance to all patients, regardless of the setting and diagnosis (see **EXHIBIT 18-4**).

This patient's responses were very provocative and explicitly hostile. There is a good

---

EXHIBIT 18-4 Nonverbal and Verbal Signs of Anger and Potential for Violence

- Body language: clenched fists, angry facial expressions, rigid posture.
- Hostile threatening verbalizations; boasts about prior abuse of others.
- Overt aggressive acts (e.g., destruction of objects in the surrounding environment).
- Increased motor activity (e.g., pacing, agitated movements, excitement, and irritability).
- Provocative behavior (e.g., hypersensitivity, argumentative, overreactive responses).

Consider the following dialogue between provider and patient in an inpatient encounter. The patient has a history of substance abuse but is hospitalized for symptoms related to HIV and his or her current opportunistic infection. The patient exhibits provocative behaviors and hostile, threatening gestures and verbalizations. The patient appears suspicious of his caregivers.

PROVIDER: "Edward, I hear you're having trouble with the food. We need to get you to eat better."
PATIENT: "Don't force me to eat!"

PROVIDER:	"We don't want to force you, but we need to supplement your diet. That's how we are going to get you better."
PATIENT:	(Emphatically) "What good is it? I'm going to die anyway!"
PROVIDER:	"We're all going to die someday, Edward."
PATIENT:	"That's bull s_____, what does it matter?"
PROVIDER:	"It matters because we can get you better. We can't cure you of AIDS, but we can certainly get you better (over this opportunistic disease)."
PATIENT:	"Where the h__ did they get you? You must be new!"
PROVIDER:	"So, what would you like to eat? Whatever, we'll try to get it."
PATIENT:	"McDonald's."
PROVIDER:	"OK. Hamburger, fries?…anything else?"
PATIENT:	"A prostitute!"
PROVIDER:	(Jumps to respond) "I'm not talking about extracurricular activities, Edward!"
PATIENT:	(Coughs several times; silent; looks at provider) "What if I spit in your eye? Would you get AIDS?" (Menacingly looks at the provider)
PROVIDER:	"No."
PATIENT:	"Would you be scared?" (Laughs)
PROVIDER:	"No….(Pause) Edward, we're really here to get you better; there's nothing more to it— that's what we're here for."

chance that the patient's anger toward the provider includes displaced feelings about his illness, particularly his prognosis. In attempting to set limits rather than to quiet the patient's agitation, this provider's response tends to increase the patient's agitation which leads to aggressive outbursts such as the patient's threat that he will spit in the provider's eye. From the patient's standpoint, the provider has no understanding of what he is dealing with.

Had the provider slowed his or her own reaction time and avoided response-matching the tone of the patient's replies, a somewhat different outcome may have resulted. Still, the wisdom of afterthought is not always available to us and one says and does what first occurs to them.

The provider's expression of acceptance despite the patient's unacceptable behavior is what seemed to turn this encounter toward a better course. Still, when dealing with patients who are clearly and presently abusing a substance or whose history includes violence the provider needs to always be cautious about presuming too much about the patient's own internal controls. With those prone to violent,

angry outbursts, certain things are unknown, including:

- How patients perceive others.
- How the environment or setting may heighten patient agitation.
- The ability of patients to control their emotional and physical outbursts.
- The extent to which patients are able to rechannel hostility into socially acceptable behaviors.
- Patients' level of tolerance for frustration.

Because these aspects are unknown and/ or difficult to judge in a single encounter, any behaviors that suggest aggression should not be underestimated. Providers who recognize the potential for every patient to respond angrily or aggressively at some point will anticipate how to minimize this possibility. Provider attitudes of acceptance (of the person, not the behavior), maintaining low levels of stimuli, and encouraging patients to verbalize feelings of frustration and to explore alternative ways of coping will assist many patients and families to control their level of anger and hostility. In cases of potential violent outbursts, prevention is always the strategy of choice. When prevention is not possible, securing one's own and the patient's physical safety and removing dangerous objects is paramount.

Complaining and Demanding Patient and Family Behaviors and Communication Barriers

The patient and/or family who complains about the care, the cost, the provider(s), and the treatment plan are clearly difficult to encounter and deal with over time. Many times, the patient and/or family member is demanding as well. *Complaining* is the expression of negativity that implies that the patient is difficult to please. Patients who complain and are demanding are thought to have unrealistic expectations. But this might not be the case. Some complaints are warranted and need to be expressed. These so-called complaints can result in important improvements in the patient's care or organization of care.

If providers judge these expectations as unrealistic, they are likely to resist any requests that seem to be out of the usual or outside what is acceptable. Ignoring this patient, though, may increase the level of demand that ensues because the patient's perception is that the provider has not heard or does not understand or value the importance of the request. So, from the patient's standpoint the request has to be repeated, and repeated again and again. They may be feeling frustrated and that their attempts are futile.

The feeling of loss of control can trigger hostility and the need to intensify demands. Under the surface, the complainer may be feeling fear and anxiety, coupled with frustration. This patient views situations as undesirable or threatening and judges that no other rational discussion of the problem will work. Demands become expressed concerns about their lack of control. By the time the patient or patient's family issues commands or demands, feelings of loss of control are usually compounded with feelings of inadequacy. As one would expect, this patient might be experiencing multiple feelings that need to be addressed separately.

Unfortunately, these concerns do not elicit analytical replies. Unless a provider is astute and is capable of examining the patient's underlying reasons, these feelings will go unaddressed. A worst-case scenario is that the patient's or family member's behavior is needlessly exaggerated because the provider withdraws, tunes out, or otherwise avoids them. Avoidance and withdrawal responses tend to increase the patient's feelings of fear, anxiety, and concerns about rejection. This awareness serves to escalate patient and even family demands.

A subcategory of the complaining patient has been identified as one of a provider's most trying patients. This is the hypochondriacal patient. The diagnosis of *hypochondriasis* has now been replaced with the diagnoses of *somatic symptom disorder* or *illness anxiety disorder* (APA, 2013). This disorder is distinguished by the presence of physical symptoms for which there are no demonstrable organic findings or known physiologic mechanisms. Additionally, there is positive evidence, or at least a strong presumption, that the symptoms are linked to psychological or psychiatric factors. These patients unrealistically interpret physical signs or sensations as evidence of physical illness and may even persist in their concerns after a clear bill of health. They are usually preoccupied with the fear or belief of having not just a disease, but a serious disease.

Unlike people who periodically wonder about small changes that they observe or experience, these patients have enduring suspicions that they have a serious disease. They tend to be chronic complainers, unrelentingly complaining of physical problems. Typically, these patients will shop for a provider or clinic who will believe them. During this search, they can become virtual invalids, impairing their social and occupational functioning and interpersonal relationships.

There is excessive preoccupation with the symptom(s) that are usually exaggerated out of proportion. For these patients, hardly one social encounter will occur without them focusing on the symptom. Most have a history of seeking assistance from numerous health care providers. Excessive use of analgesics with minimal relief of pain may be reported, and this person is vulnerable to addiction. Unmet dependency needs, anxiety, and the tendency to shop for cures while engaging many physicians, each responding to the anxiety with prescriptions of anxiolytic medications, increases the risk of drug dependency. As these patients cling to their symptoms, a pattern of broken provider–patient relationships characterize their history.

Providers often face a double-bind situation with these patients and their families. Denying the patient's symptoms and their seriousness can hinder the development of a therapeutic relationship. Even when suspecting that there is really nothing wrong with the patient, providers may be hesitant to express their opinions outright. Yet, not telling the patient that the symptoms have no basis communicates to the patient that they do have medical meaning and it is appropriate to consider medications, treatment, and even surgery.

In fact, the more that providers seem to try to help these patients, the more important the symptoms become. The irritation that providers feel is understandable. They tend to reflect on the fact that there are so many people with real problems who are truly fighting for life, while these patients seem to revel in the diseases they think they have. Encouraging patients to focus on the stressors in their lives as well as their fears of not being cared for may provide the foundation for the patient to accept a psychological or psychiatric basis for these symptoms. If there are powerful secondary gains associated with patients' experience of symptoms (e.g., a reprieve from work, childcare, or the demands of a significant other), patients can exhibit prolonged use of symptoms despite beginning awareness that there is no real medical or physiological explanation for them.

Not all bodily complaints should be dismissed even with this type of patient. There are many reasons some symptoms for some patients are experienced. For example, patients who are depressed, grief stricken, or delusional or who are experiencing conversion reactions may amplify their experiences of backaches, headaches, stomach ailments, and a variety of other minor aches and pains.

Providers' responses should avoid causing patients to react defensively. Focusing on patients' life situations and current feelings, including feelings toward the provider, are usually helpful. Arguing or debating a symptom usually results in the patient leaving the provider's care. Consider the following dialogue between an obese 35-year-old male and his physician (**EXHIBIT 18-5**).

EXHIBIT 18-5 Dialogue of Provider Responding to Unrealistic Demands

PROVIDER:	"Your hand is just fine. I don't see any reason why you can't go back to work."
PATIENT:	"But it still hurts, and it swells up on me."
PROVIDER:	"Well, J____, it might be that you're not really interested in returning to work."
PATIENT:	"What if I injure it again? Then it would really be bad."
PROVIDER:	"Well, we don't know for sure. J____ what's going on at work? How's work?"
PATIENT:	"Work s____. If I don't find a better job, I'm going to be put in some institution!"
PROVIDER:	"So maybe your job is the problem—not your hand."

In this dialogue, the physician reframed the problem, which was not the injured hand, but the problem of going back to work. Resuming activities means going back to a job this patient dislikes. Mistakes that the provider could have made would have been to (1) focus needlessly on the hand, (2) challenge the patient to prove the problem existed, and (3) engage in a power struggle over who knew the most. The value of this provider's response lies in the fact that the physician did not support the patient's unrealistic view of his hand. By establishing an interested, concerned tone, the physician actually met the patient's needs for support and caring.

The Patient and/or Family in Denial and Communication Barriers

Prolonged stages of denial are usually, but not always, indicative of maladaptive coping. Authors who address the various stages of adaptation to disease, illness, and injury describe denial as an early stage of eventual resolution and acceptance of one's diagnosis and prognosis. *Denial* is a self-protective mechanism. It defends against underlying threats that would ordinarily overwhelm the patient. Because of this, providers are always cautioned to treat denial with respect.

Problems can occur, however, when patients and/or their families exhibit prolonged periods of denial or when, in denial, they avoid actions or treatments that are absolutely necessary for full recovery. Denial can sometimes be constructed so elaborately that to maintain their denial, patients process information to negate substantial aspects of their experience. This may include denial of pain (or minimization of its intensity), fatigue, stress, and impaired functioning related to vision, hearing, or motor-sensory abilities. Patients who minimize flu symptoms, pain from an injury, a prolonged cough, the stress on the job, or their inability to accurately read street signs due to impaired vision are very common.

Patients who use denial are unable at the time to deal successfully with the reality of their condition. Although they may in fact be assisted to cope effectively, their anticipation that they will not is sufficient to cause them to deny problems that are obvious to others. Denial may be accompanied by other defenses (e.g., rationalization and blocking).

Rationalization is the process of justifying or rejecting feedback that would cause the patient to acknowledge reality. Thus, a patient may deny the risk of exposure to HIV and at the same time rationalize the process of denying. AIDS, as everyone knows, is a problem, yet a patient can translate it in the following way: "It is not a real problem and certainly not a problem that should impinge on me (my health-related behaviors). Therefore, the threat of AIDS is not something to worry about because it is not significant (denial). If it is not significant, no real changes are needed (rationalization)."

Patients who use denial to cope may also use blocking. *Blocking* is thought to be both a conscious and unconscious defensive mechanism. It operates by not allowing certain facts into one's awareness. Patients can actively put things out of their mind with the intention of having it not affect them. Patients who block awareness of new or different data may interrupt the provider, become inattentive in conversations, and change the subject. This occurs when they anticipate painful awareness of facts and prognoses.

Denial, as was previously mentioned, may initially be adaptive. Future successful adaptation may occur if people are allowed an initial period of denial and inactivity. This period protects the individual from stress and sometimes the many responsibilities and activities that are required as one actively deals with illness, disease, and injury. Denial that is adaptive can be likened to a stage of respite, a period of "calm before the storm."

Patient and/or family denial is maladaptive when it interferes with appropriate treatment. Health care providers must always assess whether the patient's denial is interfering with care and placing the patient in additional jeopardy. While some providers would argue that denial, by definition, suggests the patient and/or family is not ready to deal with realities and cannot be pushed quickly into facing the primary and secondary consequences of one's illness, other providers will argue the contrary. Arguments that denial should be addressed early are usually supported by the following reasoning:

- The patient's and/or family's fear of the reality may be exaggerated (i.e., the real facts are less threatening than the patient's anticipation of them).
- Prolonged denial contributes to unrealistic estimates of the disease and one's ability to cope.
- Providers can successfully address most threatening aspects of injury or illness.
- Future collaborative efforts between provider and patient and family require a level of reality-based problem-solving that is not forthcoming if denial is permitted to continue.

Dealing effectively with a patient in denial is complex because denial is intimately linked with a level of hope and hopefulness. Experts suggest that if denial is reduced the patient's level of hope may also be diminished. It is unwise to be so confrontational as to bankrupt the patient's ability to be hopeful. Hopefulness is recognized as integral to the process of fortifying patients' abilities to tolerate stress and pain including negative prognoses and loss of functional abilities.

Providers who are attempting to alter patient denial for the purpose of achieving better adherence or better collaborative encounters with the patient must appreciate this phenomenon and balance their approach. Patients need to be helped to confront and deal with the realities of their illness while preserving their spirit and optimism about their quality of life and their ability to manage their illnesses, disabilities, or impairments. Consider the following dialogue between a patient diagnosed with advanced metastatic cancer of the colon and the patient's physician (**EXHIBIT 18-6**).

As providers, one might question this scenario. Should the physician (1) have been so frank, (2) have said something else (e.g., "We can keep your pain under control"), and (3) have asked more about her feelings? The issues are multiple. The main idea here is that the physician presented the reality of a shortened life span to the patient in concrete, simple-to-understand terms. The patient may have anticipated a more negative outcome—some patients admit that they "know" in advance.

Nonetheless, the patient needed to be told and was perceived by the physician as able to tolerate the new findings. Additionally, other aspects of care were in place that were

---

EXHIBIT 18-6 Dialogue of Patient Having Difficulty Accepting Facts

PHYSICIAN:	"The tests don't look good, Tina."
PATIENT:	"Well, they couldn't be too bad. I've been feeling OK, really."
PHYSICIAN:	"I'd like to tell you that things are OK, but they're not."
PATIENT:	"How bad is it?"
PHYSICIAN:	"Well…we're going to run some more tests."
PATIENT:	"A year, 2 years?"
PROVIDER:	"Let's hope for the best but we might be looking at several months."
PATIENT:	(Silence) "Six months?" (Silence, begins to cry.)
PROVIDER:	"I know this is hard; you want to know exactly." (Reaches out to touch patient's hand)

potentially supportive to this patient and family. First, the physician, members of the treatment team, and patient and family have had a continuous, ongoing relationship. Second, they have had previous discussions of the gravity of the illness. Third, the patient and family trust the physician's ability to empathize and understand the unique implications of declining health. It is these elements that bolster the patient's and family's ability to manage the trauma of being told a negative prognosis.

▶ Special Considerations for Communicating with Depressed or Anxious Patients

In addition to the difficult behaviors described there are additional patient conditions that are viewed as challenging, particularly among providers who have had limited exposure to and training in mental health. The patient's psychiatric condition may be complex requiring an adjustment in standard plans of care. These patients benefit from the same therapeutic alliance afforded to patients without a psychiatric diagnosis (Dudzinski & Timberlake, 2014); but because of their depressed or anxious state should be given even more consideration. There is every reason to believe that health care providers, no matter the treatment setting (hospital, clinic, or hospice setting), will repeatedly encounter patients and/or their family members who are experiencing significant degrees of anxiety and/or depression.

In the context of any one day, providers can encounter up to 50% of patients in a primary care setting who have anxiety and depression and will require additional interventions to provide tailored support and treatment. Either depressed or anxious patients are frequently seen in primary care settings and frequently these conditions coexist (depression

with anxiety). There are multiple levels of each condition which compels us to not only assess the presence of anxiety and depression but also to identify its severity.

Depression and/or anxiety may be reactions to stress, particularly to the stressful life event of an illness or injury. Depression has been associated with many medical comorbidities, including cardiac illness. It can be secondary to many medical conditions: metabolic disturbances (e.g., hypercalcemia), endocrine disorders (e.g., diabetes), neurological diseases (e.g., Parkinson's disease), cancers (especially pancreatic cancer), bacterial and virus infections (e.g., influenza), and others.

The anxiety and/or depression the patient exhibits may be mild and time limited or may reflect a clinical psychiatric syndrome or disorder. Clinical anxiety can appear as panic disorder, agoraphobia, social phobia, obsessive-compulsive disorder, posttraumatic stress disorder (PTSD), and generalized anxiety disorder (APA, 2013). For example, adults and even children seen in emergency rooms for physical abuse, gunshot wounds, rape, or other forms of physical assault may be experiencing initial signs of PTSD that are related to how they were injured. When the condition does not subside, a syndromic condition will result. But for many, the signs and symptoms are indicative of less serious prognoses. The uncertainties surrounding who, what, and when the patient will get medical attention may be important but the driving force behind the patient's experience of emotional distress may be the recollections of events leading to the injury.

Emergency room staff are aware of the effect of such trauma and monitor patients' levels of distress looking for potential escalation of symptom severity. They have a full range of mild to moderate tranquilizers if needed. PTSD is a more-severe condition, warranting additional attention, and is characterized by the development of physiologic and/or behavioral symptoms following the psychological trauma that occurred. A PTSD-inducing event such as assault, mass shootings, and threats of hurricanes and fires would be considered markedly stressful to almost anyone and has usually been experienced with intense feelings of fear, terror, helplessness, and powerlessness. While many patients experience this phenomenon long after the event (referred to as PTSD with delayed onset), most patients show signs early after the trauma as the shock of the event subsides.

It is understandable that all occurrences of illness or injury are events that can carry anxiety for all patients and families. This anxiety may be evidenced in behavioral dimensions (e.g., expectant apprehension), vigilance (e.g., about medications and disease signs and symptoms), or perceptual scanning of the environment.

Young children do not understand a hospital environment and when combined with loss of a parent's support are prime candidates for considerable anxiety. All patients who are subjected to hospitalization where control is lost and routines are disrupted experience some level of uncertainty and anxiety. Particular treatments can also create anticipatory anxiety. Families are vulnerable to anxiety surrounding the diagnosis, treatment, and prognosis of their significant others. Anxiety is so omnipresent in the health care delivery system that it behooves providers to be very adept at recognizing, differentiating, and intervening effectively to minimize this condition.

Like all conditions, anxiety is best addressed when the provider is more fully cognizant of the sources of anxiety, can understand both real and perceived threats from the patient's perspective, and can judge the level and magnitude of the condition. Is anxiety the predominant condition or is other distress (e.g., depression) also occurring? Do certain stimuli expose the patient to elevated levels of anxiety? Is ritualistic or compulsive behavior involved in patients' attempts to curb fear and tension? Answers to these questions will help

providers assess the magnitude and complexity of the patient's emotional state.

There are clear behavioral manifestations that indicate that the patient is anxious. *Anxiety*, usually defined as a vague uneasy feeling, is different from fear where there is a specific situation or thing that is feared. Patients who are feeling anxious will not be able to state or specify the source of their discomfort.

The following signs suggest that the patient is suffering anxiety: dyspnea, palpitations, choking or smothering sensations, dizziness or unsteadiness, chest pains, feeling of losing contact with reality, hot and cold flashes, sweating, trembling, shaking, restlessness, hyperattentiveness, recurrent and intrusive fearful thoughts, and abdominal discomfort. Any combination of these signs and symptoms suggests that the patient is experiencing significant anxiety and this recognition might alter provider communication.

The highly anxious patient or family member may only comprehend the most rudimentary communication. In giving these patients orders or directions, clear, simple, and brief commands will often be reassuring. They may be more capable of responding to close-ended questions because they are less demanding. The patient's immediate environment is usually perceived as overwhelming; therefore, it is important to remain calm, restore quiet, and speak slowly. Patients with very high levels of anxiety will lack the usual abilities to care for themselves, at least temporarily. Some patients may even significantly regress for a period of time, such as becoming more withdrawn and unresponsive. While it is important for providers to encourage these patients to take care of their own activities of daily living, initially they need additional assistance from staff and family members.

Depressed patients are usually thought to be difficult to care for because they are experienced as "draining" and "time consuming." Some providers admit that caring for depressed patients and their families can make them feel depressed. Of all emotional disorders that require psychiatric labels, *depression* is the most common condition that providers are likely to confront. It has been estimated that depression in primary care settings gets diagnosed only half the time. This means that depression in primary care patients is not adequately assessed and treated.

Depression is generally viewed on a continuum from low levels (sometimes referred to as "the blues") to more enduring episodes that fit the diagnostic criteria of a syndrome or disorder. Major depressive disorder (MDD), which can be recurrent and severe, is only one class of depressive conditions that providers may encounter. There are other less-severe conditions. Individuals with certain medical conditions (e.g., diabetes, cancer, strokes, and myocardial infarctions [MIs]) can even develop a MDD during the course of their general medical condition. Patients who do experience these depressive episodes can create complex treatment conditions.

In responding to patients and/or their families who are anxious and/or depressed, communications that provide information, show empathy, respond to nonverbal clues, listen attentively, and avoid close-ended questions are critical to establishing a therapeutic alliance. Patients seek medical help and often feel out of control when it comes to their illness or health condition. This can make them feel dependent on health care providers. This awareness is likely to cause patients to feel anxious, worried, hopeless, and uncertain about their health which can be displayed as tension and negative responses toward health care providers (Hardavella et al., 2017).

Providers sometime justify that under the circumstances, anxiety or depression are understandable and will naturally dissipate over time. However, if this perspective presents a barrier to treatment because it is assumed to be normal this conclusion must be seriously questioned. Some providers feel uncomfortable dealing with anxiety and depression due to lack of training or feeling that they might be alienating patients and subsequently avoid tackling these important behaviors and conditions.

▶ Monitor and Master Provider Reactions to Difficult Patient Behaviors

Patients who display "difficult" behaviors in encounters with providers may negatively affect the ability to form a therapeutic alliance that is trustworthy. In fact, even among mental health specialists who are experienced in dealing with a wide range of behavior problems, patients with difficult behaviors are a challenge, particularly when patients seek care but are ambivalent about receiving care (Koekkoek, van Meijel, & Hutschemaekers, 2006). With these patients, health care providers find it hard to maintain a clear strategy because patients' behaviors cause concern as well as annoyance.

Researchers have questioned whether encounters with difficult patient behaviors cut short patient and physician discussions, and some have studied the effects of these behaviors on medical errors. The idea is that when providers are challenged by these behaviors the ability to employ sound diagnostic and treatment reasoning is impaired (Mamede et al., 2016; Schmidt et al., 2016). All providers need to be aware of their emotional reactions to patients and families whose behaviors are difficult for them. A primary point of departure is that providers need to respond, not react. To respond means to thoughtfully consider patients' and/or family's communications and to formulate a careful return. To react, on the other hand, means to move quickly without forethought and sometimes in opposition to what the patient is saying or trying to say.

The primary process of responding, not reacting, is the process of thoughtful consideration and sometimes is referred to as mindfulness. This response calls for active listening aiming to answer such questions as: "What is the patient or family really saying?"and "Why are they saying it?" Otherwise, the provider is looking for the underlying meaning of the patient's or family's communication. It is easier, for example, to communicate with a demanding patient or family member when providers understand that this behavior is triggered by feelings of losing control. It is easier, as well, to communicate general acceptance of aggressive patients if the provider understands that this behavior is a result of feelings of being inferior or frustration. Therefore, from the standpoint of increasing responsive statements and decreasing reactive responses it is critical that providers look inward to their own emotions and outward to the underlying meaning behind the patient's or family member's expressed behaviors. Part of the task of looking inward is to identify personal "triggers."

Most responses to difficult patient behaviors will be positive if the underlying motives are addressed and providers can control their own fears and concerns. It is recommended that providers not express negative emotions; but when they do, they should reduce the number of blaming statements they use with patients and their families. Providers who are upset with, or angry at, patients can fail even if they do address underlying motives. Patients and their family members need to feel that providers' responses are, in a sense, "neutralized." Neutrality will encourage response-matching that demonstrates mutual control.

What to Do About Feelings

The area most confusing to providers in the majority of encounters with difficult patients, difficult tasks, and difficult contexts is the *feeling dimension* of emotions. Feelings are one of the most important ingredients in the relationship between patients and providers, and the degree to which feelings should be controlled or expressed is not always clear.

Patients and families look for warmth, friendliness, and understanding under all conditions, even when their behavior is offensive. They become concerned when providers appear cold, aloof, withdrawn, or critical. They may worry that the provider does not care and will not give them good enough care. For some, the fear of "divorce" or referral out to another provider is behind their apprehension, especially if this has happened before. A simple referral to a specialist can be interpreted as a gesture of rejection even though there is a clear rationale for the referral.

There are specific instances in which feelings toward difficult patients can be problematic. These include providers' (1) lack of, or withholding of, feelings and (2) expression of too much feeling (e.g., elevated feelings of agitation, frustration, and anger). In all but a few patient encounters, human drama, and sometimes great tragedy, unfolds before the provider's eyes. The expression of no feeling tends to minimize the reality of the circumstances and the patient's experience.

Demonstration of lack of feeling or "stoicism," may be due to the provider repressing very strong feelings. Patients have absolutely no way of knowing whether they are getting through to the provider or whether the provider does not care enough. If patients think that they are not getting through to the provider, they will repeat or accentuate their behavior. Whether the behavior is repeated or accentuated, the provider is still subjected to difficult behaviors that now occur on a larger scale. In short, a vicious cycle is occurring.

The expression of too much feeling or strong feelings can be problematic as well. Expressing too much feeling can heighten conflict when there are differences of thought or opinion. Anger matched by anger (and irritation matched by irritation) can threaten the strength of the therapeutic alliance and derail open communication. One of the best means of dealing with the provider's feelings toward difficult patient behaviors is to conduct a self-examination which can include reflection and conversations with a counselor. When providers are able to understand their own feelings and control them, they will be better able to meet the needs of their patients and deal effectively with the patient's difficult behavior. It should be noted that not all providers experience difficult patient behaviors in the same way Krebs et al. (2006).

General Guidelines to Follow with Difficult Patients and/or Their Family Members

While the following discussion can apply to all provider–patient–family relationships, the concepts and principles discussed are particularly helpful reminders when it comes to communicating with difficult behaviors.

Show Respect and Compassion

Although the idea of showing respect and compassion seems obvious, it is probably one of the most seriously violated principles in health care delivery systems when difficulties are surfacing. Delivery systems can violate patients' rights for respectful treatment. This occurs, for example, when patients are left waiting for long periods, are not told what and when to expect procedures or tests, and are treated as if they are mere clogs in the wheel rather than human beings.

When providers treat any patient with disrespect, these insults affect the formation and maintenance of the therapeutic alliance. Ignoring, avoiding, and depersonalizing all tend to escalate the conflict situation to the point where communication is blocked and/or a third person, usually another provider (but possibly the patient's significant other or family), is drawn into the interaction.

Practice Unconditional Positive Regard

Unconditional positive regard or acceptance means acknowledging the patient and/or family member as a person of worth no matter what they say or do. However, although it means acceptance of the patient's way of thinking, believing, and behaving, it does not mean acceptance of destructive gestures or actions.

In many small ways, patients and their families measure the level of provider acceptance. Providers are deeply committed to sound health care practices, and patients who test providers can use this fact as the major weapon in dealing with diagnosis and treatment. For example, "If you accept me, you will accept the fact that I prefer to eat foods that are bad for me," is a challenge for the provider. The question is how can the provider show acceptance but disapprove of the behavior? Still, if acceptance is the issue that leads to adherence, the provider never wants to win the battle just to lose the war. Sometimes, bargaining for change involves persuading the patient to alter patterns with the understanding that the provider unconditionally accepts the patient.

Show Concern and Interest

The therapeutic alliance between provider and patient and patient's family members is based on concern and interest. Caring, a feeling state related to concern, can be an underdeveloped skill in a high-tech environment. It is important that providers care about patients and nurture this feeling with even the most difficult of patients by showing concern and interest as an expression of preparing to help them. Patients view providers who do not have an attitude of concern as ill-equipped, not because of their competency but because they do not have the patient's interests in mind (i.e., they cannot be trusted). Spoken or unspoken, it is the feeling of concern and interest that patients look for when choosing a provider. It is also the basis for dissatisfaction with providers and their care when it is absent.

Practice Objectivity

Just as the show of concern is critical, the practice of objectivity is also essential. Providers' feelings cannot obscure reason and good judgment. Objectivity means that the provider can stand outside the immediate situation and evaluate it from all directions. The ability to look at an encounter from all sides before responding or taking action requires awareness of self, self-discipline, and practice.

Beginning providers usually have a greater deal of difficulty stepping outside the uncomfortable encounters with difficult patients while remaining engaged. When faced with abusive remarks, they may take the criticism personally, experiencing hurt and rejection. These reactions can even immobilize them. Standing apart from the encounter and viewing the situation from different vantage points usually has the effect of increasing providers' insights while at the same time neutralizing the feelings they have about how they are being treated.

When they practice objectivity they will be in better positions to respond, not react, to difficult patients and/or their families' behaviors. Objectivity, however, does not mean being aloof and noncaring. On the contrary, a supportive empathic approach is critical. Withholding concern for a patient or patient's family while trying to maintain objectivity is both unnecessary and problematic. The skill is to show concern but remain detached enough to establish the facts as they relate to the encounter.

Enhance Awareness and Observation Skills

Being intentionally aware of patients' circumstances, including their state of wellness (symptoms and any changes) is the bare minimum. It is safe to say that a majority of difficult patient and family encounters are due to inadequate awareness on the part of the provider.

Providers come across insensitively when they are not aware of patients' conditions and their responses to their changed conditions. Being unaware and approaching a potentially difficult patient or patient's family is like walking into a minefield. The risk of unsatisfactory communications is very high. Therefore, providers have set themselves up for difficulty. Furthermore, providers' failure to become aware are clearly their fault—not the patient's.

In addition to being aware of the patient's condition, both physical and psychological symptoms and changes in the symptom picture, providers must be cognizant of the special caring needs that patients have. Does the patient want tenderness or detachment? Do they want to be informed about everything or just told the essential facts? Do they want to be alone or want to talk? Every patient has unique needs and these needs change as their health and condition changes.

Sometimes these needs are communicated clearly and directly. More often than not, they go misunderstood. In the case of difficult patient behaviors, these needs may be very obscure, and this obscurity must be matched with high levels of awareness on the part of the provider (**EXHIBIT 18-7**).

▶ Analysis

This aggressive, verbally abusive, and threatening behavior comes from a patient experiencing a great deal of distress—not only about his illness (and prognosis) but also about the functional decline that he feels is linked with his masculinity. It is manly to take yourself to the bathroom when necessary, to jump up and get going, to get your own food—to provide for yourself. His symptoms and acute infection noticeably force him into unaccustomed dependency.

He does not think that the provider understands or appreciates these aspects, and he does not want to be treated as an invalid. Unfortunately, the provider, at more anxious

EXHIBIT 18-7 Case Study: Angry and Aggressive Behaviors

Patient name: Edward S.

Age: 30 years old

Marital status: Single

Occupation: Sales—unemployed

Diagnosis: PCP—1 week ago diagnosed as HIV+ with intravenous drug abuse history

Hospitalization: To control infection

Treatment: Includes supplemental feedings, nonroutine sedative and sleeping medications, O$_2$ PRN by mask

    This patient has been and is currently a substance abuser and is suspected of continued illicit drug use. He is hospitalized for symptoms related to his HIV infection and current opportunistic infection. The patient exhibits provocative behaviors, hostile threatening gestures, and verbalizations as well as suspicion of his caregivers. The following is an expanded version of the previous conversation with this patient. Observe that in this continued discussion the patient's concerns become clearer.

PROVIDER:	"Edward, I hear you're having trouble with the food. We need to get you to eat better."
PATIENT:	"Don't force me to eat."
PROVIDER:	"We don't want to force you, but we need to supplement your diet. That's how we are going to get you better."
PATIENT:	(Emphatically) "What good is it? I'm going to die anyway!"
PROVIDER:	"We're all going to die someday, Edward."
PATIENT:	"That's bulls ____, what does it matter?"
PROVIDER:	"It matters because we can get you better. We can't cure you of AIDS, but we can certainly get you over this disease." (PCP)
PATIENT:	"Where the h____ did they get you? You must be new!"
PROVIDER:	"So, what would you like to eat? Whatever, we'll try to get it."
PATIENT:	"McDonald's."
PROVIDER:	"OK. Hamburger, fries? Anything else?"
PATIENT:	"A prostitute!"
PROVIDER:	"I'm not talking about extracurricular activities, Edward."
PATIENT:	(Coughs several times; silent; looks at provider) "What if I spit in your eye…Would you get AIDS?"
PROVIDER:	"No."
PATIENT:	"Would you be scared?" (Laughs)
PROVIDER:	"No…Edward, we're really here to get you better; there's nothing more to it—that's what we're here for."
PATIENT:	"Ha, ha, ha." (Coughing uncontrollably)
PROVIDER:	"You know we're here because we care. I'm offering to help you. Do you need help to the bathroom?"
PATIENT:	"No! I don't need help. I'm a man—f____, s____."
PROVIDER:	"I know you're a man, but you need help. I didn't say you weren't a man."
PATIENT:	"Don't get smart with me—or I'll…I'll slap you!"
PROVIDER:	"You need help, Edward. Let me help you."
PATIENT:	"I told you…I'm a man!"
PROVIDER:	"It takes a man to admit he needs help."
PATIENT:	"Don't give me that phony psychology s____."
PROVIDER:	"Edward, do you need to go the bathroom?"
PATIENT:	(Nods yes)

PROVIDER:	"OK, lie over on this side. Put your legs over the side. I'm going to help you get up so you can go to the bathroom."
PATIENT:	(Silently responds to provider's directions, somewhat confused) "Which way are you going to sit me up?" (Angrily)
PROVIDER:	"This way. How are you feeling now?"
PATIENT:	"It's cold. Why don't they turn up the heat? If they really cared, they would turn on the heat."
PROVIDER:	"The heat is on, Edward. Are you dizzy?"
PATIENT:	"I'm dizzy and I'm cold. If the heat's on, then why am I cold?!"
PROVIDER:	"You have a fever, Edward. You've got a major infection. Are you still dizzy?"
PATIENT:	"I'm dizzy and cold!"
PROVIDER:	"If you're dizzy, I want you to lie down. Lie back down, Edward."
PATIENT:	(Complies and is silent)
PROVIDER:	(Pulls up a chair by Edward's bed) "What's going on?"
PATIENT:	(Silent, curled up in bed)
PROVIDER:	"Obviously, something is bothering you a whole lot."
PATIENT:	(Mumbles) "They won't let me see my son."
PROVIDER:	"They won't let you see him? Is that because of your drug problems or your diagnosis?"
PATIENT:	"Both. I'm just tired."
PROVIDER:	"We talked before about your eating better, getting rest."
PATIENT:	"I used to be able to jump out of bed—get going."
PROVIDER:	"You'll regain your strength once we get you over this infection. Then we can see about getting your family involved."
PATIENT:	"What do you mean? What can you do?"
PROVIDER:	"We'll talk to the social worker—you have every right to see your son."
PATIENT:	"I'm so tired."
PROVIDER:	"Do you still have to go to the bathroom?"
PATIENT:	"I can't go by myself."
PROVIDER:	"I'll take you now."

(Provider successfully gains patient's cooperation and escorts him to the bathroom.)

moments, feeds into this patient's concerns by becoming directive and authoritative, perhaps making the patient feel even more infantile. The patient, facing the threat of his own loss of power, challenges the competency and sincerity of his provider. He insists on being treated respectfully but treats the provider abusively.

Abandoning the task—getting the patient to the bathroom—was needed. Focusing on feelings, "What's going on—obviously, something is bothering you a whole lot," was the primary therapeutic shift in this encounter. This intervention was punctuated by pausing. The open-ended question, "What's going on?" altered the style of communication and

expressed the provider's concern and readiness to be open and receptive to the patient. The reflection, "Obviously, something is bothering you a whole lot," expressed empathy and a desire to become more aware of the patient's situation as he experiences it. The fact that the provider did not reject this patient by leaving the room communicated a level of acceptance that the patient needed before trusting the provider with more intimate and painful details.

The provider displayed respect for both the patient's identification of his problems and his inherent rights as a patient undergoing treatment. Much of the dialogue that had occurred up to this point was affected by the provider's own reactions to the patient's accusatory and belittling comments. The provider communicated somewhat defensively to threats (e.g., "If I spit in your eye...would you be scared," and "don't give me that psychological s_____").

At either of these points, the provider could have attempted to refocus the patient on what was really bothering him. However, several factors may have prevented earlier attempts from working. This includes both the provider's and patient's awareness that a lot is going on here—this is not just a simple task of changing the patient's eating patterns or assisting him to the bathroom. Awareness of

the complexity of the situation increased the provider's level of empathy.

What is also noteworthy is that the provider's effectiveness increased in the segment of dialogue with the use of various therapeutic responses. Reflection, open-ended questions, expression of concern, showing acceptance, and enhancing one's objectivity and awareness were used effectively. They assisted the provider in this difficult encounter to compose a more therapeutic intervention.

The following case study describes an interaction with a patient displaying demanding and dependent behaviors (**EXHIBIT 18-8**).

EXHIBIT 18-8 Case Study: Demanding and Dependent Behaviors

Patient name: Marcia Y.
Age: 56 years old
Marital status: Divorced
Occupation: Secretary, law firm
Diagnosis: Acute bacterial intestinal infection acquired on vacation to the West Indies approximately 2 weeks ago. No other diagnosable problems.
Outpatient treatment: Antibiotics to control infection. Lomotil to control diarrhea. Encourage bed rest and adequate diet.

This 56-year-old legal secretary is off work and on bed rest for an acute intestinal infection acquired during a vacation to the West Indies approximately 2 weeks ago. Although she has no other diagnosable problems, she complains of a variety of aches and pains and seeks reassurance that these signs are benign. She is being followed-up in the outpatient clinic for this infection by a nurse practitioner.

PROVIDER:	"Hello, Marcia. I don't think I've met you yet. Dr. S_____ and I practice together."
PATIENT:	"Oh, yes, I've heard of you. Where is Dr. S_____?"
PROVIDER:	"He's out of the office today. So, how have you been doing?"
PATIENT:	"I guess OK. I don't feel well though."
PROVIDER:	"What's going on?"
PATIENT:	"I feel weak, tired. Sometimes I have pains...you know, last time Dr. S thought I might have something wrong with my back. I get pains between my shoulders. And..."
PROVIDER:	(Interrupts patient) "Nothing in your chart about back pain, though. Let's see how you are doing with this infection you have."
PATIENT:	"I've been feeling really guilty."
PROVIDER:	"About what?"
PATIENT:	"Being off work for so long. Everything is piling up at the office. I've worked really hard to get the job I have now, and now I can't do it."
PROVIDER:	"I think in another week you'll feel well enough to go back to work."
PATIENT:	"I don't know...do you really think so? What if this infection goes on longer than 7 more days? This is serious—I thought I was going to die."
PROVIDER:	"You were pretty sick in the beginning. Seven more days though and you'll be able to get up and feel good about going back to work."

PATIENT:	"I guess I worry too much. There is so much to worry about…You know I'm not 20 anymore. I'm weaker than I used to be."
PROVIDER:	"How do you mean, weaker?"
PATIENT:	"I can't do that much. I sleep more. When I go home, I'll probably sleep for 2 days."
PROVIDER:	"Two days? Don't think so." (Pats patient on arm)
PATIENT:	"You've been so kind. I guess I need reassurance. Other doctors don't take me seriously."
PROVIDER:	"We take you seriously."
PATIENT:	"Yes…Before you go, do you think I should have X-rays of my spine? Maybe this infection will aggravate the back problem I have. It's probably a good idea, don't you think? Women my age have bone problems, and I'm worried that I could fall down and break a hip. That's all I need—an infection and broken hip at the same time."
PROVIDER:	"Marcia, I've got to see my next patient. Let's concentrate on getting you over this infection right now. I want you to come back in a week."
PATIENT:	"OK Doctor, thank you. Will I see you next time?"

The nurse practitioner exits the room and does not respond to patient's last question. It is not clear whether the patient's question was heard or heard but ignored.

▶ Analysis

This patient's general presentation was friendly and appreciative. She appeared eager to cooperate. Less obvious was the patient's multiple requests that resulted in the nurse practitioner spending more time on fictitious problems than expected. This patient wanted attention and was able to hold the provider's attention through a series of pleas to consider and reconsider potential complaints and ailments. It is true that most of the symptoms she addressed were legitimate, with the exception of back pains, but she was not totally convinced that the back pains were insignificant.

Her expressed reluctance to return to work raised the possibility that her current illness had some secondary gain. That is, she did not want to return to work and because she was feeling guilty about not being at work, her symptoms and delayed recovery could function to legitimize her absence. Her response to the provider's reassurance that she could return to work soon was more of disappointment than relief. This patient's last request for attention, namely, her question about whether she would see this provider again, reflected her need to establish a special relationship not enjoyed by most patients.

This provider's responses were very typical with the first response being an attempt to meet the patient's need for attention. As the encounter progressed, however, it became clear that these attempts would fail to provide the level of support she was asking for. It became clear that reassurance about recovery was not what the patient sought.

As the provider became progressively aware of this patient's dependent tendencies, the provider began to withdraw. The nurse practitioner's response on departure was to virtually ignore her last attempt to engage the provider in further discussions. Although one can only guess, this provider's thoughts and feelings upon leaving the room ("Will I see you next time?") may have included "I sure hope not!" "Sorry I can't tell you that you have another problem—I know that's what you want to hear!" The end result reinforces the patient's fear, that the provider will reject her, and any continuation of a helpful, supportive relationship is unlikely. That is, what the patient feared—rejection— is what she managed to achieve through her demanding, self-pitying interaction with the provider.

This provider showed respect for the patient's experience and exhibited patience in soliciting descriptions about her various concerns. Even when the patient clearly held onto false beliefs, the provider did not challenge her, express judgment, or show irritation. Rather, reality was presented firmly, and her cooperation to work on getting better from the acute infection was presented as the appropriate objective. This focus set limits on the patient's attempts to distract the provider. Not responding to the expressed complaints in ways that would encourage a special relationship was also appropriate here.

The remaining issue here is how the provider could avert the ultimate outcome—irritation and rejection of the patient's pleas for attention. The answer to this dilemma is in the provider's reflecting exactly what seems to be going on. Initially an open-ended question may be helpful: "Marcia, what's going on? You are continuing to talk about your back pain even after I told you there is no problem." This is a reflection about the process, not the content, of the encounter.

These kinds of questions generally get through to patients at deeper levels. What will probably be discovered is that the patient's view of life is that small events can be overlooked and result in tragic outcomes. Therefore, her need to dwell on what seems to be insignificant issues is understandable. Using an open-ended question actually invites the patient to talk about world views and basic premises underlying her life events. It also allows the provider an opening to discuss the differences in the patient's views (fears) and the reality of the situation. Had this conversation actually occurred, the provider may have felt more in control and less a victim of the patient's strong dependency needs (**EXHIBIT 18-9**).

The next case study describes the interaction of a provider with a patient displaying complaining and manipulative behaviors.

EXHIBIT 18-9 Case Study: Complaining and Manipulative Behaviors

Patient name: Howard R.
Age: 48 years old
Marital status: Separated
Occupation: Institutional stockbroker
Diagnosis: Diagnostic screening, possible MI hospitalization: Bed rest, diagnostic work-up

This 48-year-old institutional stockbroker is hospitalized with a possible MI. He is on bed rest and undergoing several diagnostic tests. The provider in this case is a nurse who is caring for this patient and four others on the unit as well as supervising the care of eight other patients on the unit.

PROVIDER:	"Well Mr. R____, it looks like you can get out of bed today. The doctor wrote orders for you to get up and begin to ambulate."
PATIENT:	"Well, tell the doctor I'll get up later." (Smiles at the nurse)
PROVIDER:	"Because I need to help you, it's better we do it now."
PATIENT:	"What's the results of all those tests?"
PROVIDER:	"I don't know. I have a big assignment today—it's hard to keep up on everything… Anyway, it's your doctor who will let you know."
PATIENT:	"And who knows when that will be! Well, what about that blood test? It has something to do with my heart—what are the results of that test?"
PROVIDER:	"I know you want to hear about the results. It just isn't my place to tell you, even if I did know."
PATIENT:	"Well what is your 'place'? Who are you, just the bath lady? I'll get up when I know the results of my test."
PROVIDER:	"I'm not the 'bath lady,' I'm a nurse. I guess you think that if you hold out in bed here you'll get what you want, but really, Mr. R____, I need to get you up."

PATIENT:	"It doesn't make sense—how do I know it's OK when I don't know how my tests turned out? If I ran my business like they run this hospital, I'd be bankrupt in 6 months! Angiogram—that's what it was they did, an angiogram—how did that turn out?"
PROVIDER:	"Yes, you had an angiogram. Remember, your doctor will tell you."
PATIENT:	"You know something—you've got to tell me. You're not a robot…even though you act like one. How can you work in a place like this without knowing if it is safe to get a patient out of bed?"
PROVIDER:	"I know it is safe to get you out of bed, Mr. R_____. Now let me help you…turn your legs around now…over the side of the bed."
PATIENT:	(Sitting on the edge of the bed) "So, you do know the results. I hate to be difficult, but you know I need to know these things."
PROVIDER:	(Assisting the patient to a wheelchair) "I'm going to get a bath blanket to put across your legs—here…"
PATIENT:	"I know you're trying to help …So, my tests turned out OK, huh?"
PROVIDER:	"Yes…they're probably OK. As I said, I haven't looked at your chart yet this morning. Well, anyway, your doctor will be in to see you later this morning."
PATIENT:	"He should have seen me before I was to get out of bed!"

▶ Analysis

It is obvious from an examination of this interaction that the patient was anxious about his test results but also afraid of exciting himself in ways that would put him in jeopardy. It also appears that control is an issue for this man who is accustomed to running a demanding and successful brokerage firm. He is sensitive to how work is organized and the way things should be done to maximize profits and production. He is also customarily in control as he directs the efforts of a staff of many people in his firm.

The overall presentation of the patient was hesitancy. He also attempted to "bargain" for information, implying that he would cooperate if he got what he wanted (test results). He paid little attention to the nurse's statements about the scope of practice, suggesting that he did not want to hear the nurse's descriptions and did not really care about protocol. He used several responses to try to get what he wanted. He complained about not being informed. He challenged the basis of the nurse's actions. He bargains, "I'll get out of bed when I find out my test results." He attempted to get the nurse to elaborate by offering suspicions and waiting for the nurse to respond.

The issue in this case is not whether the patient is correct in his judgments. Rather, it is the patient's need to trust providers and hospital procedures and comply with his treatment. Patients of this type can cause an uproar on a service very quickly because they seem to have legitimate complaints and they insist that procedures be done their way.

The provider responded appropriately in several ways. First, the nurse described the role of the physician and the nursing staff. Limits were set on the patient's attempts to manipulate the nurse to tell him the test results. Further, reflective statements (e.g., "I know you want to hear about the results") were used instead of angry, hostile replies. The nurse redirected the patient to the task at hand (getting out of bed) rather than being entrapped in defensive replies to insulting remarks about, for example, being "the bath lady" or being just a "robot." The patient, however, got a partial answer by deducing that he must be "OK." And while the nurse could have expressed frustration, she conceded.

Who won here? Did the patient get what he wanted? Did the nurse get what was wanted? And, at what lengths did both need to go to get these results? While it could be said that the patient won out over the nurse, in reality, the nurse "won" because the patient eventually consented to get out of bed and into the wheelchair, thus fulfilling the doctor's order. It is likely that this patient will continue to want to direct his care and that he will utilize similar manipulative strategies to achieve this. And with other, more harried nurses, the results may not turn out as they did in this case. Patients who complain and also manipulate providers can create a great deal of irritation and resentment. Experience will show that angry or hostile remarks to these patients and/or their families will likely result in battlefield conditions where control is the central issue. Providers must remember to identify the underlying meaning before choosing an appropriate therapeutic response.

▶ Summary

Of all providers' communications, those with difficult patients, difficult tasks, and difficult care contexts are the most challenging. In the high-stress environment of health care delivery systems, the demands of providing care are complicated many times over by problems with difficult patients, families, and even difficult coworkers. These problems create feelings of frustration, tension, and sometimes stronger feelings of anger and disgust. Whether a handful of patients or many more, these patients can evoke strong responses. The most critical skills are providers' capabilities in recognizing their own emotional responses and responding out of sensitivity and knowledge to the underlying meaning of these behaviors.

Patients and their families are facing moderate-to-severe levels of distress due to the multiplicity of stressors that accompany illness and injury and their treatment. They may respond in ways far removed from their customary reactions. Even transient long-standing psychological or psychiatric problems could surface. A person who is usually cooperative, receptive, and responsible may present

as complaining, demanding, and difficult to please. Still other patients who are predisposed to reactions such as self-pity and dependency will manifest these personality tendencies in heightened ways. These individuals may actually feel frightened and helpless but the underlying meaning of their behavior may go undetected. The behaviors that patients exhibit very frequently can be difficult for providers to deal with because they are outside what is generally accepted. Patients' responses may even surprise themselves, their family, and friends as well. Likewise, providers' unchecked responses can surprise themselves and their peers as well as patients and their families.

As previously indicated, the key to dealing with difficult behaviors in therapeutic ways lies in providers' abilities to respond, not react, to the communications of these patients and their families. The crucial condition is engaging in an analysis of patients' behaviors wherein the underlying meanings (hidden thoughts, feelings, and attitudes) are uncovered and understood. Empathy is key in dealing with these patients because the provider focuses more on patients' emotions, not behavior. It is important to recognize that strong emotions directed at health care providers are often misplaced. Becoming aware of one's own tendencies to respond emotionally is also important. Providers' responses can then reflect both reluctance to response-match (e.g., anger matched by anger) and thoughtful consideration of the patients' circumstances.

Perhaps the most difficult of all difficult patient and/or family behaviors are those that provoke providers to retaliate angrily or withdraw. Examples of these behaviors are aggression, demands, complaints, and/or manipulation. Therefore, it is important to anticipate such reactions and think intelligently and objectively about what choices a provider has in responding to these behaviors. Providers can prepare for these encounters by observing conversations between providers and patients and their families and by identifying specific behaviors and attitudes that have a negative impact on them. Better yet, providers can practice responding to these scenarios in the protective and instructive environment provided by formal course work and discussions. One would expect fearful patients to behave in demanding ways, families to be critical of their relative's care, and coworkers to be on edge.

Expectations of patients, their families, and coworkers should be viewed in the context of difficult situations. Appropriate guidelines and the providers' use of therapeutic response modes should considerably decrease the toll that difficult behavioral responses have on provider encounters.

Discussion

1. Discuss whether the percentage of difficult patient encounters in primary care settings might exceed 10%. Give a rationale for whatever estimate you think is more representative of actual occurrences.

2. Identify and analyze several patient-, provider-, situation-level factors that make for a "difficult patient encounter."

3. Identify and discuss at least two guidelines in working with difficult patient encounters.

4. Discuss the possibility that difficult encounters with patients could lead to professional stress in health providers.

5. Using one of the patient–provider scenarios described in this chapter, give your analysis of what happened.

References

American Psychiatric Association. (2013). *Diagnostic and statistical manual of mental disorders* (5th ed.). Washington, DC.

An, P. G., Manwell, L. B., Williams, E. S., Laiteerapong, N., Brown, R. L., Rabatin, J. S., ... Linzer, M. (2013). Does a higher frequency of difficult patient encounters lead to lower quality care? *The Journal of Family Practice*, *62*(1), 24–29. PMID:23326819

Chepenik, L. G. (2015). Difficult patient encounters: Medical education and modern approaches. *Current Emergency and Hospital Medicine Reports*, *3*(4), 195–201. doi:10.1007/s40138-015-0084-8

Dudzinski, D. M., & Timberlake, D. (2014). Difficult patient encounters. In Ethics in Medicine, University of Washington School of Medicine. Retrieved from https://depts.washington.edu/bioethx/topics/diff_pt .html

Hahn, S. R. (2001). Physical symptoms and physician-experienced difficulty in the patient-physician relationship. *Annuals of Internal Medicine, 134,* 897–904. PMID:11346326

Hardavella, G., Aamli-Gaagnat, A., Frille, A., Saad, N., Niculescu, A., & Powell, P. (2017). Top tips to deal with challenging situations: Doctor–patient interactions. *Breathe*, *13*(2), 129–135. doi:10.1183 /20734735.006616

Hinchey, S. A., & Jackson, J. L. (2011). A cohort study assessing difficult patient encounters in a walk-in primary care clinic, predictors and outcomes. *Journal of General Internal Medicine, 26*(6), 588–594. doi: 10.1007/s11606-010-1620-6

Hull, S. K., & Broquet, K. (2007). How to manage difficult patient encounters. *Family Practice Management*, *14*(6), 30–34.

Institute of Medicine. (2004). *Improving medical education: Enhancing the behavioral and social science content of medical school curriculum*. Washington, DC: The National Academies Press. doi:10.17226/10956

Koekkoek, B., van Meijel, B., & Hutschemaekers, G. (2006). "Difficult patients" in mental health care: A review. *Psychiatric Services, 57*(6), 795–802. doi:10.1176/ps .2006.57.6.795

Krebs, E. E., Garrett, J. M., & Konrad, T. R. (2006). The difficult doctor? Characteristics of physicians who report frustration with patients: an analysis of survey data. *BMC Health Services Research*, 6, 128. doi:10.1186/1472-6963-6-128

Lorenzetti, R. C., Jacques, C. H., Donovan, C., Cottrell, S., & Buck, J. (2013). Managing difficult encounters: Understanding physician, patient, and situational factors. *American Family Physician*, *87*(6), 419–425. PMID:23547575

Mamede, S., van Gog, T., Schuit, S. C. E., van den Berge, K., van Daele, P. L. A., Bueving, H., ... Schmidt, H. G. (2016). Why patients' disruptive behaviours impair diagnostic reasoning: A randomized experiment. *BMJ Quality & Safety, 26*(1), 13–18. doi:10.1136 /bmjqs-2015-005065

Marcum, Z. A., Sevick, M. A., & Handler, S. M. (2013). Medication nonadherence: A diagnosable and treatable medical condition. *JAMA : The Journal of the American Medical Association, 309*(20), 2105–2106. doi:10.1001/jama.2013.4638

Osterberg, L., & Blaschke, T. (2005). Adherence to medication. *New England Journal of Medicine, 353*(5), 487–497. doi:10.1056/NEJMra050100

Schmidt, H. G., van Gog, T., Schuit, S. C. E., Van den Berge, K., Van Daele, P. V. A. L., Bueving, H., … & Mamede,S. (2016). Do patients' disruptive behaviours influence the accuracy of a doctor's diagnosis? A randomized experiment. *BMJ Quality & Safety, 26,* 19–23. doi:10.1136/bmjqs-2015-004109

Smith, M. E., & Hart, G. (1994). Nurses' responses to patient anger: From disconnecting to connecting. *Journal of Advanced Nursing, 20*(4), 643–651. PMID:7822598

Stacey, C. L., Henderson, S., MacArthur, K. R., & Dohan, D. (2009). Demanding patient or demanding encounter?: A case study of a cancer clinic. *Social Science & Medicine (1982), 69*(5), 729–737. doi:10.1016/j.socscimed.2009.06.032

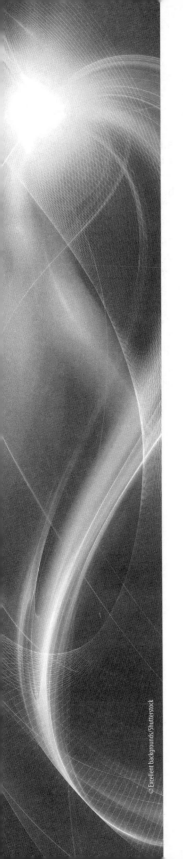

PART V

Beyond Patient–Provider Encounters: Managing Communications Within and Across Relevant Constituencies

The very dynamic that makes the health care system work is the very thing that can torpedo good communication. That is, a quality health care system is a series of layers—layers upon layers upon layers. The overwhelming number of constituents in any given case is mind-boggling. Interacting together, these layers manage a highly complex industry.

The numbers, kinds, and levels of health care providers in managed care situations are almost beyond imagination. Each provider and provider group has a commitment and responsibility to serve the patient. Their service is complicated by the fact that providers must have a common vocabulary and view situations similarly. And, if that were not enough, they must design, execute, and evaluate appropriate means or procedures for communicating across divisions and among providers and provider groups. In an amazing display of system interactions, consensus occurs and decisions are made in the spirit of providing quality patient-centered care which is also safe.

In Chapter 19, "Communications Within and Across Health Care Provider Groups," group interpersonal communication skills are discussed. Because providers make decisions in the context of the dynamics of working groups, it is important to understand the development and character of healthy group communication. Many providers will be both members and leaders of these provider teams; skill at recognizing and averting dysfunctional group communication patterns is essential.

Chapter 20, "Conflict in the Health Care System: Understanding Communications and Resolving Disputes," describes the qualities of communication that are characterized by conflict. This communication includes interactions on a continuum from minimally helpful to disruptive interactions. Negotiation and conflict-resolution skills are discussed as potential solutions to provider conflicts and as restorative steps in cases where communication seems hopelessly derailed.

Finally, Chapter 21, "Family Dynamics and Communications with Patients' Significant Others," addresses the constituency that rarely simply "sits on the sidelines." Families differ a great deal in their constellation as do support networks in their complexity. Whatever the makeup, the "family" is a relevant constituency that must be considered. It is not simply another layer. Rather, the family is pivotal in achieving successful medical outcomes. As such, providers must be concerned with how the family adapts. Significant others, particularly families, have the power to represent the patient in affairs of health and illness. Communicating effectively with families, even beyond the immediate patient–provider encounter, is critical to the outcome of care and the dynamics of the therapeutic alliance.

CHAPTER 19

Communications Within and Across Health Care Provider Groups

CHAPTER OBJECTIVES

- Describe functional and dysfunctional communication patterns in groups, especially in problem-solving or work groups.
- Identify and describe common group communication problems (e.g., conflict and delays in solving problems).
- Identify at least one example of how problems in staff or team communications can result in inadequate documentation of patient problems and consequently poor care or even no approved plan of care.
- Discuss the role of the group leader or manager in optimizing group communications.
- Conflicts can occur between groups as well as within groups; discuss problems that occur across provider groups and how these might impact coordination of patient care.

KEY TERMS

- Functional or dysfunctional group communications
- Formal groups and informal groups
- Group conflict
- Group content
- Group maintenance
- Group process
- Leadership styles (transformational and interactional)
- Stages of group development
- Types of groups

▶ Introduction

Health care organizations are composed of health care providers and teams of providers from multiple disciplines who function in a cohesive manner to provide the highly coordinated and high-risk activity of patient care (Ratnapalan & Uleryk, 2014). These providers are organized in interconnected care teams and committees to provide quality care and patient safety. Given new advances such as Internet technology, health care teams and work groups are not always meeting face-to-face. They may be communicating remotely and no more than two providers might be in a face-to-face encounter. Concepts of group behavior and group development still apply in understanding what goes on in these somewhat loose gatherings of work groups.

In health care systems, providers are always interacting in group contexts. These groups include peer, multidisciplinary, patient–family, and consumer groups. They may be homogenous teams (include only members of a particular department) or heterogeneous teams (include system-wide representation from various departments). According to Ratnapalan and Uleryk (2014), teams within the organization can be either "frontline" or "invisible." Examples of frontline patient care teams are physicians and nurses or ancillary care teams such as radiologists and laboratory technicians; those that are invisible are operating behind the scene. Examples would be a hospital's biomedical engineering team, kitchen staff, or information technology teams. These teams are interdependent and interconnected but their interrelationships are sometimes not apparent or appreciated. Every team has something in common, reliance upon sound communication processes.

There can be variability across teams in how well they function and how well they communicate with other teams or groups. It is important to understand how to assess levels of group functionality. Some communications in groups are productive. They facilitate goal and task achievement, and they meet members' needs for a sense of belonging. Other groups communicate in nonconstructive or dysfunctional ways. They display an inability to define and/or achieve goals and complete tasks. Their communication can be marked by conflict, apathy, and the inability to make decisions.

A dysfunctional group frustrates its members and expends a great deal of energy in unproductive communication. All health providers should be able to identify and assess group communication problems, interrupt dysfunctional interactions, and facilitate a shift toward more functional communication patterns.

Health professionals do at times have a less than ideal collegial relationship with health provider peers (Gadacz, 2003). As in any work group, a finely tuned team of providers can accomplish much more than the total individual efforts of its members. Professional work groups can be enjoyable and personally satisfying for most providers. The key is to better understand the nature of group relationships and avoid the traps of dysfunctional group interactions.

As previously stated, sound communication within or between provider groups and teams are important in the care of patients and their families. This is particularly the case for patients with multiple health conditions, problems in navigating the health care system, special health care needs (including children with disabilities), care needs requiring different types of providers and specialists, life-threatening illnesses, and at a greater risk of adverse patient care events. As teams, groups of providers are responsible for discussing plans for treatment, informing each other of changes in patients' health status, communicating about changes in treatment, and bringing others up-to-date on the current results of examinations and medical tests. Providers also have responsibility for ensuring that patients' health records are up-to-date and that the records follow the patient through the health care system.

When this happens smoothly, there is less trauma to the patient and family, lower risk for repeated unnecessary tests, and less possibility for mistakes or omissions in care.

▶ The Pervasive Nature of Groups

Groups involve the interactions of three or more people. Groups can be found everywhere and in all aspects of one's daily experience. Human interaction is characterized by small-group constellations with the first and primary group being the family group. We have regular contact with some groups and infrequent interaction with others. We also have "invisible" groups that do not occupy our daily activities but are present in the form of *a reference group.*

Reference groups are groups that provide a backdrop for judging our behaviors and the behaviors of others. One example of a reference group is a group of people that model behaviors that we aspire to emulate. There are many examples. Consider teenagers who practice basketball while having in mind the skills and characteristics of their favorite basketball players. These teens may not have access to basketball stars but shape their behavior, values, and goals to fit what they envision they should be if they were members of a pro basketball team. Thus, reference groups act as a frame of reference for those aspiring to become a member of this hypothetical group.

Health providers have reference groups that fit their ambitions as well. Think of those that aspire to be, for example, heart surgeons or to design a program to support a cause. While we all have reference groups, the types of groups addressed in the following sections of this chapter apply largely to work groups or teams of health providers. When considering provider work groups, it is helpful to think of them as *glue* (i.e., *the glue* that keeps this fairly diverse set of practitioners communicating well with each other on the behalf of quality care and patient safety).

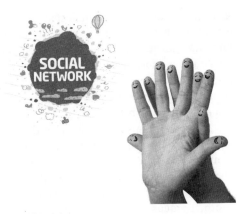

© Ra2studio/Shutterstock.

The perception of interdependency among group members keeps these individuals communicating with one another.

Types of Groups

Most people are impacted by a variety of **types of groups**. Health providers spend a significant proportion of their personal and work lives in groups. On the personal level, these include family, friends, neighborhoods, and communities. Providers also belong to a number of professional task groups. Task groups include peer or multidisciplinary teams. Task groups are work groups whose primary purpose is the completion of some objective or goal. They focus on the specifics of the task(s) at hand and on getting the job done.

Task groups can serve as reference groups but usually their affiliation is more transient. For example, health providers may be members of a quality-improvement committee. Members tend to identify with the objectives of the group and reflect the goals and values of this committee. This task group serves as a reference group when there is strong identification with the group. Such groups, however, rarely serve as permanent reference groups, and other groups (e.g., culture or religious groups) are peoples' primary reference groups because of their universal and long-standing impact on one's life.

Another way of conceptualizing groups is through the designation of "formal" or "informal" groups. **Formal groups** within an institutional setting are reflected in organizational charts, policies, and procedures. **Informal groups** function in more oblique ways such as those that influence needs, values, attitudes, expectations, traditions, group norms, and network communications (the grapevine or social network).

Informal groups are made up of three or more individuals whose purpose is primarily to meet the affiliation needs of its members. The cliché, "people need people," describes the motivation behind the establishment of informal groups. Informal groups can always be found in large organizations despite the fact that formal organized groups are more noticeable and are given importance because of their link to organizational purpose and goals.

If one were to study a formal organization such as a hospital or a large medical center, a number of loosely formed social groups could be identified. Information, support, and a sense of belonging are generally the outcomes that motivate people to form informal groups. Within the formal structure of the organization, then, are a number of affiliations that create what has come to be known as the informal channels of communication. Informal groups can cross peer and professional lines.

Because receiving and exchanging information for personal advantage is so key to these groups, informal groups rely heavily on face-to-face regular encounters wherein they share the latest gossip, speculation about administrative decisions, and information that enhances personal influence and power. Some group theorists attribute a great deal of influence to informal groups and informal channels of communication and explain that if you really want to know what is going on, study the informal communication networks.

The second type of group is the formal group, also known as a task group or work group. These groups are organized around institutional aims which include professional, moral, and ethical standards. More often than not, they have specific delineated objectives and procedures for reaching their goals,

frequently articulated in mission statements and strategic plans. They possess authority, are accountable for their actions, and are generally regarded as having both official sanction and an area of recognized influence. They also display hierarchical arrangements, governing relationships, and influence within their membership.

Phases or Stages of Group Development

Some people may find that the interactions that go on in groups are very mysterious. What makes groups decide what they decide, act as they do, come together, and dissolve? The workings of groups are both complex and easily understood. An important way to understand groups is through the concepts of task, process, and stages of development. A group's task is an important feature.

The **group content** is driven by the task that the group is working on and is usually the explicit reason that the group exists, and this purpose should be readily discernible. The second aspect to understand is the *process* of the group or **group process**. The process of the group refers to the manner in which the group works together. The process of the group may not be readily apparent because it refers to the interpersonal relationships within the group and the sequential interaction as it unfolds from meeting to meeting. It is much more than what is recorded in meeting minutes.

It is commonly understood that groups proceed through various **stages of development**. Some theorists speak of phases and subphases, others of stages and substages. Inherent in this notion about groups is the observation that groups can vary a great deal depending on how long the group has been in existence. This idea is not difficult to accept at face value. Most of us, even those who are not sophisticated in analyzing group process, would notice differences in communications. Discussions in newly formed groups are relatively superficial. Newly formed task groups may cling to the task, while established task groups are not threatened by an occasional deviation of the group's purpose.

In actuality, there are many theories that describe how groups develop over time. These theories range from complex mathematical models to theories that are grounded in the direct observation of group dynamics. Some models delineate three phases or stages (e.g., Lewin's three-stage process: unfreezing, change, and freezing [Arrow, Henry, Poole, Wheelan, & Moreland, 2005]). Other models describe more stages and specify leadership strategies that help groups move successfully toward meeting their goals. A commonly used model to describe group development in teams or work groups was originally proposed by Tuckman and Jensen (1977).

Tuckman described five discreet stages explaining small-group development: forming, storming, norming, performing, and adjourning. Member behaviors are explained by the stage of group development. For example, in the forming stage, members learn about the task and each other. This stage is identified by certain behaviors (e.g., lack of commitment and involvement, and confusion) which make the case for having a leader or coordinator to help facilitate group goals and a team-shared mental model (Manges, Scott-Cawiezell, & Ward, 2017).

The storming stage refers to the process of the group where members may argue about the structure of the group. According to Manges, Scott-Cawiezell, and Ward (2017), a leadership strategy would include helping to resolve the conflict and tension (e.g., by acting as a resource). Norming and performing depict a time when the group establishes rules and directions for achieving the group's goals (norming), and the group reaches a conclusion and implements the solution to their issue (performing). Finally, the stage of adjourning signifies the end of the group project and disbanding of the group. Each of the five stages of this model involves two aspects: interpersonal relationships and task behaviors, implying that both aspects are critical in understanding the group's development and need for specific leadership strategies.

Whether ascribing to a simple conceptual model or to a more complex model of how groups change over time and the leadership strategies needed, it is important as health care providers working on teams and in task groups to understand that communication can differ a great deal depending on the group's stage of development.

Functional Versus Dysfunctional Communication and Problem Solving in Groups

Groups, and particularly group communications, can be described as **functional or dysfunctional group communications**. In all likelihood, groups perform somewhere on a continuum of *functionality*. Some theories of group development (e.g. the Tuckman model), explain that functionality can be explained by the stage of group development. Otherwise, for example, in the norming stage, a number of dysfunctional behaviors occur: lack of involvement and commitment, confusion, and poor listening behaviors.

Usually if a group is proceeding smoothly toward its goals and if attendance and morale are high, the group is regarded as functional. Signs of functionality on a health care team would be working together to achieve common goals, recognition that each member is essential to achieving the goals of the group, clear and fluid communication across and within channels, a cross-section of skills and knowledge to achieve goals, and effective sharing of information to meet health care delivery goals and needs.

In contrast, groups that appear to be *dysfunctional* would demonstrate difficulties in goal achievement, significant membership fluctuation (due to dissatisfaction or turnover), a tendency to miss deadlines, avoiding requests for information, absenteeism, passive-aggressive behavior, gossiping, complaining, and filing grievances. These behaviors may all be indicative of dysfunction. If a task group is not successful it is not a good working group. Group members are neither communicating collaboratively nor effectively. All of these indicators can be observed at some point in most groups, but it is the degree to which they are present that distinguishes a group's functionality.

Consider, for example, a team that is established to evaluate the cost-effectiveness of using nurses to perform minor suturing in the emergency room. The hospital's administration established a task force that consists of a variety of disciplines. Only one-third of the membership, however, is truly invested in the issue. The other two-thirds of the membership believe that a task force is not necessary, does not really care about the outcomes or decisions that are reached, do not have time to meet, and/or are not directly affected by the results of any decisions made by the task force.

The group is dysfunctional because attendance is poor. It is not that the members are unable to make decisions or could not deliberate successfully and suggest a proposal; this same group of individuals may have worked extremely well together on other task forces. Nonetheless, the group at this time seems to be dysfunctional. Corresponding leadership strategies would include facilitating development of agreed-upon group goals and creating a process for the group to move forward in meeting its goals.

To summarize, although exactly what constitutes a healthy group is often unclear, organizational theorists generally agree that there are several attributes that are indicative of functional groups (**EXHIBIT 19-1**).

Whether groups go through a dysfunctional stage and reach resolution or remain stuck in dysfunctional interactions, group development issues are significant in the life of all health providers.

EXHIBIT 19-1 Attributes of Functional Groups

- Group processes encourage and enable work to be done. They do not prevent it.
- The knowledge and expertise of members may be the same or complementary, and control and influence are equally distributed.
- Members are clearly supportive of the group as a whole.
- A sufficient number of good and novel ideas and suggestions keep the group working successfully toward its goals.
- Members evaluate their relationships in the group as supportive and constructive.
- Leaders take their roles and responsibilities seriously.
- Members understand the goals and procedures that will meet the group's aims and objectives and have the resources to reach group goals.
- An appropriate level of feedback and rewards for goal attainment are experienced.
- Members' personal effectiveness is valued. Individuals grow and develop as a result of their group involvement.

▶ Identifying Group Communication Problems

Health care managers and administrators are required to have excellent communication skills, including abilities to lead and organize work groups and promote teamwork (Healthcare Leadership Alliance [HLA] model [Clement et al., 2016]). This includes a deliberate role in resolving and managing conflict within groups and teams. The ability to judge group effectiveness is critical to achieving this role and, as a matter of fact, important not only to leaders but members of work groups and teams.

Positive group behaviors have been identified as those that support the work of the group and loyal to its aims and goals. Group problematic behaviors have been described by many theorists with some focusing on team building and others on small group development. One classic conceptualization that continues to have practical relevance to work groups is described by Bradford, Stock, and Horowitz (1978, pp. 94–104). Essentially, three common group communication problems are identified: conflicts or "fights," apathy and nonparticipation, and inadequate decision-making.

Conflicts, Disputes, and Disagreements

In actuality, what is meant by conflict, fights, and disagreements in work groups is not shouting matches and fist fights; rather, what is observed in many groups are the following: disagreements, arguments, nasty comments, and unresolved passive-aggressive behaviors. These behaviors are usually indicative of some level of **group conflict**. Members' dialogue in the group might be strained and uncomfortable, and usually the atmosphere is tense.

Bradford et al. (1978) enumerated 11 ways fighting occurs in groups. They are paraphrased and listed below (**EXHIBIT 19-2**).

As these authors suggest, there may be several reasons for group dysfunctional interaction. For example, the task group may have been given an impossible goal, and members are frustrated because they feel inadequate in meeting the demands of the task. Smaller groups such as committees within larger organizations may have this problem because they have too few members to accomplish the task(s) or the specifics of what they are to do have not been sufficiently communicated to them. At other times, they may think they do not have sufficient power or influence required to implement their ideas. Any one of these predicaments can cause frustration and

EXHIBIT 19-2 Descriptions of Fighting in Groups

1. Members behave impatiently toward others.
2. Ideas are criticized before they are even completely expressed.
3. Polarization of sides occurs with refusals to compromise.
4. Members disagree openly on plans, objectives, and suggestions without resolving these disagreements.
5. Comments and suggestions are forcefully presented with a great deal of fervor.
6. Members attack each other on a personal level and in subtle ways.
7. Members discredit the group (e.g., insisting that the group does not have the ability or knowledge to accomplish tasks).
8. There are suspicions that there is something about the group (e.g., its size) that keeps it from accomplishing tasks.
9. Disagreements with the leader's ideas or suggestions occur frequently and consistently.
10. Members are openly critical of one another, particularly of their inability to understand real issues.
11. Rather than hearing and understanding comments, members hear distorted fragments of other's communications.

irritation and cause bickering and arguments within the group as well as between the group and administrators.

A second explanation is that the main purpose of members attending group meetings is not to work toward goals but to "flex some muscle." That is, members are motivated to join the group because it is a place to establish their status on the team. Consider, for example, a physician who is chief of staff and who is participating as a member in a multidisciplinary meeting. This physician feels the need to comment on every suggestion or issue before the group. It is as if the group cannot proceed toward closure on any issue before it hears from the chief of staff. The example is of a powerful physician but could as likely be a motivated health provider in another health discipline, such as nursing, pharmacy, dentistry, or physical therapy.

Members such as these may disagree with others or oppose a certain solution just to flex muscle. Once set in motion, this behavior may be seen in other members as well. Power moves begetting power moves or power struggles can preoccupy the group and stifle achievement of group goals. Formal group leaders are usually drawn into these power struggles which sometimes are an attempt to dethrone the appointed group leader.

Sometimes groups are filled with conflict because certain members are loyal to other groups that have conflicting points of view or interests. This might be the case, for example, if members of the multidisciplinary team on the emergency room task force have dual interests and are loyal to some other group. The most cost-effective solutions may not fit with the ideals and interests of the members' own professional group. If the nurses on the task force realize the best solution but evaluate it as opposing the best interests of nurses in the hospital, they may not know whether to respond as a committee member or in keeping with their professional alliance with other hospital nurses.

In the group, these members may vacillate on issues or express confusing ideals. Occasionally, their expressed alliances to groups outside the task force may be made forcefully and they may be labeled as disruptive because of their irritation or stubbornness. Blatant opposition may be interspersed with expressions of passive resentment or refusals to cooperate. One response of the group may be to "blackball" these members, recognizing that it is difficult to work cooperatively alongside them.

Still, another explanation for conflict and disagreement is the honest, high-level involvement that members feel in relation to the task and their hardworking attempts to solve problems surrounding the task or goals. Rather than feeling uninvolved in the outcome, they feel that they have a really high stake in any solutions proposed by the group. Impatience, irritability, or disagreement may reflect their overinvolvement. Interestingly enough, their behavior may appear to others as disruptive of the goal. Others may come down "heavy" on their attitudes and outspokenness.

To some extent, the group appears to be unable to handle emotions of these most dedicated and committed members. If other members engage these members in dialogue and the group moves further along in its goals, the group remains functional. If, however, interpersonal struggles take the place of needed problem-solving, the group can fall prey to ongoing dysfunctional communication problems.

Imagine a group where some members are overinvolved and are expressing irritation in the group, and suppose the leader or chairperson gets angry at these individuals and criticizes their behavior openly in the group. All group members are witnesses to the anger and criticism of the group leader. How might the group react as a whole? Not only will these overinvolved members be misunderstood but it is very likely that the group will lose confidence in the leader. Rather than express criticism, it would be important to interpret the overinvolvement of members as their having concerns and maybe hesitation. Such acknowledgment; for example, "Phil, I know you have a big investment in this issue—whatever we decide will affect just about everyone in your department." In this way, the leader addresses Phil's behavior with understanding and acceptance rather than barring his participation because it seems to be more extreme.

In assessing conflict and disagreement, leaders must decipher the underlying issues and motivation behind members' behaviors. It is these dynamics that should be addressed, not necessarily the behavioral symptoms of conflict.

Nonparticipation and Apathy

The opposite of overinvolvement in a group is, of course, underinvolvement. Underinvolvement can be evidenced as apathy, absenteeism, and nonparticipation. It is detrimental to group communication for many reasons. Frequently, dysfunctional groups are typified by high levels of apathy, which unfortunately, occurs more often than one would like to think. Individual members, as well as entire groups, may suffer from apathy. However, functional groups can also go through "dry" periods in which productivity has slowed and the group lapses into periods of inactivity and this would not be concerning. Taken to a different level, it is problematic. Apathy can appear as complete boredom or a lack of enthusiasm or a failure to mobilize energy toward the task. Some members may show a lack of consistent action and others will appear to be content with low-level performance.

If one were to walk into a multidisciplinary meeting at a medical center never having attended the group before it might be quickly apparent that the level of apathy in the group is high and is displayed in members' lack of enthusiasm. Verbal and nonverbal behaviors showing member interest might include open exchanges between many members and attempts to clarify communication. On the other hand, verbal and nonverbal behaviors might suggest apathy including silence, yawning or dozing off, distractibility, absences or lateness, restlessness, frivolous decision-making, failure to follow through on decisions, early adjournment, and reluctance to take on more responsibility.

These groups are more likely to display low levels of decision-making and responsibility. Members might even label the group as "deadbeat," "boring," or "going nowhere." It is true that apathy and boredom can overtake any group. Some groups, however, seem to be more apathetic than others. An apathetic group also reflects the absence of high-quality group leadership. Generally speaking, groups behave more positively with an upbeat, enthusiastic, inspirational leader—an individual with vision and direction—to establish and maintain interest and morale and to overcome periodic apathetic phases.

As with anger in the group, providers should treat apathy as a symptom of an underlying problem. In their early work on apathy in the workplace, Bradford et al. (1978) identify several underlying causes for apathy: (1) lack of investment in the problem or task of the group, (2) barriers to arrive at solutions to the problem, (3) inadequate approaches or procedures to address the problem, (4) a sense of powerlessness over final decisions, and (5) prolonged conflict that has significantly affected the group over time. In many kinds of situations, members feel that they have had no part in initiating a program or project, and in establishing its priority.

Under these circumstances, members approach problems as if they were imposed on them and represent meaningless busywork. Apathy can be even more pronounced if the tasks have little or no relationship to group members' perceived needs or concerns. There may be members who are more immediately involved and committed, but a core of apathetic, disinterested members can bring the whole group to a standstill.

Sometimes members are given responsibilities but feel conflicted about them. An example would be making decisions but knowing they will be unpopular. Consider, for example, clerical staff who feel resentful when asked to revise policies. If these policies are controversial, then any decision—one way or the other—will be met with disapproval from some professionals or administrators.

Very rarely will group members want to assume accountability for actions or decisions when the information or resources to solve a problem are inadequate. This situation is frequently viewed as an inadvertent or deliberate set-up for failure. If, for example, a team of cardiologists interested in establishing an adequate teaching program for their postsurgery patients assigned the responsibility to their nursing staff but could not supply the task force with essential information as to the content that should be covered or who was available to help implement the program, the group is likely to falter. This problem would be even more prohibitive if the physician group did not communicate with the task force.

Most of the time providers are assigned tasks they are capable of completing. However, sometimes they feel that they will make no real headway on the assigned problem. This may be because their recommendations are not really valued or because the real decisions have already been made. This happened to the staff on a geriatric inpatient and outpatient service. The staff was to establish a project for continued quality improvement. They met to deliberate but, over time, grew to realize that the supervisory group was really not invested in implementing their recommendations. They became suspicious that this assignment was a response to an anticipated review by the Joint Commission on Accreditation of Healthcare Organizations (JCAHO). They felt as if they were assigned to go through the motions but no serious attempt to change patient care was intended. This concern was not substantiated in remarks made by the supervisory group but the damage can occur just the same.

Status and authority differences within a group can also create the feeling that whatever contributions members make will not be heard or heeded. On occasion, one member, and it may or may not be the officially appointed leader of the group, will dominate the group process. Sometimes, rather than a single dominant member, there will be a specific subgroup that monopolizes the group's meetings. In instances such as these, other members experience group communication as restricted because only the views of a select few seem to influence group decisions.

In some cases, competition within the group can serve to provoke others to speak or may alienate quiet or passive members who may withdraw even further. Competition in a group can be healthy; however, when it is intense and prolonged, it may cause a sense of helplessness and powerlessness that leads to significant disenchantment or apathy among noncompetitive members.

Inability to Make Decisions

Decision-making in a group is not always easy because communication in groups can be quite complicated. As previously described in a summary of stages of group development, groups seem to have to progress through stages of development that correspond to members' interpersonal needs. Sometimes satisfactory decisions come easily; other times, especially early in the life of a group, they are hard to come by. Reasons for inadequate or incomplete decision-making are many. Certainly, problems such as anger and apathy influence decision-making capabilities in a group.

At other times groups are confronted with decisions that are too difficult (e.g., when members are pressured to make decisions too early or when the group has not jelled sufficiently to feel comfortable with the results of their deliberations). Certainly, no group of health care professionals wants to make what is deemed "a premature decision."

Premature decision-making is regarded as very risky. Therefore, asking a group of providers to come to a quick decision based on inadequate data stands in opposition to their customary approach to issues. These decisions may be perceived as potentially threatening. A fear of being wrong or of creating unclear and undesired consequences can be the result.

Signs that groups are manifesting an inability to make decisions include indecisiveness, repetitive discussions, or attempts to shift the decisions to some other group. The discussion may wander or be filled with hypothetical situations. Sometimes, just as the group appears to be reaching consensus, the group will argue that no real agreement exists or some members will disown responsibility for the decisions and a new task group might be established.

▶ Improving Communication in Health Care Teams and Work Groups

Fortunately, the number of conflict-resolution programs and consultants has increased, and today, most providers are expected to be trained in conflict resolution and multidisciplinary collaboration. This is important for new professionals learning how to organize groups to direct team projects or for those organizing and managing work teams of providers who are engaged in direct patient care.

Project managers are generally forming and leading groups working on administrative projects with those from risk management, compliance, research labs, revenue cycle departments, marketing, training and human resources, finance and accounting, and information systems. All of these group members are coming from different departments, not involved in patient care even though their actions can and do impact patient care indirectly. These work groups differ from direct patient care groups which are reviewing and deciding courses of action to impact patient care directly.

Whatever the focus, it is important to know and understand how to work effectively as a leader in these groups. Several important factors contribute to successful communication in professional work groups. These factors include adequate preparation, preparing meaningful agendas, and being respectful of the time and pressure group members experience when taking time away from their assigned responsibilities to work on a project or work team. They also include interpersonal awareness skills (of self and others) to improve the effectiveness of the group or team and to promote satisfaction with group process and goals.

Understanding Self and Others

Self-awareness is not only extremely important in one-to-one encounters with patients, patients' families, and other providers, it is also essential to successful participation in health care professional work groups.

Becoming a valuable contributor to a work group is important. One's leadership and membership capabilities can determine the success of the group. Providers can actively influence movement in the group through their own self-awareness. Self-understanding includes awareness of how we relate to others—the impact we have on others, our strengths and weaknesses, and how we use these in a group context.

It is critical that as providers we first understand our own personal reactions to key interpersonal issues. These are feelings and reactions about interdependency, interpersonal intimacy, and authority. For example, how do health providers react to having to work with peers that lack certain skills and knowledge? If others were to attempt to shape, direct, or control our attitudes and behavior, how would we respond? If asked to take a leadership role in a group requiring us to direct others, how would we respond? Having been assigned to work cooperatively toward a group goal, what behaviors would we exhibit in collaborating with others?

In order to evaluate one's current or potential capacities to be a contributing member or take on a leadership role, it is important to reflect on how one has responded in past relationships, particularly when in small groups. Providers' current behavior and ways of communicating in a group have been influenced by the first primary group, the family. Depending on birth order, role in the family, and training and experience in leadership positions, a person may or may not exhibit strong leadership behavior.

The dynamics within one's family can contribute to current behavior (e.g., learning to placate authority figures in order to get one's needs met might be an outcome of previous family interactions). Communication within the family could have been sparse, rigid, and guarded or communication among members of the family could be marked with openness, honesty, and trust. In either case, this experience in part shapes one's current communication styles in groups.

Providers may not be totally aware of this fact or the ways in which they act in response to early beginnings. One way of establishing self-awareness is to ask oneself some very personal questions about early communication patterns within the family as a whole and within specific dyadic relationships (e.g., between oneself and an older sibling).

A second approach to self-awareness in groups is to assess our communication in the context of role theory. Group roles have been the subject of a great deal of social science research. One model of viewing member roles is to classify these roles as either self-oriented or group-oriented.

Behaviors that primarily serve an individual's needs or interests without regard to the needs or interests of the group are *self-oriented* roles. Self-oriented members may communicate in a self-protective manner which includes withholding data or communicating defensively. They may also manifest self-importance by establishing and proclaiming self-value at whatever cost. Self-adulation, then, is a predominate feature of this member's verbalizations.

In contrast to self-oriented communication styles are behaviors that are typically relevant to the fulfillment of the purpose of the group. These behaviors may be either group-maintenance or group-task focused. That is to say, both are group-oriented but they differ in that group-maintenance roles tend to satisfy only the interpersonal needs of members. For example, giving positive feedback in the group is morale enhancing. It does not relate directly to goal or task achievement but it is the important glue that keeps the group enthusiastically centered on its task.

Behaviors such as initiating new topics, providing information, summarizing group opinion, and taking minutes are all directed at helping the group achieve its goal. Specifically, members who define problems; suggest procedures for solving problems; offer ideas, facts, or information to clarify ideas; explore alternatives; restate areas of consensus; and maintain a record of group ideas and suggestions move the group toward its ultimate goal. To what extent does a person choose behaviors or communications that maintain the group or move it toward its stated goals?

Another approach that providers can use to analyze their own and others' behaviors in a work group is to examine responses to group leadership. Whether work groups are teams, committees, or *ad hoc* task forces, the nature of leadership influences communications within the group. The leadership may be democratic or autocratic or transactional or transformational. Despite common belief, not all members will prefer democratic-participative **leadership styles** over more autocratic ones. Some group tasks are more adequately addressed by autocratic styles.

Generally speaking, the more dependent members are on a leader's direction, rules, and disciplinary action, the more comfortable they may be with an autocratic leadership style. A very autocratic leader will make decisions and define rules. Concomitantly, a member who is comfortable with an autocratic style finds it difficult to function without procedures and feedback from the leader. In contrast, a leader who encourages group decision-making and simply acts as a coordinator will be most acceptable to members who tend to be self-starters and who do not need or seek close supervision.

Just how one responds to a leader's approach will influence interaction within a group. A great deal of attention and corresponding observational studies have looked at leadership style and its ability to enhance participation and communication and correct for deficits in health care delivery and

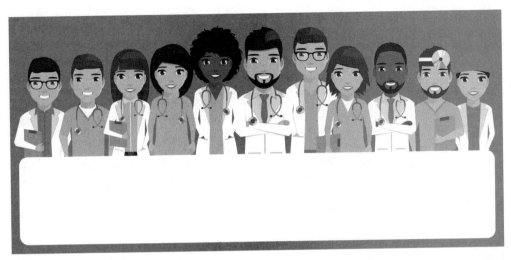

© Illin Denis/Shutterstock.

the retention of staff (Dunham-Taylor, 2000; Thyer, 2003). One such example is the relative value of "transformational" leadership over "interactional" leadership. The hallmarks of transformational leadership are its ability to influence, engage, challenge, and inspire. Transformational leadership appeals to a higher order of motivation. It seeks to raise the consciousness of members—getting them to reach beyond problems of jealousy, need for control, and power plays to work cooperatively to solve problems.

Understanding others' responses includes knowing their value systems and personal goals, their relevant skills and past experiences, what motivates them, and how they perceive others in the group. Understanding the group as a whole includes knowing the experience and capabilities of the members, the nature of the leadership, existing interpersonal relationships among team members, the cohesiveness and morale in the group, and the group's level of goal achievement.

Observe and Reflect Back to Members the Group Process

Examining communication patterns within a work group is not only a common method that is used to study group behavior, it also has

potential positive effects on a group's process and sense that the information obtained can help the group move on. Just what is important to observe and reflect back to the group?

An assessment of how well a group is functioning is determined by gathering a variety of data about the verbal and nonverbal behavior that occurs in groups (**EXHIBIT 19-3**).

Through observing these aspects of the group's communication, any interpersonal conflict and the quality of decision-making

EXHIBIT 19-3 Data to Gather in Assessing Group Functioning

- Members' verbal and nonverbal communications.
- Spatial and seating arrangements that depict attitudes toward the group or selected members.
- Common themes expressed by the group (e.g., frustration with the task).
- The pattern of communication in the group and between individuals (e.g., who talks to whom and how frequently).
- The quality of listening that occurs (e.g., member to member and leader to member).
- The level and quality of problem-solving that occurs in the group.

can be detected. Additionally, these observations will give insight into dysfunctional communication patterns.

To effectively assess, monitor, and facilitate group members' communications, it is important to understand the roles that members assume. *Role* is the position a member takes with respect to the problem-solving process within the group. Each group role has certain expected behaviors and responsibilities. Much of what one shares with the group is related to member role behavior. In addition to the identities members establish outside the group, each member exhibits behavior that is typical of one's role in the work group. For example, a member may assume or be assigned the role of record keeper.

Role selection and enactment are influenced by individual characteristics such as personality or characteristics of the member. In addition, the specific task and size of the group, the characteristics of the group interaction, and the position or status of individuals in the group, influence role assignment and role behavior. These roles are generally one of three kinds: (1) **group maintenance**, (2) group-task roles, or (3) self-oriented individual roles not related to group functioning.

There are many ways in which data can be compiled. Different kinds of observations yield different kinds of information. For example, much can be gleaned from observing who talks to whom. It is possible to diagram interactions in a group over a given period and by this method, identify problems. Consider, for example, one 15-minute segment in which 48 statements were made with the largest proportion being made by the leader of the group to the group as a whole. Few statements were made by members, and only one-eighth of the statements were members' comments to other members. Given this pattern, it might be concluded that the group was in a beginning stage of development and functioning at a low level with an autocratic leadership style.

Additionally, the kinds of contributions that were made by the leader and the members can be examined. Perhaps the majority of statements were made to challenge the advisability of the group making a decision. Based upon an appraisal of what happened in the group and the assessment of the quantity and quality of work that was accomplished, one would have a pretty sound picture of the level of group functioning, at least at this time (see **EXHIBIT 19-4**).

Groups need to include feedback mechanisms that evaluate and improve their effectiveness. Along these lines, members have a responsibility not only to observe aspects of group functioning but to give group members feedback based on these observations. This process of feedback is facilitated by directed observations. It is not enough just to make observations. The results of these observations must be fed back to the group and frequently, either the leader or minute taker will contribute to the group's assessment of itself.

EXHIBIT 19-4   Information to Gather in Determining Group Effectiveness

1. What is the group's goal? How successful is the group in keeping to the goals and/or aims of the group?
2. Where is the group in the process of decision-making: the stage of discovery, analyzing, suggesting, or testing solutions?
3. What barriers and strengths are affecting the group's task performance? How severely is the group limited by these barriers and facilitated by these strengths?
4. Is the group using the most effective measures and/or procedures to accomplish its work?
5. Is the membership participating equally in accomplishing goals and in taking actions or are a small number of individuals doing the majority of the work?
6. How are members getting along together? Are they resolving differences and disagreements?
7. What are members' opinions of and attitudes toward the group, its effectiveness, and the leadership?

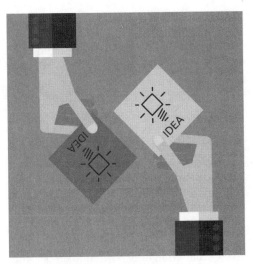

© Dmitry Guzhanin/Shutterstock.

Certain guidelines are suggested for feeding information back to the group. It is important to realize that groups, like individuals, have a low tolerance for negative feedback. Also, like individuals, they may not be receptive to feedback at the time you are ready to share your observations. Providers should be sensitive to the kinds of information that the group is ready to hear and work with and assess what will be most helpful to the group rather than what is the most telling or interesting observation.

It is important not to overload the group with observations. If too much information is presented, a group, like an individual, will not be able to put it to good use. Present one or two observations and let the group think about and digest this information. For example, it might be important to share an observation about the groups having difficulty in making a decision and the speculation that many facts are not yet known, and not knowing all the facts can prevent group members from feeling confident about any chosen direction. Once this observation is brought to the group and discussed, members will have a better understanding of their barriers to decision-making.

It is also important to gauge evaluative comments of a critical or rewarding nature. Critical, negative comments are usually received as judgments of below-standard performance. Sometimes those that make the comments are viewed as "superior" or "above it all," especially if delivered by someone with authority. On the other hand, it is also possible to praise the group so much that growth does not occur. When it comes to commenting on individuals' communication styles, it is better to discuss behaviors in general as they relate to goal attainment. It is too easy for members to perceive evaluative comments as individual attacks or favoritism. Placing the emphasis on behaviors to accomplish goals takes the emphasis off individual shortcomings or strengths.

Facilitating Group Performance Change

Early on in this chapter the topic of leadership style was discussed briefly, and the differences between types of leaders were addressed. While transformational leadership behaviors, for example, will be valued, it should be kept in mind that group changes are the business of the group members through their presentation of their views of group functioning. Once one or more members present their views of the functional capacities of the group, thoughtful consideration of what the group should do can occur. But, for this to happen, a full discussion of group strengths and limitations must come first.

The group is no different from an individual who contemplates certain weaknesses in communicating. Members should review evaluations and determine the extent to which there is group consensus about barriers in communication. The group should also be encouraged to examine the reasons for poor communication behavior. As indicated previously, many group behaviors are symptoms of larger, more profound problems (e.g., negative reactions to the organizational changes that are occurring in the institution). Finally, the group should move toward solutions. What corrective measures need to be taken or what new directions should be sought? Unless the group can successfully utilize feedback that was elicited through the observations of member interactions, the overall functioning of the group is not likely to improve. A point worth noting is that the process of members working on solutions together will increase satisfaction and motivation.

Modeling Good Group Communication Skills

What groups need most are members who can model functional communication. First and foremost, communicating effectively in groups in ways that will positively influence members depends on a particular style of interaction.

A variety of functional and effective group communication skills has been described previously. In general, they include skills in the areas of receiving, processing, and sending. Sending clear messages, speaking clearly and thoughtfully, avoiding stereotyping, maintaining good listening posture, expressing oneself honestly, listening carefully, and qualifying or clarifying vague statements are important principles of effective communication in groups. It should be noted that a climate or feeling tone in a group is extremely important because in general, supportive climates promote effective problem-solving, while defensive or aggressive climates impede effective problem-solving.

The dominant motivation behind defensive communication is power and control. Defensive communication is easily recognized because it is often designed to persuade or sway the beliefs of others. Even if the member or leader appears to be friendly and open, the basic drive is to persuade or direct others. Strategy and superiority predominate.

Supportive communications, however, promote group involvement in discussions and decision-making. The dominant goal behind supportive communication is understanding. Contrasting positions on issues are not threatening because new and meaningful outcomes can be a result of different views. Members truly seek meaningful dialogue, to listen

actively, and to explore and appreciate differences in opinion.

The results of supportive communication styles are very different from those of defensive styles. Rather than persuasion and control, members attempt to understand others' views. Empathy and mutual problem-solving characterize members' statements. Supportive climates make room for the resolution of differences that are bound to exist in any group. Active listening in a climate of mutual trust and support not only yields good communication, it is necessary for high levels of productivity and the achievement of group goals.

Although supportive communication styles seem straightforward and simple, they are often difficult to practice for many reasons. First, lack of cultural awareness and diversity training may be a major barrier. Cultural differences in the group membership may subtly impact what gets done and by whom; who will accept leadership positions and who will defer to others for leadership. Second, emphasis on competition and individual achievement, reinforced by professional values, may inhibit abilities to establish supportive climates.

Professional providers are accustomed to being rewarded for arriving at independent decisions and skills of persuasion. Although this varies across disciplines, less attention may have been given to teaching attitudes of acceptance and understanding. It is important that health care providers nurture and protect their inherent abilities for supportive communication regardless of the discipline.

If, in fact, supportive communication occurs naturally and consistently, then providers may not need to learn and model these behaviors. In addition to one's own inherent limitations, barriers exist in the context of work environments. The chief and foremost barrier is lack of time or energy. Short-cuts (e.g., Internet messaging and conference calls) have made it less necessary to have a sit-down face-to-face meeting in a group. However, the impact of the group process cannot be underestimated, not even in these groups.

Group work can be conducted online and with Internet communication and, for the most part, work well in many cases. Creating and maintaining a positive milieu takes work. The team or work group must deliberately assume responsibility for developing an atmosphere that facilitates understanding because it is often easier to respond superficially or inappropriately to what is being said or discussed. At least one member must see to it that the group responds to what is actually being said. Supportive communication also includes some risk. To the extent that one is threatened by others' opinions and communications, opinions of others will not be always perceived accurately.

Finally, it is difficult to model supportive communications when not feeling good about oneself. Feelings of anger, hostility, guilt, shame, insecurity, and self-consciousness will also affect our abilities to genuinely express and receive support. Our basic inclinations might be to response-match with criticism and negativity, which further limits mutual understanding.

There are five essentials to facilitating supportive communication (**EXHIBIT 19-5**).

EXHIBIT 19-5 Modeling and Essentials to Supportive Communication in Groups

1. An environment valuing mutual exchange must be established.
2. Active listening is important.
3. Grasping the full meaning (both fact and feelings) of what other members are saying, though not easy, must take place because discipline and role differences as well as status and authority discrepancies can create barriers to openness in provider groups.
4. Clarifying and checking out one's perceptions of messages is essential.
5. Feeding back to the group observations of communication barriers may help the group break free of stalemates.
6. By avoiding insecurities better peer-to-peer exchange is possible.

Dealing with Problem Group Members

Supportive communication is generally a sound technique in dealing with most group members. The idea is that supportive communications will facilitate group dialogue, and when response-matching occurs, supportive communication will form the basis for other member-to-member encounters. There are some instances, however, in which supportive responses are inappropriate or not useful. When observing members whose behavior is destructive in the group, interventions are needed to help members modify their behavior. One should keep in mind that simply supporting this member in such cases may reinforce behaviors that need to change.

Steps toward changing members' response patterns begin with a self-inventory. That is, as a witness to this behavior, how do you feel and what makes you feel this way? Examining your specific reactions will help define the problem behavior—is the member distracting the group from its purpose, challenging the authority of the leadership, seeking special attention, or resisting involvement? Also, what outcomes occur as a result? Is the member's behavior rewarded, punished, or simply ignored? How are other members responding to these behaviors? Are they reacting similarly or differently from you? Does the behavior warrant intervention, and if so, what kind of approach and by whom?

As in dealing with specific problem behaviors in patients, there are also specific communications that are advisable in group settings with group–member problems. In **EXHIBIT 19-6**, examples of several problematic group behaviors are listed along with examples of corrective leadership responses. These corrective responses are offered as potential strategies; they are not to be used as must dos. Problem behaviors included here are: (1) the aggressive, (2) the silent/withdrawn, (3) the shy to fragile, (4) the domineering/dominating, (5) the attention-getter/clown, and (6) the bored/detached member.

EXHIBIT 19-6 Problem Behaviors and Examples of Corrective Leader Responses

Problem Behavior	Potential Corrective Responses
Aggressive	Avoid negative confrontation.
	Encourage member to be concrete about personal feelings.
	Ask for a private conference, share feelings and ask for cooperation, point out harmful effects on others, or ask the member to leave the group.
	Assign aggressor the helpee role on a "personally relevant" topic. (Look for clues to the aggression from the person's self-disclosure.)
Silent/withdrawn	Avoid negative confrontation.
	Invite responses.
	Assign nonthreatening roles that require responding but do not demand self-disclosure to the whole group.
Shy to fragile	Avoid negative confrontation.
	Reduce risk level by supervising one-on-one interactions and avoid group exposure.
	Arrange a private conference to investigate reasons for member's behavior.
Domineering/dominating	Avoid negative confrontation.
	Avoid eye contact.
	Reward only very significant contributions.
	Ask for a private conference and assess the person's sensitivity/awareness of the problem; ask for cooperation.
	Arrange for a presentation to the group that requires appropriate, extended verbalizing.
Attention-getter/clown	Avoid negative confrontation.
	Respond to insecure feelings if present.
	Assign serious roles.
	Ask for a private conference and assess reasons for the behavior.
	Assist members to identify inappropriate humor.
Bored/detached	Avoid negative confrontation.
	Assign responsible roles.
	Provide options for creative involvement.
	Support involvement.

▶ Intergroup Problems

While communication problems clearly appear, disappear, and reappear within a specific group, these problems transcend group boundaries. Intergroup (between more than one group) communication difficulties are frequently reflected in patient care problems. Sometimes the tension within a group is also brought to interactions across groups. For example, the inability to make a decision in one group can also be seen in communications between the group and other groups or teams within the same medical center or health care organization. Thus, intergroup problems can mirror communication difficulties occurring inside the group (intragroup conflicts).

Organizations are composed of many groups; some are specific coalitions or alliances that compete with one another for resources. Discrepancies between expressed goals and values, even ethics and morals, fuel a number of communication difficulties among groups as do issues of esteem, control, and affiliation previously mentioned in describing communications within groups.

Consider, for example, a disagreement between a task force that has been assigned to choose a computer-based patient health record system, the administrative group that will purchase the system, and the service center that will pilot the new system. The staff on the pilot unit wishes to be recognized for their valuable practical ideas. The administrative group is concerned that the task force is exaggerating needs which will drive costs too high. The task force questions the sincerity of the administrative group stating that the administrators are not interested in quality tracking systems when they criticize the task force. Conflict and mistrust exist and are acted out in the relationships between the pilot group and the task force and between the administrative group and the task force.

The conflicts and disagreements between these groups may not be expressed openly. They may be acted out through various ambiguous communications and disjointed information exchanges. Information from the task force to the administrative group may be withheld or may be rigidly guarded. The pilot unit staff may express their opinions obliquely, but at other times, aggressively and all but boycott the decisions of the task force. The observable aspects of these intergroup conflicts are manifested in these communication responses.

Reflecting on this example, one can see that all the ingredients of conflict are present. First, an observable struggle exists in which opposing groups come together periodically to interact or do so through representatives. Second, there is a clear element of interdependence. The task force relies on the pilot unit, the pilot unit on the task force, and the administrative group on both the pilot unit and task force. Third, areas of contention arouse feelings. Because of the need for control, affiliation, and esteem are involved, the arousal of strong feelings is inevitable. Finally, the differences felt between these groups are deemed incompatible or are feared to be incompatible.

Incompatible beliefs, values, and goals form the content of these struggles. Desires for control and status, however, may also underlie the intergroup communication exchanges. Concerns about the unequal distribution of power among groups can affect many aspects of a provider's working life including motivation, job satisfaction, absenteeism, stress, and turnover. It is understandable that these internal struggles may have significant effects on members and when providers are under outside pressure, their performance of patient care activities could be compromised.

Conflicts between groups can be avoided or resolved using the same strategies or interventions that are appropriate within a single group. Supportive communication can replace defensive communication in these situations as well. In capacities of leadership, modeling supportive communication is essential but not enough. Recognition of the problems and their underlying dynamics, including the basis for contention, is paramount. It is important to understand the political struggles that also underlie intergroup communications. Kazley et al. (2016) address the need to promote a collaborative leadership model in health administration education. The idea is that rather than allow conflict to continue it is important to shift to the enhancement of health care management through collaborative interactions in and between work groups. Otherwise, administrators should seek a synergistic work environment.

Recognizing and factoring in the feelings that are motivating intergroup conflict will help tailor responses to the feelings of members within the groups. Rather than focusing exclusively on superficial manifestations that are revealed in the content of disagreements, group leaders should also recognize and respond to the interpersonal struggles between groups. Finally, transformational leadership perspectives may enhance the groups' abilities to rise above smaller issues and pull together to arrive at the common good.

▶ Summary

Whether they want to be or not, every health care provider is a member of different kinds of work groups. Whether they are aware of it or not, as group members they have a significant impact on the functioning of these teams which have the responsibility to deliver quality care to a wide range of patients and families. The health care workforce is unique in that there is wide disparity in knowledge, influence, and control among members.

Conflicts and resolutions of problems are always executed in this context which already assumes an uneven playing field. By far, group dynamics are inherently important in understanding member communications, in judging functional and dysfunctional communications, and in coming to resolutions.

There are a variety of factors that predispose a group to communicate in a particular way. The type of group (formal or informal) and the maturity (stage of development) of a group are critical factors influencing the way a group communicates. The internal functioning within any group—and this is true of professional work groups—is a result of the dynamic interaction of all members. It also includes the relationship of the group within the context of the larger institutional setting because the goals and resources available to a group are contingent on this interdependency with the external work environment. Communication within groups can be said to be either functional or dysfunctional. In truth, most groups lie somewhere on the continuum of effective functionality. Some theorists explain that all small work groups can be dysfunctional in the early phase of their development.

Group communication problems are manifested in a variety of ways. Conflicts, arguments, disagreements, nonparticipation, apathy, and/or the inability to make decisions effectively are diagnosable features of poorly functioning groups. Improving communications within groups not only includes knowing yourself and others but also reflecting knowledge and observations back to the group so that corrective processes can begin. Practicing and facilitating supportive communications is helpful not only in dysfunctional groups but also in maintaining a state of high-level functioning in work groups that are proceeding successfully toward their goals.

Intergroup communication problems are frequently reflective of communication problems in a larger context. Power differences, autonomy struggles, insufficient inter-professional understanding, unshared meanings, differences in perception, and interpretation of others' behavior contributes to intergroup conflict.

Intergroup and intragroup communication difficulties are everyone's concerns. Providers must work together effectively in small groups to provide both quality and safe care to patients and their families. The spirit and practice of collegiality makes quality care possible. Without it, we run the risk of putting both patients and ourselves in jeopardy. Problems with communications in and between work groups are frequently linked to adverse events in medicine (Wright et al., 2009) and health care. These include failure to communicate vital assessment information, misdiagnoses, and failed follow-up of patient treatments. Because providers typically work in groups or teams a good deal of attention and effort should be given to teaching students and practitioners how to assess and foster productive group and team communications.

Discussion

1. Distinguish between work groups and informal groups.
2. Identify both supportive and destructive group behaviors.
3. Discuss several ways of evaluating the effectiveness of a work or task group.
4. How might problems in patient care be a result of poor working relationships within a team or work group?
5. What observations about leadership in the group would provide insight into the leadership style and members' needs?

References

Arrow, H., Henry, K. B., Poole, M. S., Wheelan, S. A., & Moreland, R. L. (2005). Traces, trajectories, and timing: The temporal perspective on groups. In M. S. Poole & A. B. Hollingshead (Eds.), *Theories of small groups: Interdisciplinary perspectives* (pp. 313–368). Thousand Oaks, CA: Sage.

Bradford, L. P., Stock, D., & Horowitz, M. (1978). How to diagnose group problems in communication and group process. In L. Bradford (Eds.), *Group development* (pp. 94–104). Washington, DC: National Training Laboratories, National Education Association.

Dunham-Taylor, J. (2000). Nurse executive transformational leadership found in participative organizations. *Journal of Nursing Administration, 30*(5), 241–250. PMID: 10823177

Gadacz, T. R. (2003). A changing culture in interpersonal and communication skills. *American Surgery, 69*(6), 453–458. PMID:12852500

Kazley, A. S., Schumacher, E. J., DelliFraine, J., Clement, D., Hall, R., O'Connor, S., … Stefl, M. (2016, Winter). Competency development and validation: An update of the Collaborative Leadership Model. *The Journal of Health Administration Education, 33*(1), 73–93.

Manges, K., Scott-Cawiezell, J., & Ward, M. M. (2017). Maximizing team performance: The critical role of the nurse leader. *Nursing Forum, 52,* 21–29. doi:10.1111/nuf.12161

Ratnapalan, S., & Uleryk, E. (2014). Organizational learning in health care organizations. *Systems, 2,* 24–33. doi:10.3390/systemes2010024

Thyer, G. L. (2003). Dare to be different: Transformational leadership may hold the key to the nursing shortage. *Journal of Nursing Management, 11,* 73–79. doi:10.1046/j.1365-2834.2002.00370.x

Tuckman, B. W., & Jensen, M. A. (1977). Stages of small-group development revisited. *Group Organizational Studies, 2,* 419–427. doi:10.1177/105960117700200404

Wright, M. C., Phillips-bute, B. G., Petrusa, E. R., Griffin, K. L., Hobbs, G. W., & Taekman, J. M. (2009). Assessing teamwork in medical education and practice: Relating behavioural teamwork ratings and clinical performance. *Medical Teacher, 31*(1), 30–38. doi:10.1080/01421590802070853

CHAPTER 20

Conflict in the Health Care System: Understanding Communications and Resolving Disputes

CHAPTER OBJECTIVES

- Describe the signs and types of conflict that might be observed in health care settings.
- Define and differentiate among conflict, tension, and disputes.
- Describe the process of resolving interpersonal conflicts through the mediation process.
- Differentiate between positional bargaining and interest-based bargaining.
- Identify key factors in reaching resolutions (e.g., active listening and reframing).

KEY TERMS

- Active listening
- Bargaining
- Compromise
- Conflict
- Conflict resolution

- Consensus
- Deadlocks, stalemates, or impasses
- Disagreements, tensions, and disputes
- Mediation
- Reframing

▶ Introduction

Interpersonal conflict is neither abnormal nor irreversible. In fact, it has been said that in the midst of conflict, flickers of agreement and unity can be seen and felt. That being said, the mere mention of the word "**conflict**" strikes fear in most people. "Conflict!" and red lights flash. The English definition of the word means war, battle, or fight. In all instances, it means that a struggle has ensued as a result of differences, usually incompatible needs, values, drives, wishes, or demands. The notion of conflict resulting in someone's getting hurt is vivid. There are needs for softer words and softer ways of framing the phenomena of conflict. This is the case in the health care arena as it is in most work environments.

It may help to know that conflict is inevitable. Striving to avoid conflict of any kind is futile and unnecessary. Conflict can occur within an individual (e.g., a conflict between what one wants and should accept or between individuals). It is predictable that two or more individuals will, at some point, express **disagreements**. In any one relationship, disagreements will recur, although they may differ in content. Some of these disagreements will go incompletely resolved. Conflicts that go unresolved lead individuals to a "deadlock" in decision-making, and the quality of communications can be severely curtailed.

Chronic communication difficulties between two or more individuals are usually evidence of unresolved conflict. In the patient–provider relationship, conflicts can result in patient dissatisfaction, the patient leaving treatment, and/or lack of adherence to treatment or impaired communications with patient and families about treatment dilemmas. Conflict in health care organizations is common; in part, a consequence of the continuous change and transformation in health care placing providers under pressure to respond quickly and effectively. Their response calls for new and changing interactions with other providers who may not be clear or confident with changes in the workplace. Reports have shown that while conflict can have positive effects, it is also clear that conflict can exert negative effects on providers in health care settings.

It is the purpose of this chapter to focus on several key concepts and principles that are used not only to describe conflict but also to describe the process of **mediation** that will resolve these communication difficulties. In some cases, providers will be a party in the **disputes** (e.g., between a patient and themselves or between a patient's family and themselves). At other times, they may not be one of the disputants (persons involved in a disagreement or dispute) but they are intimately affected by the presence of the conflict. In some instances, they may have a role in mediating a dispute between others (e.g., between physician specialty groups, between pharmacists and physicians, or between teaching staff and administrators). Dealing successfully with conflict requires specific communication skills. Everyone needs to be familiar with the dynamics and skills of **conflict resolution**.

As previously stated, good or bad, in our society, conflict is inevitable. Disputes can happen at any time and are observed everywhere—in interpersonal relationships as well as in small and in large groups. Sometimes the disputes are quite apparent but they can also be latent or emerging. In the workplace, disputes arise at all levels—between patients and providers; among coworkers, managers, and supervisors. On occasion, they involve many other departments directly or indirectly. Because the costs of unresolved conflicts are very high and result in potentially tremendous litigation expenses, more and more attention is placed on early resolution of conflicts, or better yet, on preventing them in the first place.

Certain work situations might appear to be "magnets" for conflict. Environments in which conflicts occur very frequently are those where major changes have occurred and where unclear or overlapping roles, ambiguous lines of authority, and inadequate communication occur. These conditions may produce conflict and/or worsen conflict that already exists. Issues of diversity (e.g., gender, age, status, ethnicity, and race) are sometimes at the base of the conflict. In other instances, these factors provide a unique context for the central issue around which conflict exists.

▶ Conflicts and Communication

Conflict is omnipresent. Everywhere we turn, we can observe conflict in interpersonal relationships. Conflict can occur between individuals, groups, and organizations. Most individuals grow up witnessing and participating in conflict with siblings, parents, friends, and neighbors.

When conflict occurs in the workplace but is modified by rational responses, it appears as if there are no disputes or conflicts; or, if conflict does exist, it is minimal, circumspect, and transient. In health care delivery systems, it is assumed that conflict is minimal or minimized because it needs to be. Also, clinical work is an empirically defined practice and requires predictability and control. One would think that there would be a very low tolerance for conflict. Still, in health care delivery systems, disputes and conflicts arise regularly for different reasons.

On occasion, these conflicts spill over to individuals or groups who are not parties in the dispute but who are affected directly or indirectly by the actions of the disputants. As in many other industries, health care systems become involved in large litigation suits between parties who cannot agree. Problems in the delivery of quality care may be a result of conflict. At other times, conflict results from perceptions that inadequate care was provided.

Health providers generally find support from their encounters with other providers.

These relationships often offer different points of view, new information, and a sense of affiliation. They also offer a respite or break from the stressful experience of giving care and when behaviors of patients or families are difficult to address. Still, conflict occurs even when providers strive to avoid it.

Recognizing the potential for conflict to derail delivery of quality care in health care organizations, Hetzler, Messina, and Smith (2011) emphasize that it is important to recognize the vital role of communication and conflict skills. They explained that these skills are likely to be the primary predictors of the organization's ability to advance improvement in quality care and patient safety. Furthermore, they add that if these important developments are put into place a wide range of critically important organizational outcomes may occur with lower turn-over, less burnout, increased patient loyalty, and lower rates of medical errors.

Conflicts in health care organizations can be found at all levels as provider groups interact in interdependent ways.

They occur within and across provider groups and as the following example shows can manifest in aggressive and passive-aggressive behaviors. Consider the following event describing staff conflict. The nursing staff on a postpartum unit had felt long-standing **tensions** toward the nursing staff in the neonatal-care division. Generally,

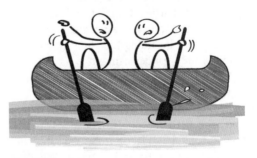

© Trueffelpix/Shutterstock.

the postpartum staff believed that the nursery department was staffed more generously and did not work as hard. One evening shift, a staff member from the postpartum staff observed that the nursery staff had left a newborn unattended. No one was around, and this staff member assumed that the nursery staff was on break. Angered at this apparent neglect, the nurse commented to her peers, "I'll show them." She proceeded to take the newborn from the nursery and hid the infant at the postpartum nursing station. The nursery staff returned but did not find the baby where they left him. They realized that this was a retaliatory action and became enraged.

At this point the conflict is localized and impacts the nursing staff on the unit and any supervisors responsible for patient care on the two units. Although the parents did not learn of this occurrence, one can imagine how they might have reacted—which would then have brought the parents into the conflict situation.

It is sometimes hard to believe that conflict and workplace aggression would escalate to these proportions in any health care setting bent on rational practices. But because providers are human, these episodes, though rare and quite dramatic, do happen. Regardless of whether providers are directly involved in the dispute or indirectly affected (e.g., a member of the physician team or the administrator in this hospital), they will soon know about the incident. Likely, those providers directly or indirectly associated with the disputants will be somewhat confused about how to handle their relationships and communications with the "at war" parties. Conflict and its behavioral and communicated aspects can affect the entire system including the patients, patients' families, and legal department.

Historically, conflict and tension were viewed as inevitable and as such, people just waited for resolution with expectations that in time, the tension would dissipate. Administrators would be called in to instruct staff and levy punitive responses if needed. With the escalation of potential conflict, multicultural work environments, and a new look at the costs of conflict, there has been renewed interest and commitment in attempting to prevent and control interpersonal conflict in the workplace.

Studies have shown that the cost of replacing nurses and other provider groups lost to unresolved conflicts is far greater than training and educating staff in crisis resolution. Health care institutions cannot afford to let conflict go without explicit intervention. Concomitantly, with various new approaches to conflict management, it has been shown that conflict and disputes can be resolved differently and, in some cases, better.

Conflicts in Health Care Teams

Much attention has been given to identifying the sources of conflict within health care teams of professionals and across multiple professional groups. Bochatay et al. (2017) conducted a multilevel analysis of professional conflicts with health care teams. They conducted semistructured interviews with health care professionals directly involved in first-line patient care in four departments of a university hospital system. Those interviewed were nurses, nursing assistants, nurse supervisors, medical residents, and fellows in medicine. They discovered six sources of conflict with disagreements on patient care tending to be the primary trigger for conflict.

Interestingly, sources related to poor communication contributed to escalation of conflict without triggering conflict. These authors stressed the importance of using a multidimensional framework in understanding health care team conflict. They emphasized that only understanding the sources of conflict was inadequate. The consequences and reactions to conflict situations are interrelated and also associated with the initial sources of conflict.

Reactions to conflict can impact health care providers, teams, organizations, as well as patient care. Attention has been and continues to be directed toward understanding the multidimensional nature of conflict in order to prepare students entering the work world and strengthening current health care professionals' ability to identify and respond in helpful ways to conflict in health care teams.

Differences Between Disagreements, Tensions, Disputes, and Conflict

The chief vehicle by which conflict is initiated, nurtured, and resolved is interpersonal communication. This does not mean that all conflicts or disputes are evidenced in verbal encounters. Many conflicts get played out nonverbally (e.g., in the deliberate absence of communication, in withdrawal and separation, and in posturing and facial expressions). Thus, two parties can be in conflict but this may not be evident because many individuals hide or disguise their conflictual feelings, attitudes, and opinions.

Conflict that has escalated out of control frequently gets played out in silence. "She or he is giving me the 'silent treatment'" means that the tension has escalated to the extent that an impasse has occurred and one or more parties is no longer sending or receiving verbal messages.

Disagreements and *tensions* are different from conflict. Although many conflicts might have started as disagreements, they may not always escalate to conflicts. *Disputes* are conflicts in which the parties have dealt directly with their differences but are unwilling or unable to resolve the issues. Usually these problems or disagreements move into a more public forum becoming the topic of a meeting and frequently, they involve a third party. These third parties may simply observe and monitor the quality of communication or they may facilitate the resolution of problems through specific mediation and negotiation strategies, and describe conflict in cases where provider work teams are called into action.

The first basic principle of conflict manifestation explains why conflict takes place.

Conflict arises when individuals (or groups of individuals) have incompatible, or seemingly incompatible, values, ideas, or interests. Conflict would not occur if these individuals or groups of individuals were separate, distinct systems and independent of one another. Individuals, groups, and even nations, can coexist without conflict despite vast disparity in values and beliefs if they are not related in some way to one another. When the relationship changes, however, and these parties become reliant on one another, the potential for conflict surfaces when previously there was no basis for dispute. This principle is important to understand—conflicts are more likely to occur when there is interdependence.

Janss, Rispens, Segers, and Jehn (2012) address the characteristics of interdependence in *ad hoc* medical action groups often found in emergency or urgent care settings. These groups may or may not have been previously interdependent but come together to address an emerging medical problem. They are interdependent and then split apart. Janss et al. list three types of conflict impacting these *ad hoc* groups: (1) disagreements in ideas and opinions about the task before them, (2) relationship conflict or personality clashes, and (3) process conflict arising out of logistical or delegation issues such as who is responsible for assembling necessary equipment or transporting a patient.

Ad hoc medical teams differ from other types of teams in that they can be formed on an *ad hoc* basis where teams exist only for the duration of the task and then split up. Janss et al. explain that *ad hoc* medical action teams have preexisting perceptions of intra-team power and conflict relationships based upon former work experiences with different team members, in different team compositions, and in different task contexts. This complex history becomes apparent in their interactions when they are called to work together.

The second basic principle is that conflict can be either positive or negative. Up to this point, the potential negative results of conflict have been addressed. Although the destructive consequences of conflict are feared (and there is good reason to fear them), conflict does not always have a negative outcome. Positive outcomes can and do occur and can result in better communications, enhanced problem-solving, and growth in the individuals involved. Still, the positive results of conflict are not necessarily forthcoming in a timely fashion. The position that conflict ignored will result in mostly negative outcomes is now widely accepted. And much of what is taught today is influenced by this notion. To minimize destructive consequences and elicit positive outcomes from conflicts, deliberate strategies must be employed based on a thorough examination of the cause(s) of the conflict.

Not only is the cause of a conflict important, the behaviors in reaction to conflict are also extremely important. Tension and stress always accompany any kind of conflict. In fact, it is these emotional components that frequently produce the negative results of conflict. If one were to interview the nursing staff in the example previously discussed, it is likely that one would learn something about the feeling and stress levels about all nurses involved. Tension and stress often predate angry outbursts. Some might say, "they really stressed me out," "how are we ever going to be able to trust them again," and "what were they thinking!"

Tension and stress are affective (feeling) responses to conflict. If continued over time, they can result in somatic symptoms, such as headaches, backaches, or just heightened body sensitivity. They have been associated with job tension but also job dissatisfaction. Left untreated, they tend to have direct and more significant impacts on individual behavior. Poor abilities to concentrate as well as decreased abilities to express oneself and respond rationally can all occur as a result of the tension and stress of conflict. The staff's use of poor judgment in the scenario that was presented exemplifies how tension due to conflict can eventually erupt in exaggerated expressions of discontent.

Incompatibilities in views and values among these nurses together with their inabilities to resolve differences seemed to reach escalated proportions and one member acting as if it was a last resort took it upon himself or herself to end the tension and stress.

Consider for a moment that you are either a hospital administrator or medical director and that you are responsible for addressing the dysfunctional communication on the postpartum and nursery units. The specific conflict issues are unknown but disputes about staffing and cooperation between the units seem to be involved. These disputes have gone into a more public forum in the shape of unit and division meetings but have not been resolved.

While human resource arbitration or even outside mediation is a possibility, you prefer to facilitate the problem-solving and closure process without bringing in additional parties from outside the hospital. To skillfully handle this conflict and the underlying disputes, some of which may involve you directly, you must determine how to maximize the probability of increasing both parties' willingness and abilities to resolve their differences. In essence, you attempt to modify the dispute, where possible, by providing facts and support so that the participating parties will negotiate a resolution within the ranks. You move a dispute toward successful resolution, maintaining the parties' faith in themselves that they have the power to resolve their differences.

Behavioral Displays and Signs of Conflict

If 100 people were asked how they know they are in a conflict situation, at least 75% would mention anger or irritation as a sign. It stands to reason that in dealing with people under tense circumstances, when individuals are expected to cooperate but have conflicting values or beliefs, anger and frustration may result.

Consider, for example, the number and kinds of words used to describe a situation fraught with conflict (**EXHIBIT 20-1**).

EXHIBIT 20-1 Kinds of Words Describing Conflict Situations

- "He (She) is upset with me."
- "She's (He's) hot about that!"
- "Let them 'cool off' for a while."
- "Give them a 'time out' and they'll settle down."
- "He (She) is 'seeing red'!"
- "Blind rage—that's what it is."
- "He (She) is 'psycho.'"

These descriptions suggest everything from mild irritation to irrational anger or a stronger feeling of anger that is difficult to control (e.g., rage). In conflict, as well as in other encounters where anger is displayed, the emotion of anger is secondary to other more basic emotions (e.g., disappointment, fear of loss of control, sadness, hurt, confusion, and guilt). It follows then that behavioral expressions of conflict may reflect either the primary feeling of anger or the secondary feelings of hurt and confusion that underlie anger.

What does anger look like? There are many verbal and nonverbal clues about anger and conflict. They include but are not limited to, defensive responses, verbal battles, and even withdrawal into silence. They also include nonverbal defensive or aggressive posturing. What must also be recognized is that these clues can be complicated by expressions of other feelings (e.g., fear of lack of control). In fact, primary feelings of anger may predominate but expressions of disappointment, sadness, hurt, confusion, and guilt may also be communicated.

Part of the difficulty that parties have in responding to conflict is that they must sort through and prioritize among several affective states. If they choose to respond to one (e.g., anger), they may suppress feelings of disappointment and confusion. While it is critical in conflict resolution to appreciate all the facets of human experience, it becomes unwieldy to address every emotion. The tendency is to reduce the phenomenon in order to make the situation resolvable. This tendency toward reductionism, however, is the very thing that can lead to negotiation failures because there is always the possibility of missing something that is very important in conflict resolution.

Recognizing conflict through multiple cues about primary and secondary affective states and carefully registering verbal and nonverbal aspects of communication is only half the story. What providers must also remember is that individual parties will go to great lengths to hide their true feelings and reactions, therefore, be cognizant of the fact that conflict is often masked.

But, even individuals who are masking conflict will display certain behaviors that are clues to their feelings. They may avoid direct eye contact, remain superficial or curt in their remarks, and display politeness or courteous behaviors that are not really required. They may appear "cool" or "cold" and mask their feelings for a variety of reasons. First, they may not want the opposing party to know that they are vulnerable. Second, they want to hide the specific kinds of feelings they have (e.g., hurt or sadness). They may be willing to let the other party know that they are angry but not willing to let them know about their feeling hurt and sad.

The adage, "Don't get angry, just get revenge," implies that the better way to deal with conflict and betrayal is to hide or suppress feelings and take action that will ultimately hurt the other party. This approach can lessen the possibility that conflict will be resolved adequately and in a timely manner. A third reason for suppressing feelings associated with conflict, especially if this is an administrative situation, is the fear that revealing their true feelings will result in disfavor. For them, talking it out (e.g., sharing unmet expectations) is ill-advised. The idea is to litigate versus resolve issues. So, you may find that the individual will prepare a letter or memo to express that their rights have been violated, the system is treating them unfairly, or there is prejudice in the decision-making process.

Verbal and nonverbal masks of anger and conflict usually minimize or exaggerate because the real stimulus, not the apparent stimulus, is what the individual keeps hidden. Therefore, being overly polite may actually express the opposite. One might not feel like being polite, therefore, they will force it and the other person will never know. This line of thinking is faulty because underlying feelings are always accessible, to some extent, to others. The other sees that the politeness is a feigned gesture. What is actually communicated is, "I don't feel like being nice, but I will be," and "you won't know" is the false assumption behind the thought.

Types of Conflict

Conflicts frequently arise out of providers' differences in beliefs, attitudes, and values. These may be actual differences or merely perceived differences. Conflict does not always reflect reality. There can be a great deal of distortion in conflictual relationships about what other groups or individuals think and feel.

These differences can serve as strengths or limitations in group functioning. They are not likely to result in intense conflict unless they are deemed to be in opposition. For example, if you want to ask for the opinion of the physician before you ambulate a patient or begin an exercise program, but the physician reacts as if it were a superfluous issue, this may create a sense of conflict. Otherwise, differences in point of view about what is important can create disagreement, whether open or masked. Within group or intragroup conflict can be either ask-related or relationship-related, or both.

Task-related conflicts occur when group members argue about the task of the group. Relationship conflicts result from interpersonal discord not necessarily related to the group's function. While these types of conflict can appear simultaneously, one type of conflict might have predated the other.

While conflict is either relationship-related or task-related, there are subtypes of conflict within these broad categories. For example, technologic conflicts, a type of task-related conflict, are those opposing ideas about the procedures, steps, and equipment to be used to achieve the aims of the group. They involve knowledge and perception of the scientific basis behind a situation and an awareness of the standards, policies, and capacities to apply technology to a given patient situation.

Providers disagree frequently about the necessity of treatment, the best treatment, and the best surgical or medical intervention to achieve the desired results although providers do not necessarily openly disagree. If one party, however, is more familiar or more knowledgeable and the less knowledgeable party does not yield, conflict can ensue.

Relationship conflicts are the most common type. They are highly influenced by providers' values, attitudes, previous experience, and beliefs. For instance, in the context of social relationships, one person may want a committed relationship and the other may not. For relationships to survive, both parties must perceive that a significant number of their personal interests are addressed in the relationship. This may be impossible if the real source of conflict is not an issue in the relationship (e.g., equality, authority, or superior/subordinate stances) but is actually a conflict stemming from ideological differences.

Relationship conflict in task groups can be created by differences in interpersonal styles and philosophies. For example, one staff member may be comfortable with small talk as a precursor to the work of the team. Other team members may prefer to get right to the issue facing the group. These members may behave in opposite ways in the group and eventually wrestle for the chance to project their way of doing things onto the group. Relationship conflicts frequently reveal differences in values, interests, or needs.

Conflicts may be either task-related or relationship-related or some subtype of either category. Some aspect of technologic, ideological, or relational conflict can be found simultaneously in provider work groups. Sometimes issues have their origins in one source (e.g., task-technologic) and proceed to additional domains (e.g., relational). Further, relational conflicts can fuel conflicts in other areas (e.g., the task-technological area). The cardinal rule is to analyze conflicts carefully keeping in mind the various types or categories of conflict that may exist and the reasons behind these conflicts.

Conflict Resolution Styles

Much attention has been given to identifying the potential responses to conflict among different health care professional groups. An early landmark study on the similarities and differences in conflict resolution styles among allied health professionals was conducted by Sportsman and Hamilton (2007). These researchers studied the conflict management styles of students in allied health professions. They used the Thomas-Kilmann Conflict Mode Instrument (TKI) which asked students to choose behaviors most characteristic of their response in cases of conflict.

The prevalent style of conflict management among the nursing students was **compromise** followed by avoidance. Avoidance, followed by compromise and accommodation, was most prevalent in allied health students. The trend in data analysis also showed that more than half of these participants chose two or more conflict management styles, commonly avoidance and accommodation. These findings are important because avoidance of conflict, in particular, results in poor resolution.

What happens when conflicts are unresolved or under-resolved? Some authors early on described the history of unresolved conflict resulting in frustration and even destructive outcomes. Saltman, O'Dea, and Kidd (2006) suggest that the process leading to destructive outcomes has four stages: (1) frustration, (2) conceptualization of the cause (an early attempt to clarify the cause of the problem), (3) expressed solution where a number of

actions are directed toward what the problem is thought to be, and finally, (4) destructive outcomes.

It is usually not difficult to judge when conflicts are unresolved or under-resolved because the tension that originally surfaced may be only somewhat alleviated or may erupt in significant ways without much provocation. Typically, communication styles remain the same. The disputants may exhibit evasive or avoidant gestures, express themselves rationally but also irrationally, use both direct and indirect messages, and display either rigidity or inconsistency.

Unresolved conflicts usually occur when different parties have reached a **stalemate** or **impasse**. *Impasse*, synonymous with *stalemate*, suggests the inability of the parties to move forward and settle their differences. A characteristic common to many instances of unresolved conflict is that one or both parties attempt to resolve issues through a series of positions that are presented as solutions to the issue.

These positions may be presented sequentially—the first position is less demanding than the second, and so forth. If parties are fixed on one position and display rigidity in their ability to negotiate with respect to new data, then positional bargaining is a negative process. Stalemates connote inflexibility and rigidity with respect to positions on an issue is bound to lead to stalemate. Parties who participate in positional bargaining generally come to a win—lose outcome. They perceive that the goal is "to win" and that they need to take a position. The only right solution is their solution, and conceding to the other person or party is a sign of weakness. It can be inconceivable that both parties will benefit because their goal is to come out on top.

Negotiations may worsen conflicts when the roles of each party are confusing. Sometimes third-party negotiators have a stake in the outcome. When roles are confusing the outcome is likely to be unsatisfactory. Consider for a moment that you are the outside third party in a conflict between the nursery and the postpartum staff.

Assume that you have also disliked members of the nursery staff and felt they were not to be trusted. Your attitudes and previous history may have a significant impact on the process of resolving this conflict. If your job is to facilitate the negotiation, then you may be biased and this will show. If your job is to decide for these groups what should be done, then your decisions will be suspect. Much will depend on your official power base which you may or may not choose to use. Confusion about your use of positional power may lead to an impasse and unsatisfactory negotiations.

In health care delivery systems, the primary approach to identifying unresolved conflict is to examine what went wrong. Because "what went wrong" is due to a fault in the system, not in particular individuals or groups, the analysis is complicated. Also, because conflict "spreads," there is a need to examine primary and secondary causes. System-level conflicts are not only complicated and costly, they are costly to resolve. The personal resources and energy expended as a result of conflict is high, and the costs of errors due to conflict is also high. So, when establishing the need to resolve conflicts, providers must also recognize the costs of not resolving conflict.

▶ Assessing One's Conflict Management Style

Because interpersonal conflict in health care organizations is widespread, considerable attention has been given to assisting clinicians and students evaluate their personal responses to conflict situations in the workplace. The idea is that in order to participate in conflict resolution, either as a leader or member of the team, one needs to understand how one feels about workplace conflict and how they are likely to respond in conflict situations. In the field of pharmacy, a measure for assessing

responses to conflict was designed and tested in a number of medical practices.

The following is a sample of some of the questions asked of respondents about what works best for them. The measure is the conflict management scale (Austin, Gregory, & Martin, 2009). Students and clinicians are asked to answer whether certain experiences characterize their response to conflict (either in the workplace or personal life) and respond "usually," "sometimes," "rarely," or "hardly." Items include "I am willing to compromise in order to get a resolution," "I feel it is my responsibility to reach a compromise," and "It is important to raise all issues immediately and get them out in the open." The items, when grouped in clusters, are able to inform students and clinicians about whether they are likely to behave in the following ways in conflict situations: imposing, settling, avoiding, and thwarting.

Concerned about the effect of conflict to affect the quality of care provided to patients, Gregory and Austin (2017) used this scale with a community pharmacy practice group that included pharmacists, technicians, and assistants. Their aim was to identify the conflict management style of these clinicians. The results of the study indicated that four key themes that explained conflict: (1) role misunderstanding, (2) threats to self-identity, (3) differences in conflict management style, and (4) workplace demotivation (a lack of motivation).

Further, the impact of conflict in their workplace was reported to be significant, adverse, and multifactorial. In fact, conflict was said to be an important reason for demotivation. These researchers concluded that effective collaboration requires providers to have conflict management and conflict resolution skills to not only resolve conflict but to help de-escalate and prevent conflict. Role misunderstanding and ambiguity can trigger conflict situations, and when the scope of practice and roles are changing, this can place escalate conflict because of the impact on providers' personal and professional self-identity.

▶ The Process of Conflict Resolution

Can you imagine a workplace that is totally conflict free? Not likely. This was never true of growing up in families and certainly not likely in the workplace. Most of us would agree that a workplace without conflict does not exist and cannot be found. However, certain workplace environments can appear conflict free but a thorough and up-close appraisal would suggest that this is only temporary and not likely to remain conflict free indefinitely.

Understanding that conflict cannot be totally eradicated is important when considering what is meant by conflict resolution. In fact, many times the goal is not to eradicate conflict but to manage conflict situations or minimize the escalation of conflict behaviors. Conflict management skills are equally important.

Resolution means to modify differences between individuals and bring disputes under control. Saltman et al. stress that conflicts have a history and this history influences the resolution process. This history may include various attempts to deny a problem, compete for the choice of solutions, and accommodate to minimize the circumstances of the conflict. Modifying differences does not mean forcing one party's views on the other or even forcing a third party's view on the disputants. Resolution means facilitating parties to realize that their existing differences, which will not change, can coexist in harmony. This important principle—that incompatible values can coexist—underscores the work of many mediators or counselors who practice mediation.

When speaking about conflict resolution, one is referring to eradicating a dispute or conflict. Conflict management is the containment of conflict or preventing it from escalating and causing further adverse outcomes in the workplace. Thus, conflict management implies that the conflict may still exist but is sufficiently controlled.

Many times, conflict arises from conflict about professional role behavior. Valentine, Godkin, and Varca (2010) explain that role conflict occurs when a job possesses inconsistent expectations incongruent with individual beliefs and can result in considerable frustration as well as other negative work outcomes. These authors describe the usefulness of mindfulness and adherence to organizational ethics.

Mindfulness is the psychological process of attending to what is going on in the present to develop self-knowledge and wisdom. The results of their study indicated that mindfulness was associated with decreased role conflict, and that perceived ethical values and a shared ethics code were associated with decreased role conflict and increased mindfulness. Mindfulness has the potential to promote thoughtful response to conflict in contrast to knee-jerk reactions out of frustration.

While it is most important that individuals and groups learn to resolve and minimize the consequences of conflict, they frequently need outside assistance. When outside assistance is needed, a third party (individual or group) could be asked to take part in order to either mediate or arbitrate the conflict. Successful negotiation involves a problem-solving process requiring each party to discuss their differences and reach a joint decision about their common concerns.

The health care literature provides many examples of stepwise approaches to resolving conflict in health care organizations. In fact,

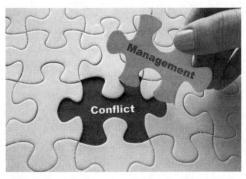

© Rei and Motion Studio/Shutterstock.

these approaches include anywhere from 1 to 10 steps. All approaches include the initial step of identifying the source of conflict. This is followed by the process of "looking beyond the incident" or clarifying any disagreements.

Next is the step of either establishing a common goal for the group or individuals involved and requesting solutions from all parties involved. The ways of meeting common goals and identifying solutions that both parties will support precedes the formulation of an agreement and acknowledging that an agreement is in place. The following discussions of strategies are those typically seen in conflict resolution situations.

▶ Steps in Conflict Resolution

Entering disputes: Most providers, if given a choice, would go out of their way to avoid being involved in conflicts—and for good reason. Conflictual relationships produce a great deal of confusion and frustration, and make working conditions difficult. Still, before any resolution occurs, some individuals will be drawn into the dispute and others will voluntarily become involved because of their concern and commitment to resolving the conflict.

There are various ways providers enter a dispute or conflict. In fact, at one time or another all providers will be drawn into a dispute between ourselves and others or where two or more parties are involved but we are not, at least, initially, only indirectly affected. It is important to differentiate roles in conflict situations—the disputants themselves, the third party who may be a "volunteer," and the officials who have been designated to mediate or arbitrate (see **FIGURE 20-1**). These groups function within the larger context of the particular health care arena.

Involuntary involvement in disputes is complicated. Because one would rather not have anything to do with the dispute, there are

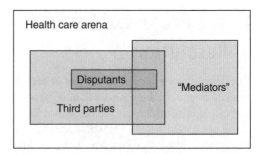

FIGURE 20-1 Roles in Conflicts and Disputes.

very strong feelings about involvement, and resentment and irritation about being brought into a conflict tend to confuse the issues further. Examples of involuntary involvement in the health care workplace could include disputes between members of the staff and patients or between staff and patients' families. They may also include conflicts and disputes between staff as well as within and between disciplines or departments.

Frequently, outsiders do become embroiled in the dispute or conflict. Not only is there anger about being drawn in involuntarily but the tendency to withdraw from others' conflict may also play a role in the manifestation of the conflict or dispute and its resolution. The cost of merely witnessing conflict is sometimes just as frustrating. Silent witnesses suffer; the extent to which they suffer is intangible and difficult to assess but it could lead to workplace stress and dissatisfaction.

When providers enter a conflict or dispute voluntarily, they do so for several reasons. First, providers may understand that, quite unintentionally, they are a part of the problem. Second, providers may realize that their work and/or their personal lives are affected by the conflictual relationships and communications. They may perceive that quality and safe patient care are jeopardized by the conflict. Both these reasons motivate them to get involved in the conflict and resolution process. A third compelling reason to enter a conflict or dispute is the personal investment an outsider has in its resolution. However, just because one voluntarily involves themselves in the process of conflict resolution does not mean that they are the person(s) who are qualified and able to negotiate a compromise or arbitrate a solution. The skill of mediating disputes and conflicts requires both specialized skills and neutrality.

Securing a Mediator

While it is hoped that disputing parties will resolve their own conflict or at least bring the conflict under control, the fact is that more often than not, specialized intervention will be needed. This fact reflects our lack of preparation in resolving conflicts, our tendency to avoid versus pursue resolution, and the overriding impact that our feelings and attitudes have on our communications and judgments. Given this understanding, it will not be difficult to comprehend that the mediation process must be impartial.

It stands to reason that successful mediators will not only be those who are skilled but also those who can maintain neutrality. One reason that authority figures are not regarded as effective in negotiation is that they have power that could be used to punish one or both disputants. Even if the authority person promises to be neutral and is capable of maintaining neutrality (a very difficult task indeed), the disputing parties may perceive (or worry about) the bias of the authority figure. Although administrators and directors have traditionally been viewed as good "referees" in disputes, in many cases today, they are viewed as inappropriate mediators.

Good communication is critical in health care work roles but not enough when conflict occurs. Disputes and conflicts cannot be addressed using just basic communication skills (Kayser, 2015). Competency in the processes of negotiation and conflict resolution is essential in the training of health care providers, particularly those who hold administrative roles and who interface with parties that may be affected (e.g., patients and their families,

as well as health care single discipline and interdisciplinary teams).

When we speak of *mediation*, we may mean mediation with a small or big *m*—informal or formal. That is to say, mediation with a small *m* is an informal process performed with and around people who are at an impasse. Mediation with a big *M* is a standardized formal approach to a dispute in which an official mediator is asked for or appointed to help the disputants overcome their stalemate.

When mediation at any level occurs, certain interpersonal and communication skills are necessary. These include nondefensive responses, **active listening**, and negotiation and/or **bargaining** skills. The need for these skills in formal mediation procedures remains the same. The difference is that formally appointed mediators have specialized training in negotiation, undergoing extensive education and receiving some form of certification.

In a classic statement about the process of mediation, Christopher W. Moore, with Communication/Decisions/Results (CDR) Associates (1986), defined the formal process of mediation as the intervention into a dispute wherein an acceptable, impartial, and neutral third party, who has no authoritative decision-making power, assists the disputants to voluntarily reach their own, mutually acceptable settlement. Each of these elements of mediation is necessary if the disputants are to arrive at an amicable resolution.

Acceptability refers to the fact that both parties agree to the presence and even the choice of the mediator, which is important if the parties are to follow the mediator's direction and guidance. *Impartiality* and *neutrality*, referred to earlier as a critical element, means that one individual or group (party) will not be favored over the other. While it is not possible to be totally opinion free, mediators are expected to control their preferences, attitudes, and biases. Mediators do not have authority or power so the tendency of disputants to feel threatened is lessened considerably.

Mediators assist the parties in reaching mutually agreeable outcomes—neither the event of mediation nor a decision to resolve the issue is forced upon the disputants. Mediation, whether informal or formal, is a valued process. It is expected that if the consequences of conflict can be better contained, settlements are reached more quickly, parties are more satisfied with the outcome, and regardless of the agreement, compliance is more likely. Mediation is extremely important in situations where the parties are expected to have an ongoing working relationship.

Moore (1986) carefully outlines several conditions that have led to successful mediation. These conditions—or, in some cases, preconditions—make successful mediation more possible. Their absence does not make successful mediation impossible but their absence and the number of unmet conditions will, however, considerably decrease the odds that positive outcomes will be reached (**EXHIBIT 20-2**).

Identifying and Clarifying the Root Cause of the Conflict

Once all parties are identified and a leader of negotiations is named, the next responsibility is defining and describing the cause of the conflict. The literature consistently emphasizes the inherent need and value of identifying the root cause of the conflict. Clearly the leader

or facilitators will make sure all parties stay focused and voice their ideas and thoughts.

While leadership takes a formal role in identifying the root cause, every coworker should take responsibility to identify all issues not raised. Coworkers or team members are influenced by a number of factors that can help or hinder this fact-finding stage. Just how well one fulfills this responsibility for others varies and depends on several factors (e.g., their investment in the issue or potential solutions, their personal attitudes and opinions about the situation, and beliefs about the disputing parties).

What is also clear is that each participant helping to identify the problem has a particular conflict management style and philosophy. Participants may be primarily collaborators, compromisers, accommodators, controllers, or avoiders, and these characteristics will determine how they define the problem. Collaborators will frequently view conflict as multifaceted and be accepting of others' views of the problem or conflict. Controllers, however, may not be as comfortable with views expressed by several participants.

For example, while avoidance would seem to be negative because issues may never get addressed, there are some potential uses for it. When arguments or demands get heated, avoidance sometimes provides the respite that everyone needs to reassemble their thoughts (and emotions) and come back together for more positive negotiation attempts. Similarly, compromising would seem to be a positive conflict management style. Yet, compromising may lead to situations in which solutions do not please either party and the main issues lose their value and importance.

Establishing Common Goals: Changing from Positional- to Interest-Based Negotiations

Once the source of the conflict is understood, the most important next step is to properly address it (Kalambo & Parikh, 2017). In most situations, this involves changing the current kind of negotiation styles that have been used. For example, most reasons why groups or teams have not resolved their differences and decided on a course of action is a result of the kind of negotiations they have used.

Positional bargaining is a style of negotiation that stakes participants up against each other based upon their position relative to the issue. When parties establish positions and stay fixed in these positions not a lot will happen. However, if they shift to an interest-based negotiation style, where all participants share their perceptions and ideas, much more is possible.

Positional bargaining strategies are more familiar. Classically, it is compatible with notions of being assertive. If we are assertive we will verbalize our position, and verbalizing our position will increase the odds that we will have our needs met. Positional bargaining is a strategy used by one or more parties in a dispute to maximize the gain likely to benefit them the most. By stating a preferred outcome up-front, the parties hope to minimize concessions. Usually they view each other as opponents where a win is a loss for the other. Using positional bargaining strategies on the part of one party usually begets positional bargaining by the other party. The disadvantage of this mode is that compromise is not valued, and parties often reach a standoff where no resolution is immediately foreseeable.

In contrast, *interest-based bargaining* is a negotiation strategy that attempts to satisfy as many interests or needs of the disputing parties as possible. It is a problem-solving technique that is used to reach a mutually satisfying solution rather than to determine an outcome in a win—lose manner. Although compromise may occur, the intent is not to compromise but to construct a solution to address the specific needs and interests of both parties. When parties are cooperative problem solvers, they do not behave as opponents. In interest-based bargaining, win–win solutions are sought. This is very different from win–lose scenarios created by positional bargaining strategies.

How can others be assisted to change from one strategy to another? It was explained that interest-based bargaining is, in many ways, better. **Deadlocks**, stalemates, and impasses are less likely to occur with interest-based bargaining. The process of changing positional- to interest-based bargaining includes a sophisticated analysis of conflict situations. For example, in any potential conflict, three elements are always present. Each conflict contains issues, interests, and positions. Dealing with positions alone decreases the potential for resolution because there is less to discuss and more temptation to polarize.

Consider this example of a group discussing the issue of whether health care providers should support assisted suicide. "What is your position? Do you believe in it and support it? Or do you oppose it?" If someone says, "I support the concept," the automatic response is to agree or disagree with the position—"I don't" or "I do support it, as well." However, if one discusses the situation from the standpoint of issues (e.g., "Is assisted suicide appropriate for only some medical cases?" or "How do we define assisted?"), there is much to discuss. Because there is more to discuss, there is a greater chance that these providers will arrive at a **consensus** to articulate in a professional position paper.

In another example, consider the issue of having fewer patients to care for (better provider to patient ratios). If this potential area of conflict among staff and administrators is discussed by members of the group holding onto their position, one outcome is possible. If the conversation changes to an interest-based discussion more related issues could be discussed. These might include establishing staffing ratios using indicators (e.g., patient acuity, quality care, and cost constraints). Then, there is a great deal to discuss. If the subject of personal interests is discussed in reference to the issue, the dialogue can be expanded further and has more of a chance to satisfy all parties. For example, needs or interests of the staff may include fears that they will deliver unsafe care or that their patients may be harmed and that they will be held accountable.

From the management or administrative side, interests may include wanting staff to feel supported but knowing that an already out of control budget must be kept in line. Mediators will generally treat positions as incomplete. They may even ignore them to avoid coming to solutions too early. In successful negotiations, issues, interests, and positions are relevant. Arguments and compromises that adequately reflect these elements are more likely to be acceptable to both parties.

Reaching and Acknowledging Agreement

One hopes for the best when seeking resolution of conflict. In the workplace scenario presented, one would hope and expect that the postpartum and nursery staff would realize how senseless and futile their behaviors were and that each group was in some way responsible for the event. One would also hope that realizing all this and having compromised on other issues, they will change and may even become model communicators. Such a thought is more fantasy than reality. In truth, the potential for further problems is high. However, so is the potential for successful resolution.

In actuality, there is a host of potential resolution outcomes. In reality, however, more partial resolutions are reached. Settlements, compromises, and decisions to drop all or most of the issues are all possible products of resolution. The settlements or solutions may be partial or temporary.

Sometimes disputing parties will just decide to drop the issue because the time, energy, and resources needed to face the issue are too overwhelming. In those instances, no resolution is perceived to be more advantageous than a partial resolution. In those instances, stalemates may be initiated by one or more parties. Sometimes one party will initiate an impasse hoping that time or resources will change things and that they will be at a better place down-the-line to compromise.

While the level of agreement or disagreement at resolution is important, of equal importance are the attitudes and feelings of both parties. Both sides must feel that they have had an adequate opportunity to explore their issues, interests, and positions. They also must believe that although they disagree with one another, they are better able to understand and to be understood by the other party. If this is not the case, whatever resolution occurs, partial or complete, the attitudes of participants are sufficiently problematic as to undermine any future cooperative activities.

▶ Communication Guidelines in Conflict Resolution

While providers need training and preparation in both effective communications and conflict management skills, to some extent, conflicts are synonymous with dysfunctional communication and the strategies used are the same or very similar. Associations between dysfunctional communication responses and level of conflict are quite strong. Does faulty communication, however, lead to conflict, or does conflict lead to faulty communication?

The answer is that both are true. In fact, conflict can be interrupted by changing communication patterns. It is also true that by improving communication, conflict can be avoided or at least resolved more quickly. Brown et al. (2010) list a number of facilitative communication strategies to enable individuals to resolve conflicts. They include open and direct communication, a willingness to find solutions, showing respect for others, and humility in the process of coming to solutions to conflict in health care teams.

The following discussion describes three strategies providers can use in moving closer to open, respectful communication in conflict situations. These strategies have been used to improve dysfunctional interpersonal communication and are also vital in avoiding conflict and resolving disputes. They include: (1) active listening, (2) reframing, and (3) assertive versus aggressive styles.

Active Listening

Active listening is a strategy or technique that is very familiar to mental health professionals. A large part of what therapists do is engage in active listening with their patients. *Active listening* entails paying attention to all aspects and levels of communication—the verbal and nonverbal elements and the report and metacommunication aspects of messages. Active listeners not only perceive the explicit content of messages but also the implied emotions and views of how individuals perceive their relationships with one another. Providers involved in efforts to resolve or manage conflict situations need to identify the source of the conflict, and by using active listening they observe and establish core issues more completely.

Active listeners also use other strategies useful in assessing core issues in conflict situations. They use empathy to enable disputants to feel more comfortable in sharing their concerns and underlying issues behind conflict situations. They are capable of reading beyond the expressed idea and into the feelings, attitudes, and beliefs of individuals. They are also able to articulate these perceptions in ways that increase learning and insight and validate experience.

Because this strategy tends to legitimize the communication abilities of the other person, the process of active listening often encourages disputants to disclose more than they have revealed so far. With more disclosure comes better understanding, and better understanding minimizes the chance of conflict and controls the destructive aspects of conflict.

EXHIBIT 20-3 Steps to Achieve Effective Communications During Disputes

- Listening to and carefully observing the overt content of each party's message.
- Perceiving the feelings, values, beliefs, and attitudes behind disputants' spoken messages.
- Identifying both the verbal and metacommunication aspects within the personal or interpersonal context for this conflict situation.
- Putting oneself in each individual's shoes—noting discrepancies in messages, feelings, and context.
- Expressing understanding in meaningful ways.
- Feeding back to the parties what was observed and what it might mean.
- Listening for the parties' clarification and responses to these observations.
- Assisting parties to form new conclusions based on the entire process.

Active listening includes a number of smaller steps to achieving more effective communication during disputes (**EXHIBIT 20-3**).

Active listening, like most other strategies, can be both taught and learned with relatively high rates of success. Active listening can significantly affect the outcome of conflict situations and the speed with which disputes can be resolved.

Reframing

Among all other conflict resolution strategies, the process of **reframing** has been advocated in a variety of settings from a small group to community-wide conflict resolution. *Reframing* is a term that describes the process of redefining the issues, the importance of the issues, the investments of the parties in the issues, and the value of one or more perceived solutions.

The act of reframing can redefine the issues and make them appear as if they are resolvable. It can also convince the disputants that they are capable of resolving the problems. Zola (2016) describes the use of reframing to support community-level decision-making where defensiveness is minimized and hopefulness is restored. Zola recommends placing the word "how" in front of closed-ended proposals. For example, a closed-ended proposal would start with the word "should" (e.g., "Should the community invest in first aid CPR training for directors of all community facilities serving the recreational services to the elderly?")

The alternative might be, "How can directors of community facilities be prepared to deal effectively with emergencies in their membership of elderly residents?" Zola explains that by removing the word "should" and replacing it with the word "how," the proposal encourages a broad range of responses around the interests of members of the group, not just their positions on the issue at-hand. Essentially, debate is replaced with open discussion. Once similar interests are revealed in the group it is much easier to reach a solution or resolution that appeals to a larger number of members. Thus, the initial conflict inherent with close-ended statements is relaxed with reframing, and the group has the ability to move ahead to a commitment shared by most of the group.

Reframing in conflict resolution also occurs when an outside third party describes a problem or issue in a different manner from how the parties are accustomed to perceiving it. Cognitive behavioral theories suggest that the way in which we cognitively construct our situations constitutes our reality. Therefore, when offered a revised definition of a problem or issue, we are actually offering disputants new realities.

Sometimes the manner in which a conflict situation is described or defined is detrimental to providers' ability to negotiate solutions. For example, with the conflict between the nursery and postpartum unit staff raised earlier in this chapter, an attitude or conclusion detrimental to these parties' abilities to resolve their differences would be, "I'm not surprised; I expected something crazy would happen—they're 'psycho.'" This conceptualization of the problem limits resolution, and no material that has been presented is worth discussing. Solutions to the conflict are deemed hopeless, and one has the feeling of "What's the use?"

When attitudes, beliefs, issues, or interests, or even the context of the conflict, interfere with conflict resolution, reframing can be very helpful. Individuals and whole groups develop definitions and beliefs about situations according to their independent or collective realities. From earlier discussions of the principles of human communication, we know that people perceive based on need and thus do not always perceive accurately the stimulus that is presented.

A part of managing conflict, then, is presenting a different reality, a reality that might more accurately reflect the situation and one that diminishes perceptions of competition, antagonism, and hopelessness. A good deal of what occurs in teaching people motivational skills is teaching them to redefine and re-conceptualize the problem. Insurmountable problems are small glitches, and difficult people are people who are behaviorally compromised. Notice that when we describe the staff of the postpartum and nursery units as "energized" instead of "crazy," we have altogether different attitudes about their actions and the prospects of their resolving conflicts.

Assertive Versus Aggressive and Passive-Aggressive Stances

A lot of literature over the years has suggested that being assertive is good and being aggressive is not. Theorists have attempted to dichotomize these behaviors and project consequences if individuals behave in either manner. In truth, both aggressive and assertive behaviors make use of aggressive energy.

It can be said that even passive responses are aggressive. This notion is borne out in descriptions of those behaviors that are labeled passive-aggressive.

At one level, it was believed that individuals could be classified or typed according to certain personality attributes (i.e., they were either passive-aggressive or aggressive personalities). Assertive individuals are those who state their thoughts and opinions while being respectful of others. Aggressive people ignore or challenge others' opinions in critical ways frequently to fortify their own positions. Historically, assertive individuals were perceived to be healthy, well-adapted individuals taking advantage of life's challenges but never at the sake of another's interests.

The issue of assertive versus aggressive behavior and the relative preference for assertive communications over either passive-aggressive or overtly aggressive styles is still an issue today. When it comes to a discussion of conflict and negotiation of differences, it is generally believed that being assertive without being aggressive (disrespectful of others' needs) is important in negotiating solutions that favor all parties. Most providers dealing with conflict resolution would agree, but why?

One reason is that *assertive* individuals bring their issues, interests, and positions to the bargaining table. They are open but not pushy, patient but not avoidant. Furthermore, *aggressive* individuals behave as if their issues, interests, or positions are the only ones or, at least, are the most important. For these reasons, they are not sufficiently open nor flexible enough to entertain alternatives and incorporate others' ideas.

Conflicts with a low probability of resolution generally involve one or more disputants who are either passive-aggressive or overtly aggressive. Also, resolution failures are frequently complementary where one party is aggressive and the other is passive-aggressive. Some authors argue that the symmetry or complementary nature of relationships and communications rules out the possibility of assertive behavior when one party is either overly aggressive or passive-aggressive. But this idea may undervalue the human capacity to avoid dysfunctional patterns. The idea that aggressive or passive-aggressive styles once learned can never be altered is not true.

These styles can be changed, and there are many training programs that prepare individuals to become assertive in both their personal relationships and their work settings. Needless to say, conflict mediators are very interested in the capacities of parties to relinquish aggressive and passive-aggressive styles and take on more assertive, respectful stances.

▶ Summary

Conflict is a growing concern among staff and administrators because of its negative impact on all involved and the consequences of low productivity, poor patient care, and staff dissatisfaction and turnover. Although conflict is inevitable, positive as well as negative consequences can occur but depend largely on how conflict is managed (Overton & Lowry, 2013).

Communicating with people in conflict requires providers to have a substantial awareness of conflict as a human condition. This awareness includes knowing what spurs conflict as well as what resolves conflicts and disputes. Each provider may formulate a unique conflict management style based upon both personal style and known conflict management strategies.

Whatever the style and approach, there are always limitations as well as advantages in a given approach to managing conflict. Specific tactics to use in conflict situations are those that reframe situations in helpful ways and engage disputants in active listening. A general problem-solving process that encourages providers to stay grounded in the issues is important.

EXHIBIT 20-4 Effective and Noneffective Conflict Resolution Skills

Effective Conflict Resolution Skills

Active listening.
Identify conflict triggers and conflict consequences.
Establish common goals.
Use reframing.
Accommodate varying points of view.
Compromise when appropriate.
Reach agreement.
Acknowledge agreement.

Noneffective Conflict Resolution Skills

Avoidance of conflict when it exists.
Expressing anger and aggression toward others.
Passive-aggression blocking identification and resolution of conflict.
Threatening reprisal.
Agreeing but not agreeing to compromise or resolution.
Undermining the attempts to compromise or resolve the conflict.

In summary, in the current health care climate, conflict is inevitable. These conflicts are played out in professional and bureaucratic differences, in differences in perceptions of institutional goals, and in conflicts over roles and responsibilities (some of which may be competing). While it is possible that work conflict will reflect personality differences, there are many more potential sources of conflict. Usually, there are multiple causes behind workplace conflict, and a more complete understanding of its complexity increases the likelihood that any solutions that are reached will be more than just partial settlements resulting in under-resolved conflicts (**EXHIBIT 20-4**).

Discussion

1. What is meant by the statement, "amidst conflict harmony and unity can be found?"
2. Identify at least three negative outcomes that could result from unresolved conflict in health care organizations.
3. What is the difference between interest-based and position-based bargaining?
4. Identify key strategies to lessen the impact of conflict on a work team.
5. How does relational conflict differ from interactional conflict?

References

Austin, Z., Gregory, P., & Martin, J. (2009). A conflict management scale for pharmacy. *American Journal of Pharmaceutical Education, 73*(7), 122. PMID:19960081

Bochatay, N., Bajwa, N., Cullati, S., Muller-Juge, V., Blondon, K. S., Junod Perron, N., ... Mathieu, R. (2017). A multilevel analysis of professional conflicts in health care teams: Insight for future training. *Academic Medicine, 92*(11S), S84–S92. doi:10.1097/ACM.0000000000001912

Brown, J., Lewis, L., Ellis, K., Stewart, M., Freeman, T. R., & Kasperski, M. J. (2010, August 26). Conflict on interprofessional primary care teams—Can it be resolve? *Journal of Interprofessional Care, 25*(1). doi: 10.3109/13561820.2010.497750

Gregory, P. A. M., & Austin, Z. (2017). Conflict in community pharmacy practice: The experience of pharmacists, technicians and assistants. *Canadian Pharmacists Journal, 150*(1), 32–41. doi:10.1177/1715163516679426

Hetzler, D., Messina, D., & Smith, K. (2011). Conflict management in hospital systems: Not just for leadership. *American Journal of Mediation, 65,* 5. Retrieved from www.americanjournalofmediation.com/docs/Conflict%20Management%20in%20Hospital%20Systems.pdf

Janss, R., Rispens, S., Segers, M., & Jehn, K. A. (2012). What is happening under the surface? Power, conflict and performance of medical teams. *Medical Education, 46*(9), 838–849. doi:10.1111/j.1365-2923.2012.04322.x

Kalambo, M., & Parikh, J. R. (2017). Building relations with radiology administrators. *Diagnostics, 7*(2), 33. doi:10.3390/diagnostics7020033

Kayser, J. B. (2015). Mediation training for the physician: Expanding the communication toolkit to manage conflict. *Journal of Clinical Ethics, 26*(4), 339–341. PMID:26752391

Moore, C. W. (1986). *The mediation process* (pp. 1–87). Boulder, CO: Communication/Decisions/Results (CDR) Associates.

Overton, A. R., & Lowry, A. C. (2013). Conflict management: Difficult conversations with difficult people. *Clinics in Colon and Rectal Surgery, 26*(4), 259–264. doi:10.1055/s-0033-1356728

Saltman, D. C., O'Dea, N. A., & Kidd, M. R. (2006). Conflict management: A primer for doctors in training. *Postgraduate Medical Journal, 82,* 9–12. doi:10.1136/pgmj.2005.034306

Sportsman, S., & Hamilton, P. (2007). Conflict management styles in the health professions. *Journal of Professional Nursing, 23,* 157–166. doi:10.1016/j.profnurs.2007.01.010

Valentine, S., Godkin, L., & Varca, P. E. (2010). Role conflict, mindfulness, and organizational ethics in an education-based healthcare institution. *Journal of Business Ethics, 94,* 455. doi:10.1007/s10551-009-0276-9

Zola, Y. B. (2016, July). *Reframe community proposals to reduce conflict.* East Lansing, MI: Michigan State University Extension.

CHAPTER 21

Family Dynamics and Communications with Patients' Significant Others

CHAPTER OBJECTIVES

- Discuss how the family is a major dynamic constituency in health care.
- Identify potential functional and dysfunctional communication patterns in families.
- Discuss providers' responses that would be helpful in building alliances with family units to engage them in shared decision-making when appropriate.
- Describe the process that families experience in adapting to their family member's injury or illness.
- Discuss the concept of "caregiver burden" in a family coping with giving care and communicating with an ill or injured member.

KEY TERMS

- Caregiver burden
- Families in crisis
- Family engagement in health care
- Family and kinship
- Functional and dysfunctional aspects of families

- Patient-and family-centered care (PCFC)
- Plain language
- Significant others (SOs)

▶ Introduction

Providers cannot adequately care for patients without knowing their loosely formed or formal family groupings that reflect specific cultural values and beliefs. This includes the cultural norms and religious beliefs of patients and their families that interface with health care approaches and policies. Not only patient but **family engagement in health care** is essential in formulating, implementing, and evaluating health care interventions and programs.

The *family unit*, however large or small (narrow or extended), is very important in assessing, planning, delivering, and evaluating health promotion and medical treatment of health care problems. Current thought about the nature of comprehensive care would view blatant disregard of the patient's family, culture, and social networks as tantamount to health care neglect. Note that in this chapter while the term "family" is used, the contents of the chapter are inclusive of many types of family units and social networks that act in capacities to help patients and participate in decisions about health promotion and medical care.

Patient- and family-centered care (PCFC) approaches, described as patient and community engagement projects, are being advanced not only in the United States but in Canada, Europe (United Kingdom), and Australia (Burns, Bellows, Eigenseher, & Gallivan, 2014). Clearly, patient engagement encompasses activities to enhance patients' understanding of their care, their condition, treatments, care plans, partnership, and involvement in decision-making and evaluation of care outcomes but also engages patients' families in similar ways as well (Bucknall et al., 2016).

The family and **significant others (SOs)** of patients are the most important social network in patients' management of and recovery from illness and injuries. In children, this is not just for colds, flu, and chickenpox but serious conditions such as childhood cancers, attention deficit disorders, autism spectrum disorders, cystic fibrous, diabetes (type 1), and chronic and severe asthma. In adults and elders, it is not just for upper respiratory illnesses and minor injuries but for life-threating cancers, Alzheimer disease, heart failure, diabetes (type 2), substance abuse disorders, and mental illness. Most families have wide exposure to illness or the threats of illness, and this exposure can extend more than 5 years for each illness afflicting a family member.

Whether it is the family unit or some other form of social unit, others are acting in capacities to help patients. The dominant ways in which families interact with health care providers and their sick family members are often unique but do show some common threads. Whatever the structure, the goals of family units are similar and include some aspect of maintaining the equilibrium of the family system. The unity and viability of any family system is threatened when illness and injury occurs even if anticipated.

Despite the fact that patients are many times treated separately or in isolation it is important to recognize that patients function in families and community systems. Patients' families and support networks form an intricate pattern of relationships not always easy to understand because of their interrelated parts and facets. Who is in charge of what and under what conditions is often obscure and may change over the course of care management.

A knowledge of cultural and religious beliefs and family dynamics is critical to all providers before they enter practice. Additionally, to provide culturally responsive care to patients and their families it is vital that providers be aware of their own attitudes, beliefs, biases, and assumptions about what families are, how they function, and how they may interact with health providers on issues related to patients' health care and recovery. Some families might resist the input of outside influences including traditional medical practices and others might retreat from caregiving decision-making ("…that's the doctor's/nurse's/health provider's job, not mine"). Still other family units might be more insistent

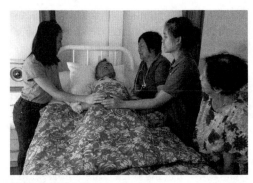

© Aodaodaodaod/Shutterstock.

about having a significant role in the patient's care and resent any sign of being "left out."

The importance of adequate patient–provider family communications is addressed extensively in the literature. Providers are sometimes accused of forgetting or ignoring the importance of family members in all phases of the caregiving process: their role as potential informants in the assessment phase, as decision makers in the planning phase, as caregivers in the implementation phase, and as reporters in the evaluation phase.

Family-system theories suggest that what happens to the patient happens to the family. While family members may not suffer the same ways patients do, they can and often suffer. The family may not feel the physical pain of the injury or disease but frequently experience the social, psychological, and financial consequences of illness or injury impacting their family member.

Family members, including parents of patients, can become fearful, anxious, and frustrated as a result of witnessing the injury or disease that afflicts their child or family member. They may understand health risks but not how they can create healthy living for their family. If they adapt successfully, they are likely to be stronger for the experience. If they do not, they might experience prolonged feelings of helplessness and powerlessness. In many instances, their relationships and communications are characteristically "dysfunctional." Providers can do much to alleviate

the emotional pain and effectively modify the communications of family members to put them at ease. Thus, it is important to learn to communicate compassionately and effectively with the family unit—the patient's major constituency.

The classical work of Miller (1992) attempted to describe provider–family clinical encounters in primary care and identified three discrete types of encounters. Thinking of family encounters in the context of type can help providers integrate family system concepts into practice. These three encounters are: (1) *routines*—clinical encounters that are simple, single, and brief; (2) *ceremonies*—rituals that involve covenantal style; and (3) *dramas*—a series of visits concerning situations of conflict and emotion that include families' psychosocial problems. "Routines" were simple, single, and brief visits in which the biomedical model was used. "Ceremonies" were linked rituals. "Dramas" were a series of visits concerning situations of conflict and emotion. The family was often convened for dramas.

Extending this framework further one can understand how these types might also be seen in hospital encounters with patients and families. *Routines* would be encounters while taking vital signs or administering medications. *Ceremonies* could include family-initiated, culturally or religiously based gatherings or meetings that are witnessed by health providers. *Dramas* could occur when the seriousness of the patient's illness is more evident to all and when feelings are heightened and conflicts across family members emerge.

The idea that providers witness and participate in multiple ways requires providers to shift focus from *just the patient* to the *patient and family as a whole*. The following discussion includes a more in-depth description of family dynamics and family member communication and participation patterns. The importance of understanding the cultural and religious beliefs of patients and their families are highlighted in selected descriptions.

▶ The *Family*—A Major Dynamic Constituency

Throughout time, *families*—whether formal or informal units—have played a crucial role in the care of the injured and critically and chronically ill patient. These patients are infants, children, adults, and elders. In actuality, a family's history of caregiving may have extended over very long periods of time and with a few or many family members.

The family's experience and knowledge can vary significantly with some family members being very savvy about disease prevention, health promotion, and treatment of illness while others may have very little experience and knowledge. Their preparation is also strongly influenced by the willingness to participate and the hardships placed upon them by their roles as family caregivers.

In the field of family medicine there is a strong emphasis on caring for the patient within the context of the family, and while family members may not be physically present, they have a significant influence. Additionally, maintaining a focus on the patient and at the same time gaining support of family members can be difficult. With this being said, it is our task to understand patients' families in the context of their cultural backgrounds and the dynamics of their family life. The following discussion revisits the *family* as a social unit and its role in health care.

Definitions of Family and Social Network

The concepts of **family and kinship** have been revised extensively in American society. It used to be that families were units comprised of children and biological parents living together under the same roof. Today, families are defined in a variety of ways to encompass many variations of the traditional family unit. We have single-parent, blended, nuclear, and three-generational household families.

There are families that are significant social networks by virtue of their membership in religious and/or cultural groups. Some of these groups have blood ties to the patient, such as members of indigenous groups worldwide or American Indian cultures in the United States. We have *families* not bound by any legal or blood ties that function in ways similar to traditional families and that are linked together in a system of exchange of resources and role reciprocity. In some single-parent households, there is no definable family unit per se but the community or tribal group assumes various roles as needed.

In addition to changes in notions of what constitutes a family, the family network has also been described as *fluid*. That is, it will change over time somewhat like an accordion; it may become expansive and then narrow and so on. Not only do affected family members and family structures change over time, some change dramatically over the course of the patient's life. It is possible that individuals can be children in a divorced family, grow up in a blended family, establish a nuclear family of their own, and end up in a divorced-family situation. Multiple generations of families form the structure of still other family systems. Additionally, the *in-law family* is a family unit that influences its members. Culturally prescribed roles and social norms shape the nature of primary and collateral family units.

The complexity of kinship and family has been further described in the notion of *everyday family* which may transcend households and extend to communities. The everyday family typically consists of persons who are not related by blood or marriage, who are of different ages, who live in the same neighborhood or community, and who trust one another as if they were family. These families provide varying degrees of contact and intimacy. Social networks are frequently comprised of loosely or tightly bonded everyday families who serve the functions of traditional, primary family units. Although these families are not bound legally or financially because of religious or cultural beliefs, they have a significant impact on their members. These groups influence the perceptions, feelings, attitudes, decisions, and behaviors of its members in everyday living and in other matters involving the members' quality of life and life transitions.

Functional and Dysfunctional Characteristics of the Family Unit

Families in some ways act similar to groups. Families can be regarded as collections of individuals with subsystems. Families, like groups, are not just individuals, they are more or less cohesive systems organized for a specific purpose. Families are also affected by the supra-systems, culture, and genealogical structure in which they are imbedded. Thus, to understand the **functional and dysfunctional aspects of families** one must first understand these rather basic principles. In the previous chapter, we looked at the unit (group), also using a system's perspective.

It is not the purpose of this text to delve deeply into theories of family dysfunction and teach about families from the perspective of a family therapist. There are separate sources that provide elaborate details about family pathology. Rather, family function and dysfunction is described here from the perspective of family stress theory. Family stress theory views the family in evolving stressful situations where stressors occur and resolve throughout the life of the family. These stressors affect how a *family* will adapt to illness and disease.

Unresolved stress over time produces chronic strain in a family that, in turn, causes dysfunction in the family unit. A theory particularly useful in understanding the family's ability to adapt to illness in the family is the classic resiliency model (McMillan & Mahon, 1994). This model supports the idea that by intervening to help families, providers can have a positive impact on the resilience of the

> **EXHIBIT 21-1** Early Perspectives on the Family and its Role in Illness and Recovery
>
> - Family as a resource (protective).
> - Family as a deficit (contributor or threat to illness).
> - Family and the course of illness (adaptive or maladaptive responses).
> - Family and the impact of illness (burden and stress).

family, enabling the family to regain homeostatic balance while decreasing the possibility of a buildup of unresolved stress. A family's functioning can be, and has been, categorized to include various tasks that fulfill relational, communicative, and survival needs. Whenever the physical and emotional resources of the family are insufficient, the performance of critical family tasks and functions are threatened and families are said to be more or less functional or dysfunctional.

Conceptual frameworks that have made landmark and significant contributions to understanding families facing illness are those utilized to analyze families' coping and adaptation to acute and chronic illness. Four different perspectives have been represented in the literature: (1) the resource perspective, (2) the deficit perspective, (3) the course perspective, and (4) the impact perspective (Steinglass & Horan, 1987). These perspectives are briefly summarized in **EXHIBIT 21-1**.

Each of these perspectives is briefly discussed here.

The Family as a Resource

Families are frequently the primary source of support and resource to the patient in accessing health care and adhering to a prescribed treatment. Thus, the first perspective on family functioning conceptualizes the family as a resource to individuals who are coping with illness, particularly with chronic illness.

Families are frequently the primary source of social support and comfort. As such, families can potentially serve a preventive, protective, and healing role.

The family can strengthen the patient's capacity to overcome the effects of illness, and is a major influence in patient adherence once a medical regimen has been established. For example, families can act in tangible supportive roles to patients by reminding them to take their medications, preparing a special diet, or transporting them to and from medical appointments. They can monitor patients to see that the regimen is followed correctly and consistently. They can also give emotional support during the course of difficult times with medication side effects and weariness about long drawn-out treatment.

Evidence for this aspect of the family's role comes from a series of studies indicating that family qualities such as empathy, as well as the family's own coping resources, have been associated with both improvements in the patient's medical condition and adherence to medical treatment.

Of significant importance to providers is the potential for the family or significant other to be supportive. Social support, typically derived from close social relationships, is felt to buffer or mediate the stress that is associated with chronic and/or life-threatening illness. Because most people use social support to cope with all kinds of stress, including the stresses of illness, the mere perception that adequate support is available can be as important as the actual support itself. Families have played a crucial role in the care of injured or ill members but most recently the technology of health care and treatment required has been perceived to limit family participation in health care decision-making and patient care (Davidson et al., 2007).

The Family as a Deficit

The family as a deficit refers to the disabling role the family might play in the patient's health maintenance, disease prevention, and recovery from illness. As previously explained, the *family* can be both a potential helpful resource but also a potential negative contributor. In this case, the main influence of the family is not its protective, buffering capability but rather its tendency to weaken or jeopardize patients' effective coping and even increase the debilitating aspects of their health condition.

One example is the family member who urges the patient to be mobile faster than what is recommended. Another example is the family that ignores the order of a low-fat diet and prepares meals high in fat and sodium. A final example would be family members who fail to recognize their role in discouraging substance abuse in the patient who is struggling to maintain sobriety. Families may fail to recognize the power of their negative contributions. In short, family members may intentionally or unintentionally encourage the alcohol-/drug-abusing behaviors of the patient.

These kinds of undermining behaviors on the part of family members is often found to be a result of a dysfunctional, rigid, and/or a very stressful family system that is incapable of recognizing and meeting the patient's needs. In summary, any support system, including the family, might not always be supportive. Thus, their impact can be of no value or negative value. Families might not always be supportive nor facilitate healing.

Before leaving the topic of unhelpful aspects of the family, it is important to point out the fact that family members, particularly caregivers, may suffer their own health problems from the continuous demands that affect their care duty tasks. Several studies of caregiver strain and health have shown a relationship between the health of family caregivers and the capacity of families to assist their ill family member. Caregiver stress is taken up again in this chapter under the topic of the family and caregiver experience.

▸ Families over the Course of Care Management

Families are also believed to influence the course of illness. This notion does not address the roles of families during the onset of illness but it does focus on the ways families influence the course of illness. Because the course of chronic illness can vary, some analyses of the differences in patients' abilities to cope effectively and recover in a timely manner are attributed to the role and interaction with family members. Thus, an important factor is the role of the family.

The idea is that different illness consequences and phases of illness place different demands on the family unit. The manner in which families respond to these challenges, then, may have a substantial impact on the patient's adaptation to illness and its course over time. This perspective analyzes the interface between family behavior and patient illness characteristics which are considered to reinforce one another. Questions that often get asked are, "What aspects of family behavior serve to maintain or delay patient adherence to treatment and early recovery?" or "What illness factors (symptoms and demands for care and attention) provoke certain dysfunctional behaviors in families?"

For example, family resistance to cooking low-fat meals might delay needed dietary control and prolong disease or make a condition worse. On the other hand, symptoms (e.g., uncontrolled diabetes or hypertension) might put added stress on the family and the homeostatic balance they strive to maintain.

The Family and the Impact of Illness

The fourth and final perspective described by Steinglass and Horan (1987) focuses less on the way families influence the onset or course of illness and more on the impact of the illness on the family. Chronic medical conditions, in particular, can drain families of emotional and financial resources. These conditions can significantly divert the family from its usual operating agendas and deprive them from the time and energy required to function effectively in their work roles. Studies of the indirect costs of chronic debilitating disease address the significance of this type of burden on the family.

One poorly understood behavior associated with family burden is, for whatever reasons, overinvolvement, not underinvolvement. Overinvolvement is of concern because it threatens family resources. Overinvolvement with the patient (or the treatment) can threaten the family's broader social life. Also, when the patient's needs predominate over all else, someone else in the family may be neglected. In the case of an adult patient, a child or spouse may suffer, and in the case of a child patient, a parent or sibling may not have certain needs met. And as previously explained, the depletion of these resources may result in negative psychological states in family members (e.g., suppressed anger, frustration, and guilt). These states are ultimately communicated to and influence the patient in negative ways.

Family burden has been linked with family perceptions of the seriousness of the illness, whether or not the illness is as bad as the family pictures it to be. Reactions such as worry, fatigue, guilt, anger, ambiguity, depression, alterations in eating and sleeping patterns, and decreased socialization can occur when families become preoccupied with their ill or potentially ill family member. Sometimes they harbor fears that are fueled by not having enough information. Families might tell providers that they have lost their appetite, do not feel like having a social life, and have difficulty sleeping. They might worry about the health and welfare of their ill family member but also their own health or that of other family members such as their infants or young children.

The ability of families to overcome the impact of illness on themselves and their ill family members relies to a certain degree on their supportive resources but also their capacity for resilience. *Resilience* is the ability to recover quickly from difficulties. The American Psychology Association (cited in Jagannathan, Varghese, & Vasava, 2015) defines resilience as the process of adapting well in the face of adversity, trauma, tragedy, or even significant sources of threat. Resilience is as important to the family as to the ill family member's recovery from threat and adversity of illness. Thus, in these cases, providers should think about both the resilience in patients and their family members.

▶ Families, Illness, and Providers

Notions of the Impact of the Family

Families, like patients, express changing needs depending on the events that occur. Because family members influence patient recovery, failure to address their needs may hinder patient recovery. One such concern of families that is often expressed when caring for acutely ill patients is the stress they experience in interactions with hospital personnel.

Originally, the stress of illness on the family was seen to be a byproduct of the specific disease itself. That is, the stressors on the family when a member had cancer were unique to the disease and different from the stressors imposed by cardiovascular disease or diabetic conditions. Potential stressors were perceived to be a function of the specific disease itself. The underlying assumption was that the family lay victim to the demands and stresses associated with the particular illness. As a result, there were separate family educational and support programs for many different conditions such as renal failure, arthritis, diabetes, stroke, cancer, and AIDS.

A more recent approach to the study and design of support and educational programs for families recognizes the commonalities across various categories of disease: chronic or life-threatening illness or short-lived injury. That is, families might be grouped together based on the characteristics of the onset, course, or prognosis of the condition. For example, some conditions based on acute onset and subsequent incapacitation, such as with AIDS and some cancers, have similar psychosocial challenges for the patient and the family. Epilepsy or asthma, however, has acute onsets but is not as incapacitating or as life threatening. Still other illnesses like Alzheimer's disease and late-onset multiple sclerosis are characterized by a gradual onset and a progressive debilitating course.

In summary, illnesses vary in type of onset (acute or gradual), course (progressive, constant, or episodic), and degree of incapacitation. The prognostic time frame (crisis, chronic, or terminal) is still another variable that differentiates illnesses from one another. Illnesses in turn differentially challenge families, requiring different resources, strengths, attitudes, and behavioral changes. The overall extent of readjustment may be similar but the manner and pace of those adjustments can be quite different. Because family adaptation is fluid and dynamic, the degree to which the family meets these challenges can affect not only patients' adjustment to illness but the strength of the psychosocial stressors that affect the family.

Much of this approach of looking at families presumes illness to have negative effects on families. It is also known that illness can and does bring out the best in families. It has been reported that families sometimes grow closer, stronger, and more peaceful and even talk about more important things. Like individual patients, families can perceive the illness to be a challenge and then not only meet the challenge but even surpass expectations for coping. Just what makes the difference between high-level coping and low-level coping in families is not altogether clear but is probably accounted for by many factors relating to the family, the patient, the disease burden, the contributions of the health care team, and the demands of the treatment program.

Communication Challenges with Families

In order to give sensitive patient- and family-centered care, it is critical that providers cultivate an awareness of the sociocultural norms and religious beliefs of patients and their families, particularly as they apply to those families they frequently encounter in selected communities and geographical areas. One of the most important challenges to communicating effectively with families is cultivating an awareness of families and their relationships with their patient family members.

With researching and experience, providers learn about the different types of families that they may encounter and develop a communication style suited to each. Nonetheless, their comfort in initiating interaction with families may vary a great deal. Most providers will engage families in communication but some providers avoid direct interaction with family members—at least, as much as possible. They may not feel at ease in communicating with families and may even delegate this task to another team member.

This discomfort is not altogether surprising. There is a certain ambiguity in encounters with families. Family members are or have participated in the illness process as the protector, the enemy, and/or the confounding variable in the onset and course of the illness. On the other hand, the family is as much the victim as is the patient. So, how are providers to view the family, and how do providers converse when there are so many possible interactions between patients and their families? Should they trust the family, be suspicious, engage them compassionately, or some combination?

In addition to this ambiguity, there are other reasons that communicating with the family may be difficult. Not all providers are trained to communicate effectively with family members or with the family as a whole and can even feel threatened. What would seem to be easy, speaking in **plain language** so families understand them, is not so with many providers. They may be unsure about their role and what they should and should not divulge about the patient. When their competency or knowledge is challenged by family members they may feel uneasy. They may worry that families will make requests that they cannot fulfill because these requests fall outside their standard of practice and doing so might ultimately lay them open to malpractice litigation.

Other providers may resent the time it takes to establish contact and talk with the family, especially if it is not clear that this effort makes a difference in patient care. This becomes even more the case when they find that they are repeating what they told a family member over and over again.

Providers who lack recognition and understanding of the cultural and religious beliefs of the family may feel ill-equipped to effectively communicate with family members. It is important that they understand how family cultural and religious beliefs fit the traditional medical model which could run counter to the needs and preferences of these groups. Some families have been known to be hostile or rude and mistrust providers.

A final explanation for provider discomfort is that families may become another difficult variable with which to deal, and providers do not want to complicate an already challenging treatment situation. Is it plausible that some providers, on seeing the family from a distance, might feel like walking the other way to avoid them? Despite these concerns and hesitation, health care delivery systems take an effort to design, implement, and evaluate programs for families. Unfortunately, families who need attention are not always those that are able or who choose to participate.

Provider and family communications are a two-way street, meaning that they involve mutual or reciprocal actions. Families frequently express difficulties communicating with providers. Two common complaints from families are having only minimal contact with providers and poor or controlled access to information about patients' health status.

These complaints are associated with each other since minimal contact with providers also means that families may not be getting sufficient information. Even when information is posted on patient health record online portals, families may not be able to obtain enough information about the patient's health status and treatment plan. What is missing is dialog; dialog or conversation between family and providers that comfort the family and enable exchange of detail and expression of concern.

With limited contact and controlled access, families frequently feel unsupported by providers. On the whole, providers generate strong feelings in family members. Providers are the source of help and hope, and when the patient gets worse or better, providers' behaviors or lack of response are considered to be the reason. When things go wrong, providers are safer to blame than the patient and they are more tangible than the disease.

Because family members are the patient's primary constituency, they feel compelled, in some cases, to fulfill the role of advocate to the maximum degree possible. The stress they experience in their advocate role can place additional strain on their communications with providers. Providers need to offer appropriate reassurance, referrals, and factual information in a caring and empathetic manner with adequate follow-up in order for families to feel relief from any worry and stress they may be experiencing. Examples of family comments and their possible underlying requests for help are displayed in **EXHIBIT 21-2**. Providers who use the communication skills of active listening and empathy will be better able to uncover these types of concerns.

Family Adaptation to Injury and Illness

The perspectives and reactions of families to a health concern or illness to their family member are highly contingent upon the specific cultural and religious beliefs of the family unit in question. In principle, any health condition that threatens the functioning and well-being of the patient also threaten the family. As indicated previously, a number of illness- and treatment-related stressors can affect families. They may experience actual or potential losses (e.g., alterations in their everyday activities, loss of independence, loss of support, affection, and leadership from the ill family member, and potential loss of financial security and stability if the patient must suspend employment). Just as patients need the support and compassion of providers, so do their family members.

It is important to understand that the family's response to the patient's condition is highly influenced by the family's previous experience with and beliefs about the patient's health and illness. If the family is not organized to support those intimately impacted by their family member's illness or the community as a whole is ill-equipped to help them, health providers can serve important roles in helping families through each phase of an impending or actual illness or injury.

Families may experience crisis at the first sign of a serious illness or injury. Depending upon the strength and resources of the family and community some families will experience this first stage as a major crisis. Principles that apply to working with patients in crisis, in large part, also apply to families. Families facing chronic, debilitating, or life-threatening illnesses are also believed to progress through grief-like stages in response to the illness. The family can exhibit signs of the grief process even at the same time the patient is experiencing the very same process: denial and disbelief, anger, bargaining, depression, and acceptance.

EXHIBIT 21-2 Family Members Comments and Questions and Underlying Needs

Selected Family Members Comments and Questions	Request Value of the Statement or Question
"Is he/she OK?"	Reassure me; is everything OK?
"How is he/she doing?"	Educate me about this disease and tell me what I can expect.
"How did he/she get it?"	Was it something I did or did not do? (Will I get it? Prepare me for what I have to face.)
"Will he/she die?"	Tell me I can trust you to do what needs to be done when it needs to happen. Will the worse possible outcome happen?
"Why hasn't his/her tray come/bath been given/medicines or treatments been started?"	What is going on? Is my family member getting the care that is needed?
"Can I talk to you for a minute?"	I really need more time; can you talk to me? I need answers and a chance to really connect with you.

The similarities in patient and family adaptive tasks are so great that the phenomenon of adaptation is frequently attributed to both. The assumption here is that the patient and family progress through an illness process in parallel fashion. Although this is generally the case, there are exceptions and the gap between patient and family seems to widen with time. For example, an initial diagnosis may cause disbelief in the patient and the family and the length of time it takes to move on may be similar. By the point of acceptance, however, the gap may have widened. The patient may have reached acceptance but the family, or selected members of the family, may not have. The reverse may also be true. That is, the family may be in resolution but the patient may be primarily angry or in the bargaining mode. Reasons family members have a delayed response or accelerate through the grieving process depends on many factors including specific characteristics of the family and the patient.

Assessing Family Health and Family Relationships

Taking a health history relies not only on the patient's self-report but also on the information that family members as informants give the provider. This information can be broken down into roughly four categories: (1) the family's previous experience and beliefs about the patient's condition, (2) their knowledge and understanding of the health condition, (3) actual health and medical concerns of other family members (through generations), and (4) family relationships and roles.

This information is first gleaned from patient reports because the patient is frequently the first line of inquiry. Families, however, are often brought into the assessment process because patients cannot or will not report certain data. In other cases, patients have given providers their information but they are judged to be poor historians so family members are utilized to clarify, extend, and corroborate data derived directly from the patient or indirectly from records and charts.

While many families want to hear from providers about what they perceive to be the health concerns of their family member and do want to hear providers' advice and recommendations not all families can be comfortable with or accept provider input. Providers should anticipate that their conversations with family members could be met with resistance. The family's previous experience and beliefs surrounding the patient's condition is the first major category in the health history. Some cultural and religious groups may perceive the practices and approaches of traditional medical care to be foreign to or antithetical to their views and practices in treating and supporting their ill family member. Still, whatever family members can share will be of value.

The family's report on the patient's current condition provides a window into the family's knowledge and understanding of the patient's condition, the second important category of information. The family's level of health literacy will become apparent. The report reveals how the patient's illness or injury is perceived from outside the patient but inside the family. This report may also reveal the patient's tendency to minimize or exaggerate symptoms. It also reveals the family's level of awareness and their own tendencies to minimize or exaggerate changes in the patient's appearance, behavior, or demeanor.

Essentially, the provider wants to know what family members know, what they have observed about the patient, and how they interpret their observations. This is particularly important in evaluating the nature of any relevant signs and symptoms and the degree of disability or impaired functioning the patient is experiencing. Providers also want to know how the family has observed and processed patient information, and how members of the family have been affected by the patient's condition and/or treatment requirements.

Actual health and medical concerns of other family members is the third category in the family history. As suggested, families are informants. Providers need to identify which family members have knowledge of the family's history with health and medical concerns. Senior members of the family might possess a wealth of information about the family's health concerns. Elderly caregivers, because of their previous roles in giving care to family members, might have a good deal of valuable information. Family members who are older, who have had recent experiences with illness themselves, and who are (or have been) interested in health issues and familial problems are likely to be fairly good historians. Some family members are hypervigilant about disease prevention and are able to report major illnesses (heart disease, cancer, strokes, etc.) as many as three generations back.

Providers need to progress systematically through information provided about histories of major illnesses, injuries, and deaths. Where hereditary, infectious, or familial conditions are concerned, extending the list of significant others beyond the immediate family are important. While most family members are generally good informants, some are not. Those who have no recent contact with the patient and have not been told about problems by the patient may not have enough important information. Also, those with memory or cognitive deficits may not be able to share the kinds of information providers are looking for.

The fourth category of data needed by providers is information about family roles and relationships in the family and community support network. Beyond identifying who to contact in case of emergency or who has the power of attorney, more circumstantial information is needed. Providers need to identify which community and family members assist patients the most and are important to the patient.

The health and level of functioning of these family members is important because it will have the most bearing on patients' current and future health status (who usually helps the patient with everyday activities and who helps with issues about health and disease treatment) Inquiring, "Who lives with the patient?" and "Do they have health problems? If so, what kind?" generally picks up on any non-familial relationships that the family member may have forgotten to mention. Full information about the patient's current life situation is important. There are several basic categories of information about family relationships about which family health care providers want clarity. They include:

- Quality of communication between the patient and specific designated responsible parties.
- Patient's role in the family and alterations in role functioning as a result of the onset or progression of illness.
- Factors that may inhibit communication in the family.

There are numerous strengths and problem areas inherent in family relationships that can be revealed in this dialogue. Evidence of patient isolation or alienation from family members may surface. Evidence of impaired verbal communication, altered family functioning, and compromised family and parental role performance can be determined. Clues about actual or potential abuse or violence directed at patients may also surface. Additionally, family-role conflict, ambiguity, role reversal, and role overload may become apparent from these initial conversations.

It is expected that families can elaborate on details, especially in areas where the patient was vague or where independent corroboration is needed. It is not unusual that a provider will get more information from family members than from patients themselves. This is obviously the case when patients are suffering communication and cognitive deficits or when they are not able from a developmental standpoint to communicate with providers as with young children. Also, even when able to communicate, patients may be unaware of or reluctant to expand their answers to providers' questions. For example, patients may not be aware that they had a seizure or exactly how an accident occurred and they may not understand that their behavior was irrational or bizarre.

Sometimes patients not only minimize or exaggerate symptoms but they distort them in other ways as well. Providers may find that the patient was more acutely ill than the patient reported. Families can fill in important details and give an additional perspective. They also have access to friends and neighbors of the patient that can share observations of the patient's recent behavior.

Families are also helpful when providers are collecting data about patients' reactions and responses to treatment. Sometimes providers will need to secure the entire history from a family member. As previously mentioned, this is the case if the patient is incapacitated or unable to communicate for reasons of being very critically ill, demented, delirious, unconscious, psychotic, cannot speak and/or hear, or for other reasons.

Repeated brief contacts with family members, particularly if they are assuming caregiving functions, is important. These contacts not only allow providers to follow patients' disease course but also reveal more about family concerns. Throughout the course of illness, families' involvement can change—caregivers and their caregiving duties can change. For example, it is common for female siblings to shift responsibilities for the care of their elder from one sibling to another.

Such information is essential in planning the patient's care and managing the patient's illness. On some occasions, providers will meet conjointly with family and patient to discuss the patient's condition and plan of care. These sessions can be very valuable but are not always possible unless the treatment program is specifically designed to actively involve family in shared decision-making opportunities. A more common occurrence is periodic family contact and very brief conjoint encounters, a structure that permits only limited education and support.

The confidentiality of family communications is very important. Personal information about other family members is not communicated to the patient. Also, patients need to be protected from conflictual data that are obtained from the family unless their condition requires it.

Patients' Requests with Respect to Families

As if to make the process of communicating even more difficult than it inherently is, there are other circumstances that complicate the picture. These circumstances are defined by patients themselves and include formal and informal requests.

Patients typically define their own family unit. They identify a responsible person, a next of kin, and/or a parent/guardian but these individuals are not always the same person. These individuals may not even be those persons who actually and/or legally fill these roles.

In addition to this complexity, patients establish the boundaries of communication with either their significant others or their next of kin. These boundaries include what the patient wants and does not want the family member to know. "I don't want them to know," or "I don't want them to be told," is not a rare occurrence. In some cultures, however, the role of family prevails. Some patients, typically those of Hispanic or Asian cultures, expect the family to know everything and take a major role in decision-making. To maintain trust, their requests to share or withhold data from family members must be respected or negotiated with the patient if needed.

Professional judgment may override patient requests. Professional judgment can dictate the necessity of sharing information with family members if it relates directly to the well-being of the patient. For example, the family may be instrumental in helping the patient make a decision or obtain resources. Another reason professional judgment may prevail is that discussing the patient's condition with the family or a family representative may prevent reinforcing the patient's avoidance of health care problems.

Providers aim to avoid supporting maladaptive coping strategies (e.g., by helping patients not accept an illness and subsequent need for treatment), especially if it includes life-threatening nonadherence to treatment. Providers do not want to be placed in positions of conflict in their own clinical attempts to help patients acquire adaptive coping strategies.

For providers to be released from obligations of confidentiality, both patient and provider should negotiate compromises. Patients who openly express preferences do not make requests without reasons and it is critical that providers understand the basis of the request. Providers cannot take these requests lightly. Still, by observing the patient with the family and by discussing the patient's reasoning, the consequences that are feared are usually clarified under most situations. Providers are not released from their promises of confidentiality until the patient has stated the circumstances (when and how) under which this confidence is to be suspended.

There are instances in which the patient's request becomes more imperative. Certain diagnoses and prognoses carry with them social consequences. A positive diagnosis of HIV infection, for example, produces stigma, fears, and responses that can lead to social isolation and even alienation and discrimination. While families may not, in reality, react negatively to information about the patient's diagnosis, patients' concerns may be deep-seated. Violation of patient confidence, even (or especially) with family, is prohibited in such cases.

If patients do not negotiate the release of confidentiality, the responsibility rests on the provider to determine if withholding information would jeopardize patients' well-being. Sometimes these decisions are exceedingly complex. Consider, for example, the issue of teen pregnancy. If the teen (patient) requests that her next of kin (mother) not be told of her pregnancy, her well-being may be jeopardized. Also, withholding information about current or potential conditions from the patient's mother could be a violation of the mother's parental rights because it would significantly hinder her from fulfilling her parental responsibilities.

There are other instances in which the interface between patient and family becomes complicated. This problem can occur in caring for terminally ill patients. It is generally known that caring for terminally ill patients requires effective communication with the families. Effective communication must become a regular part of the treatment. Decisions to support patients do not always have equally good outcomes for families and conversely, decisions favoring families may not be good for the patient.

Providers may find themselves in a dilemma. If they, on the one hand, do what appears to be best for the family, they may violate rights or ignore the needs of the patient. On the other hand, if they address specific needs of individual patients, they may weaken the family unit. Examples of these dilemmas also include acting on the information that patients report about the alleged abuse they have experienced at the hands of a family member or significant other. Note that both child and elder abuse are instances of mandatory reporting regardless of what the patient, caregiver, or family members wish.

Families, Family Difficulties, and Provider Responses

Families encountered by providers bring with them a series of life circumstances which impact their readiness and ability to deal with

and management significant health conditions and illness in their members. Obvious examples would be those families that experience imposed separation or divorce, those dealing with homelessness, and those facing bankruptcy or significant legal problems. Some families experience these life circumstances simultaneously.

Life problems that families bring to encounters with providers can make effective communications more difficult. Frequently, these families who already have high stress levels also have difficulty communicating with providers. Most providers will observe that if they try to understand the family dynamics, they will personally experience less stress and more satisfaction, will achieve better overall treatment outcomes, and will lower the potential for conflicts and disputes.

In this section of the chapter, families in crisis and chaotic families are discussed.

The following discussion highlights basic principles and concepts that are important in communicating with these difficult families.

The Chaotic Family

According to the classic framework of Howell and Schroeder (1984), chaotic families are usually characterized by having multiple problems. They might also have multiple caregivers as others have stepped in to help the family. They may appear to lack structure, to have no goals, and to have no designated person in authority. In neuroscience terms, they seem to lack executive functioning. Their communication can be erratic and disjointed. This family looks to providers for guidance and structure but is uncertain about its needs.

Because of the continuous chaotic lines of communication and members' self-defeating encounters with each other, it appears that little effective problem-solving will take place. And while the provider may diligently seek the origin of each problem and offer suggestions, the family has a temporary plan and structure to follow but is not likely to adhere to the plan laid out for them. In this case, providers must recognize the character of these families and set limited and realistic goals.

Guidelines to structure communications with the chaotic family in conjoint sessions would be to (1) structure the topics, direction, and duration of the interview; (2) speak clearly and gain and maintain control of the flow of communication and discussion; (3) appeal to the designated leader(s) of the family to follow up on recommendations; and (4) establish definite timelines for follow-up.

The Family in Crisis

A second important category of family is the family in crisis. **Families in crisis** are generally experiencing incapacitating trauma. In addition to the stress brought on by a severe and debilitating injury or illness, they are undergoing trauma of a different kind. Like chaotic families, those in crisis also appear to have limited executive functioning. The major reason that providers have difficulty communicating with these families is that communication is boundless.

Typically, they may not synthesize instruction or information in a rational manner (Howell & Schroeder, 1984). Because family members vary in their responses, providers may have multiple responses to deal with simultaneously that may or may not have anything to do with the diagnosis and treatment of a health condition. These include anger, rage, fear, panic, blame, and guilt. Providers can be flooded by the number of responses as well as by their intensity from a variety of family members.

The primary therapeutic response is to allow family members time to express their emotions even when they may not directly pertain to the health problem of their family member. Similar to organizing the care of families in chaos, it is preferable that a central organizing figure (primary health care provider) be assigned to deal with this family's responses and needs. Further, feedback to the family needs to be provided in an empathic, supportive manner.

In summary, families in crisis and chaos present additional communication challenges to providers. It is important to remember that all behaviors displayed by families are not necessarily related to the current health concern of the family. Life stressors appear in every aspect of the lives of family members and need to be understood and taken into account in shared decision-making approaches.

An important additional concern that is pertinent to either families in crisis or those in chaos is the level of cooperation that can be elicited. Uncooperative families clearly are problematic if they exhibit very little or no real concern for the patient. They may also be very resistant to speaking with providers as well as carrying out any suggestions or recommendations. Some uncooperative families virtually abandon the patient, leaving the patient to fend on their own. This type of family may also not be helpful in the assessment and history-taking process and may even be secretive and somewhat paranoid about being addressed in an official capacity.

Establishing communication with these families requires careful analysis of underlying issues and assessment of how the family responses will affect the outcome of the patient's care and treatment. Establishing an alliance, communicating fully what care is planned, and how the family may be helpful are constructive measures to make an otherwise uncooperative family more cooperative.

▶ The Family and Caregiver Burden

Families are traditionally those resources expected to assume caregiving responsibilities for patients who are members of their family unit. Since inpatient, rehabilitation, and extended care residential centers make up only a fraction of the services received by patients with severe injury, illness, and recovery, families are needed to take up the slack, and they do.

According to findings of the 2015 National Academies Caregiving Survey, 43.5 million adults in the United States provided unpaid care for an adult or child in the prior 12 months. Nearly 1 in 10 caregivers was 75 years of age or older and 3 in 5 themselves had a long-term physical condition. More than a third had a short-term physical condition, and a quarter had a memory problem.

These caregivers assist patients with activities of daily living (bathing, dressing, toileting, feeding, dealing with incontinence or diapers, and helping patients in and out of beds and chairs) but also medical/nursing tasks, such as giving medications including injections, tube feedings, and wound care. Many also assist with transportation, grocery shopping, housework, preparing meals, managing finances, monitoring the patient's health, communicating with health care professionals, and arranging outside services. One in three caregivers reported having no other help, paid or unpaid. About half said they had no choice in taking on the responsibility of caregiver. The average time spent was 20 or more hours per week and the average number of years was 4.3. Finally, 38% reported feeling highly stressed in their role as caregiver.

Children are also caregivers in the home. More than 1 million children ages 8–12 provide care to someone in the family. This kind of role reversal (children caring for parents/grandparents instead of parents caring for the needs of children) create role conflict for children, change the dynamics in the family, and can lead to emotional and physical issues in these children caregivers.

Over time, a shift in concern about caregivers has occurred. Initially, the concern was whether family members were adequately prepared to assume the caregiver role. As experiences of family caregivers became more transparent there was concern for the health and well-being of these caregivers. Some providers readily identified the stress on families

because they identified similar stressors in giving care to these patients. While clearly more attention has been given to the value of family caregivers, accumulating data is an accelerating concern for caregiver well-being when the caregiver is actually a patient as well.

Recent literature specifies more dramatically the fact that many of these caregivers are in fact 'care recipients in their own right' (Sherman, Austin, Jones, Stimmerman, & Tamayo, 2016). Family caregivers have spoken up and providers have sought clarification of their opinions and expressed needs. Sherman et al. attempt to move family caregivers out of the shadow of the patient to more fully understand who they are, their burdens and benefits in care giving, and how to communicate with these vulnerable family caregivers. They recommend a comprehensive family caregiver assessment along with interventions to lessen the negative health consequences of family caregiving and to promote and protect their health, well-being, and quality of life over time.

These interventions should include multiple sources of support—financial, psychological, social support services, tangible task support, and education to assist them to perform their activities. Engaging caregivers as partners with patients and health professionals is still another important step in securing protective health services and quality of life for these patient–caregiver dyads.

The stress of professional caregiving has been reported in a wide variety of literature addressing the professional stress syndrome and burnout. An increasing emphasis has been placed on the stress of caregivers who are not professionals. With the advent of changes in the health care delivery system, including more care being carried out at home by family members, **caregiver burden**, as previously explained, is growing significantly.

Becoming more concerned about caregivers is appropriate because their health has been linked to the health, welfare, and successful rehabilitation of persons, especially those with chronic illness. The problems of informal caregivers are not the same as those for the professional. Professional caregivers have been educated and trained, and it is presumed this knowledge and skill helps them cope with the stresses of caregiving. Informal family caregivers typically lack the skill, knowledge, and experience that providers have.

These informal caregivers receive variable amounts of support and education to accomplish similar tasks. While their responsibilities are typically limited to one patient at a time (but this is not always the case), these responsibilities can be 24 hours a day, 7 days a week. This may be in the context, however, of caring for 2 children under the age of 5 and a nephew age 16. Professional and family informal caregivers experience stress and burnout perhaps for different reasons, but the expressions of stress are similar.

First, families experience stressors unrelated to specific caregiving tasks. Some of the most compassionate reports of caregiver stress have appeared in the last decade and come from family members of cardiac, cancer, HIV, and Alzheimer's disease patients. These family stressors are many and occur in significant magnitude to place the family at high-risk for further problems and afflictions. These include social and emotional costs, physical exhaustion, financial drain, and, in some cases, stigma and alienation.

In most cases, the stressors related to the patient's illness and treatment are also many. But among those that are of most concern to families who are giving care are the cognitive and emotional changes both in the patient and, potentially, in themselves.

Cognitive impairment in patients can include memory loss, disorientation, impaired concentration and judgment, impaired perception, confusion, mental slowing, and the inability to engage in abstract thinking. These problems can occur in patients with senile dementia, HIV, depression, and in patients with mental and addictive disorders.

In addition to cognitive impairment, emotional changes and disturbances occur in patients who have mental illness, the elderly, persons with HIV, substance abusers, and with patients with medical illnesses such as cardiac disease and cancer. Patients who experience these disturbances can be bothered by sleep and eating disturbances, fatigue, generalized apathy, irritability, low self-worth, hopelessness, and even suicidal or homicidal ideation and/or risk.

Informal caregivers must learn to give instrumental care (administer medications, treatments, etc.) and emotional support, and these must be accomplished in cases where the patient's ability to cooperate or render self-care may be minimal, unpredictable, and variable. Family caregivers must organize these responsibilities in and around their own activities. Thus, the social and occupational lives of family caregivers are threatened, sometimes considerably.

Family caregivers' reports of emotional exhaustion indicate that the burdens that they experience are significant and not easily modified. To better understand the informal family member's experience of emotional exhaustion, a list of potential reactions is included in **EXHIBIT 21-3**. Typically, informal family caregivers are faced with the same situations that confront the professional but may not

EXHIBIT 21-3 Caregiver Burden: Emotional Exhaustion in Family Caregivers

- Physically and emotionally drained from caring for the patient.
- Angry and frustrated by the prospect of endless caregiving responsibilities.
- Frustrated about the program of caregiving and the numerous demands without clear signs of patient improvement or progress.
- Powerlessness over the disease, its course, and their ability to make changes for the better.
- Angry at the patient for significantly altering their personal independence and autonomy and, therefore, quality of life.

have sufficient respite periods to regroup and refresh. In a study of caregivers of patients with leukemia, caregiving for a patient receiving chemotherapy for leukemia influenced their quality of life and well-being. The study highlighted the need for better nurse–caregiver communication and education, particularly in the areas of medication administration and symptom management (Tamayo, Broxson, Munsell, & Cohen, 2010).

▶ Summary

Knowledge of patients is incomplete without knowledge of their cultural and religious beliefs and their social networks including their family by birth or family by choice. Working with families during times of patient illness is both challenging and rewarding. Illness can present an altered set of circumstances for which patients and families are ill prepared. In some instances, illness or injury is unexpected and catastrophic while at other times, expected and progressive. In either case, patient and family coping responses may be strained and their adaptive capacities depleted.

Providers have a significant role in addressing the needs of families and responding in supportive ways. This role includes thorough assessment of family functioning to determine how they can be effectively engaged in sharing decision-making. In cases where patient caregivers are also vulnerable in their own right, careful assessment and supportive interventions are needed over time to ensure the health and safety of both the identified patient and caregiver. Adequate intervention always includes an evaluation of the patient but the resources within the family unit.

Families are not just "those people" who "ask stupid questions" or "get in the way." They are special patient constituencies who significantly affect and are affected by the patient, the treatment, the provider–patient relationship, and the treatment setting. Providers need to enlist families in formal and informal ways.

Because of their importance, it is critical that providers understand family communications and how best to converse with family members.

A small part of this time will be spent in taking a social or family history. A much larger portion of the investment will be learning how to engage the family in shared decision-making processes and teaching family members what is going on and what will happen during the course of treatment.

Family functions and roles have been associated with both the occurrence and outcomes of diseases, particularly chronic conditions, in a number of ways. Studies have documented instances in which families contribute to the progression of disease and worsening of the patient's quality of life. More often than not, this occurs due to deficits in health literacy of family members.

Research has also focused on the protective role of families, particularly in their ability to buffer illness-related stressors. More recent research has addressed the interdependent nature of the patient's illness and adaptive capabilities of the family. Finally, in this chapter, a model that addresses the significant burden that families endure as a result of an ill family member was discussed. Within the broad range of possibilities—to help or to hinder and sometimes both simultaneously—the family needs to be approached with appropriate respect and caution.

Families who are regarded as most difficult to communicate with (e.g., the anxiety-ridden, guilt-ridden, or uncooperative families) can be managed. The key is to understand that the behavior is amenable to change if the underlying issues are approached and resolved in supportive and compassionate ways. Behind the family members' resistance might be the cultural and religious beliefs that shape family views of health and illness.

With medical advances and the rapid increase in our aging population, the leading cause of death has shifted worldwide from infectious disease to chronic illnesses. There are certain health conditions that are expected to challenge our health care system. These include cancer, dementia, obesity-related conditions, and diabetes. Injuries due to falls are expected in a frail and aging population. Families are currently and will continue be faced with burdens of caregiving that they may never before expected to see. This is, in part, an outcome of the many delivery system changes that have moved caregiving from inpatient intensive care and recovery centers to outpatient facilities and the home.

The needs of long-term, critical care patients' families seem not to subside. The number of hours and years of supportive care expended is high and likely to grow. Family caregivers' desire for information remains the number one need expressed. This is not the time to abandon the family because it is difficult to communicate with family members or the unit as a whole. Rather, providers must embrace the family with all its rough edges, strengths, and limitations.

Next of kin, parents or guardians, responsible persons, and everyday families (broader social units acting like families) are a part of the picture. Patients may need to rely on these constituencies for extended periods. Many, but not all, will deliver aspects of care. As such, they constitute the largest potential health care resource today and in the future. Data shows that many aspects of medical/nursing care of patients are attributed to family members and happen without any outside paid or unpaid help. In spite of the growing recognition of the importance of family caregivers and the time needed to communicate and educate family members a void exists.

The ability to reach families in meaningful and supportive ways falls short of what is needed. More research and piloting of interventions to meet the needs of family–patient units are required. In a recent report of the National Academies of Sciences, Engineering, and Medicine (2016) it was stated that *the nation's family caregivers provide the lion's share of long-term care* for older adults in the United States. Furthermore, the report stresses that the need to recognize and support caregivers is among the least appreciated challenges facing health care in the United States.

Discussion

1. Examine potential bias and assumptions about behaviors of families in caregiving settings, and discuss how these biases and assumptions could either facilitate or inhibit culturally responsive care to patients and their families.

2. What is the difference between patient-centered care and patient-centered family-centered care?

3. Identify characteristics of the family in crisis and how families might be helped by proactive measures.

4. Discuss caregiver burden and its potential effects on quality care and patient safety.

5. Discuss family and provider caregiver burden and the needs to thoroughly and continually assess the health and well-being of caregivers in one or more of the following situations: patients in intensive care units, end of life care, and management of progressive and debilitating illness. Identify how caregiver burden could be alleviated in each scenario.

References

Bucknall, T. K., Hutchinson, A. M., Botti, M., McTier, L., Rawson, H., Hewitt, N. A., … Chaboyer, W. (2016). Engaging patients and families in communication across transitions of care: An integrative review protocol. *Journal of Advanced Nursing, 72*(7), 1689–1700. doi:10.1111/jan.12953

Burns, K. K., Bellows, M., Eigenseher, C., & Gallivan, J. (2014). Practical resources to support patient and family engagement in healthcare decisions: A scoping review. *BMC Health Services Research, 14*, 175. doi:10.1186/1472-6963-14-175

Davidson, J. E., Powers, K., Hedayat, K., Kamyar, M., Tieszen, M., Kon, A. A ... Armstrong, D. (2007). Clinical practice guidelines for support of the family in the patient-centered intensive care unit: American college of critical care medicine task force, 2004–2005. *Critical Care Medicine, 35*(2), 605–622. doi:10.1097/01.CCM.0000254067.14607.EB

Howell, J. B., & Schroeder, D. P. (1984). *Physician stress: A handbook for coping.* Baltimore, MD: University Park Press.

Jagannathan, A., Varghese, M. M., & Vasava, T. (2015). Concept of 'resilience' in promotion of mental health: Importance and feasibility in clinical settings. *Austin Journal of Psychiatry and Behavioral Science, 2*(3), 1044.

McMillan, S. C., & Mahon, M. (1994). Measuring quality of life in hospice patients using a newly developed Hospice Quality of Life Index. *Quality of Life Research, 3*(6), 437–448. http://www.jstor.org/stable/4035312

Miller, W. L. (1992). Routine, ceremony or drama: An exploratory field study of the primary care clinical encounter. *Journal of Family Practice, 34*(3), 289–296. PMID: 1541955

National Academies of Sciences, Engineering, and Medicine. (2016). *Families caring for an aging America.* Washington, DC: The National Academies Press. doi:10.17226/23606

Sherman, D. W., Austin, A., Jones, S., Stimmerman, T., & Tamayo, M. (2016). Shifting attention to the family caregiver: The neglected, vulnerable, at-risk person sitting at the side of your patient and struggling to maintain their own health. *Journal of Family Medicine, 3*(7), 1080.

Steinglass, P., & Horan, M. E. (1987). Families and chronic medical illness. In F. Walsh & C. M. Anderson (Eds.), *Chronic disorders and the family* (pp. 127–142). New York, NY: Haworth Press.

Tamayo, G. J., Broxson, A., Munsell, M., & Cohen, M. Z. (2010). Caring for the caregiver. *Oncology Nursing Forum, 37*(1), E50–E57. doi:10.1188/10.ONF.E50-E57

The National Alliance for Caregiving (NAC) and The AARP Public Policy Institute. (2015). *Caregiving in the U.S. 2015 executive summary.* Retrieved from www.caregiving.org

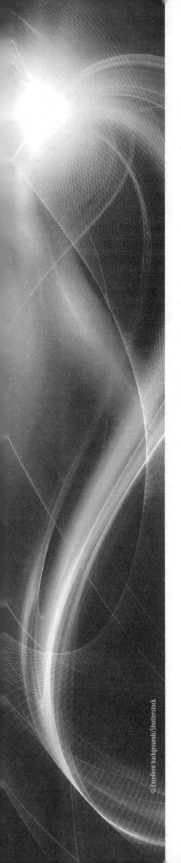

PART VI

Ethics and Communications in Health Care

Instruction in the skills and concepts of applied communication in health care would be incomplete without a discussion of the important ethical and legal concepts that shape and limit providers' communications with patients, their families, and other health care organizations. Stipulations about the nature of professional patient–family–provider communications underscore a good deal of what is considered ethical. Some rules and norms are not only standards of professional practice, they are addressed in statements of patient rights, in statutes, and in laws. It is important to understand the issue of patient rights in its fullest. While much of what is important in health care communications involves the role of families, ethical standards and statutes most often focus on patient rights.

Patient rights stipulate the ethical standards and practices in patient-health professional communications as well as the transmission of patient information via medical records and health information technology within and between health care organizations. They govern what patients have a right to know and what protections they have against unauthorized sources gaining access to their medical history and important health information—essentially what will be communicated to them but not to others.

In Chapter 22, "Patient's Rights to Informed Choice and Consent in Health Care Decision-Making," the concepts of truth-telling, informed consent, and informed choice are discussed. These concepts are applied to research- and nonresearch-based clinical practice situations. They are basic concepts in intent but their assurance is far from simple, thus problems in securing informed consent and informed choice in clinical and research contexts are identified and discussed.

In addition to patients' basic rights to informed consent and informed choice, there are specific stipulations, rules to be followed, that protect patient communications and records from unauthorized exposure. One such stipulation governs issues of confidentiality—that which providers can ethically and legally divulge, to whom, and under what conditions. In Chapter 23, "The Privileged Nature of Patient–Provider Communications: Issues of Confidentiality, Anonymity, and Privacy," the rules around confidentiality are presented. Two related concepts, that of anonymity and privacy, are also discussed.

It has been said that today, health care providers need to be more concerned than ever before with the ethical and legal foundations of health care communications. The U.S. Department of Health and Human Services established the Health Insurance Portability and Accountability Act of 1996 (HIPAA) to protect the use and disclosure of individuals' health information. Still, for various reasons these standards are sometimes not adequately met.

Twenty or more years later there are still examples of flagrant abuse of patients' rights. Even when unintended these problems can be observed in many health care arenas and in many different ways even after the establishment of the HIPAA. With the advent of m-Health and health information technologies (HIT) new concerns arise. These include the quality of HIT devices used, whether they meet established standards, the possibility that they may impede lawful information sharing, and whether there is adequate matching of patient data to the correct patient.

Policies that protect patient rights and afford patient control must be uppermost in the minds of providers. Certainly, the disrespect of patient confidentiality is among the most serious infractions. Providers' commitment to ethical practices in communications to and about patients and their families must be fostered, monitored, and reinforced. This applies to what is communicated during conversations, written documents shared, and what is transmitted via online messaging and electronic sharing of patient data and communications.

CHAPTER 22

Patient's Rights to Informed Choice and Consent in Health Care Decision-Making

CHAPTER OBJECTIVES

- Discuss the concept of truth-telling as it applies to patient-informed choice.
- Describe the process of obtaining patient-informed consent in the context of health care encounters.
- Discuss providers' legal duty to care for patients.
- Identify and discuss selected instances in which patients do not have personal choices about health care communication.
- Identify which factors make informed consent difficult to obtain.

KEY TERMS

- Informed choice
- Informed consent
- Patient's Bill of Rights

▶ Introduction

The privileged nature of patient–provider communications is played out in specific encounters with patients and patients' families but also in many different instances within the industry and practice of health care.

Today digital technology has transformed how health care information is acquired and transmitted. Health care organizations as is the society at large are becoming more adept with information without paper. Becoming paperless in health care can make patient information easier to retrieve and transmit but does not

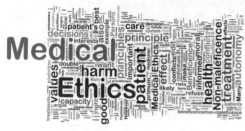

relinquish providers and health care institutions from determining what information is appropriate to disclose and judging the risks of doing so. The following discussion lays out the important principles in adhering to major guidelines for the protection of patient health care information.

It is understood that patients who enter into relationships with providers are protected by a set of laws and regulations that outline, at least in part, how the roles of provider and patients are to be enacted and exactly what privileges and responsibilities are afforded in these roles. The reality of practicing as health care providers includes risks as well as rewards. In this era of malpractice controversies and the emerging legal considerations of health information technology (HIT), these risks become more than just hypothetical circumstances or philosophical debates. The rights and privileges of patients regarding their care and communications with providers should be taken very seriously.

Many kinds of legal and ethical issues impact the professional practice of health care providers. These vary from what seem to be straightforward issues of informing patients of their diagnosis to more complex issues related to extending patients' lives. From a legal and ethical standpoint, we are concerned with patient safety, liability, incident reports, and malpractice litigation. From a communication perspective, we are concerned with the basic challenge of effectively communicating with patients to maximize their privileges of choice and execute our responsibilities. There are several sources of pressure that influence our actions. Licensure and accreditation of health care facilities support practices that are

respectful of patients' rights and sanction those that are not. These sanctions range from very severe sanctions to merely warnings. Providers' own professional licensure requirements, however, strongly enforce adherence to basic fundamental patients' rights.

Additionally, legal systems have evolved in elaborate ways to address the complexity of provider–patient encounters. Federal and state laws regulate practice through professional practice acts. Each state must assume the responsibility for developing these guidelines and for providing regulatory measures to ensure that professional standards are upheld. Certain federal regulations support and extend these standards of care. This legislative authority is both ethically and legally binding. It is important to note that providers are expected not only to practice within standards but they are also expected to protect patients from abuses within the health care system. It is this latter area that can create dilemmas that are not easily resolved. Many providers are clear about their own level of practice. However, when the system and/or other providers are involved and place the patient at-risk, indirectly or directly, the fundamentals of practice and of protecting health care systems become complex. These conflicts raise a number of professional consequences that can create confusion and stress in providers. Thus, the role of providers in protecting patient rights is influenced by many factors. These problems are addressed in many ways through in-house conferencing, professional training, and close monitoring. The communication and interpersonal competencies of providers are intimately connected to safeguarding patients' rights.

▶ Issues of Provider– Patient Privilege

A sacred premise behind fostering an effective provider and patient relationship is the need to empower patients to be fully informed sufficiently enough to enable them to play a role in shared decision-making about their care and treatment. The American Medical Association (AMA) Code of Medical Ethics (2012) states that the patient's right of self-decision can be effectively exercised only if the patient possesses enough information to enable an **informed choice**. This premise suggests that patients are told the full extent of their illness, prognosis, and treatment options. However, the process is more complicated than what it appears to be. Cultural and religious beliefs have a significant affect on patients and families as they are asked to engage in health care choices and decision-making. For example, informed choice is internationally recognized and accepted as an important aspect of ethical health care (Ahmed, Bryant, Tizro, & Shickle, 2012). Still, some populations and groups, based upon culture and religious beliefs, may value this ethical consideration differently.

In a cross-cultural study of informed choice in antenatal screening, these authors reported that women interpreted informed choice in different ways, challenging policy assumptions that all women want autonomous choice. Some women, particularly from minority ethnic groups, wanted health professionals to give them advice and make recommendations. This situation does not require patients to abdicate their rights entirely but does point out that protection of patients' rights may not be as straightforward as one would expect. Such findings raise the issue of whether and how much providers' advice is wanted and needed. Other researchers studying the roles of health providers in shared decision-making situations with these patients make important recommendations. They stress that providers should cultivate an awareness of sociocultural norms and family dynamics when supporting non-Western patients in making decisions about care, particularly in making decisions about such serious health conditions as cancer treatment choices (Lee et al., 2015).

Truth-Telling

The Patient Self-Determination Act (PSDA) is a federal law that informs patients of their rights regarding decisions surrounding their medical care. Compliance is mandatory. It is the purpose of this federal law to ensure that patients' right to self-determination in health care decisions be communicated and protected.

Patients' rights for self-determination include protection from deception. Deception in health care is a type of manipulation that subverts patients' capacities to exercise rational and deliberate choice. Kirlin (2007) explains that when a physician fails to tell the patient the truth about diagnosis, prognosis, or even risks and benefits of alternative treatments, it has the effect of making a unilateral decision to deny the patient his or her right to participate autonomously in care decisions.

Truth-telling is defined as the avoidance of lying, deception, misrepresentation, and nondisclosure in encounters with patients as related to patient care. The ethical principal of patient autonomy is protected by patients' abilities to determine the course of care and treatment. But withholding vital information from patients or deceiving them limits their decision-making capability.

Health providers have not always been upfront with patients about their diagnoses. Providers have been particularly sensitive to cases where the diagnosis is serious and there appears to be no real treatment options available. Health providers' concerns about what this information will do to the patient are also shared with many families and patient caregivers. In some cultures and societies, families fear that patients' hearing unfavorable outcomes will be too upsetting and may make them feel hopeless and depressed.

Discussions about death with patients and families in some societies are met with resistance. For example, there are specific cultural and religious beliefs held by ethnic minorities and indigenous groups that influence how news about impending death is to be handled.

For these reasons, the cultural and religious beliefs of these patients and their families must be taken into consideration and planned for accordingly. Providers must be cognizant of the fact that many immigrant and cultural groups are being treated within the context of the mainstream culture. It may be that patients and their families want information but prefer to use their own words and customs to convey this information to their sick family member. Providers should be aware that approaches to these patients and their families must take their religious and cultural beliefs into consideration when planning and carrying out these kinds of discussion.

In the medical field, withholding information is paramount to misrepresenting the facts or nondisclosure. Truth-telling is a standard that takes precedence. Absence of truth-telling can and usually does have negative consequences. Deception or lying to the patient is unethical, may create mistrust in the health care team, and may lead to the need to withhold still more information. It should not be assumed that patients do not know about their diagnosis and prognosis. Patients frequently sense what is not being said, their family members may tell them, and other providers on the team may inadvertently give clues to the results of tests or procedures.

Provider Discomfort in Truth-Telling

There are several reasons why providers prefer to not fully disclose information. These reasons may be similar to those of the patients' family. First, they do not want to give patients a diagnosis and prognosis if they are not entirely certain. Second, they may be unsure of patients' emotional stability and the appropriate time to share information with them. Third, they have not yet had a conversation with the patient where they have discussed what the patient did and did not want to know, or when they wanted to be told. Parallel to these issues is patients' preferences about what family members are told.

There are a few exceptions to the rule of truth-telling. First, patients may tell the physician or team members they do not want to be told their diagnosis or prognosis. Second, patients may be cognitively, emotionally, or mentally unable to receive the information. This includes situations where the patient is unconscious or otherwise incapable of consenting and harm from failure to treat is imminent. Additionally, not all health care team members are authorized to give the patient this kind of information. Even if they are asked for the information, it is their duty to say they are not authorized to give the patient the information but will inform their physician that they want to know. Ideally this is followed up by a note in the patient's chart, a secure Internet-transmitted message or phone call. This allows the physician or provider some background about the concerns of the patient and/or family.

It should be noted that if patients later change their mind and inform providers that they want to know more, they are entitled to the information. In no case should it be assumed that the patient prefers nondisclosure; or for that matter, full disclosure. Both how much and when the patient wants to know, if at all, is best gleamed from conversations with patients and questions e.g. "While we are waiting to find out the results of the tests, what if anything would you like to know when we get the results?" And, "Do you prefer I ask you at that time what you want to know?"

The AMA notes that physicians should sensitively and respectfully disclose relevant health care information to patients and the quantity and specificity of this information should be tailored to meet the preferences and needs of individual patients. Some information may be given initially and then more information given at a later time based upon the patient's needs and capacity. Respect for the patient's particular cultural and religious beliefs is important when assessing patient needs and capacities, planning an approach, and charting the approach for other providers to follow.

Still another special circumstance surrounding truth-telling is the extent to which different words are used to describe the patient's condition when medical terminology is either too harsh or difficult for patients to understand. The idea is not to either *sugarcoat* bad news or give the news harshly and without regard to the emotional impact on the patient.

In a documentary about framing troublesome diagnoses, Geppert (2011) uses the example of talking to a patient about a diagnosis of seizures of nonneurological origin. This terminology may confuse the patient and lends no additional information. A preferred term may be *functional seizures* because it avoids the mistake of implying nondiagnosis of medically unexplained conditions and side steps the issue of whether the condition is of psychological origin. Providers face this kind of dilemma when being fearful that the exact diagnosis will create emotional stress and may even cause patients to exit the care of the provider before therapy can be started. Generally, all providers are sensitive to and aware of adverse effects of unloading information without regard for the emotional impact on the patient and family.

Truth-Telling with Vulnerable Populations

As mentioned, it is critical to consider the capacity of the patient to receive certain information. The former example addressed issues of truth-telling with patients who may be upset emotionally. There are still other patients who have a separate psychiatric or mental health diagnosis which impacts what approach providers should take in truth-telling. When patients have comorbid psychiatric conditions the concern for the emotional impact of a troublesome diagnosis is even more complicated.

When patients are judged to be emotionally or mentally unable to receive and process the information, consultation from a mental health professional about the circumstances

of disclosing unfavorable news is warranted. When patients are cognitively incapable of receiving important information (e.g., patients receiving care for dementia or Alzheimer's), a critical part of truth-telling is engaging family caregivers. Gitlin and Hodgson (2016) suggest that with these patients reaching out to these family caregivers is a moral obligation out of concern for the caregiver and the patient. Reaching out to family caregivers can mean revealing details about the patient that was previously not available to them or the patient. However, as Gitlin and Hodgson suggest, when a provider engages the family in these discussions, they are working under the umbrella of family-centered care which is not only appropriate but ethically and morally warranted.

Special Consideration in the Case of Minors

Consideration of the impact of truth-telling on patients is also important in reviewing the rights of children and adolescents. In the strict sense of the doctrine, patients have the right to know. One can argue that some children (early teens) or adolescents have the cognitive capacity and maturity to be provided sufficient relevant information to make a rational decision or participate in shared decision-making. However, minors are in a category which would not afford them the right to health information of significance, especially if the treatment approach is uncertain or impinges significantly on their welfare.

In most cases, there is little doubt that deferring rights to know to surrogate decision-makers such as parents or legal guardians is the appropriate practice. The proper involvement of underage children is to gain their assent, not consent, for treatment. Still, a lack of clarity can exist. Do minors, particularly older ones, have a right to know which is foundational to shared decision-making? And, does this right to know take precedence over parents wishes or preferences not to tell their minor about their illness and the potential impact of treatment? (See **EXHIBIT 22-1.**)

Physicians and providers faced with the situation in this case can feel torn between on the one hand, their beliefs that the child has a "right" to know about a probable side effect that could profoundly affect him in his adult life and on the other hand, the desire of his parents to "protect" him. Should the parents be pursuaded to enable Adam the opportunity of having a procedure to produce a semen sample? The final outcome of these deliberations was that the parents' wishes must prevail. The reasoning was that Adam resides in a state that does not have a mature minor law but there was also uncertainty about what approach (disclosing or not disclosing) would cause Adam the most psychological distress, immediately and in the future.

EXHIBIT 22-1 Case Study: Addressing the Need to Know in Minors and Teens

Rosoff (2017), in a commentary in the *American Medical Association Journal of Ethics*, discusses the case of a 13-year-old patient (Adam) diagnosed with Ewing's sarcoma (a cancerous tumor that grows in bones and surrounding soft tissue). The dilemma faced by the attending physician and medical student caring for Adam involved deciding what information this teen should have about the affects of his treatment. Essentially, this teen needed to be treated immediately and the treatment was likely to cause infertility. Additionally, Adam might not have time to use a sperm bank because of the necessity to start treatment immediately. The parents clearly stated that they did not want Adam to be told about this treatment's side effect.

This should be a clear and uncontested decision to honor the parents' preferences but the medical student (Jenny) while talking to Adam hears Adam say, "I can't wait to have a big family one day." This medical student discusses the possibility that Adam could suffer psychologically if he realizes later he was uninformed about the treatment's infertility risk. Does he need to be informed of the risk? Does he have a right to know about this side effect? In his commentary, Rosoff adds that in at least 14 states (mature minor) laws exist to empower certain children who demonstrate evidence of the capacity to understand their medical condition and potential benefits and harms of the proposed treatment to act as authorities over issues related to their treatment.

▶ Informed Choice and Informed Consent

Informed choice and **informed consent** require that patients are fully informed about their illness, the available treatments, the side effects of any treatment, and the anticipated prognosis given the chosen treatment. The practice of truth-telling is intimately linked to patients' informed choice and consent. The underlying assumption behind the issues of informed choice and informed consent is that in health care arenas, the balance of power seems to rest with providers. After all, the patient is ill or otherwise incapacitated and is at the mercy of the system's definition of when, where, what, and how actions will be taken.

By virtue of this actual or perceived inequitable power distribution, patients' rights for self-determination must be protected. Inherent in this objective is the standard to act and communicate in ways that respect the dignity and worth of every patient. Above all, patient autonomy is to be protected and respected. Health care providers are ethically and morally obligated to respect the individuality of all patients who are recipients of their care, and this includes patients' and families' unique perceptions of their rights to informed choice and consent.

An entire science of bioethical decision-making has emerged to assist providers with complexities surrounding patient autonomy in health care situations. In a summary of the history of truth-telling in American medicine, Sisk, Frankel, Kodish, and Harry Isaacson (2016, p. 77) explain that although the patient's right to know is supported, *it is difficult to know exactly what they ought to know, and how to best share this information.* These are critical questions that are worthy of study. The truth about truth-telling is that it is an unfinished history that continues to evolve.

Informed Choice

In each and every health care situation, providers have a duty to provide patients choices and participation decision power germane to their care and treatment. Informed choice refers to the process patients use to arrive at a decision about health care. It is based upon access to and full understanding of available information about one's diagnosis and treatment. Informed consent refers to the communication patient and providers have after patients have been provided information needed to make health care decisions.

Providers are the conveyors of available choices. They explain what health care options are available and why certain choices are not available. These choices reflect the medical technology and resources available at the treatment setting and at the time. For example, providers cannot offer an alternative surgical procedure if the procedure is contrary to hospital policy or is not available due to lack of medical and professional resources. Also, they may not be able to offer a certain kind of surgical intervention because the patient's insurance does not consider it to be an approved procedure.

Providers are, however, obligated to describe the alternatives that are available, and if asked, other options that exist but are not available at the particular health care setting. Informed choice requires providers to clearly communicate about treatment choices but also about other less-favored approaches or alternatives.

Do Not Resuscitate Orders

A commonly reported area in which discussion of choices may not be handled adequately is in do not resuscitate (DNR) orders. The idea is that patients or their legally appointed guardian are to be consulted before orders to not resuscitate are made, added to, or changed in the patient's medical record. In many cases where patients' rights have been violated, the courts have ruled in favor of patients and their families, sending a clear and strong message to providers and the health care setting that patients have a legal right to be informed and consulted in relation to DNR decisions. The provider excuse that patients might get upset by this discussion is not a valid excuse. Providers are clearly warned not to exclude patients and/or their guardians from these decisions even when their involvement might distress them.

Robinson et al. (2012) studied the awareness of outpatients about the term DNR and their preferences: when, where, and with whom they want to have DNR discussions. The results of their survey reported that of those were surveyed and had heard of the term, only a small number (8%) of those who reported being aware of DNR orders reported ever discussing the subject with a health care provider. On the whole, patients preferred to have these discussions early with their family physician and in an office setting.

In another pilot study of the DNR education needs of patients in a multidisciplinary lung cancer clinic, Ahmed et al. (2015) found that patients expressed a limited degree of understanding of DNR even though providers perceived patients to understand DNR most of the time. Both caregivers and patients believed that the physician was responsible for choosing the appropriate time or opportunity to initiate the discussion of DNR. The results of these studies suggested that patients may not have discussed DNR prior to becoming critically ill and those who were experiencing a critical illness had only a limited understanding of DNR while their providers thought they understood DNR most of the time.

Advanced Care Directives

The issue of DNR orders brings up a related concern, the patient's advanced directive. The Patient Self-Determination Act (PSDA) set the stage for clarifying patient informed choice. On November 5, 1990, Congress passed this measure as an amendment to the Omnibus Budget Reconciliation Act of 1990. It requires providers to give adult individuals at the time of inpatient admission or enrollment certain information about their rights under state laws governing advance directives, including (1) the right to participate in and direct their own health care decisions, (2) the right to accept or refuse medical or surgical treatment, (3) the right to prepare an advance directive, and (4) information on the provider's policies that govern the utilization of these rights.

The act also prohibits institutions from discriminating against a patient who does not have an advance directive. The PSDA further requires institutions to document patient information and provide ongoing community education on advance directives. Whereas attitudes toward advance directives are generally positive, some providers have little knowledge of the Durable Power of Attorney for Health Care Act and are poorly equipped to discuss it with patients, not only out of ignorance, but because of their own personal discomforts.

Provider Discomfort with Informed Choice

While providers must promote and insure informed choice, a number of factors influence the process, including the historical and technological treatment patterns as well as the philosophical and even religious background of providers. These factors often explain why providers may hold different attitudes about the same issue and why certain providers are

more comfortable in their communications with patients than others.

Some providers come from cultural and religious backgrounds that do not place high value on principles of autonomy and self-determination. One might expect these providers to understand and practice informed-choice procedures somewhat differently. Without accusing or critically evaluating these providers, we can say that their approach to informing patients of treatment choices may be influenced by their underlying belief system. For example, they may fail to address all potential treatment choices or they may overemphasize their authority in directing patients' choices.

Provider authoritative views and opinions can influence the degree to which patients perceive they truly have a choice in the matter. On a more subtle level, these providers may verbally present choices but nonverbally suggest that their opinions should be followed. Hopefully not, but in some cases their encounters with patients and families may suggest that if provider advice is not followed, there may be negative repercussions. Whether real or perceived, patients and families are not always able to negotiate a different outcome. Along these lines not only providers but, as previously explained, patients and families may hold cultural or religious beliefs that place less emphasis on autonomy in directing medical care. These patients and families frequently prefer the leadership of health professionals in making decisions about their care.

Despite this subtle, and not so subtle, interplay between providers' preferences and patients' choices, one thing must be clear, the patient, although this can be delegated to a legal guardian, has the right to be the primary decision-maker. With the advancement of the science of bioethical decision-making, there has been a renewed concern for patients' individual roles in their care and their personal freedom to direct this care. It is generally maintained that patients are critical participants and should retain significant control over health care decisions that affect their welfare, and they can only do this if the communications between the provider and patient is open and fluid.

Choice Is Not Absolute

In 1983, the President's Commission for the Study of Ethical Problems in Medicine and Biomedical and Behavioral Research issued a recommendation with regard to patients' roles in health care decisions. This document supported the important concept that patients with the capacity to make decisions be permitted to do so. The Commission, however, indicated that the process is based on mutual respect and shared information, although this choice is not absolute. For example, patients and their families cannot expect health care providers to render services that violate standards of practice or the providers' moral beliefs. This document also touched on the issue of reasonable rights; that is, the patient and family cannot insist on services that draw on limited resources to which the patient has no binding claim.

For example, expensive one-to-one nursing care at the expense of the hospital, although desired by some patients and families as a routine aspect of their care, is outside the realm of possibility—the patient and family have no binding contract with the facility to receive this type of care. This clarification of the limits of patients' choice in health care is made on a case-by-case basis. The institution's rights may predominate but this is not just an issue of providers maintaining power over patients or their families. Rather, it provides some protection to the health care facility and provider groups as they attempt to balance patient autonomy with instances in which it is inappropriate to let patients or their families to make the final choice.

What remains critical here is that regardless of the request, respectful discussions, in which information is provided in ways the patient and family can comprehend, must be ensured and is a prerequisite to informed consent.

Informed Consent

Informed choice and informed consent are overlapping concepts. Both rely on patients and/or their legal guardians to be adequately informed of the patient's condition and treatment choices. That providers are competent in ethical decision-making is no longer a given but must be nurtured on an ongoing basis. Clearly, recent changes in health care delivery have profoundly changed the way in which providers and patients and providers and families communicate. As patients and their families now assume two identities—health consumers or customers and active participants in medical decision-making—they are more and more concerned not only about symptoms, disease, and treatment but equally preoccupied with issues of quality, access to, and cost of health care. Informed consent requires confidence in providers as well as the health setting to deliver the best care possible.

Legislation and policy have addressed multiple concerns of surrounding informed consent in today's health care marketplace. Among these policy documents is the Institute of Medicine's landmark 2001 report on *Crossing the Quality Chasm*. The Institute of Medicine (IOM) listed "patient-centered care" as one of the six fundamental aims of the U.S. health care system. The IOM defines patient-centered care as

> Health care that establishes a partnership among practitioners, patients, and their families (when appropriate) to ensure that decisions respect patients' wants, needs, and preferences and that patients have the education and support they need to make decisions and participate in their own care.

Such policies reinforce the expectation that patients must have access to information and most importantly, be offered the opportunity to make decisions based on information they receive. The issue of informed consent is derived from the value of self-determination wherein information is the prelude to informed choice. That is, under normal circumstances informed patients are capable of making decisions about their care.

Barriers to Informed Consent in the Clinical Setting

There can be many difficulties in achieving patient-informed consent and these difficulties cause us to consider how well-informed consent can be secured in every instance. Patients, families, and providers frequently come to decisions with dissimilar values and beliefs. This is particularly the case if patients and families come from minority groups or non-Western cultures that may resist open discussions about issues of life and death related to health care choices. Even if these values and beliefs appear compatible, their translations may be quite different. For example, both patient and families and provider may want the best possible surgical intervention and on the outside their views seem compatible. When these views are translated to specific steps and "surgical cuts," however, providers' views tend to be more radical.

Because patient- and family-held values and beliefs are always subject to individual interpretation, they are best presented explicitly by the patient and family and not simply inferred from previous conversations. If the patient and/or family is unable to verbalize the specifics, then providers can address gaps in understanding by qualifying or clarifying patient and family views.

Time to discuss patient preferences can be limited. Knowing the views of the patient and/or family requires time, time in the context of a therapeutic relationship. Does the provider have the time that is required to learn the views of the patient and patient's family? Some providers feel that too much time spent in extracting patients' and families' views may inhibit decision-making rather than facilitate it. They are concerned that the process can

get bogged down when decisions need to be made. In extended communications of this sort, it is common that patients and families ask about many options. Sometimes these options are impractical or have never been tried before.

As previously explained, providers worry about a phenomenon referred to as *patient overwhelm*. Bester, Cole, and Koish (2016) discuss factors that commonly overwhelm patients' decision-making capacity in clinical settings. In summary, too many options can contribute to the confusion about what decision to make. The patient, family, and provider may have already had difficulty with only two options for action, and now the situation is complicated with still additional choices. These authors differentiate between emotional overwhelm and informational overload. They argue that in these situations the provider's primary duty is prevention of harm and suggest the basis for discharging patient obligation.

They use the example of genetic sequencing testing which involves both scientific and technical information that may compromise the decisional capacity of patients because this information in not easily understood by patients and families. Furthermore, these authors discuss several alternative approaches to obtaining informed consent in clinical situations. These include surrogate decision-making and shared (provider evidence sharing) decision-making. They rebut the objection that these could lead to paternalistic practices.

On the whole, providers would agree that the time spent in learning to understand the patient and family concerns, religious beliefs, and cultural beliefs is very worthwhile. There are many of us who would say that this process is not only valuable, it is an imperative. Providing the best care possible rests on knowing patients and their families well. Earlier in this chapter truth-telling was addressed in the process of informed choice. Truth-telling is also critical in the process of gaining informed consent. Deception, when translated into specific acts, includes withholding information, deliberately making the information unclear or difficult to understand, minimizing important aspects, and presenting an unbalanced picture.

These actions when applied to ensuring informed choice or informed consent are unethical. It is currently held that with each act of deception, however minor, there is a corrosive effect on the patient–provider relationship. The trust that is necessary in patient–family–provider relationships suffers with even the most minor instances of deception. Patients cannot consent to care or procedures under these conditions.

Informed Consent to Participate in a Research Study

The process of informed consent becomes even more deliberate when patients are involved in research studies. Research studies are usually of two kinds: (1) those focused on specific medical experiments (e.g., studies involving experimental drugs or devices) and (2) those focused on nonmedical research (e.g., studies in the social and behavioral sciences that study attitudes, beliefs, and behaviors through the use of surveys and interviews).

Research studies involve several issues around patient's rights and, therefore, undergo a great deal of scrutiny in institutional review boards (IRBs) and human subject protection committees (HSPCs). Issues of concern to review committees include notification of patients about: (1) risks (minimal and major) of physical and/or emotional injury; (2) freedom to withdraw without consequences to care and treatment; (3) physical and/or emotional (mental) discomfort or pain related to the research process; (4) loss or invasion of privacy, dignity, and/or autonomy by consenting to participate; and (5) the time and energy required to participate.

In any research study, these issues must be addressed clearly and truthfully by researchers. Under review, these issues are extensively examined, including the clarity of the investigators' descriptions. An approval issued by an IRB or HSPC always evaluates the risks of participation in the study relative to the benefits. Any conditions placing the patient at risk are explained and provided for and that all this information has been adequately communicated by the investigator.

Additionally, IRBs will expect to be assured that specific issues related to subject recruitment, procedures for obtaining informed consent, and protecting confidentiality are addressed. They are concerned with how subjects will be selected and contacted as well as what subjects will be told on the first contact. IRBs are concerned about whether subjects and data about subjects will be identifiable by name and, if patients are identified by name, what procedures will be used to collect, process, and store data that will protect patient identity.

Review boards expect patients to be informed of the purpose of the study; the expected duration of their participation; and the reasonably foreseeable immediate and long-term discomforts, hazards, risks, and potential consequences. Every consent must include certain guarantees. These vary from institution to institution but generally include stated reassurances that (1) the patient may refuse to participate or may withdraw from participation at any time without any negative consequences; (2) no information that identifies the patient will be released without the patient's separate consent (except as specifically required by law); and (3) if the study, design, or use of data is changed, patients will be informed and their consent reobtained.

The written informed consent forms (ICFs) tell the patient and family who to contact with concerns or questions about the research study and how to proceed if this avenue does not satisfy them. A copy of the written consent along with a statement of the **Patient's Bill of Rights** is provided to each subject. In the case that a subject is unable to sign (e.g., in the case of minors), a signature (and date) is obtained from a parent or guardian. If the patient cannot sign because of physical disability or illiteracy but is otherwise capable of being informed and of giving verbal consent, a third party not connected with the study (a next of kin or guardian) would be asked to witness the discussion, sign, and state the reason for standing in for the patient. When a research participant's native language is one other than English (or the person is poorly versed in English), an accurate translation must be used.

Studies of a medical nature involving treatment of disease or illness (e.g., those involving experimental drugs or medical devices) must provide additional information to patients. Studies of this kind must include a statement that describes any appropriate alternative procedures or treatment that might be advantageous, including both the risks and benefits of these alternatives.

▶ The Legal Status of the Patient–Provider Relationship

Health care providers are confronted with many legal and ethical issues but advancing medical technology is not the sole reason for this circumstance. Health care delivery has become exceedingly complex. The emerging system of managed care and provider medical groups brings countless important issues to the surface that includes who decides, who gives care, and who, ultimately, is accountable for outcomes. A good deal of this complexity is played out in one-to-one encounters with providers. Accountability, responsibility, and, subsequently, liability, is understood or misunderstood in the specific context of patient–provider relationships.

Just about every ethical and/or legal issue raised reflects the inadequacy of patient–family–provider communication and the trustworthiness of the relationship. Refusal or withdrawal of treatment, for example, occurs in the context of mutual understanding of one another's roles and beliefs. Patient and family dissatisfaction and/or the decision to pursue litigation reflects, in large part, the poor quality of communication.

Legal Duty to Provide Care

Duty to the patient, including a breach of duty, underlies standards of practice for all health care professionals. When health care professionals enter into a relationship with patients and/or families, a duty or obligation is established and is recognized as an ensuing legal relationship. This legal relationship holds the professional accountable for practicing within established standards of practice. When this duty includes providing care as well as protecting patients from harm, the legal relationship becomes even more complex. Consider instances of complexity when the provider delivers substandard care and is also charged with protecting the welfare of the patient. Unfortunate outcomes in these cases generally provide legal grounds for malpractice claims.

Providers, however, are also commonly confronted with situations that impinge on, or have the potential to impinge on, patients' rights. The four basic consumer rights outlined by the American Hospital Association (AHA) are (1) the right to safety, (2) the right to be informed, (3) the right to choose, and (4) the right to be heard. What happens if the provider witnesses infractions of these rights by others in the health care system?

Most clearly, the legal duty of all providers includes protecting patients from harm and from any violation of their rights even when they are not the primary provider for the patient. Consider, for example, a particular patient who is not warned of the consequences of a research protocol or drug trial. Let us also say that another provider, or even a group of providers, is aware of this problem.

It is obvious that the provider who is prescribing the treatment is wrong and at risk for malpractice through negligence. Still, are the providers who are aware of the problem and who do not intercede also negligent? One could argue convincingly that this is the case. In many cases, malpractice claims are levied against the institution as well as the individual practitioner in charge of the patient's care. The issue here is that other professionals in the institution were aware of the situation and did not correct it. As providers within the clinical setting, they had a moral, ethical, and legal duty to intervene.

Providers Who Refuse to Provide Care

Ethical standards state that providers cannot refuse to provide care because of any prejudice, discrimination, or dislike of a patient or family. It is not publically or widely known that providers can refuse to give care under certain circumstances. Essentially, providers do have the right to refuse to provide care under selected instances. The most common objection would be that the providing care would violate a personally held moral or religious belief. If the interventions to be used stand in opposition to the provider's ethics or values refusal is generally supported. When providers practice in institutions (e.g., hospitals or public clinics) any conflicts of this kind are usually communicated early on to avoid circumstances of singling out a specific patient or family. Additionally, if the provider feels incompetent to care for a patient, this refusal is supportable. On the flip side, if providers assume care that they are not competent to perform, they may be disciplined for incompetence or negligence.

There are other circumstances that may cause providers to refuse to give care: (1) physical risk (when there is strong evidence to suggest more than minimal risk to the providers themselves), (2) the care to be given violates patient autonomy and rights to self-determination, and (3) religious and/or moral issues that cause the provider to object.

Most institutions will support a provider's personal objections provided that these are stated well in advance and result in no harm or negative consequences for patients. The following statement adopted by the AMA addresses the physician's right to refuse.

> A physician shall, in the provision of appropriate patient care, except in emergencies, be free to choose whom to serve, with whom to associate, and the environment in which to provide medical care.
>
> (Adopted by the AMA's House of Delegates, June 17, 2001)

While the duty to provide care is quite clear, providers' refusals to provide care are not infrequent. Early on in the AIDS epidemic, many providers expressed their fears, and even distaste, about caring for patients with AIDS. These fears, expressed as fear of AIDS contagion, were questioned because the chance of a provider contracting HIV infection was extremely small. These fears were often worsened by conflicting values and underlying prejudice against persons or groups who practiced risky behaviors. With time this initial fear and reservation changed. In a study regarding stigma against those with HIV/AIDS (Kinsler, Wong, Sayles, Davis, and Cunningham, 2007) the concern that provider bias could result in serious consequences was raised. Essentially, stigma can affect health care utilization, and lack of access or delayed access to care may result in late presentation to receive care (i.e., until more advanced stages of HIV disease). These authors called for interventions to reduce stigma in health care settings which might include modeling non stigmatizing behavior during education of health care professionals.

A provider's reluctance to care and refusal to care can be communicated to patients even when the patient is not told about the provider's reluctance explicitly. Such hesitancy may be blatant (e.g., in refusal to enter a patient's room, exaggerated protective measures, and even direct comments to patients, implying that they have some form of character weakness). It may also be covert (e.g., in little time spent with the patient and minimal communication responsiveness). Historically, provider refusal to provide care was viewed as unethical. Ethical codes focused on patients' rights, ignoring providers' values and beliefs, but times have changed. The shift toward recognizing providers' limits to providing care have largely been regarded positively because forcing them to provide care could be detrimental to both patient and provider.

Limitations on Patients' Personal Choices

The doctrines of personal choice and informed consent originated largely from malpractice litigation. Historically, patients' rights to informed consent were blatantly violated. Patients knew little of the nature of their treatment, outcomes, or alternative procedures (and/or the outcomes of no intervention).

There was no conceivable way in which patients could enter into a personal cost–benefit analysis. To correct this situation, numerous changes occurred but the outcomes of these changes did not respect the limitations of patient decision-making. The President's Commission for the Study of Ethical Problems in Medicine and Biomedical and Behavioral Research (1983) recognized that patients' choices were not absolute. This limitation was described as irregularities in patients' requests such that they violated standards of practice or overtaxed clinical resources.

There are specific circumstances where providers' recommendations clearly need to be heeded in spite of contrary beliefs of patients and/or their families. In these cases, it is appropriate for providers to make the final decision for action. Perhaps the most obvious situation is when the patient clearly and directly requests the provider to make the decision. In this case, it is important for providers to understand why the patient or patient's family has requested that the provider decide. There is at least one problem area in respect

to the traditional deference given to providers. Some cultural groups are more likely to defer to authority figures. When their request is an unnecessarily dependent one, the provider has an obligation to engage the patient or patient's family more actively in the decision-making process. In any case, providers should not take the relinquishing of decision-making by the patient and/or family lightly.

▶ The Problems with Informed Choice and Informed Consent

In the previous discussions of difficulties in achieving informed choice and informed consent, several issues were raised, many of which do not appear at first but become more obvious with time. It is important to understand some basic principles behind the processes of informed choice and informed consent in further judging patients' capacity to participate in these processes and how they might need to be adjusted to meet the particular needs and readiness of patient groups.

Assumptions About Patients

The concepts of informed choice and informed consent are based on the important assumption that the patient (and/or family) is adequately informed. Prerequisites are patients willing, capable, and competent to receive and process the information provided to them. Questions that must be satisfied appear in **EXHIBIT 22-2**.

Special Problems with Certain Patient Groups

It is important to recognize that all patients have handicaps in one or more of these areas: perception, processing, and expressing their thoughts and preferences. Patients' unwillingness to be informed, their inability to receive

EXHIBIT 22-2 Questions That Must Be Satisfied to Ensure Patients Are Adequately Informed

- Does the patient have the ability to hear or read?
- Is the language used respectful of the patient's preferred language and level of understanding?
- Is the method used to present the information tailored according to the patient's age and educational level?
- Is the patient's attention span and memory sufficient enough to adequately comprehend and process the information provided?
- Is the patient likely to clarify information that is not clear to them or is there a need to explore this with them in additional further discussions?
- Does the patient understand his or her rights to decide even if their decisions run counter to providers' advice or recommendations?
- Does the patient have the capacity to clearly communicate his or her decisions and preferences?

and to process data, and their incapacities to express themselves are due to many factors. These factors include their particular symptoms and illness, the effects of treatment, their psychological responses to illness, any trauma and crisis resulting from the awareness of a guarded prognosis, recency of diagnosis, and other personal demographic factors (age, education, and sociocultural background).

Historically, certain groups have been recognized because of their special limitations. These groups include the mentally impaired and developmentally delayed, prisoners, the mentally ill, children, and the elderly. These groups are known to have limitations in one or more areas of communication (reception, processing, and/or expression of thoughts and feelings). A group that is particularly

vulnerable to infringement of personal choice are those individuals who are institutionalized or imprisoned. In these cases, the freedom that patients can exercise in making choices, even if they are fully informed and communicate competently, can seem severely restricted.

Coercion, in the form of implied or expressed threat, is considered to be a factor in restricting choices and, therefore, is an actual or potential threat to individual rights in prisons. Prisons, for security reasons, exercise nearly total control over their residents' lives. In situations outside of correctional institutions, the right to consent to care brings with it the right to refuse care. The right to informed consent and refuse medical treatment is also a right of prisoners (*Prison Legal News*, 2017). While a required provision in prisons as well, some question the true provision of prisoners rights to choose or refuse treatments.

First, many prisons do not have the full range of treatments that are found in public and private community health centers. Additionally, surrogate decision-makers are appointed to manage the medical treatment needs of prisoners who are incapacitated or ambiguous about treatment. However, the National Commission of Correctional Health Care (2009) clarifies that written informed consents are required and a single "blanket" consent for medical treatment is not in keeping with standards of care. Furthermore, this involves not only major illness but even in cases where invasive diagnostic tests and use of psychotropic medications (e.g., for anxiety, depression, and posttraumatic stress disorder [PTSD]) are used.

Patients may represent multiple groups who have known impairment. Patients can belong to one or more than one of the following groups: the elderly, mentally ill, and children with mental impairments. These individuals are known to not be able to participate in the informed consent, informed choice processes. Usually, family or court-appointed guardians representing the patient are included in the informed consent process.

▶ Summary

A lack of effective communication between providers and patients is at the root of the violation of patients' rights. Whether the problem is one of violations of the standards of informed choice or informed consent, a lack of effective communication can lead providers into serious ethical, moral, and legal problems. Providers have an obligation to care and also to protect patients from harm. When the problems in communication are not a result of their interactions but involve encounters with other providers, there remains the obligation to intervene and change existing circumstances. If a patient does not know about treatment options, is not aware of the consequences of a chosen treatment, or feels that the choice provided is not a "real choice," patients' rights are in jeopardy.

Communications are increasingly important in cases of informed choice and informed consent because of concerns about truth-telling and the medical and legal implications of denying patients these opportunities. Providers have not always been convinced of the patient's need for or desire to be told the details of their diagnosis, prognosis, or even alternatives for treatment. However, current Western medical practices place a high value on providing adequate and accurate truthful information to patients and/or their families. This is indicative of the commitment to patient autonomy and participation in shared decision-making.

Above all else, professionals are members of an ethical and moral community. This community is made stronger by the support of and adherence to standards of practice that protect patients' rights. The privileged nature of patient–family–provider relationships derives meaning from the morality of the health professions and health care system as a whole.

Discussion

1. What are the ethical standards for truth-telling in matters concerning patients' health status and needs for treatment?
2. Are there exceptions about truth-telling. If so, what are they and what about truth-telling is questionable?
3. Discuss the statement that informed choice is a prerequisite to informed consent.
4. Identify barriers providers may experience when providing patients opportunities for informed choice.
5. Identify groups for which obtaining informed consent for medical or research study purposes is difficult to achieve.

References

Ahmed, N., Lobchuk, M., Hunter, W. M., Johnston, P., Nugent, Z., Sharma, A., … Sisler, J. (2015). How, when and where to discuss do not resuscitate: A prospective study to compare the perceptions and preferences of patients, caregivers, and health care providers in a multidisciplinary lung cancer clinic. *Cureus, 7*(3), e257. doi:10.7759/cureus.257

Ahmed, S., Bryant, L. D., Tizro, Z., & Shickle, D. (2012). Interpretations of informed choice in antenatal screening: A cross-cultural, Q-methodology study. *Social Science & Medicine, 74*(7), 997–1004. doi:10.1016 /j.socscimed.2011.12.02

AMA. (2012). The AMA Code of Medical Ethics' opinions on informing patients. *Virtual Mentor American Medical Association Journal of Ethics, 14*(7), 555–556. Retrieved from virtualmentor.ama-assn.org/2012/07 /coet1-1207.html

Bester, J., Cole, C. M., & Kodish, E. (2016). The limits of informed consent for an overwhelmed patient: Clinicians' role in protecting patients and preventing overwhelm. *American Medical Association Journal of Ethics, 18*(9), 869–886. doi:10.1001/journalofethics.2016.18.9.peer2-1609

Geppert, C. (2011). Commentary. Clinical case: A virtue ethics approach to framing troublesome diagnoses. *Virtual Mentor American Medical Association Journal of Ethics, 13*(12), 861–865. doi:10.1001/virtualmentor.2011.13.12.ccas3-1112

Gitlin, L. N., & Hodgson, N. A. (2016). Commentary. Who should assess the needs of and care for a dementia patient's caregiver. *AMA Journal of Ethics, 18*(12), 1171–1181. doi:10.1001/journalofethics.2016.18.12.ecas1-1612

Institute of Medicine. (2001). *Crossing the quality chasm: A new health system for the 21st century.* Washington, DC: The National Academy Press. Retrieved from www.nationalacademies.org

Kinsler, J. J., Wong, M. D., Sayles, J. N., Davis, C., & Cunningham, W. E. (2007). The effect of perceived stigma from a health care provider on access to care among a low-income HIV-positive population. *AIDS Patient Care and STDS, 21*(8), 584–592. doi:10.1089/apc.2006.0202

Kirlin, D. (2007). Truth telling, autonomy and the role of metaphor. *Journal of Medical Ethics, 33*, 11–14. doi:10.1136/jme.2005.014993

Lee, Y. K., Lee, P. Y., Cheong, A. T., Ng, C. J., Abdullah, K. L., Ong, T. A., & Razack, A. H. A. R. (2015) To share or not to share: Malaysian healthcare professionals' views on localized prostate cancer treatment decision making roles. *PLoS ONE, 10*(11), e0142812. doi:10.1371/journal.pone.0142812

National Commission on Correctional Health Care. (2009, June). Informed consent. *Correctional Care, 23*(3), *Summer 2009.* https://www.ncchc.org/informed-consent

Prison Legal News. (2017). *Prisoners have right to informed consent and to refuse medical treatment.* Retrieved from prisonlegalnews.org

Robinson, C., Kolesar, S., Boyko, M., Berkowitz, J., Calam, B., & Collins, M. (2012). Awareness of do-not-resuscitate orders: What do patients know and want? *Canadian Family Physician, 58*(4), e229–e233. PMID:22611610

Rosoff, P. M. (2017). Commentary. Ethics case: Do pediatric patients have a right to know? *American Medical Association Journal of Ethics, 19*(5), 426–435. doi:10.1001/journalofethics.2017.19.05.ecas2-1705

Sisk, B., Frankel, R., Kodish, E., & Harry Isaacson, J. (2016). The truth about truth-telling in American medicine: A brief history. *The Permanente Journal, 20*(3), 74–77. doi:10.7812/TPP/15-219

CHAPTER 23

The Privileged Nature of Patient–Provider Communications: Issues of Confidentiality, Anonymity, and Privacy

CHAPTER OBJECTIVES

- Describe and discuss the regulations surrounding the principle of protecting patient–provider confidentiality.
- Explain the ways in which provider–patient communications are privileged.
- Identify the strengths and limitations imposed by the principle of confidentiality.
- Describe how anonymity and privacy can be maintained.
- Discuss the inability to provide absolute protection for confidentiality of patient–provider communications.

▶ Introduction

The issue of confidentiality of patient and/or family communications with providers has not always been debated but in recent times the legality of divulging patient information has received more attention. In the past 40–50 years, a great deal of attention has centered around the meaning and limitations of privileged communications in relationships between patients and providers. The majority of this discussion has been sparked by two important and related issues: the confidentiality of the clinical and research process and infractions of patients' rights that reached the level of litigation.

The issue of **privileged communication in health care** is extremely important in regard to patient–provider relationships. Many states have granted statutes that guarantee privileged communication for health care professionals; that is, these professionals are not compelled to provide information in courts of law because the information is privileged. Still, these statutes have been challenged by arguments against privileged communication because what is "right" in most cases can be terribly wrong in others. The following cases raise the concern about withholding information that would protect the common good.

One case centers around the threat of societal exposure to HIV. The argument addresses the issue of social good versus individual rights. That is, it is deemed essential to reveal certain health information that would otherwise be held confidential because reporting it is essential to protect society. A different and most notable example, where the rights to confidentiality were challenged, was in a landmark case in California (*Tarasoff v. Regents of the University of California*, 1974) (**EXHIBIT 23-1**).

▶ The Sacrosanctity of Provider–Patient Communications

The communications between providers and patients are considered to be sacrosanct. The **sacrosanctity of provider-patient communications** means that these communications are so vital and important that nothing should interfere with patients' rights to trust that what is revealed is protected.

When patients and families seek medical intervention, they might reveal very intimate details about themselves and their families. In fact, effective patient–family–provider relationships rely on their willingness and ability to talk frankly and openly about their situations. The information may be denunciatory or incriminating. For many patients and/or families, this information is placed in the realm of secrecy. It is data that may not have been shared with any other individual, even another family member or a member of their tight network of close confidants in their communities.

Many times, the information that patients and/or families divulge, because it is related to problems, causes them distress. They might worry about how the information will be used and if it will be held against them in any situation, not only by the health care setting but also in other social and legal contexts if the information was shared or inadvertently revealed to other nonauthorized persons.

EXHIBIT 23-1 Rights to Confidentiality and *Tarasoff v. Regents of the University of California*, 1974 and 1976

This was a case in which the <u>Supreme Court of California</u> upheld the order that mental health professionals have the duty to protect persons who are or might become threatened with bodily harm by a patient they have counseled. The original 1974 decision mandated warning the threatened individual. However, in 1976 a rehearing of the case by the California Supreme Court called for not only warning a potential victim but protecting the intended victim. Protecting the potential victim was defined as one or more of the following: notifying police, warning the potential victim, and/or taking steps to protect the potential victim.

This case set an important precedent in the United States and many other parts of the world. The critical incident involved a therapist who knew that a patient had homicidal thoughts toward another person but did not warn the person who was in danger. The situation resulted in the stabbing death of the targeted person. The patient (Mr. Poddar), seen at the college student health services, had confided to his psychiatrist, Dr. Moore, that he was going to kill Ms. Tarasoff when she returned from summer break.

Dr. Moore subsequently informed the campus police that he felt Poddar was dangerous and that he should be hospitalized involuntarily. The police picked up Poddar but after questioning felt he had "changed his attitude" and released him after he promised to stay away from Tarasoff. He did not and Ms. Tarasoff was not informed of the threat. It was also argued that the patient (Poddar) should have received involuntary hospitalization because of his threat to others.

This landmark case established that despite the preservation of patient–provider communications, it was the therapist's duty to warn endangered parties if the patient intended to harm them. Thus, providers can be held liable for failing to inform others at risk if their patient reveals a risk to self or against a specific-named person.

In truth, the issue to disclose or not and the doctrine to protect individuals' rights versus what would be societal rights is not as straightforward as one would expect it to be. Each individual case must be evaluated with respect to the particular facts and consequences that surround the case. Absolute confidentiality, anonymity, and privacy cannot be guaranteed. However, protection of patient information must be respected and provided. Practices that do not reflect a conscious effort to provide for these rights are subject to severe ethical and moral scrutiny and in some cases, legal action.

It is generally recognized that professional health care providers have an explicit obligation to hold all information in confidence with the understanding that the patient's welfare and trust could be jeopardized by the disclosure of this confidential information. The Privacy Rule or Standards for Privacy of Individuality Identifiable Health Information establishes a national set of security standards for protecting certain health information. These standards apply not only to the immediate primary care provider but also who are indirectly or secondarily involved and have access to the patient's information (e.g., providers giving consultation, specialists referred to the case, and those supporting diagnostic or treatment procedures).

Providers also have the responsibility to evaluate the risk of unveiling any aspect of treatment and communication about the patient. Additionally, they must protect against reasonably anticipated threats to the security of patient information. **Protection of patient privacy** is critical in every health care setting and across all health care provider groups.

Confidentiality

Confidentiality as it relates to professional patient–provider communications has the sole purpose of protecting the patient from unauthorized disclosures as determined by standards and regulations.

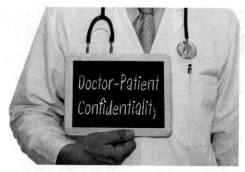

© Docstockmedia/Shutterstock.

Confidentiality establishes that professionals who have access to patient information, patient records, or communications hold this information in confidence. State and federal laws and regulations governing the confidentiality of patient information have existed for some time and long before this information was transmitted in electronic form (e.g., with physician order entry systems, electronic health records, radiology, pharmacy, and laboratory systems). The Security Standards for the Protection of Electronic Protected Health Information (the Security Rule) establishes a national set of security standards for protecting certain health information that is held or transferred in electronic form (U.S. Department of Health and Human Services [HHS], Health Information Privacy, 2011).

Whether information is communicated in verbal exchanges, written documents, or transmitted electronically, it is the patients' basic right to have their privacy respected. This privacy cannot be breached. Only patients have the authority to release information stored in their medical record. Any breach in confidentiality, no matter how minor, can be construed as grounds for mistrust and potential litigation and disciplinary action (American Medical Association, 2007, May 7).

This ethical principle is concerned with privacy, with secret knowledge, and with knowledge known only to a select few. A *confidential communication* refers to personal or private matters that are revealed to a provider who cannot be compelled by law to repeat this communication or be a witness against the patient. Codes of professional ethics address the issue of confidentiality explicitly. Essentially, patients and/or families should be able to assume or be explicitly assured that their private communications with the professional will not be passed on to others, except in a few specific situations. Exceptions include the need for professionals to seek other professional opinions about the patient in consultation but even these communications are subject to the same standards governing confidentiality of patient information.

A field of practice that has addressed the issue of privileged communication in detail is that of mental health. There are precise stipulations governing conditions under which information can be disclosed. As previously explained in the discussion of *Tarasoff v. Regents of the University of California*, 1974, in specific situations (e.g., psychiatrist–patient encounters), the provider must disclose any threats that the patient has made to the mental health provider, or to others.

Generally, however, the guideline is that providers should disclose that which is needed and specifically requested. That is, the provider should and is allowed to keep in confidence those disclosures that are immaterial or irrelevant (Stern, 1990). Thus, unless otherwise specified, information about the patient's sexual preferences, fantasies, or fetishes would not be disclosed if deemed irrelevant to the issue at hand.

On the issue of confidential written records, the provider has the obligation and duty to maintain patient records in a manner in which there is no reasonable chance of their getting lost, stolen, or falling into the hands of unauthorized persons. With the advent of e-records and emails between provider and patient, interpretations and guidelines are spelled out more specifically in the document entitled The Security Standards for the Protection of Electronic Protected Health Information (the Security Rule). Readers are encouraged to refer to this document for the very specific guidelines and rules which need to be followed, including evaluating the likelihood of threats to confidentiality; the implementation of appropriate security measures to address risks identified in the risk analysis; documentation of security measures and their rationale; and maintenance of continuous, reasonable, and appropriate security protections.

Confidentiality, it would seem, is like anonymity, privacy, and other such phenomena. There are specific differences, however, and these differences have been addressed in the literature. Essentially, confidentiality protects the patient from unauthorized disclosures of any sort by the professional who has not obtained informed consent of the patient. The federal **Health Insurance Portability and Accountability Act (HIPAA) privacy rule** pertains to the right to privacy of information.

Examples in which providers are or are not at liberty to reveal details to family members are cases of interest. Consider, for example, a terminally ill male patient who expresses a desire to commit suicide or a woman who, unbeknown to her husband, admits that she has had two therapeutic abortions. What is the provider's obligation to keep this information confidential and, confidential with whom and for what purposes?

The ethical codes of professional organizations aim to safeguard the patient's right to confidentiality even though it could be argued that the patient's significant other(s) may have an equal right to know this information. Professional ethics would support the sanctioning of any health care provider who violated the patient's rights to confidentiality in these instances, even if this meant only sharing this information with selected family members.

Other specific instances in which rules of confidentiality are taken extremely seriously include cases in which patients are human subjects of research studies. In research studies, the issues of confidentiality are clearly stated. Research subjects should not be identifiable (e.g., by name, social security number, or medical record number). Rather, another

procedure (e.g., a code number) should be used that is impossible to link with the subject.

On the chance that identifiable data (name, medical record number, address, and phone number) are obtained, the researcher must explain the specific procedures that will be used for collecting, processing, and storing this data, including who will have access to the data and what will be done with the data when the study is completed.

The HIPAA privacy rule sets the standards for protecting individuals' medical records and other personal health information. It gives patients more control over their health information and sets boundaries on the use and release of health records, holding violators accountable with civil and criminal penalties that can be imposed if providers violate the patient's right to privacy. HIPAA requires that patients be notified of their privacy rights and of how their information may or may not be used.

Privileged Communication

Historically, the doctrine of *privileged communication* simply meant that patients have a legal right by law to have their communications protected. The history of privileged communication dates back to early English law where the responsibility to testify in a court of law was the issue. Despite the stated duty to provide witnessed data, it was argued that some relationships were of sufficient importance and that communications originating in these relationships should be privileged.

Recent cases have reaffirmed the need for strict statutes pertaining to privileged communication. Arguments in favor of privileged communication include the need to promote patient disclosure, not only to adequately care for the patient but to ultimately reduce the threat to others. Taking this argument into account, it is logical to understand that the provider–patient interaction be protected to inspire trust and confidence both for the good of the individual and society at large. Under these conditions, confidence in providers is nurtured and a full account of symptoms is made available to the providers.

This protection is also specific. That is, patients have the legal right where that right exists to not have their confidences revealed publicly from a witness stand during legal proceedings without their expressed permission. Through judicial interpretation, this protection can be extended to legislative and administrative proceedings as well. Privileged communication statutes exist to govern patient–provider communications in many, but not all, states in the United States.

Furthermore, there are differences across states depending on the law of the applicable jurisdiction. For example, in one state there may be only a limited physician–patient privilege in criminal proceedings and the privilege is limited in civil cases as well while in other states, physician–patient privilege is not as limited. In any case, the type of crime, the injury incurred, and other aspects of potential danger to others might impact the application of the statute. In states without such statutes, the right to privileged communication can be affirmed by common law on a case-by-case basis.

What is meant by patient–provider privilege is that the privilege is assigned only to the patient. They alone have the right to employ it. The privilege does not extend to a family member or provider. For example, providers must withhold information and cannot relinquish the information even to protect themselves. It cannot be used in any way to enhance the well-being of another. For example, if physicians are engaged in litigation about a certain surgical procedure and their abilities to perform this procedure, they could not provide the attorney with information about other patients they treated and if the results were good because this would be an unauthorized use of the data. When a patient dies it is usually the case that the person that represents the patient (e.g., in a wrongful death case) is given the power to waive the physician–patient privilege.

As has always been the case, the issue of privileged communication involves striking a balance between two important social values: (1) society's right to access information critical to fact-finding and (2) the individual's right to privacy. But, as has been previously discussed, these principles are far from simple to apply in selected instances.

Anonymity and Privacy

Anonymity refers to the right of patients to have their identity protected from its being known to others. *Privacy* more generally refers to the right of patients to limit any knowledge about themselves to become known to others. Infractions with both would result in both patients' identities and particular health data (e.g., diagnosis and treatment being known to others not involved in patients' care and treatment). It has been maintained that the right to privacy was upheld and first recognized by the U.S. Supreme Court. It was first deemed an independent constitutional right in the landmark case of *Griswold v. Connecticut*, 381 U.S. 479 in 1965 (Shah, 1970).

This case concerned the unsuccessful attempt by the state of Connecticut to prevent (by statute) anyone from using contraceptive devices, including married couples. The Connecticut Comstock Law prohibited any person from using any drug or medicinal article or instrument to prevent conception. In their decision against Connecticut, some of the Supreme Court justices invalidated the Comstock Law on the grounds that it violated the right to marital privacy. This and other cases supported the right to privacy as a right to protect from governmental intrusion and claimed that the right to privacy was not to be found in any specific constitutional amendment but in the implications cast by several amendments (First, Third, Fourth, Fifth, and Ninth Amendments).

The right to **privacy** and anonymity presents itself in both formal and informal situations. The obvious is a provider revealing patient data to another without the explicit permission of the patient. How many times have health care providers themselves witnessed infractions of the principle of patients' rights to anonymity and privacy in even informal gatherings?

Consider, for example, the pharmacy assistant who speaks loudly to a person in the presence of several other people standing in line to pick up medications at the pharmacy: "Mr. Smith, your Trizivir is not ready for pickup. Can you come back in 20 minutes?" Trizivir is an anti-HIV medication in a category called nucleoside reverse transcriptase inhibitors (NRTIs) that prevents the development of new virus and decreases the amount of virus in the body as a whole.

This specific information is about medications but it also includes something about the patient's diagnosis, explicitly or implicitly revealed in the conversation with the patient waiting for his medication. Additionally, if the pharmacy tech also reveals any other aspect of the patient's identity (e.g., the spelling of his first and last name), the infraction is flagrant. This would be a violation of the patient's rights even though no one in line might recognize that it is prescribed because the patient has HIV/AIDS.

Consider also the medical resident or student nurse who discusses the details of a patient's case (revealing the patient's name) in a clinic or hospital elevator in the presence of other providers. If you are a witness to such events you may see the other providers pull away and become silent or whisper. Other persons than the staff may even turn their heads and look down or look away. People are aware that this data about another patient is privileged and they are not entitled to know this information.

When these situations occur, most people feel angry and concerned but are not sure how to deal with the situation. People waiting in line for their medications worry that this will happen to them and they may speak softly or withhold verbalizing information in hopes of decreasing any violation of their own right to privacy and confidentiality. Assertive providers,

such as the bystanders in the elevator scenario, may pull the inappropriate provider aside and reprimand him or her for their misconduct.

In either case, the patient could file a case against the provider and the health care institution for a violation of patient rights. Every patient who experiences a violation has the opportunity to file a health information privacy complaint with the Office for Civil Rights (OCR). There are many examples of this same infraction. Consider the patient in an outpatient clinic who is awaiting diagnostic-testing procedures. The receptionist broadcasts the name of the patient to the room of six to seven patients and family members. Having not obtained all the information initially, the receptionist requests the patient to call back to him or her (behind the desk) the reason for the diagnostic test, where the patient lives, and home and work phone numbers.

Can one say that the information that is revealed publicly in these situations does not have to be confidential? Not so, given the rights of patients for anonymity and privacy. These infractions are serious ethical errors and necessitate not only reprimands but potential defense against legal action.

In general terms, the concept of privacy acknowledges the freedom of patients to pick and choose for themselves the time, circumstances, and, particularly, the extent to which they wish to share or withhold information about themselves. This data not only includes health care information but their identity, attitudes, opinions, beliefs, and current, past, or future behaviors. The right to privacy is not just being entitled to have the curtain pulled during a physical exam or medical procedure, it is an affirmation of the importance of the uniqueness and individuality of patients and their desired freedom from unreasonable intrusion by others.

Responsible actions by providers need to reflect the fact that with issues of privacy, confidentiality, and the privileged nature of patient–provider communications, dilemmas will always arise. In fact, as stated earlier, these issues are not translated into absolute terms.

The particular facts and consequences of each individual case must be considered. Additionally, patients' bills of rights, professional codes of ethics, and the legal statutes of a specific state will influence the resolution of the dilemmas. However, the HIPAA regulations rule over any state codes; they are national standards.

▶ Summary

Patients and their families who seek health care or medical treatment reveal important intimate information that is known to very few or, often, to no one else. Some of this information or the meaning of the information may be out of the patient's and/or family's immediate awareness. Thus, patients and families could be revealing not only data no one else knows but also data previously unknown or not understood by them. Because the provider uses techniques to promote patient self-disclosure, the chances of patients and/or their families revealing personal and private information are very high. Many times, the contents of this private and personal communication can be distressing or even self-incriminating.

Therapeutic relationships with providers rely on both the patient's and family's willingness to self-disclose as well as provider's skill in promoting self-disclosures and their ability to secure the privacy of what is shared with them. HIPAA, the first-ever federal privacy standard, regulates the disclosure of medical record information and other health information.

There are inherent professional obligations in patient–provider encounters. Patients' communications, both written and verbal, including those transmitted electronically must be held in confidence. Although not absolute, these principles of confidentiality, anonymity, and privacy characterize professional–patient–family relationships. The patient's and family's welfare and trust may be severely compromised by the disclosure of information provided in confidence or by the disclosure of identifying information to others outside the immediate circle of health care providers responsible for the patients' care. Exceptions do occur, particularly when the welfare of others is in question (e.g., when the patient is an immediate threat to himself or herself or a specific other) but these exceptions are relatively few compared to the times and situations in which respect and protection of privacy and anonymity should be uppermost in the minds and actions of providers.

A full and detailed discussion of the principles and skills of therapeutic communications is appropriately closed by the affirmation of the special professional obligation that underlies the treatment of patient self-disclosures once they are effectively elicited.

Discussion

1. Identify the similarities and differences between the terms confidentiality, privacy, and anonymity.
2. Describe and discuss the regulations surrounding the principle of protecting patient–provider confidentiality.
3. Using your own observations of an actual or potential breach of privacy, describe the situation and explain what rights were (or might have been) violated.
4. Identify cases in which a court of law might support a provider's breach of patient confidentiality.
5. Discuss one or more inherent difficulties in ensuring confidentiality of patient data transmitted electronically.

References

American Medical Association. (2007). *Patient confidentiality. Division of Health Law.* Retrieved from http://www.ama-assn.org/ama/pub/category/4610.html

Shah, S. A. (1970). Privileged communication, confidentiality and privacy: Privacy. *Professional Psychology, 1,* 243–252. doi.org/10.1037/h0028790

Stern, S. B. (1990). Privileged communication: An ethical and legal right of psychiatric clients. *Perspectives in Psychiatric Care, 26*(4), 22–25. doi.org/10.1111/j.1744-6163.1990.tb00321.x

U.S. Department of Health & Human Services. *Health information privacy: Your rights under HIPAA (Available in multiple languages).* Retrieved from hhs.gov

U.S. Department of Health & Human Services. (2011). Privacy, security, and electronic health records. Retrieved from HealthIT.gov

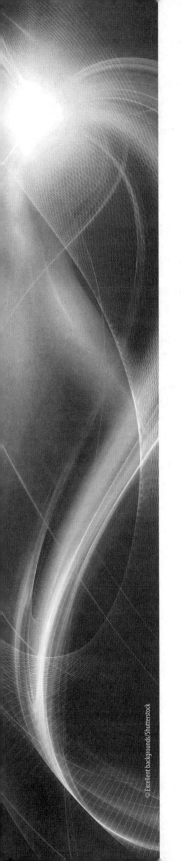

PART VII

Transforming Health Care Through Changing Patient Behaviors and Systems of Care

Successful professional role development depends on one's grasp of advanced issues in the use of health care communications. This section, "Transforming Health Care Through Changing Patient Behaviors and Systems of Care" provides insight into how behavioral change theories can be incorporated in communication encounters with patients and their families. Knowledge of systems and organizational theory enable providers to meaningfully alter systems of care to enhance health care communications.

Theories of behavior change explain the use of communication principles in the context of a theoretical or conceptual framework. Knowledge of behavior change theories can serve as an advantage in understanding how general communication skills and concepts fit within paradigms of knowledge.

The role of health care systems in shaping health communications is clearly outlined. The structure of the health care system is less studied for its impact on the nature of communications between patients and providers and providers with one another. However, the structure of systems of care clearly influences communications and, subsequently, quality of care. The content and issues presented in this section of the text are compelling and will encourage the reader to further examine possibilities for affecting changes in communications they observe in a variety of health care arenas.

Chapter 24, "Health Communications to Enhance Behavior Change," describes the role of communication in supporting behavior change in patients and families. This chapter describes and discusses specific theories guiding health promotion and disease prevention in individuals, groups, and populations. Essentially, the message is that interventions or communication strategies to change behavior may be significantly more effective if backed by one or more theoretical models.

The models selected for discussion in this chapter include the social learning theory, the theory of reasoned action (TRA) and theory of planned behavior (TPB), the health belief model (HBM), the Transtheoretical Model of Change™ (TTM), and the social ecological model (SEM).

Each framework encompasses several principles that encourage behavioral change. Providers, friends, and family are sources of interpersonal influence that can encourage health promotion behaviors. When these influences are in agreement and are coupled with patients' sense of self-efficacy (believing they can make the change), patients are more likely to change their behavior in positive ways. When these sources of interpersonal influence offer conflicting views, even if patients feel they can make a change, change may not occur, or if it does change, change might not be sustained.

Chapter 25, "Altering Systems of Care to Enhance Health Care Communications," examines the many ways systems of care delivery influence and shape communications between patients and health care providers. Independently or collectively, providers are often in a position to make at least minor changes in the organization of care delivery to enhance therapeutic communication.

This chapter discusses various system-level factors that promote therapeutic communication (e.g., the impact of continuity of health care services improves therapeutic alliances between providers and patients). Examples of variations in delivery systems, such as transitional care, telephone-based continuing care, and systematic care are discussed and their potential impact on communication between provider and patients/families are detailed.

CHAPTER 24

Health Communications to Enhance Behavior Change

CHAPTER OBJECTIVES

- Identify key theoretical models that explain behavior and behavioral change in health care.
- Compare and contrast the transtheoretical model (TTM) of change and theory of reasoned action (TRA).
- Compare and contrast the health belief model (HBM) and social ecological model (SEM).
- Identify concepts common across theoretical models.
- Consider obesity as a public health problem, and differentiate the approaches each theory might recommend to support behavioral change in at-risk individuals and communities.

KEY TERMS

- Cues to action
- Generalized self-efficacy (GSE) scale
- Health belief model (HBM)
- Person-centered approach
- Self-efficacy

- Social cognitive theory
- Social ecological model (SEM)
- Subjective norms
- Theory of reasoned action (TRA)
- Transtheoretical model (TTM) of change

▶ Introduction

A good deal of what health providers seek to do is to communicate in ways that promote behavioral change. Helping patients change behaviors is an important aspect of the role, yet few providers have an understanding of the dynamics or processes that elicit patient behavior change. Historically, patient–provider communication to achieve behavior change was been viewed as an art resulting from the unique nature of a particular patient in response to the approach of the provider. But what is this this "art" and how can it be understood in the context of the reality that multiple interacting factors promote or deter the change process?

Over the past several decades a number of social behavioral theories or analytical models were proposed to educate providers in what facilitates change and how providers can be adequate motivators for behavior change. Most providers would be surprised to know that more than 10–20 theories have been suggested. Davis, Campbell, Hildon, Hobbs, and Michie (2015) in their review of theories of behavior and behavior change across the social and behavioral sciences cited 82 theories relevant to their review. The bulk of the articles describing these 82 theories addressed four models: (1) the **social cognitive theory** (SCT), (2) the theory of planned behavior (TPB), (3) the information–motivation–behavioral skills (IMB) model, and (4) the **transtheoretical model (TTM) of change.**

In this chapter, these theoretical frameworks or models are described and discussed. One additional theory is added because of its relevance to behavior change at the community level, the **social ecological model (SEM)**. These theories are not altogether different from one another, but there are usually a number of assumptions or principles that set them apart. Among an extensive list of behavioral change models, of particular importance are those that include implications for guiding communications between patients and providers. These models cover a wide range of topics to promote lifestyle changes, encourage health promotion and disease prevention, and improve patient compliance to medical care.

Similar to those listed by Davis et al., the social behavioral models discussed in this chapter include: social cognitive theory (SCT) or social learning theory (SLT), the **theory of reasoned action (TRA)** and the theory of planned behavior (TPB), the **health belief model (HBM)**, the TTM, and the SEM. Within each paradigm are certain concepts and principles that guide providers in promoting behavior change.

Providers and researchers have developed an array of interventions that spring from theories of behavior change and target social support, provider–patient interaction, self-efficacy, and coping. These interventions have a basis in a wide variety of behavioral change theories, some of which clearly overlap. The following is a description of the frameworks and models and how they may impact providers' interacting with patients.

▶ Theoretical Frameworks and Models of Behavior Change

Most Americans have at least some idea about what to do to stay healthy and prevent the lifelong effects and mortality from chronic and life-threatening diseases. Exposure to health messaging is noted in the wide variety of media sources that stress health promotion and disease prevention. There are many public health announcements and alerts on television and in schools, public places, and on billboards in many communities. The public health message is: *eat healthy, exercise, stop smoking, don't use drugs, and practice safe sex*. But, have Americans gotten these messages and are they doing what they know they should do? The answer to both questions: *not nearly enough*.

As previously noted in this text, the rate of serious chronic disease and illness (heart disease, stroke, cancer, type 2 diabetes, obesity, and arthritis) are among the most common, costly, and preventable health problems in the United States (CDC, cdc.gov). Obesity is a serious concern and is expected to skyrocket in coming years. Arthritis is the most common cause of disability and diabetes is the leading cause of kidney failure, loss of limb, and adult blindness. Human behaviors associated with these serious health concerns include tobacco smoking, alcohol consumption, poor diet, and inadequate physical activity. It is not totally clear in all cases but assumed that even small changes in these behaviors can reverse these trends.

Healthy People 2010 proposed two overarching goals: (1) to increase quality and years of healthy life and (2) to eliminate health disparities among different segments of the population. The first goal—to help individuals of all ages improve their life expectancy and quality of life—has direct implications for providers to implement and evaluate their approach to helping individuals and families change unhealthy behaviors.

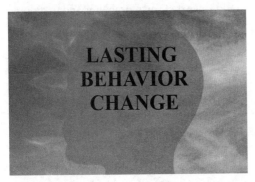

LASTING BEHAVIOR CHANGE

© Hafakot/Shutterstock.

Examining the report card on the efforts so far, one can understand that new vision needs to be applied to these old problems. Davis et al. add that behavior change programs and interventions have generally had only modest effects but they are likely to be more effective if grounded in appropriate behavior change theories. Theoretical or conceptual models provide answers that can guide providers' communications with patients and their families.

Integral to understanding theories of behavioral change are general principles of change theory. The following is a list of key points (**EXHIBIT 24-1**).

EXHIBIT 24-1 Behavioral Change Theory General Principles

1. Change happens incrementally. It is rarely a single event or something accomplished over a specific period of time. Change is ongoing, and it is of particular importance to consider that providers are communicating with patients at a specific point in an ongoing process.

2. Permanent change is not likely to occur if the motivation to change is not internalized. Thus, simply telling the patient that they *must* or *should* change their behavior is not likely to result in the change that is needed.

3. Reinforcement motivates individuals either to continue or discontinue behavior and behavior change. Reinforcement can be negative or positive. For example, telling patients they did a good job in starting to make behavioral changes is likely to motivate them to continue or sustain the changes they have made.

4. Individuals' motivation to change is integrally bound to their perceptions of the need to change. Providers, in part, are agents for cues to action. When talking to patients about the need to change, providers bring to the forefront a new perspective and urgency.

5. Patients' social environment (social network, culture, and social support system) has a direct impact on their desire to change and maintenance of behavioral change. Patients' changes are reinforced not only by the provider but social environment. If the provider and social network agree in the need to change, the patient is more likely to attempt a change. Dissension or disagreement between the provider and the patient's social support figures is likely to cause confusion and ambivalence about making needed changes.

6. Patients must believe in their ability to execute behavior change if they are to form intentions to change. Self-efficacy (belief in one's capacities to change) motivates patients to try or continue a behavior change. Expressed support and confidence in the patient to change will also enhance behavior change.

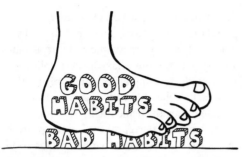

© iQoncept/Shutterstock

As each of the theoretical models is discussed, it will become apparent that there is a good deal of similarity in the models of understanding and motivating behavioral change. A background in behavioral and social sciences to include psychology, sociology, public health, and education provides a foundation for understanding current models.

▶ Humanistic Psychology

The study of behavioral change has a long history dating back to early thoughts of eradicating the problem. Psychology and psychiatry, particularly those models of personality theory, are most credited for early behavioral change theory. Among these theorists is Carl Rogers (1902–1987), an American psychologist who was also credited with advancing the field of humanistic psychology.

The principles of Rogers's personality change theory (1959, 1961, 1977, 1994 [posthumously, with Freiberg]) have affected providers' approaches to patients and can still be observed in providers' responses to patients. Rogers's view of behavior change evolved from his overriding belief that humans have an underlying *actualizing tendency* and will approach change as a natural result of this tendency. Several theorists subscribing to this model would agree that self-acceptance is key to growth, and unconditional positive regard nurtures change. Rogers's **person-centered approach** is most obvious today in the belief that motivation to change requires

individualized approaches to patients. In 1982, *American Psychologist* ranked Carl Rogers number 1 out of the 10 most influential psychotherapists.

Rogers put considerable faith in the individual's experiential learning which he thought could be facilitated by the provider's approach. Rather than thinking he could solve the problems for the client, he believed that clients could solve their own problems and that doing this creates the change to make the client better (**EXHIBIT 24-2**).

One of Rogers's most well-known techniques is *rephrasing*. Rogers believed that knowledge comes from within and providers are present to unveil this awareness. Otherwise, instead of answering a patient's question directly, he would rephrase the question and ask the patient what he thought. Not only would he ask patients the question, he would then ask them how they felt about the answer. (Retrieved from http://www.enotes.com/psychology-theories/rogers-carl-ransom.) Rogers devoted his time to improving communications between patients or clients and health care providers. The following is a brief

---

EXHIBIT 24-2 Rogerian Theory of the Role of Provider in Facilitating Behavior Change

The role of provider as facilitator (or teacher as Rogers described) would include:

1. Setting a positive environment for learning.
2. Clarifying the purpose of the learning with the client.
3. Organizing and making available learning resources.
4. Balancing both intellectual and emotional aspects of learning.
5. Sharing thoughts and feelings with clients without dominating the conversation (retrieved from http://www.tip.psychology.org/rogers.html).

EXHIBIT 24-3 Rogerian Dialogue to Facilitate Behavior Change

I. Focus on the actualizing tendency

Instead of:

"Well I don't seem to convince you that if you don't control your diet, things are going to get worse." *Consequence:* Patients feel hopeless and shameful that they are unable to satisfy the provider's expectation.

Use:

"I know you are moving toward changing your diet…it's what you want to do…but, it is taking time…I believe you will find a way." *Consequence:* Patient may ask for resources and explore small steps which are more realistic.

II. Rephrasing

Instead of:

"What do you mean you can't change your diet?" *Consequence:* Patient feels inadequate and unconvinced about being able to change their diet.

Use:

"You are saying you can't change your diet." *Consequence:* The provider paraphrases what the patient has said and the patient takes ownership of the problem and is encouraged to explore the reasons.

list of the major concepts and how they would translate to conversations (**EXHIBIT 24-3**).

While Rogers's work influenced the early development of humanistic psychology, the literature addressing his theory and the empirical evidence is limited. Still, Rogers's approach to client-centered counseling is considered foundational and important in counseling for behavioral change. Current theories of planned behavioral change explore the importance of internal motivation and the potential of individuals to make changes in light of perceived internal and external barriers and facilitators. This discussion continues with a description of social learning and social cognitive theory.

▶ Social Learning and Social Cognitive Theory

Social learning theory maintains that change occurs in the context of an individual's cost–benefit analysis where the positive outcomes of changing offset any negative consequences that result from the change. Environmental factors, personal factors, and attributes of the behavior itself all affect the process of behavior change. These factors act both independently and interdependently on the change process. For example, patients' social environments, including social resources and culture, have a direct impact on patient behavior change. Social resources and patients' personal skills and knowledge in turn affect behavior change.

Social cognitive theories combine social learning theory and cognitive behavioral approaches. Social cognitive theories emphasize the importance of considering individuals' subjective perceptions of situations and their interpretations of the meaning of events. Individuals are inherently influenced by the norms, beliefs, and ways of behaving consistent with their social reality. Behavior change can be approached or avoided depending on the support of groups with which the individual affiliates. Lack of support and encouragement may cause individuals to be uninterested in change.

A critical principle of social learning theory is the concept of **self-efficacy**. *Self-efficacy* refers to the belief individuals have that they can actually perform a certain behavior or behavior change. Self-efficacy—a sense that one has control over one's environment and behavior—is said to predict intention to change and maintenance of change after it is implemented. In Bandura's vision, "Self-efficacy is the belief in one's capabilities to organize and execute the sources of action required to manage prospective situations" (Bandura, 1986). According to Bandura (1997), a personal sense of control enhances behavioral change. Self-efficacy also affects how goals will be set, with persons having a low sense of self-efficacy expressing goals in hopeless ways. Individuals with high levels of self-efficacy may create more challenging goals because they feel competent to pursue more lofty expectations.

Bandura did not describe the presence of a general sense of self-efficacy. Rather, self-efficacy was observed in the context of a specific situation (e.g., the ability to increase one's physical exercise or lose weight). However, it is possible to think about self-efficacy in a more global context. To measure general self-efficacy, a provider might ask patients how confident they feel—"I am certain that I can do most things"—is an example. And, response choices could range from "definitely not" to "exactly true." An example from the **generalized self-efficacy (GSE) scale** (Schwarzer & Jerusalem, 1995) would be, "When I am confronted with a problem, I can usually find several solutions."

However, to make the measurement more situation specific, providers would ask patients to respond to such items as: "I am certain that I can lose weight, even if I have periods where I eat unhealthy things" or "I can manage to stick with healthful foods, even if I have to try several times until it works" (the nutrition self-efficacy scale; Bagozzi & Edwards, 1998). In the literature there are numerous specific self-efficacy measures each addressing a target for change such as smoking cessation self-efficacy, condom use self-efficacy scale (Brafford & Beck, 1991), physical exercise self-efficacy measures (Fuchs, 1996), and an alcohol resistance self-efficacy scale.

For social cognitive theorists, two essential aspects of the behavior change must be tracked over time: (1) the intention to change a behavior and (2) the actual behavior which is to change. These are not always congruent in that someone may have high intentions to change but the behavior suggests the intention is very low. Self-efficacy is important to both

because self-efficacy is said to influence intentions to change as well as resultant behaviors.

According to Bandura (2000), the path of influence through which perceived self-efficacy affects other social cognitive factors is complex. For example, self-efficacy might have a direct impact on behavior but factors such as *outcome expectations*, goals, and sociostructural factors (facilitators or impediments) would mediate the relationship of self-efficacy and goal setting. For example, perceived impediments might dominate patients' views of behavior change. This would influence the goal-setting actions of these patients and weak goals or no goals at all might be the result.

The role of the provider in influencing how patients perceive the need to change, the goals they set, and their attitudes toward impediments to change is critical. Provider communications can express openness to consider patients' points of view. When there is just the right amount of empathy and understanding, providers can help patients navigate the change process. Perceived self-efficacy plays a role in the beginning when the patient is developing goals for behavior change and in the maintenance stage when self-efficacy to maintain the change is critical.

Using principles of social and cognitive behavioral learning, providers might select from a number of communication strategies that would build on patient self-efficacy and assess how feelings of self-efficacy might fluctuate over time. For example, an area of assessment would be the patient's beliefs about being able to change an unhealthy behavior, how the unhealthy behavior plays a role in everyday life, and what the *impediments* and *facilitators* are in adapting behavior changes (**EXHIBIT 24-4**).

This line of inquiry when carefully paced can demonstrate empathy and understanding and can help patients feel they will have support in the change process. Additionally, providers' continued interest may reduce patients' feelings of being overwhelmed by the barriers they face.

EXHIBIT 24-4 Dialogue to Promote Self-Efficacy

"Tell me about your overeating; tell me something about your pattern of overeating."

"How much do you believe you can control overeating?"

"What might stand in the way of your being able to control overeating?"

"How much do you want to stop overeating?"

"What can help you to keep on track?"

A number of studies have examined the use of social cognitive behavioral learning and the prediction of behaviors which could be aversive (e.g., excessive alcohol use, poor physical activity or exercise, and condom use). College students' alcohol consumption is of concern because of the incidence of problem drinking.

The Substance Abuse and Mental Health Services Administration (SAMHSA) has shown concern for college student alcohol consumption noting that this is a vulnerable time for these young adults. In a SAMHA report by Lipari and Jean-Francois (2016), 60% of college students aged 18–22 were reported to drink alcohol in any given month and when compared to others their age, full-time students are far more likely to binge drink or drink heavily.

Both positive and negative expectancies or consequences of drinking were found to contribute to alcohol use. Positive expectancies (fun and socializing associated with drinking) and drinking refusal self-efficacy (lacking capacity to curb drinking) were strongly related to college student alcohol use (Young, Connor, Ricciardelli, & Saunders, 2006). Otherwise, the greater the positive expectancy the lower reported self-efficacy in refusing to drink. A more recent study of alcohol drinking in college students showed that experiencing any positive consequences predicted more

favorable overall evaluations and perceptions that drinking was worth it, and perceptions of drinking as worth it was associated with an increased likelihood of drinking the next day (Fairlie, Ramirez, Patrick, & Lee, 2016).

The use of social cognitive theory has also been useful in understanding exercise behavior in both college-aged students and adults. Parents facing barriers to exercise and having high levels of inactivity were studied in order to test a social cognitive model of parental exercise (Mailey, Phillips, Dlugonski, & Conroy, 2016). This study showed that efforts to increase exercise in parents should focus on improving confidence to overcome exercise barriers, reducing perceptions of barriers, and helping parents make specific plans for prioritizing and participating in exercise routines.

▶ Theory of Reasoned Action and Theory of Planned Behavior

A major concern of all behavioral change theorists is *why do people behave the way they do and how do we influence them to change.* The theory of reasoned action (TRA) was first developed in 1967 by Martin Fishbein and then revised and expanded by Azjen and Fishbein in 1975, 1977, and 1980. The roots of this theory are from social psychology with an emphasis on how individuals' attitudes affect behavior. The major premise is that attitude and behavior are positively correlated. An individual's belief that a behavior leads to certain outcomes and positive attitudes about these outcomes influence attitudes toward the behavior, which in turn influence performance of behavior. Only some attitudes are influential in this way, and these are referred to as *salient attitudes* formed from salient beliefs toward an outcome. Attitudes, **subjective norms**, intentions, and behavior are the primary concepts of TRA.

Attitudes are influenced by the opinions of others, and *intentions* shape behavior. Intention is the probability that the individual will perform a behavior which is influenced by both attitudes and subjective norms. *Subjective norms* are what the individual perceives others will think of the behavior. For example, subjective norms about illicit drug use among substance abusers are that drug use is OK. Other substance abusers form the normative beliefs of the individual and the degree to which the behavior change will occur. Otherwise, if the norms are to *use*, then drug-using behavior is in concert with the individual's norms. Intentions are the individuals' reported statements of the likelihood that they will perform desired behaviors.

Although Fishbein recognized that other factors may influence behavior (e.g., demographic characteristics), he believed that those factors would not be important in the context of experience unless they affected individuals' attitudes or normative beliefs. Any given behavior is a product of intention to action influenced by individuals' attitude about the behavior and anticipated outcomes of performing these behaviors. That is, the person with an intention is likely to perform the behavior provided that the attitude about the behavior and subjective norms support the behavior. **EXHIBIT 24-5** is an example of the relationship of intention and behavior change.

Perhaps the most noteworthy strength of this model is that it is simplistic and has been shown to support interventions for behavior change in a number of populations (e.g., weight loss, condom use, and preventing sun exposure). A major weakness of this theory is the presumption that behavior is under volitional control, and that there is a reasoning process that occurs that is systematic and always follows a particular route.

Behaviors that are spontaneous and not thought out are not explained by this framework. Also, the pattern of variance in behavior

> ### EXHIBIT 24-5 Theory of Reasoned Action: Relationship of Intention to Behavior Change
>
> | | |
> |---|---|
> | **ATTITUDE:** | "I think eating and not exercising is bad for me." |
> | **SUBJECTIVE NORM:** | "Other people I know tell me I need to lose weight." |
> | **INTENTION:** | "I want to do things to lose weight." |
> | **BEHAVIOR:** | "I am going to start an eating and exercise program to help me lose weight. And, if that doesn't work, I will ask my health care providers for advice." |

is not fully addressed in this framework. To correct for these limitations, Ajzen revised the model to incorporate other variables (e.g., how difficult the behavior change is and whether individuals perceive that they will be successful in changing).

The revision of the original TRA model is described as the TPB (Schifter and Ajzen, 1985). Thus, TPB, which appeared in the 1980s, is an extension of TRA. TPB views behavior change as a result of the interaction of three constructs: attitude, subjective norms, and perceived behavioral control (self-efficacy as interpreted here). Subjective norms are the perceived social expectations about what is valued or accepted in the individual's social network.

Studies by Quo et al. (2007) and Sable, Schwartz, Kelly, Lison, and Hall (2006), using different populations and different target behaviors, illustrate the application of the TRA model. In the study of smoking behavior in Chinese adolescents by Quo et al., the applicability of TRA and TPB were tested. Although TPB was thought to be superior to TRA, these authors also found that TRA can better predict smoking among students with lower (rather than higher) perceived behavior control. The independent effects of attitudes about smoking and perceived norms about smoking behavior were partially mediated by intention, pointing to the utility of TRA factors in predicting behavior.

Sable et al. examined physician behavior in prescribing contraceptives to a largely female population seen in emergency room settings. They found that high intentions to prescribe contraceptives were positively associated with attitudes toward doing so and with the perception that their colleagues and professional groups support prescribing condoms. The proper circumstance to promote behavior change is also taken up in the HBM.

▶ The Health Belief Model

The HBM originated from the work of Rosenstock, Strecher, and Becker (1988) and at the time was considered a social learning model that contributed an expanded view of the role of motivation to change. It incorporated beliefs and perceptions of individuals that speak to motivation as an underlying propelling element which is affected by a logical examination of the need for change.

The HBM rests on general principles of behavior change in response to perceptions of the likelihood of illness. There are four critical areas: (1) perception of the severity of a potential illness or disease, (2) individual's perceived susceptibility to a given illness, (3) the benefits of taking action, and (4) the barriers to taking action.

The HBM also includes a concept—**cues to action**—that is important in eliciting and maintaining behavior change. Cues to action may be as simple as a note posted on the refrigerator to remind a person about eating vegetables and fruit or more complex such as the cues subtly played out in a social situation in which everyone is slim and is avoiding the unhealthy foods attractively set at the table.

Perceived threat is activated by cues to action. The concept of self-efficacy, discussed earlier in the discussion of the social learning theory, has been added to the HBM. Self-efficacy beliefs in this model help explain why when severity and susceptibility to health problems are believed to be high, benefits are clear, and behavior change is more likely.

The distinct approach of the HBM is that behavior is seen as a result of individuals' rational appraisal of needs, benefits, and barriers. It presumes that individuals do not act but through the logical analysis of disease and illness and by using an empirical process. High perceived threat, low barriers, and high perceived benefits will increase the likelihood of health promotion and disease prevention behavior changes.

There is some disagreement about whether susceptibility is more important than perceived threat because perceived severity has a weaker association with taking action than the perception that one is at risk. The essence of this model is that all elements interact to result in action or no action. Consideration of other important mediating factors (e.g., age, socioeconomic status, and other sociopsychological variables) does not have an active place in this theory.

Using the HBM, Lin, Simoni, and Zemon (2005) wanted to examine its utility in predicting sexual behaviors in Taiwanese immigrants. Students completed an online survey which asked them about several health-belief factors and their sexual behaviors. HBM variables, as a set, predicted participants' sexual behavior (number of partners and frequency of intercourse). Although the study had several limitations in measurement, the authors suggested that self-efficacy be targeted in this group and that both measures and interventions be culturally sensitive.

Hazavehei, Taghdisi, and Saidi (2007) reported on a study to increase use of osteoporosis prevention among young females. Osteoporosis is a serious problem potentially leading to hip fractures in the elderly, yet, it is important to begin primary prevention at an early age since the majority of bone growth occurs during childhood and adolescence. These authors tested a prevention program for middle school girls modeled after HBM.

Research participants were assigned to one of three groups, one of which was an educational program using the principles of HBM. Their findings showed increased knowledge about osteoporosis, perceived susceptibility, perceived severity of the condition, perceived benefits of reducing risk factors, and most importantly, perceived benefits of taking health action. Mean scores in the education group not modeled after HBM showed significant improvement only in knowledge and perceived susceptibility but not in perceived severity, perceived benefits of reducing risk factors, or in taking health action. Those in the third group without a specific education program in osteoporosis showed no significant changes on the HBM components. The authors were optimistic about the use of a theory-based HBM educational program to induce behavior change for osteoporosis prevention in this group.

▶ Transtheoretical Model of Change

The TTM of change, first described by Prochaska and DiClemente (1983), Prochaska, DiClemente, and Norcross (1992), Prochaska, DiClemente, Velicer, Ginpil, and Norcross (l985), Prochaska, DiClemente, Velicer, and Rossi (1993), and Prochaska and Velicer (1997), is also known as the stages of change model (Zimmerman, Olsen, & Bosworth, 2000). Like many of the behavioral change models, this model can be used as both a model to describe behavior as well as change behavior. There are two major constructs in this model: stages of change and processes of change.

Essentially, the TTM theory proposes that change occurs as spiral processes of change. This model has been used in a variety of

EXHIBIT 24-6 Transtheoretical Model: Stages of Change

1. Precontemplation: Uninformed or ill informed about the need to change. Individuals are not intending to take action in the near future.
2. Contemplation: Individuals are clearly thinking about and intending to change in the near future. They are aware of the positive reasons for change as well as the negative consequences of not changing.
3. Preparation (for action): Individuals are intending to act soon and may have already taken action in the past. They have a plan of action and can engage in action-oriented programs.
4. Action: Individuals are making changes, and these actions are evident and measurable.
5. Maintenance: The changes made are in place, and individuals may adapt plans to prevent relapse of undesired behaviors.

treatment and prevention programs including alcohol and drug abuse, obesity, and smoking cessation programs. TTM stages include those listed in **EXHIBIT 24-6**.

The TTM has been widely used in the literature to describe and track patients' readiness to change. In keeping with this model, providers need to use stage-specific approaches to help patients make behavior changes. That is, if someone is in the pre-contemplation stage, they are just beginning to be exposed to information about the need to change but have not yet considered that this information really applies in their situation.

It is the task of the provider to point out how this information does, in fact, apply to them. Additionally, when patients are taking action to change unhealthy behaviors, it would be inappropriate to focus solely on helping patients consider changes when they have begun the process already. The more appropriate approach would be to acknowledge that patients are taking action to change, and that there may be unanticipated barriers that could interfere with their progress. Thus, the communication between the patient and provider is stage specific.

Teaching skills and providing knowledge are important in every stage of change but the actual content can also be stage specific. Once the patient has taken action to change a behavior, then appropriate knowledge and skill would be controlling triggers that could reverse the change and bring on negative behaviors.

This model is most useful in exploring the underlying components of long-term changes related to the prevention and management of chronic illness. It is recognized that providers may find it difficult to use the model for a variety of reasons. First, providers may not see themselves as the only or only ongoing provider that will make the difference, and second, the prospect of creating long-term changes may appear overwhelming to them. They also may be concerned that they might overestimate the steps that need to occur to cause even the most minor change.

An offshoot of the TTM is an interviewing process called *motivational interviewing (MI)*. Rather than a distinct theory, MI describes an approach based on theories of change stages (Miller & Rollnick, 1991). Like the TTM, MI looks at changing behavior in stages. It is an approach to facilitating patient change with the understanding that providers are interacting with patients who are at some level of the change process. It is critical for providers and patients to understand that change is contingent on motivation but motivation is not sufficient to create change.

The application of MI can be problematic in that a single statement from the patient about the desire to change does not always mean that the provider and patient is ready to move on. Consider for example, individuals addicted to opioid prescription pain medication who approach providers expressing the desire to change. Perhaps they have been confronted by a family member or have been accused or arrested for obtaining this medication illegally. At this time, patients may feel both panic and motivation to change. Taken simply, providers using MI might view this state as positive because the patient expresses motivation to make a change. However, providers may come to the realization that this is not readiness to change, rather this expression of motivation is short-lived.

Miller and Rollnick (1991, 2002) developed a template for appropriate interactions with patients based on change stages, and it is perhaps most useful in the early stage of change when motivation is critical. MI is most important in promoting motivation for change and relies on specific approaches to achieve changes in a wide variety of life issues beyond the specific targeted change. Three specific concepts are inherent in providing motivation for change: (1) *expression of empathy*, (2) *developing discrepancy*, and (3) *rolling with resistance*. Like many behavioral theories, this model was developed out of recognized deficiencies in current alternative models. The idea that health providers should confront patients with the worst possible scenario to cause change is alien to this approach. Scaring patients to provoke behavior change is an older concept not fitting this motivation-centered model.

In keeping with TTM of change rather than confrontation or persuasion, providers need to foster an environment in which individuals are encouraged to engage in self-exploration and contemplation of change. The outcome is improved motivation to change because the perception of the need to change comes directly from the patient rather than the health provider.

The idea is that together, the patient and provider are examining the need for change and that without bringing the patient along in decisions about change, there can be no effective long-standing approach to the targeted behavior change. A study that supported the relative effectiveness of TTM and MI over a brief health risk intervention was conducted by Prochaska et al. (2007). They were able to demonstrate that MI and TTM out-performed the HRI-only group by showing significant multiple behavior changes.

As with other behavioral change models, TTM has been used to predict and substantiate the usefulness of intervention programs based on the theory. Di Noia, Schinke, Prochaska, and Contento (2006) studied the fruit and vegetable consumption behaviors among economically disadvantaged African American adolescents.

The results of this study gave support to the fact that the stages of *action* and *maintenance* were different from beginning stages. Participants found to be in the action-maintenance stages reported higher levels of pros and lower cons as well as higher self-efficacy and greater consumption of fruits and vegetables than participants said to be in the pre-contemplation and contemplation-preparation stages. Thus, it was shown that changes were more serious in the later stages of the change process. These investigators suggested that with replication, the TTM could be appropriate in designing interventions to increase fruit and vegetable consumption among these youth. Johnson et al. (2006) examined the usefulness of an intervention designed on the basis of TTM to improve adherence and increase exercise and diet in an adult population receiving treatment.

They substantiated the effectiveness of the program in moving intervention subjects from the pre-action stage to the action and maintenance stages for adherence at the end of the 18-month randomized clinical trial. Furthermore, those who were in the treatment group were more likely to progress to the action and maintenance stages for exercise and dietary fat reduction.

▶ Social Ecological Model

The evolution of behavior change theory has been heavily influenced by a concentration on the individual (perceptions, attitudes, beliefs, intentions, personal norms, and self-actualizing capacities). SEM, sometimes referred to as the behavioral ecological model, differs in that it takes into consideration a wide range of both individual and environmental factors that impact behavior change. SEM was articulated early on by McLeroy, Bibeau, Steckler, and Glanz (1988) who hypothesized that multiple factors have to be considered in the change process, and some of these are beyond the level of the individual.

It was believed that emphasizing the importance of the individual level can create bias and blinding to factors that are critical in considering behavior change and program interventions (e.g., sociocultural and physical environmental factors that also influence behavior change). SEM places these factors on a scale equal to individual skills and knowledge and intentions to change. Otherwise, physical and sociocultural support systems have much to do with producing change in individuals' behaviors. For example, exercising is more likely if there are places to exercise (free gyms, parks, and bicycle paths). Environmental conditions can significantly influence exercise behavior.

The advantage of SEM over individually driven models is the meaningful inclusion of multiple factors working for and against change. SEM enhances our understanding of the multiple and interactive effects of the many personal and environmental factors that influence health behaviors at several levels: individual, family, community, public policy, and population.

The basic premise behind SEM is that change is more likely if the approach is at both a macro and micro level where attention is placed simultaneously on the physical and cultural environment and individual level factors. Effective interventions would include consideration of multiple levels of intervention as well (e.g., transportation, accessibility of programs, motivation to enroll, family support to enroll, and racial and cultural factors).

The following are studies selected to illustrate the application of SEM. These articles include either database research or policy implications. Patrick, Intille, and Zabinski (2005) provide a compelling exposé about the impact of computer-supported interactive media on the etiology, prevention, early detection, treatment, and posttreatment survival. SEM's multiple levels and interactions are key, and it is this theory that is more inclusive of many elements of the environment both at the micro and macro levels. Patrick and colleagues cited the example of tobacco use and the many important elements that need to be addressed to target this problem.

Debate and Pyle (2004) used the behavioral ecological model to assess what predicted women's early use of the women, infants, and children (WIC) program. Their findings indicated that cultural, intrapersonal, and interpersonal contingencies and perceived systemic barriers influenced WIC enrollment. They urged that in building programs of this kind, attention should be given to not only personal, cultural, but also environmental influences.

Interventions that simultaneously influence these multiple levels may be expected to lead to greater and longer-lasting changes and maintenance of existing health-promoting habits. SEM has significant implications for future interventions. Using this model, communications at a much larger level (governmental, community level, and wide-scale broadcasting of health promotion messages) would be important in influencing patients' desires, intentions, and actions to modify unhealthy behaviors.

▶ Summary

Theories of behavior change can give significant direction for the timely use of behavior change communications. They are very useful to providers in both understanding patients' behaviors and approaches needed to facilitate change in behaviors that entail health risks. In this chapter the models frequently used in health promotion and disease prevention were described and discussed.

Many of these theoretical frameworks overlap. For example, the concept of self-efficacy is addressed in the social cognitive theory but again in TPB, TTM, and TRA. In each theory, the role of self-efficacy may play a more or less prominent role. The fact that self-efficacy appears in multiple cases should not be a criticism. It may be indicative of the importance of the phenomenon across several domains of behavior change and different populations. In fact, Davis et al. suggested that an important next step is to investigate the connectedness of theories with one another.

Behavior change theories and models are critical to interventions and programs for patients and their families. Fishbein and Cappella (2006) emphasize that behavior theories are useful because they explain behavior and identify essential elements needed in communications with patients to achieve behavior change.

However, despite their importance, there may be a number of reasons that theories or conceptual frameworks are not applied. First, there is some support for these theories but in several instances the findings are mixed. Second, because behavioral theories overlap, providers may think that there are no unique theories, just a few major principles that seem to reappear. Third, providers may have difficulty using these theories because they do not address the full scope of behavior change as they see it in various patient populations.

Prior criticisms of behavioral theories were levied at the lack of consideration given to situational variables, physical, social, and economic factors (e.g., poverty and poor access to care). A framework that has emerged from this criticism is SEM which maintains that many factors influence behavior change, not just psychosocial phenomena, which are somewhat difficult to observe and measure. In certain populations, environmental factors may have as much or more influence than behavioral science variables. Providers should be concerned that any model used does not limit one's understanding of behavior change needs and approaches. Of particular concern is that theories may limit our vision to the extent that we ignore problems that do not fit the theory in question (**TABLE 24-1**).

TABLE 24-1 Social and Behavioral Theories of Behavioral Change

Theoretical/ Conceptual Framework	Key Concepts and Principles	Patient Behavior Change Targets	Studies Using Framework
Social and cognitive behavioral model		Perceived self-efficacy	Physical activity	Mailey et al. (2016). Parents' physical inactivity and barriers to exercise.
		Behavioral intentions Outcome expectancies (negative and positive)	Alcohol use	Fairlie et al. (2016). Alter college students' alcohol drinking patterns. Young et al. (2006). Alter college students' heavy alcohol use.
TRA and TPB		Attitude toward behavior	Smoking behavior	Quo et al. (2007). Smoking behavior in Chinese adolescents.
		Behavioral intentions	Physician contraception prescription practices	Sable et al. (2006). Physician intention to prescribe emergency contraceptives.
		Subjective norms control beliefs		
HBM		Perceived susceptibility	Building osteoporosis prevention programs	Hazavehei et al. (2007). Osteoporosis prevention education among Iranian middle school girls.
		and perceived seriousness of disease		
		Perceived benefits of behavior change		
		Perceived barriers to change	HIV risk behaviors	Lin et al. (2005). Predicting HIV risk behaviors among Taiwanese immigrants to the United States.
		Cues to action		

TTM of change	Five stages of change	Unhealthy eating	Di Noia et al. (2006). Changing fruit and vegetable consumption among economically disadvantaged adolescents.
	Linear stages of change occur in linear fashion		
	Specific patient behaviors evidenced in each stage	Lipid lowering	Johnson et al. (2006). Lipid lowering through intervention to increase exercise and diet and improve treatment adherence among adults.
	Stage-specific interventions		
Ecological model	Interaction of physical and social contingencies	Communicating about cancer	Patrick et al. (2005). Implications for communicating about cancer and the ecological framework.
	Entry into pregnancy programs		Debate and Pyle (2004). Understanding women in their first trimester and entry into WIC.
Intrapersonal factors			
Interpersonal processes and primary groups			
Institutional factors			
Community factors			
Public policy			

There is a movement nationwide to construct theories of change that will be useful in an analysis of change over time not just in isolated short-term increments. Management of chronic illness, for example, requires a long-term perspective on multiple behavioral changes required over time. Shortcomings of current theories include their inability to be sufficient in predicting and guiding behavior change over time. Many of these theories stop short of the initial step of taking action while others address the action stage but do not address maintenance of change over time. There are exceptions. For example, TTM subscribes to stages of change and includes specific analysis of the maintenance stage. Still, this model has been criticized because it suggests that distinct behaviors are associated with each particular stage. TTM has been criticized because conceiving of behavior in stages may constrain our expectations and notions of what interventions will work best.

With that said, the purpose of theories is to shed light on why things occur, in what sequence, and under what conditions. They can either add simplicity or complexity. They are preferable to common sense or, in some cases, experience. They focus and organize thinking in systematic ways and provide not only content but structure to phenomenon. Rather than producing a great deal of trivia, theories organize data in meaningful ways that allow for duplication and application in a number of situations. In this chapter, the major focus was on behavioral and social science theories of change. The chapter did not address physiological phenomenon important in changing behaviors where indeed these factors are critical to behavior change, such as physical activity, dietary patterns, and smoking and drug use. In addition to understanding the psychosocial and environmental factors that influence such behaviors, making clear the particular physiologic influences and how they interact with psychosocial and environmental factors is important but beyond the scope of the purpose of this chapter.

Discussion

1. Discuss the differences between HBM and TTM of behavior change.
2. Identify reasons why using a theoretical model may be helpful in designing behavioral change interventions or programs.
3. Which models most reflect your understanding of motivating behavioral change for behaviors (e.g., inactivity, poor oral hygiene, nonadherence to exercise protocols, substance abuse, and obesity)?
4. What principles from the model(s) you chose are key to understanding these behaviors?
5. Identify questions that need to be studied in understanding the usefulness of theoretical frameworks.

References

Ajzen, I., & Fishbein, M. (1977). Attitude-behavior relations: A theoretical analysis and review of empirical research. *Psychological Bulletin, 84*, 888–918.

Ajzen, I., & Fishbein, M. (1980). *Understanding attitudes and predicting social behavior.* Englewood Cliffs, NJ: Prentice-Hall. doi:10.4018/978-1-4666-8156-9:ch012

Bagozzi, R. P., & Edwards, E. A. (1998). Goal setting and goal pursuit in the regulation of body weight. *Psychology and Health, 13*, 593–621. doi:.org/10.1080/088704498407421

Bandura, A. (1997). *Self-efficacy: The exercise of control.* New York, NY: W.H. Freeman. doi:10.1111/1467-8721 .00064

Bandura, A. (1986). *Social foundations of thought and action: A social cognitive theory.* Englewood Cliffs, NJ: Prentice-Hall.

Bandura, A. (2000). Exercise of human agency through collective efficacy. *Current Directions in Psychological Science, 9,* 75–78. doi:10.1111/1467-8721.00064

Davis, R., Campbell, R., Hildon, Z., Hobbs, L., & Michie, S. (2015). Theories of behaviour and behaviour change across the social and behavioural sciences: A scoping review. *Health Psychology Review, 9*(3), 323–344. doi:10.1080/17437199.2014.941722

Debate, R., & Pyle, G. F. (2004). The behavioral ecological model: A framework for early WIC participation. *American Journal of Health Studies, 19,* 138–147.

Di Noia, J. D., Schinke, S. P., Prochaska, J. O., & Contento, I. R. (2006). Application of the transtheoretical model to fruit and vegetable consumption among economically disadvantaged African-American adolescents: Preliminary findings. *American Journal of Health Promotion, 20*(5), 342–348. doi:10.4278/0890-1171-20.5.342

Fairlie, A. M., Ramirez, J. J., Patrick, M. E., & Lee, C. M. (2016). When do college students have less favorable views of drinking? Evaluations of alcohol experiences and positive and negative consequences. *Psychology of Addictive Behaviors, 30*(5), 555–565. doi:10.1037/adb0000190

Fishbein, M., & Ajzen, I. (1975). *Belief, attitude, intention, and behavior: An introduction to theory and research.* Reading, MA: Addison-Wesley.

Fishbein, M., & Cappella, J. N. (2006). The role of theory in developing effective health communications. *Journal of Communications, 56,* S1–S17. doi:10.1111/j.1460-2466.2006.00280.x

Fuchs, R. (1996). Causal models of physical exercise participation: Testing the predictive power of the construct "pressure to change". *Journal of Applied Social Psychology, 26,* 1931–1960. doi:10.1111/j.1559-1816.1996.tb00106.x

Hazavehei, S. M., Taghdisi, M. H., & Saidi, M. (2007). *Application of the Health Belief Model for osteoporosis prevention among middle school girl students, Garmsar, Iran.* Education for Health. Retrieved from http://www.educationforhealth.net/

Johnson, S. S., Driskell, M. M., Johnson, J. L., Dyment, S. J., Prochaska, J. M., & Bourne, L. (2006). Transtheoretical model intervention for adherence to lipid-lowering drugs. *Disease Management, 9,* 102–114. doi:10.1089/dis.2006.9.102

Lin, P., Simoni, J. M., & Zemon, V. (2005). The health belief model, sexual behaviors, and HIV risk among Taiwanese immigrants. *AIDS Education and Prevention, 17*(5), 469–483. doi:10.1521/aeap.2005.17.5.469

Lipari, R., & Jean-Francois, B. (2016, August 16).Trends in perception of risk and availability of substance use among full-time college students. The CBHSQ Report. Center for Behavioral Health Statistics and Quality, Substance Abuse and Mental Health Services Administration, Rockville, MD.

Mailey, E. L., Phillips, S. M., Dlugonski, D., & Conroy, D. E. (2016). Overcoming barriers to exercise among parents: A social cognitive theory perspective. *Journal of Behavioral Medicine, 39*(4), 599–609. doi:10.1007/s10865-016-9744-8

McLeroy, K. R., Bibeau, D., Steckler, A., & Glanz, K. (1988). An ecological perspective on health promotion programs. *Health Education Quarterly, 15*(4), 351–377. PMID:3068205

Miller, W. R., & Rollnick, S. (1991). *Motivational interviewing: Preparing people to change addictive behavior.* New York, NY: Guilford Press. doi: org/10.1002/casp.2450020410

Miller, W. R., & Rollnick, S. (2002). *Motivational interviewing.* New York, NY: Guilford Press.

Patrick, K., Intille, S. S., & Zabinski, M. F. (2005). An ecological framework for cancer communication: Implications for research. *Journal of Medical Internet Research, 7*(3), e23. Retrieved from http://www.jmir.org/2005/3/e23

Prochaska, J. O., Butterworth, S., Redding, C. A., Burden, V., Perrin, N., Leo, M., … Prochaska, J. M. (2007). Initial efficacy of MI, TTM tailoring and HRI's with multiple behaviors for employee health promotion. *Preventive Medicine, 46*(3), 226–231. doi:10.1016/j.ypmed.2007.11.007

Prochaska, J. O., & DiClemente, C. C. (1983). Stages and processes of self-change of smoking: Toward an integrative model of change. *Journal of Consulting and Clinical Psychology, 51,* 390–395. PMID:6863699

Prochaska, J. O., DiClemente, C. C., & Norcross, J. C. (1992). In search of how people change: Applications to addictive behavior. *American Psychologist, 47,* 1102–1114. PMID:1329589

Prochaska, J. O., DiClemente, C. C., Velicer, W. F., Ginpil, S., & Norcross, J. C. (1985). Predicting change in smoking status for self-changers. *Addictive Behaviors, 10,* 395–406. PMID:4091072

Prochaska, J. O., DiClemente, C. C., Velicer, W. F., & Rossi, J. S. (1993). Standardized, individualized, interactive and personalized self-help programs for smoking cessation. *Health Psychology, 12,* 399–405. PMID:8223364

Prochaska, J. O., & Velicer, W. F. (1997). The transtheoretical model of health behavior change. *American Journal of Health Promotion, 12,* 38–48. doi:10.4278/0890-1171-12.1.38

Quo, G., Johnson, C. A., Unger, J. B., Lee, L., Xie, B., Chou, C., … Pentz, M. A. (2007). Utility of the theory of reasoned action and theory of planned behavior for predicting Chinese adolescent smoking. *Addiction, 32*(5), 1066–1081. doi:10.1016/j.addbeh.2006.07.015

Rogers, C. R. (1959). A theory of therapy, personality and interpersonal relationships, as developed in the client-centered framework. In S. Koch (ed.), *Psychology: A study of science* (pp. 184–256). New York, NY: McGraw-Hill.

Rogers, C. R. (1961). *On becoming a person.* Boston, MA: Houghton Mifflin.

Rogers, C. R. (1977). *Carl Rogers on personal power.* New York, NY: Delacorte Press.

Rosenstock, I. M., Strecher, V. J., & Becker, M. H. (1988). Social learning theory and the health belief model. *Health Education Quarterly, 15*, 175–183. PMID:3378902

Sable, M. R., Schwartz, L. R., Kelly, P. J., Lison, E., & Hall, M. A. (2006). Using the theory of reasoned action to explain physician intention to prescribe emergency contraception. *Perspectives on Sexual and Reproductive Health, 38*(1), 20–27. doi:10.1363/psrh.38.020.06

Schifter, D. E., & Ajzen, I. (1985). Intention, perceived control, and weight loss: An application of the theory of planned behavior. *Journal of Personality and Social Psychology, 49*, 843–851. doi:10.1037//0022-3514.49.3.843

Schwarzer, R., & Jerusalem, M. (1995). Generalized self-efficacy scale. In J. Weinman, S. Wright, & M. Johnston (Eds.), *Measures in health psychology: A user's portfolio. Causal and control beliefs* (pp. 35–37). Windsor, UK: NFER-NELSON.

Young, R. M., Connor, J. P., Ricciardelli, L. A., & Saunders, J. B. (2006). The role of alcohol expectancy and drinking refusal self-efficacy beliefs in university student drinking. *Alcohol and Alcoholism, 41*(1), 70–75. doi:10.1093/alcalc/agh237

Zimmerman, G. L., Olsen, C. G., & Bosworth, M. F. (2000). A 'Stages of Change' approach to helping patients change behavior. *American Family Physician, 61*(5), 1409–1416. PMID:10735346

CHAPTER 25

Altering Systems of Care to Enhance Health Care Communications

CHAPTER OBJECTIVES

- Identify needs for change in the health care delivery system to advance quality care and patient safety.
- Identify barriers to effective health care communications at the health care delivery system level.
- Discuss how certain pilot projects have affected the nature of patient–provider and provider–provider communications, and their corresponding implications for quality care.
- Describe strategies and programs that would be both feasible and effective in changing the health care system to improve communications.
- Identify the specific measurable outcomes of these programs that would provide evidence of the effectiveness of these strategies or programs to improve health care communications.

KEY TERMS

- Access and utilization of health care systems
- Comprehensive care
- Continuity of care
- Coordinated care
- Fragmentation of health care delivery
- Health care delivery system
- Informational continuity
- Integrated delivery system (IDS)
- Interpersonal continuity
- Management continuity

▶ Introduction

The U.S. health care system has been described as *broken*. The degree to which our health care system continues to be broken is not altogether clear. An optimistic view would be that this system once criticized as unhealthy, uncaring, complex, poorly organized, and costly is now sufficiently organized, integrated, patient-centered, and less costly. But this is too optimistic. All signs indicate that we are still struggling to identify, describe, and implement a better system. Undoubtedly, steps to reverse these tendencies may have made significant inroads. But the question remains, has there been sufficient reorganization of the U.S. health care system to rectify these serious problems? In the U.S. the problem of quality of care differs across geographical areas with some states outperforming others (AHRQ, 2017). What is clear is that lack of access to health care is intimately linked to the quality of care our citizens are likely to receive.

Along these lines, the World Health Organization (WHO) has described a good health system as one that *delivers quality services to all people, when and where they need them.* That the U.S. **health care delivery system** could reach the point of being so strongly criticized is both troublesome and confusing. We have amassed an army of highly qualified health professionals across all health care services and departments. The United States is a leader in health sciences and medical research. Its health information technology capabilities are highly evolved. As a country, the United States leads efforts to decrease disease morbidity and mortality. Yet, a 2008 Commonwealth Fund Report revealed that the United States ranks last among developed countries in quality of health care dispensed. Additionally, this system which is a mix of private and public institutions is the most expensive in the world.

Health care leaders and policymakers have accepted the central driving principle to make changes for the sake of quality care and

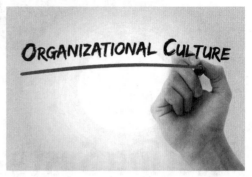
© Dizain/Shutterstock.

patient safety for all. This mission requires a change in organizational structure.

In order to make these changes, attention is given not only to technology of care but to the systems in which this care is carried out. Many providers and consumers alike, independently or collectively, are in a position to make at least minor changes in the organization of care delivery to enhance patient–provider communications. Systems of care can cause barriers to effective communications but can also set in motion processes that facilitate and improve communications between patients and providers and within provider groups.

Problems in health care systems of care have been rigorously explored, with recognition that communication problems do not occur in a vacuum. There are many factors that both enhance and impede communications and these refer to how systems of care are organized. The most well-known global issues include equitable **access and utilization of health care systems** for all. Access and utilization of health care was initially addressed in Chapter 1 of this text. These concepts will not be readdressed here but readers are encouraged to refer back to Chapter 1 if helpful.

This chapter discusses various system-level factors that promote therapeutic communications (e.g., the importance of continuity of care in building therapeutic alliances between patients and providers). A report of findings from selected research studies and descriptions of programs are offered. Programs such as transitional care, telephone-based continuing care, and systematic care are discussed and the methods of communication between provider and patients/families are detailed.

The primary aim of these programs has been to enhance continuity and coordination of care communications in hopes that quality of care will be advanced. There are several examples included in this chapter that illustrate what various health care settings are doing to improve communications and reduce communication barriers. First, it is important to understand what is meant by systems of health care delivery.

▶ Overview: Systems of Care

Systems of health care delivery refer to the major way health care is provided. Aspects of a delivery system would include inpatient, outpatient, and home care programs. It is the organization of people, institutions, and resources that deliver health care services to meet the health needs of selected populations and communities.

WHO refers to *health systems* as the combination of goods and services designed to promote health, including preventive, curative, and palliative interventions for individuals or populations (WHO, 2000). It is important to note that the term health care system is not the same as health system. Fineberg (2012) explains that health care system generally refers to the *formal system of care designed primarily to treat disease* while health system refers to solutions for health in a more general sense.

In most developed countries and in some developing countries, health care is provided to all regardless of their ability to pay. However, not all health care is delivered by a single system. For example, the United States, while it has many forms of private and public care, is the only developed country that does not yet have a viable universal health care system.

Even within the United States, there is a great deal of variability in how health care organizations operate.

Differences can be found in inpatient, outpatient, and partial care services at every phase of the prevention–treatment and palliative care cycle. For the most part, health care centers and hospitals have exercised considerable autonomy in structuring care delivery, and it is the particular way health care delivery is structured that account for many differences in what care is accessible, the quality of care given, and the degree to which it meets standards of care criteria.

It would seem that thinking logically about the differences in health care systems, we would want to identify what structural features create the best care outcomes while curbing the costs of this care. An important step is to identify what structural problems are troublesome and build new systems of care that avoid these pitfalls and, in fact, this is what has happened. One of the most notable problems is **fragmentation of health care delivery**. This is not merely multiple providers who may have little to no contact with one another. It is much more pervasive. It is fragmented due to many factors: misalignment of incentives, lack of coordination, and inefficiency. These consequences have also been linked to poor quality outcomes and high costs.

Fragmentation within the health care system is not a newly recognized phenomenon. A related issue is the splintering of health care professions which is seen in the various specialties and subspecialties that exist. Splintering is not altogether negative; for example, specialization within the health profession results in more precise and effective care yielding improved health outcomes. Honing in on key medical problems such as heart disease and noninvasive valve repair, cancers and noninvasive treatment technologies, and behavioral modification programs to treat addiction disorders are all examples where specialization has made a significant positive effect on disease management and health promotion.

Despite all reasons for promoting diversification and specialization, faulty foundation for health care services continues to be *fragmentation of health care delivery*. Fragmentation is observed in lack of continuity and coordination of care and the absence of care that is comprehensive enough to address health care issues from a variety of angles. Without proper continuity and coordination of care, patients can experience painful transitions over the course of a single illness and throughout their lifetime without the needed support and guidance to overcome these complexities. This is particularly important as the burden of chronic illness continues to rise not only in the United States but worldwide, sending many more individuals into the chaos of managing their own care without support.

Lack of system coordination and continuity puts the onus on patients and their families when rightfully this burden should be on providers and systems of care. It has been shown that not all patients and families are equipped to meet these challenges. Because of increased awareness of care fragmentation and disparities in both health care utilization and health status across communities and populations, these problems in the delivery system have made leaders and policy makers more attuned to understanding what the problem is and taking steps to correct it.

The problem of care fragmentation is not only felt by patients and their families, it is also experienced by providers. One key example is the inadequate flow of information across providers and within and between external partners in care. Financial disincentives contribute to the problem of lack of coordination and continuity. All of this results in, either directly or indirectly, poor quality of care and compromised communications. The following is a discussion of the basic principles of designing delivery systems to enhance communications between patients and providers and also to enhance providers' communications with one another and with external partners in care.

▶ System Characteristics to Enhance Health Care Communications

System characteristics that promote quality care and patient safety can be listed in a variety of ways; those discussed here pertain to the problem of health care system fragmentation. These principles, or 3Cs, are *coordination, continuity*, and *comprehensiveness* of care provided. The concepts of accessibility and utilization of health care services are also important to quality care but were presented in Chapter 1 of this text.

Readers are advised to refer to this section of the text to further understand the interplay of the 3Cs and access and utilization of health care. These guiding principles first codified by the Institute of Medicine (IOM) outline the essentials of sound primary care practices but are also germane to health care services in a variety of settings. Better patient care outcomes are associated with these organizational properties and the way in which these elements of care affect processes of care and communications.

▶ Coordination of Care

To achieve *coordinated care*, all health care providers involved are required to practice as a coherent, harmonizing team with shared responsibility for patient care outcomes to achieve the most effective health care results.

The Agency for Healthcare Research and Quality (AHRQ) defines care coordination as the deliberate organization of patient care activities and sharing of information among health providers concerned with patients' care to achieve safer and more effective care (AHRQ, 2016a). Coordinated care relies on the durability and effective interaction of many and is managed by the exchange of patient information among these providers

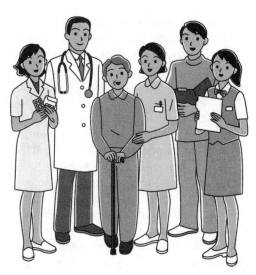

© Alphabe/Shutterstock.

for different aspects of care. With the recognition of the patient being a member of the health care team, coordination also relies on coordinated efforts with patients and patients' families to achieve the best care possible. Effective provider–provider and patient–provider communication is essential to providing coordinated care.

Coordinated care services depend upon good transitional care. Lack of coordination is problematic when trying to secure quality patient care and patient safety. Such behaviors as taking care of patients and then leaving them at the doorsteps of the hospital or health center at discharge when they clearly have unanswered questions, or being nonchalant about issues they may have when having to transfer to a new provider, is problematic if not also unethical.

The goal of successfully handing off the patient in these circumstances is to provide good transitional care. Good transitional care whether from provider to provider, hospital to home, or between health care facilities requires coordination of care. It also requires adequate communications to ensure quality of transfer.

In the landmark work of Coleman, Mahoney, and Parry (2005), concerns about the quality and safety of patients during

transitions of care remain and are growing. These investigators developed and tested a performance outcome measure based on the patient's perceptions participating in focus groups.

The potential problem areas identified were information transfer, patient and caregiver preparation, self-management support, and empowerment to assert preferences (Coleman et al., 2002). Coleman et al. created a 15-item measure called the care transitions measure to clarify deficiencies in care during discharge from hospitals and to serve as a quality improvement measure. The National Quality Forum subsequently mounted a three-item version. Coleman, Parry, Chalmers, and Min (2006), in describing their randomized controlled trial of a care transitions intervention, summarized the literature and suggested that quality and patient safety were compromised during periods of transition due to the high risk for medication errors, incomplete or inaccurate transfer information, and lack of appropriate follow-up care.

The program developed for transition of care at hospital discharge discusses more effective transitional care including improvements in communication between inpatient and outpatient providers, reconciliation of prescribed medication regimens, adequate education of patients about prescribed medications, closer medical follow-up, engaging social support systems, and greater clarity in patient–provider communication needs.

Coordinated care is important not only at times of patient transfer from one setting to another but it is also critical in the provision of primary care in physician–hospital or medical group partnerships. Typically, transfer of patient information (e.g., test results and visit notes) may not be completely transmitted and in a timely fashion. In a six-country study supported by the Commonwealth Foundation, patients' transitional care experiences following hospitalization were reported (Schoen et al., 2005). These respondents had recently been hospitalized, had surgery, or had health problems and were interviewed by telephone between March and June 2005.

As stated in the report, while the United States performed better compared with other countries on the hospital transition measure, the United States had the highest rate of problems in coordination during patient visits. These problems were reported to be providers not getting test results or records at the time of the visit or physicians performing duplicate tests. These findings suggested inefficiency in care delivery and misuse of patient and physician time. In other developed countries, the rates of this type of coordination problem were much lower, 10–15% lower than the U.S. rate of 33%. In all countries, having an accessible "medical home" that helps coordinate care is associated with significantly more positive outcomes (Schoen et al., 2007).

Failure to coordinate care during transitional points due to or resulting in poor communication has significant consequences for quality of care. Coordination problems can negatively affect patient satisfaction, patient acceptance of and adherence to medical regimens, and eventually utilization of the very care that is offered. In the Commonwealth Foundation's cross-national study (Schoen et al., 2005), at least one-fifth of those surveyed reported gaps in communication between them and their providers, and one-sixth expressed the need to have greater involvement in decisions about their care. It was concluded that to address such problems policy innovations were needed; essentially, changes would have to go beyond current payment structures and the way health care delivery systems are configured today.

Coordination of care is important in primary care settings, and is the target of a survey developed by AHRQ (2016b) to identify adult patients' experiences with care coordination in primary care settings. It builds on previous AHRQ work to develop a conceptual framework for care coordination and is used in primary care research and evaluation with potential applications to primary care quality improvement.

Patients were asked about their experiences in seeking care in the last 12 months and the characteristics of their experiences. For example, how many different primary care professionals at their primary care provider's office had they seen for a health reason, how often did they know what aspects of their care they were responsible for, how often did they get to talk to the primary care professional that knew them best, and if they saw a health care professional outside their primary care provider's office how often did their primary care provider know about the tests or results from these visits. This survey is conceptually strong covering essential experiences in primary care practices and is used in primary care research and evaluation studies.

▶ Continuity of Care

Continuity of care, like **coordinated care** and **comprehensive care**, is concerned with the quality of care. It is achieved when patients and providers or provider teams work cooperatively to ensure uninterrupted care over time. Continuity of patient care has been and continues to be associated with professional medical practice. For patients and their families, the perception that someone is in control of their care, is knowledgeable about them and their health care needs, and will follow them over time, is the experience of continuity.

Continuity of patient care, defined more broadly, signifies "coherent health care with a seamless transition over time between various providers in different settings" (Biem, Hadjustavropoulos, Morgan, Biem, & Pong, 2003, p. 1).

Management of services to achieve seamless transitions has also been referred to as "continuance of care" (Preen et al., 2005), "continuum of care" (Wright, Litaker, Laraia, & DeAndrade, 2001), or "continuing care" (McKay et al., 2005). It has been described as either a structural dimension (Kibbe, Phillips, & Green, 2004) or a process indicator

(Saultz, 2003; Saultz & Albedaiwi, 2004). Guthrie and Wyke (2000) stated that there are at least two conflicting definitions of continuity. The first stresses the patient seeing the same health care provider at each visit (personal continuity). The second stresses consistency of care from the perspective of organizations, guidelines, and electronic medical records (care continuity), irrespective of whether the patient sees the same or a different provider.

Saultz (2003) speaks of a hierarchy of dimensions including different aspects of care continuity: informational, longitudinal, and **interpersonal continuity**. Similar to Saultz et al. (2003) others examined continuity but with a multidisciplinary perspective. They identified informational, management, and relational (similar to interpersonal) continuity of care. **Informational continuity** refers to the "use of information on past events and personal circumstances to make current care appropriate for each individual" (Haggerty et al., 2003, p. 1220).

Management continuity refers to "a consistent and coherent approach to the management of a health condition that is responsive to a patient's changing needs" (p. 1220). Finally, relational continuity of care refers to "an ongoing therapeutic relationship between a patient and one or more providers" (p. 1220). The dimension of relational continuity is said to be important because it provides patients and their families with a sense of predictability and coherence. Haggerty et al. also point out that management continuity is particularly important in chronic and complex diseases when care is provided by several providers who could potentially work at cross purposes. They also explain that processes designed to enhance continuity, such as care pathways and case management systems, do not mean that continuity is ensured. Rather, it is the experience of care as "connected and coherent" that signals the presence of continuity of patient care.

Continuity of care is not absolute. Patient care may be more or less continuous. Kristjansson and colleagues (2013) emphasize that patients place a high value on continuity. They explained that there are several components that impact continuity; they span patient, provider, and practice factors. Because there are multiple factors ensuring continuity is complex, and just how much continuity of care is needed to promote quality care is not fully known. Saultz and Lochner (2005) concluded that it is likely that a significant association exists between interpersonal continuity, improved preventive care, and reduced rates of hospitalization. The perceived value of and commitment to care continuity transcends all professions in health care.

▶ Comprehensiveness

Comprehensive care is the third C element describing how health care services are structured. The concept of comprehensive care has evolved over time to mean different things. Initially, it was used to describe a treatment perspective in which patients would be seen and treated as holistically; not as a condition, disease, or surgical challenge, but as a "whole person." This meant that the wide range of physical, psychological, social, and spiritual needs of patients should be appreciated and considered in patient care. Like continuity and coordinated care, comprehensive care is also regarded as a professional value and essential in the design of patient-centered care delivery systems.

Most recently, comprehensive patient care has been referred to as a number of resources "bundled together" to produce a "one-stop-shop" service (e.g., case management, nutritional services, pharmacy, dental, women's health, and medical care representing the range of services available at a single treatment facility). Another interpretation of comprehensive care is the combined function approach based upon the disease phase: assessment, diagnosis, treatment, case management, and all indirect services for all complications.

These services are contained under a single provider or provider team. Integrated care systems have also been associated with comprehensive care. The idea that integrated care systems should include continuity, coordination, and comprehensive care is clearly detailed in the IOM report, *Crossing the quality chasm: A new health system for the 21st century* (2001). Integrated care systems entail complex communication linkages. This option is taken up in the next section of this chapter.

▶ Approaches to Providing Integrative Care

As previously suggested, *managed care* was a precursor to what is now described as integrated delivery systems (IDSs). Managed care was introduced as a solution to poorly coordinated care that lacked a comprehensive care focus. In fact, managed care (and health maintenance organizations [HMOs]) was introduced to reverse fragmented service delivery and control costs of care. In 1973, The Health Maintenance Organization Act was passed and from there HMOs grew rapidly.

This was *the medicine* for a poorly coordinated system of care that lacked a focus on comprehensive care. Exemplary models of managed care delivery systems were found in the health care organizations most capable of using managed care effectively such as the Veterans Administration (VA), Kaiser Permanente, and a few smaller enterprises. HMOs tended to restrict the choice of a provider and only approve a specialist after patients saw their primary care provider. A further criticism of HMOs was that a procedure or surgery would have to be submitted for review and approval from the insurer with the possibility that expensive or experimental treatments and procedures would not be covered. Thus, a woman's access to a provider in network may not help a great deal if the

procedure itself, by this care specialist, is not covered. The patient may still be treated by the specialist but a less costly and more invasive procedure would be the one and only choice.

A less restrictive version of the HMO managed care system is the preferred provider organization (PPO) which enables patients to have more choice over what providers they would see but within a network of providers. While HMOs dominated into the 1990s, there was an upsurge of dissatisfaction coming from both patients and providers. Along with this disenchantment of limited choice was the rising awareness that care was too costly and did not meet standards of quality care.

Integrated Delivery System

In a backdrop of dissatisfaction and even anger towards managed care, further attempts to reduce fragmentation and costs of health care emerged. Many believed that the solution was and is greater integration of health care delivery and at reduced costs via the **integrated delivery system (IDS)** model .

An IDS is an organized, coordinated, and collaborative network that links various health care providers to provide coordinated health care services to a particular patient population or community. The system is built on the foundation of what primary care has to offer but adds the coordination of services to achieve a high level of quality over the continuum of care. As IDS approaches appeared, HMOs have fallen away.

IDS approaches were seen as better solutions to the problem of fragmented health care. IDS systems can be found at Veterans Health Administration (VHA) health centers, Kaiser Permanente, and the Mayo Clinic. More loosely organized hospital–physician and medical groups now offer care that is integrated but also more comprehensive in care delivery including health promotion, disease prevention, mental health/substance abuse, and even alternative medicine. IDSs are accountable for both clinical and cost outcomes. They are designated by the community served and are committed to improving care in the community.

Enthoven, Professor Emeritus at the Graduate School of Business at Stanford University explains that no single approach or public policy will fix the fragmented U.S. health care system but IDSs represent an important step in the right direction (Enthoven, 2009). Enthoven adds that it would be a mistake to move from managed care to a system where patients choose the best doctor for their condition. Adopting IDS then was seen to be a step in the right direction and a more encompassing form of managed care.

Hwang, Chang, LaClair, and Paz (2013) conducted a systematic review of the literature reporting on the results of evaluations of various IDSs. Their purpose was to examine IDSs and changes in costs and quality of care. They summarized findings from 21 peer-reviewed articles and 4 nonpeer reviewed papers. Twenty of these studies reported an association between increased integration and quality of care. For example, there were positive associations between IDS and lower hospital admission rates per patient, a shorter length of stay per hospital admission, and an overall lower rate of adverse health outcomes. They also reported that their review indicated improvements in evidence-based practice use among physicians, and some studies reported improvements in preventive care. One paper reported no changes in quality, and none of the studies reviewed directly measured reductions in costs.

Despite the fact that IDS is recognized as an important approach to minimizing the problem of fragmentation, there are barriers to adoption of IDS programs. In fact, 100 IDSs were identified in May 2013 and were listed in a computer search throughout the country. Barriers to converting to IDS are many and include no incentives to make changes, lack of cooperation between and across health providers, physicians' and health care institutions' fears of losing autonomy over their practice, lack of clear understanding of what IDSs' entail, inadequate resources, and limited data to indicate these programs are effective (Maruthappu, Hasan, & Zeltner, 2015). Goodwin (2016) suggests that IDS may be best suited with patients who have medically complex or long-term care needs; and while the concept is evolving and being debated, there is a commitment to improving the quality of care through improvements in our delivery systems.

Accountable Care Organizations

In their conclusions, Hwang et al. reflect on a concept involving integrated care delivery: accountable care organizations (ACOs). ACOs are groups of doctors, hospitals, and other health care providers who join together (sometimes voluntarily) to give their Medicare patients coordinated high-quality care.

The purpose of an ACO is to reduce the cost of care by eliminating duplication of efforts while increasing the quality of services. A major contribution of ACOs is that they help ensure that patients, especially the chronically ill with long-term care needs and multiple medical conditions and treatments, get the right care at the right time. ACOs strive to avoid unnecessary duplication of services and prevent medical errors.

Patient-Aligned Care Team and the Patient-Centered Medical Home

Another important off-shoot from IDS is the patient-aligned care team (PACT). The VHA rolled out this innovation in 2010 (Rodriguez et al., 2014; Yano, Bair, Carrasquillo, Krein, & Rubenstein, 2014). The PACT model is built on the well-known concept of the patient-centered medical home (PCMH) staffed by high-functioning teams. A PACT involves each veteran working together with health care professionals to plan for the whole-person care and life-long health and wellness. The purpose is to provide patients a patient-centered medical home.

The VHA proposal was put into place to meet the challenges to health care but in particular, primary care. The primary care medical home, also referred to as the PCMH, advanced primary care, and the health care home is a promising model for transforming the organization and delivery of primary care. PACT transforms veterans' care by providing patient-driven, proactive, personalized, team-based care focused on wellness and disease prevention.

The results are seen in a number of important outcomes: improvements in veteran satisfaction and improved health care outcomes (e.g., decreased rates of unavoidable hospitalizations and emergency room use). Tuepker et al. (2014) add that this model is data-informed and provides highly accessible care that is continuous and coordinated across the spectrum of care. They also describe challenges to the implementation of PACT which occur with many kinds of innovations of this magnitude: inadequate staffing and unclear roles within teams.

▶ The 3Cs and Integrated Health Delivery System Outcomes

The provision of continuous, coordinated, and comprehensive care and doing this through the mechanism of IDSs is exactly how improved quality care was to happen and is something to be emulated in the design and delivery of health care services in the future. The following is a brief summary of reports of the impact of the 3Cs and IDS on quality patient care.

The concept of continuity of patient care has been repeatedly linked with quality care. Also, the reverse or absence of continuity has been linked to adverse events (e.g.,

medication errors and increased risk for re-hospitalization). Literature reporting these findings is found in studies of a variety of patient care settings from outpatient primary care practices, inpatient units, extended care, and hospice services.

Continuity of care (defined as sustained contact with a primary provider) has been associated with early diagnosis of chronic disease (Koopman, Mainous, Baker, Gill, & Gilbert, 2003) and improved quality of care (Parchman & Burge, 2002). Gill and Mainous found that after controlling for demographics, number of ambulatory visits, and case mix, higher provider continuity was associated with a lower likelihood of hospitalization for any condition. Parchman and Burge reported that patients with type 2 diabetes who had seen their usual providers within the past year were significantly more likely to have had an eye examination, a foot examination, two blood pressure measurements, and a lipid analysis.

In a follow-up study by these investigators, as the length of the relationship increased between patient and provider, scores on communication and accumulated knowledge of the patient by the physician and trust in the physician also increased (Parchman & Burge, 2003). In an extensive review of clinical studies altering systems to influence desired outcomes, several commonalities were noted. What these continuity of care interventions had in common was a focus on improving provider–provider and/or provider–patient/family communications.

It should be noted that not all studies reported positive findings. For example, Gill, Mainous, Diamond, and Lentard (2003) stated that while continuity might benefit some aspects of the care of diabetic patients, provider continuity was not associated with completion of diabetic monitoring (receipt of a glycosylated hemoglobin test, a lipid profile, or an eye examination) in patients treated under a private national health plan.

The following is an overview of selected studies reporting on the impact of system changes. In general, the interventions piloted and described here were designed to improve patient care transitions which would also improve communications, satisfaction, and coordination of care. Categories of outcome variables included in these studies were patient-level health and treatment behaviors, resource consumption, and provider influence.

Virtually all focused on some aspect of affecting patients' health status and/or their satisfaction with care. Quality of life (either generic or disease specific) was a frequently cited outcome measure (Fjaertoft, Indredavik, Johnsen, & Lydersen, 2004; Naylor et al., 2004; Neilsen, Palshof, Mainz, Jensen, & Olesen, 2003; Preen et al., 2005; Reynolds et al., 2004; Samet et al., 2003). Others addressed patient well-being and/or health status measures. For example, indicators included: (1) patient satisfaction well-being, unmet needs, and health status (Byng et al., 2004); (2) symptom severity and symptom relapse (Atienza et al., 2004; Fjaertoft et al., 2004); (3) adverse events (Crotty, Rowett, Spurling, Giles, & Philips, 2004; Atienza et al., 2004); and (4) worsening condition or mobility (Crotty et al., 2004).

Of those addressing costs of care, some focused on the nature and magnitude of resource use such as overall or total direct costs of care (Atienza et al., 2004; Byng et al., 2004). Others addressed hospital, urgent care, or emergency visits and the number and causes of readmissions (Atienza et al., 2004; Cowan, 2004; Harrison et al., 2002; Reynolds et al., 2004); extent and speed of communications between hospital and practitioner (Preen et al., 2005); hospital length of stay (Preen et al., 2005); and efficiency or number of patients missed on rounds (van Eaton, Horvath, Lober, Rossini, & Pellegrini, 2005).

Provider or caregiver factors (when associated with patient outcomes) were infrequently mentioned but included caregiver strain (Fjaertoft et al., 2004), communication and coordination of activities (van Eaton et al., 2005), processes of care (Byng et al., 2004), caregiver satisfaction (Byng et al., 2004), and

physician knowledge of patient's disease and treatment (Neilsen et al., 2003). There was no single pattern of outcome measurement. Patient outcomes were examined most often, followed by some measure of resource consumption. An overview of selected studies is provided in **TABLE 25-1**.

In conclusion, the principles of coordinated, continuous, comprehensive, and integrated care are viewed positively at all levels: across patients, families, providers, and policymakers but the outcomes of these approaches are not easily evaluated. Studies of integrated care systems are in their early phases. These projects and studies have made progress in refining these concepts and establishing appropriate measures to capture data in health care settings. However, resources to support studies of quality care outcomes require a good deal of coordination between and across health care settings and researchers to reliably capture this kind of data. Still, the commitment appears to be strong and the need for evaluation data is recognized by all involved. Until further evaluation studies can be funded and implemented conclusions about how altering systems of care can reliably transform and enhance health care communications remains hypothetical despite promising findings.

▶ Summary

Rising costs, worrisome variations in health care quality across communities, and expanding patient needs for both health promotion and disease management programs have created a health care delivery system crisis, one with serious consequences. These problems have been rigorously explored with recognition that communication problems do not occur in a vacuum. There are many factors that both enhance and impede communications, and these refer to how systems of care are organized. Fragmentation of health care delivery systems is the most recognized problem which is neither new nor resolved. In this chapter, there was ample description of the

TABLE 25-1 Selected Studies Evaluating Coordination, Continuity, Comprehensive, and Integrated Care

Author(s) and Date of Publication	Study Purpose and Design	Intervention or Independent Variable(s)	Study Population/ Setting and Measures	System Elements	Major Outcome(s)
Herrel et al. (2017)	Retrospective cohort study to examine the associations between the level of health care integration and quality of prostate care.	*Post hoc* retrospective analysis of level of integrated care as defined by top 100 integrated care delivery systems and measures of quality prostate care.	Surveillance, epidemiology, and end results (SEER)-Medicare (Parts A and B) data retrospective cohort study of 72,411 with newly diagnosed prostate cancer between 2007 and 2011.	***Integrated care*** as defined by top 100 integrated care delivery systems. Included receiving pretreatment counseling from radiologist and urologist; and avoiding unnecessary imaging or treatment when life expectancy is less than 10 years, and unnecessary hospitalization at end-of-life.	Integrated health care systems are associated with improved adherence to prostate cancer quality measures. Further examination of factors associated with quality care is advised to determine which factors or combination of factors drives quality.
Chen et al. (2016)	Evaluation study to assess the utilization of and satisfaction with ophthalmic health care provided by IDS and vision-related quality-of-life of patients receiving IDS.	Survey of community residents eligible for follow-up for ophthalmology disease (e.g., dry eye, cataracts, or glaucoma). Also multidisciplinary poststroke care program for patients after discharge in the acute phase.	Anonymous face-to-face interviews; 841 eligible patients completed the survey and 61.0% sought ophthalmic care for eye disease under IDS in past year.	***Ophthalmic care utilization under IDS***: care needs met when patients consulted care for eye discomfort (e.g., blurred vision, aching, itching, or burning sensation).	The rate of satisfaction with care under IDS program was high. Patients with high quality-of-life were less likely to be satisfied with care under IDS.

Naylor et al. (2004)	Randomized controlled trial to examine the effectiveness of a transitional care intervention delivered by advanced practice nurses to elders with heart failure.	A follow-up program of patients after hospital discharge.	Academic and community hospitals; elder patients hospitalized for heart failure transitioning to home care.	Collaboration with physicians; advanced practice nurses provided input to nursing staff regarding discharge needs of patients, thus improving **coordination** and communication among staff. Face-to-face interactions with patient's physician during hospital and initial discharge visit. Program follow-up with advanced practice nurses within 24 hours of discharge. **Continuity** of care visits conducted with the same nurses.	Improvements in time to first readmission, number of readmissions, and total costs. Short-term improvements in patient quality of life and satisfaction.
Neilsen et al. (2003)	Randomized controlled trial to determine the effect of a shared care program on the attitudes of newly referred cancer patients concerning the health care system.	Shared care program included transfer of knowledge from oncologist to general practitioner, improved communications, and active patient involvement.	Cancer patients referred to a university department of oncology practice.	**Coordination** and **continuity** of care through transfer of knowledge of patient needs from oncologist to general practitioner; discharge summary letters and information to patients' general practitioners. Shared care program with three elements: knowledge transfer, communication channels, and active patient involvement.	Improvements in patients' attitudes toward the health care system, and perceptions of cooperation between primary and secondary health care sectors (especially general practitioner's knowledge of their disease and treatment). Patient health-related quality of life improved.

(continues)

TABLE 25-1 Selected Studies Evaluating Coordination, Continuity, Comprehensive, and Integrated Care *(continued)*

Author(s) and Date of Publication	Study Purpose and Design	Intervention or Independent Variable(s)	Study Population/ Setting and Measures	System Elements	Major Outcome(s)
Simon, Ludman, Unutzer, and Bauer (2002)	Randomized trial evaluating a systematic program to improve quality and continuity of care for patients with bipolar disorder.	Multifaceted program including collaborative treatment plan, monthly telephone monitoring by a dedicated nurse manager, feedback of monitoring results, and algorithm-based medication recommendations to treating mental health professionals, as needed, outreach and care coordination, and a structured psychoeducational group program delivered by nurse case managers.	Population-based sample of patients with varying levels and subtypes of mood disorders.	***Continuous and Coordinated*** collaborative treatment plan to enhance communication and sharing of information about patients. Program with multifaceted intervention to enhance coordination of care and monthly telephone monitoring by dedicated nurse managers. Increased knowledge of and communication with patient.	Areas of improvement: acceptance of regular telephone monitoring, contact with nurse case manager, completion of Life Goals Program, and attendance at structured group sessions.

problem, its relationship to problems of care continuity, coordination, and comprehensiveness; and, further, what this means in terms of communication problems between not only providers and patients, but between providers.

According to the IOM report *Fostering rapid advances in health care: Learning from system demonstrations* (2002), the patient has the right and the provider the responsibility to ensure that patients receive safe, effective, patient-centered, timely, efficient, and equitable care. Major changes in health care delivery systems are ongoing. In addition to system changes, profound changes in the role of the patient are occurring with the idea that patients will be collaborative partners in the health care delivery system enterprise.

More research is needed to evaluate the effects of the organization and delivery of comprehensive, continuous, coordinated services on the health and utilization of services across a variety of patient populations and health care settings.

Systems of health care delivery refer to a commitment that institutions, organizations, and networks are mandated by the values and goals of the society and national health care policy. Systems of care include the organizations, processes, and methods by which health care is provided. Research is needed to create and evaluate models of care. Some models to improve the continuity and coordination of health care promise enhanced communication for both patient and provider. Still, these pilot projects have not been disseminated to a large degree and the full value to those receiving community-based care is yet not fully known. In response to the problem of health care services fragmentation, there are a series of important strategies afoot. These include PACT and PCMH. What differs most when comparing former systems of care to what is needed now is the new responsibilities for communication that are far more complex.

System reforms occur either top-down or bottom-up. This means that reform can begin at the provider and patient level (bottom-up) as well as the national policy level (top-down) and some patients might require different levels of care. It is important to heed the wisdom of writers such as Guthrie and Wyke (2000) summarizing the literature on continuity of care and quality care outcomes.

These authors warned that current attempts to reorganize care delivery systems with an emphasis on technology to promote the development of general practice might, for example, reduce continuity of care. If continuity is lost in the rush of adding new technologies (e.g., health information technology), it may be difficult to get back this important aspect of humanistic patient care. Coordinated, continuous, and comprehensive care is necessary to ensure high-quality outcomes. While few would argue with the need to enhance these aspects of patient care, providing and ensuring them might place considerable pressure on health care systems and communities.

An important area of future research is the question of whether these elements are needed for some but not equally for all patient populations. Along these same lines, for example, is continuity a clinical necessity or a patient preference or both? Reynolds et al. (2004) explain that such systems may be more beneficial to those whose social network is not strong, particularly if health providers are the main source of support for patients. The idea that continuity-enriched programs may be both more important for some and not all is an important question. In principle, the more clinically complex, the higher the likelihood that some continuity-enriched program is essential to achieve quality care and ensure patient safety.

In summary, how best to improve desired health outcomes by altering systems of care is still to be determined. Furthermore, how these changes will impact providers' needs for improved communication skills is to be explored and summarized in the professional literature.

Discussion

1. Describe the problem of fragmented health care services in the United States.
2. Identify ways in which fragmented care can impair communications between patients and providers.
3. Discuss how fragmented care can impair communications within and across health care settings.
4. Discuss the role of the 3Cs in improving both quality care and health care communications.
5. Describe one or more organizational strategies or programs that would be both feasible and effective in improving communications within and across health care settings.

Acknowledgment

This chapter utilizes with permission excerpts from van Servellen, G., Fongwa, M., & D'Errico, E. M. (2006). Continuity of care and quality care outcomes for people experiencing chronic conditions: A literature review. *Nursing and Health Sciences*, 8, 185–195. https://doi.org /10.1111/j.1442-2018.2006.00278.x

References

AHRQ. (2017). National Healthcare Quality & Disparities Reports. Agency for Healthcare Research and Quality, Rockville, MD. http://www.ahrq.gov/research/findings /nhqrdr/index.html

AHRQ. (2016a). *Care coordination, quality improvement: Structured Abstract. Closing the quality gap: A critical analysis of quality improvement strategies: Volume 7— Care Coordination.* Retrieved from ahrq.gov

AHRQ. (2016b). *Care coordination quality measure for primary care (CCQM-PC).* Survey for Primary Care Available at: Care Coordination Quality Measure for Primary Care (CCQM-PC): Formatting Guidance for Mail Surveys. Content last reviewed December 2017. Agency for Healthcare Research and Quality, Rockville, MD. http://www.ahrq.gov/professionals /prevention-chronic-care/improve/coordination /ccqmpc/formatting-guidance.html

Atienza, F., Anguita, M., Martinex-Alzamora, N., Osca, J., Ojeda, S., Almenar, L., ... PRICE Study Group. (2004). Multicenter randomized trial of a comprehensive hospital discharge and outpatient heart failure management program. *European Journal of Heart Failure, 6*(5), 643–652. doi:10.1016/j.ejheart.2003.11.023

Biem, H. J., Hadjustavropoulos, H. D., Morgan, D., Biem, D., & Pong, R. W. (2003). Breaks in continuity of care and the rural senior transferred for medical care under regionalization. *International Journal of Integrated Care, 3,* 1–16. PMID:16896374

Byng, R., Jones, R., Leese, M., Hamilton, B., McCrone, P., & Craig, T. (2004). Exploratory cluster randomized controlled trial of shared care development for long-term mental illness. *British Journal of General Practice, 54*(501), 259–266. PMID:15113492

Chen, L.-J., Chang, Y.-J., Shieh, C.-F., Yu, J.-H., & Yang, M.-C. (2016). Accessibility of ophthalmic healthcare for residents of an offshore island—An example of integrated delivery system. *BMC Health Services Research, 16,* 261. doi:10.1186/s12913-016-1501-8

Coleman, E. A., Mahoney, E., & Parry, C. (2005). Assessing the quality of preparation for posthospital care from the patient's perspective: The care transitions measure. *Medical Care, 43*(3), 246–255. PMID 15725981

Coleman, E. A., Parry, C., Chalmers, S., & Min, S. J. (2006). The care transition intervention: Results of a randomized controlled trial. *Archives of Internal Medicine, 166*(17), 1822–1828. doi:10.1001/archinte.166.17.1822

Coleman, E. A., Smith, J. D., Frank, J. C., Ellertsen, T. B., Thiare, J. N., & Kramer, A. M. (2002, April–June). Development and testing of a measure designed to assess the quality of care transitions. *International Journal of Integrated Care, 2,* e02. PMID:16896392

Crotty, M., Rowett, D., Spurling, L., Giles, L. C., & Philips, P. A. (2004). Does the addition of a pharmacist transition coordinator improve evidence-based medication management and health outcomes in older adults moving from the hospital to a long-term care facility? Results of a randomized, controlled trial. *American Journal of Geriatric Pharmacotherapy, 2*(4), 257–264. doi.org/10.1016/j.amjopharm.2005.01.001

Enthoven, A. C. (2009). Integrated delivery systems: The cure for fragmentation. *American Journal of Managed Care, 15,* S284–S290. Retrieved from www.ajmc.com

Fineberg, H. V. (2012). A successful and sustainable health system—How to get there from here. *The New England Journal of Medicine, 366*(11), 1020–1027. doi:10.1056 /NEJMsa1114777

Fjaertoft, H., Indredavik, B., Johnsen, R., & Lydersen S. (2004). Acute stroke unit care combined with early supported discharge. Long-term effects on quality of life. A randomized controlled trial. *Clinical Rehabilitation, 18*(5), 580–586. doi:10.1191/0269215504cr773oa

Gill, J. M., Mainous, A. G., Diamond, J. J., & Lentard, M. J. (2003). Impact of provider continuity on quality of care for persons with diabetes mellitus. *Annals of Family Medicine, 1*, 162–170. doi:10.1370/afm.22

Goodwin, N. (2016). Understanding integrated care. *International Journal of Integrated Care, 16*(4), 6. doi:10.5334/ijic.2530

Guthrie, B., & Wyke, S. (2000). Does continuity in general practice really matter? *British Medical Journal, 321*, 734–736. doi:10.1136/bmj.321.7263.734

Haggerty, J. L., Reid, R. J., Freeman, G. K., Starfield, B. H., Adair, C. E., & McKendry, R. (2003). Continuity of care: A multidisciplinary review. *British Medical Journal, 327*, 1219–1221. doi:10.1136/bmj.327.7425.1219

Herrel, L. A., Kaufman, S. R., Yan, P., Miller, D. C., Schroeck, F. R., Shahinian, V. B., & Hollenbeck, B. K. (2017). Health care integration and quality among men with prostate cancer. *The Journal of Urology, 197*(1), 55–60. doi:10.1016/j.juro.2016.07.040

Hwang, W., Chang, J., LaClair M., & Paz, H. (2013). Effects of integrated delivery system on cost and quality. *American Journal of Managed Care, 19*(5), e175–e184. Retrieved from www.ajmc.com

Institute of Medicine. (2001). *Crossing the quality chasm: A new health system for the 21st century.* Washington, DC: The National Academies Press. doi:10.17226/10027

Institute of Medicine. (2002). Committee on rapid advance demonstration projects: Health care finance and delivery systems. In J. M. Corrigan, A. Greiner, & S. M. Erickson (Eds.), *Fostering rapid advances in health care: Learning from system demonstrations.* Retrieved from www.nap.edu

Kibbe, D. C., Phillips, R. L., & Green, L. A. (2004). The continuity of care record. *American Family Physician, 70*, 1220–1223. PMID:15508532

Koopman, R. J., Mainous, A. G., Baker, R., Gill, J. M., & Gilbert, G. E. Continuity of care and recognition of diabetes, hypertension, and *hypercholesterolemia. Archives of Internal Medicine, 163*(11), 1357–1361. doi:10.1001/archinte.163.11.1357

Kristjansson, E., Hogg, W., Dahrouge, S., Tuna, M., Mayo-Bruinsma, L., & Gebremichael, G. (2013). Predictors of relational continuity in primary care: Patient, provider and practice factors. *BMC Family Practice, 14*, 72. doi:10.1186/1471-2296-14-72

Maruthappu, M., Hasan, A., & Zeltner, T. (2015) Enablers and barriers in implementing integrated care. *Health Systems & Reform, 1*(4), 250–256. doi:10.1080/23288604.2015.1077301

McKay, J. R., Lynch, K. G., Shepard, D. S., & Pettinati, H. M. (2005). The effectiveness of telephone-based continuing care for alcohol and cocaine dependence: 24-month outcomes. *Archives of General Psychiatry, 62*(2), 199–207. doi:10.1001/archpsyc.62.2.199

Naylor, M. D., Brooten, D. A., Cambell, R. L., Maislin, G., McCaulety, K. M., & Schwartz, J. S. (2004). Transitional care of older adults hospitalized with heart failure: A randomized, controlled trial. *Journal of the American Geriatric Society, 52*(5), 675–684. Erratum in: *Journal of the American Geriatric Society* 2004, *52*(7), 1228.

Neilsen, J. D., Palshof, T., Mainz, J., Jensen, A. B., & Olesen, F. (2003). Randomised controlled trial of a shared care programme for newly referred cancer patients: Bridging the gap between general medical practice and hospital. *Quality and Safe Health Care, 12*(4), 263–272. Retrieved from www. qshc.com

Parchman, M. L., & Burge, S. K. (2002). Residency research network of South Texas investigators. Continuity and quality of care in type 2 diabetes: A residency research network of South Texas study. *Journal of Family Practice, 51*(7), 619–624. PMID:11802086

Parchman, M. L., & Burge, S. K. (2003). The patient-physician relationship, primary care attributes, and preventive services. *Family Medicine, 36*(1), 22–27. PMID:14710325

Preen, D. B., Bailey, B. E., Wright, A., Kendall, P., Phillips, M., Hung, J., … Williams, E. (2005). Effects of a multidisciplinary, post-discharge continuance of care intervention on quality of life, discharge satisfaction, and hospital length of stay: A randomized controlled trial. *International Journal for Quality in Health Care, 17*(1), 43–51. doi:10.1093/intqhc/mzi002

Reynolds, W., Lauder, W., Sharkey, S., Maciver, S., Veitch, T., & Cameron, D. (2004). The effects of a transitional discharge model for psychiatric patients. *Journal of Psychiatric Mental Health Nursing, 11*, 82–88. PMID:14723643

Rodriguez, H. P., Giannitrapani, K. F., Stockdale, S., Hamilton, A. B., Yano, E. M., & Rubenstein, L. V. (2014). Teamlet structure and early experiences of medical home implementation for Veterans. *Journal of General Internal Medicine, 29*(Suppl 2), 623–631. doi:10.1007/s11606-013-2680-1

Samet, J. H., Larson, M. J., Horton, N. J., Doyle, K., Winter, M., & Saitz, R. (2003). Linking alcohol-and-drug dependent adults to primary medical care: A randomized controlled trial of a multi-disciplinary health intervention in a detoxification unit. *Addiction, 98*, 509–551. PMID:12653820

Saultz, J. W. (2003). Defining and measuring interpersonal continuity of care. *Annals of Family Medicine, 1*, 134–143. doi:org/10.1370/afm.23

Saultz, J. W., & Albedaiwi, W. (2004). Interpersonal continuity of care and patient satisfaction. *Annals of Family Medicine, 2*, 445–451. doi:10.1370/afm.91

Saultz, J. W., & Lochner, J. (2005). Interpersonal continuity of care and care outcomes: A critical review. *Annals of Family Medicine, 3*(2), 159–166. doi:10.1370/afm.285

Schoen, C., Osborn, R., Doty, M. M., Bishop, M., Peugh, J., & Murukutla, N. (2007). Toward higher-performance health systems: Adults' health care experiences in seven countries. *Health Affairs, 26*(6), w717–w734. doi:10.1377/hlthaff.26.6.w717

Schoen, C., Osborn, R., Trang Huynh, P., Doty, M., Zapert, K., Peugh, J., & Davis, K. (2005). Taking the pulse of health care systems: Experiences of patients with health problems in six countries. *Health Affairs.* Published online. doi:10.1377/hlthaff.w5.509

Simon, G. E., Ludman, E., Unutzer, J., & Bauer, M. S. (2002). Design and implementation of a randomized trial evaluating systematic care for bipolar disorders. *Bipolar Disorders, 4*(4), 226–236. doi:10.1034/j.1399-5618.2002.01190.x

Tuepker, A., Kansagara, D., Skaperdas, E., Nicolaidis, C., Joos, S., Alperin, M., & Hickam, D. (2014). "We've not gotten even close to what we want to do": A qualitative study of early patient-centered medical home implementation. *Journal of General Internal Medicine, 29*(Suppl2), 614–622. doi:10.1007/s11606-013-2690-z

van Eaton, E. G., Horvath, K. D., Lober, W. B., Rossini, A. J., & Pellegrini, C. A. (2005). A randomized, controlled trial evaluating the impact of a computerized rounding and sign-out system on continuity of care and resident work hours. *Journal of the American College of Surgeons, 200*(4), 538–545. doi:10.1016/j.jamcollsurg.2004.11.009

WHO. (2000). *Health systems.* Retrieved from www.who.int/topics/health_systems/en/

Wright, L. K., Litaker, M., Laraia, M. T., & DeAndrade, S. (2001). Continuum of care for Alzheimer's disease: A nurse education and counseling program. *Issues in Mental Health Nursing, 22*(3), 231–252. doi:10.1080/01612840117980

Yano, E. M., Bair, M. J., Carrasquillo, O., Krein, S. L., & Rubenstein, L. V. (2014). Patient aligned care teams (PACT): VA's journey to implement patient-centered medical homes. *Journal of General Internal Medicine, 29*(Suppl 2), 547. doi:10.1007/s11606-0142835-8

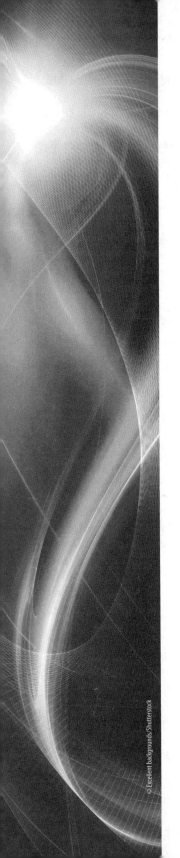

PART VIII

Evidence Supports the Importance of Effective Communications

In this final section of the text, several interventions and programs impacting health care communications are discussed. These interventions and programs aim not only to improve communications but also health care services and health outcomes. Each chapter addresses an intervention or program and the implications for promoting effective communications between health providers, health systems, and the people they serve. These interventions and programs have been evaluated, and the results of these evaluations are published in the peer review journals cited in these chapters.

For the purposes of this review, strategies are isolated and discussed for their potential impact on health care concerns. In truth, health care outcomes are a product of multiple strategies and interventions working together to meet the needs of patients and families. Many are directed at improving access to care while others address one or more barriers in disease management that are struggles for both patients and providers.

In Chapter 26, "Bringing Health Care Provider Communication to the Patient, Not Patient to Provider," the potential benefit of home visit programs for underserved at-risk prenatal women are discussed. Home visit programs can bring health care services and health promotion closer to the patient and family while respecting patients' perspectives of their needs and goals. They can promote continuous patient–provider alliances throughout the course of pregnancy and thereafter. These alliances facilitate ongoing assessments of patients and build trusting relationships that provide education and support. There is evidence that home visitation (HV) programs are linked to improvements in birth outcomes (e.g., fewer low birth weight newborns and fewer preterm births). This chapter discusses the evidence and corresponding limitations to generalizing study findings.

In Chapter 27, "Communications to Promote Behavior Change," the role of motivational interviewing (MI) in health promotion and treatment programs is discussed. MI was originally developed for use with patients impacted by addictions, particularly alcohol and drug abuse. Since its introduction, MI counseling and therapy have been used with a variety of conditions and populations. Typically, MI approaches are delivered in individual counseling sessions with a trained provider. However, there is some evidence that MI principles have shaped the scope and content of group counseling approaches. MI studies document how these programs may out-perform more traditional approaches.

MI, either extended or brief approaches, have been used in health promotion programs in primary care and public health outreach efforts to, for example, encourage weight loss, exercise, and healthy eating as well as alcohol intake. In this chapter, we discuss the application of MI approaches to the management of patients with diabetes. Patients with diabetes have multiple lifestyle behaviors to manage in order to achieve their highest level of wellness. These include glucose control, medication adherence, general dietary adjustments, weight control, and exercise. There is evidence that the use of MI principles and communication approaches may improve disease self-management and health outcomes with these patients.

In Chapter 28, "Collaborative Care to Promote Treatment Adherence and Effective Mental Health Care," the challenges of ensuring effective mental health care are discussed. Treatment adherence is a critical element of mental health care and particularly mental health medication adherence. Lack of adherence can undermine the efficacy of our many medications that are able to curb symptoms of

depression, anxiety, and other mental health conditions.

This chapter addresses the important concept of collaborative care as it applies to treatment in general and mental health services in particular. Collaborative care models impact communications in at least two important ways: linking mental health specialists with primary care health care providers and providing patient access to mental health specialist care. Depressive disorders are common worldwide and it is clear that any one intervention is not going to be adequate. However, collaborative care in treating mental health conditions, particularly depression, is important because it aligns mental health specialists with primary care practitioners. Most people with depression are first, and maybe only, seen in primary care settings. For a variety of reasons, primary care settings are not able to fully assess and/or manage depression.

Collaborative care models have been adapted to a wide range of mental health conditions including depressive and anxiety disorders. This chapter discusses examples of research that document the positive impact of collaborative care on the treatment of depression in primary care settings. Future directions for providing collaborative care depression care to underserved populations are raised.

Finally, Chapter 29, "Communications for Advance Care Planning," the topic shifts to a discussion of evidence supporting the importance of effective communications in advance care planning. This final chapter serves as a capstone to the series of chapters addressing evidence to support the importance of effective communications in various stages of illness and disease self-management.

There are many instances in which compassionate communication is appropriate and necessary in assisting patients and their families, and this chapter presents arguably one of the most important cases where effective communications are needed. In this chapter advance care planning and end-of-life care decision-making are discussed in detail. Uncomfortable emotions often felt at this time in the care process, although natural and expected, are eased when health care providers can engage patients and their families in compassionate ways. Sensitivity to cultural diversity is critical because some religious and cultural beliefs may counter the standards of care outlined in clinical practice guidelines and policies. For example, some patients and families may react very differently to basic needs for information and shared decision-making.

This chapter covers the wide range of concepts frequently addressed in discussions of advance care planning but also targets specifically the role of various barriers to effective communications. One important barrier is decisional conflict. The challenge of decisional conflict is addressed, and various strategies to minimize this barrier are described. It should be noted that some ethnic and cultural groups, rather than being at the center of decision-making, would prefer family members to make treatment decisions, rather than patients themselves.

The topic of evidence-based studies in this chapter is the use of decisional aids in easing the process of advance care planning. Evidence has shown that decisional aids can provide structure to uncomfortable discussions, increase patient knowledge and readiness to participate in shared decision-making, and in some instances, can minimize decisional conflict. Future directions for establishing the feasibility, acceptability, and efficacy of decisional aids are discussed.

In summary, in this series of four chapters there are examples of health care intervention where various phases of care and treatment are addressed from the perspective of early prevention to secure quality birth outcomes by implementing HV programs to promoting effective communications in advance care

planning by using decisional aids to guide the discussions of patients, families, and health care providers.

While the evidence for each of the several interventions discussed (e.g., HV programs, motivational interviewing, collaborative care, and decisional aids in advance care planning) have shown to result in positive outcomes for patients, families, and even health care providers, it is important to keep in mind that studies to date have been conducted with selected populations, and results are not easily generalized to other groups, communities, or populations.

The studies and reports discussed are published in peer-reviewed journals. It is recommended that these studies and reports are read in full to understand their scope and methodology. The generalizability of positive outcomes from these published studies, at least in part, are limited to the populations studied, the methods chosen to measure outcomes, and the specific elements of the programs, some of which are not sufficiently detailed. This is not a reason to minimize the value of these interventions or programs or their reported outcomes; it is however a reason to apply the findings cautiously.

With this in mind, read and discuss these chapters using critical thinking as one should in reading the results of any published research study. In this series of chapters there are several new additions to support your learning and comprehension of the content. These include boxed "Cited Studies" (examples of evidence-based evaluations), "Evidence for/ More to Know" boxes which synthesize the findings of the studies discussed and the various *take-home* points, and "Must-Read" boxes which summarize important, sometimes landmark, reports on the topic of the chapter. These additions should not only ease understanding of chapter content but also guide important discussions of chapter subject matter.

CHAPTER 26

Bringing Health Care Provider Communication to the Patient, Not Patient to Provider

CHAPTER OBJECTIVES

- Identify key barriers to communication for underserved patient populations.
- Discuss the home visit by paraprofessionals approach to enhance underserved communities access to health care communications.
- Identify potential benefits and drawbacks of home visit paraprofessional approaches.
- Analyze the results of an evidence-based evaluation of a home visit paraprofessional approach.
- Discuss the results of two or more evidence-based evaluations to examine the support for this approach to improving provider communications with underserved populations.

KEY TERMS

- Disparities in health care access
- Health promotion programs
- Home visitation (HV) programs
- Paraprofessional health care providers
- Perinatal health care outcomes

▶ Introduction

As stressed throughout this text, effective communications between patients and health professionals are the foundation for quality patient care. Effective communications refer not only to the exchange of information but the process of connecting patient and family with provider on a deeper level. Patients and their families can fail to secure quality communication in their contacts with health providers for many reasons.

Accessibility of providers and limitations (on time and opportunity) significantly impact verbal exchanges between patients and providers. And, potential barriers can be unevenly distributed across communities and populations. Underserved communities are at risk for poor access to health care provider communications.

A pervasive concern and the direction of public health care programs target underserved groups and communities that are known to experience health care disparities and have shown to need further assistance in using and navigating the complex and confusing health care system. These populations tend to be poor and less educated, and frequently mistrust or lack knowledge of medical services. In some cases, as in American Indian and Native American groups, a long and ongoing history of marginalization and cultural dislocation contributes to their health disparities and unequal access to care. A major question is to what degree are these communities deprived of communications that would otherwise enhance the quality of their health care and eliminate health disparities.

▶ Underserved Communities and Their Risk for Poor Access to Effective Communications

There are many reasons why underserved communities are at risk for poor access to needed provider communications. Research on health disparities indicate that these factors overlap: gender, race and ethnicity, existing language barriers, lower education and poor health literacy, low income, geographical inaccessibility, lack of cultural familiarity, and legal and regulatory policies that deter or facilitate access to health care professionals and health care services.

All of these factors are associated with disparities in health care and health outcomes. Additionally, to add to the complexity of multiple patient and family, provider, and system-level factors is the consequence that poor access to health care providers may contribute to any previous lack of trust in and motivation to seek out advice from health and medical professionals. All in all, the issue of poor patient–provider communications is a conundrum reflecting an intricate and difficult problem which continues to challenge national health care policy. Bringing health care communications to the patient, not the patient to health providers is an approach that seems to offer significant promise and is the topic of this chapter.

The Institute of Medicine's landmark report, *The chasm in quality: A new health system for the 21st century* (2001) informs that quality of care is

> The degree to which health services for individuals and populations increase the likelihood of desired health outcomes and are consistent with current professional knowledge.

Since this landmark report, a number of quality care reports followed to identify the scope of the problem and what policies are warranted to alleviate quality care deficiencies. As information accumulated it became clear that gaps in the provision of quality care was a result of multiple factors that could be categorized as the health care system; the structure of health care services; the processes of care, including provider–patient relationship; and individual patient characteristics.

Among several important documents describing the gap in quality care was several illuminating accounts of the **disparities in health care access** and quality across populations and communities. Select indicators from recent reports, particularly *The National Healthcare Disparities Report, 2008* (AHRQ, 2009), summarized the evidence about persisting disparities in health care quality and access to care. The report identified various improvements in eliminating disparities but also areas where disparities have remained the same or worsened. For example, it was stated that for African Americans, large disparities remain in new AIDS cases and hospitalizations for lower extremity amputations in patients with diabetes.

Lack of prenatal care for pregnant women in the third trimester was also an area of distinguishable disparities. Indigenous peoples, particularly American Indian and Alaskan Native women, experience significant disparities in prenatal care. Disparities in access can mean that for some groups all those factors impacting access (gender, race and ethnicity, existing language barriers, lower education and poor health literacy, low income, geographical inaccessibility, lack of cultural acceptance, and legal and regulatory policies) disproportionately impact these groups. In this chapter we examine the potential impact of **home visitation (HV) programs**, particularly prenatal programs in hard to reach populations, and the literature reporting on the impact of home visits on **perinatal health care outcomes**. Persistent disparities to at-risk women and children have remained a concern among health care policy makers.

▶ Structure of Patient–Primary Care Provider Visits Influence Quality Communications

The extent to which adequate face-to-face contact with health professionals influences effective communications has been repeatedly addressed. The issue of having enough time with the provider is particularly important in the context of the patient and primary care (PC) provider because this relationship is pivotal to future treatment including effective

health promotion, disease assessment, and referral to specialists if needed.

It is generally believed that a certain amount of face-to-face contact is needed to build a trusting patient–family–provider alliance, conduct in-depth clinical assessments, and explain and reinforce health care plans. It is also known that health messages and interventions are more successful when representatives of the community or specific population are engaged in planning, conducting, and evaluating these programs.

The key question is how much face-to-face contact and by whom is needed to ensure quality care, and how does this amount vary by patient, patient's condition, stage of the patient–provider relationship, and system constraints (e.g., insurance reimbursement guidelines)? In a recent *USA Today* expose, the topic of doctors rushing patients through visits was described. An example of a patient visiting an ear, nose, and throat specialist revealed that the physician was not in the exam room with her for more than 3 or 4 minutes. Further, the patient relates that when she started protesting the doctor's choice of medication, he cut her off. She stated that she had never been in and out from a visit faster.

This article goes on to explain that it is not unusual for PC visits to be scheduled at 15-minute intervals with some hospitals asking providers to see patients every 11 minutes. The article summarizes the fall-out: short visits take a toll on the doctor–patient relationship increasing the probability that the patient will leave the office frustrated. These experiences are clearly not what many poor and underserved populations are looking for even if they could access these inadequate encounters.

Typically, under usual circumstances we might address the issue of how much time is needed from the perspective of what groups use services. Time allotted to an office visit and to any one topic discussed varies. It is usually believed that an indicator of face-to-face encounter time is best understood in relationship to the topic of discussion. For example,

Tai-Seale, McGuire, and Zhang (2007) stated that it is not unusual for PC patient office visits to be very brief. They videotaped visits of elderly patients with their PC providers in multiple PC practices and reported that the visits could last from 1.1–5 minutes in length depending upon the topics discussed.

They reported that the median office visit was 15.7 minutes covering a median of 6 topics. Furthermore, the longest topic discussed lasted 5 minutes and the remaining topics lasted 1.1 minutes. These investigators also wanted to identify the factors that seemed to influence time allocations and supplemented this data with patient and physician survey reports. They concluded that many factors impact visit length including both patient and provider time pressure as well as financial incentives that may limit the time spent.

The majority of the topics discussed pertained to biomedical issues while other topics included mental health (2.9%), personal lifestyle and habits (7%), psychosocial matters (12%), discussions about the patient–physician relationship (3%), and small talk (4%). It is unknown how the disease and health status of the patients seen, the presence or absence of a family caregiver, and the duration of the patient–provider relationship has made a difference in time spent. These authors concluded that they could not help to wonder how much is accomplished during these brief exchanges. Future research should assess whether these encounters did or did not facilitate effective information exchange and patient-centered care.

"Patient-centered" is a clinical philosophy that stresses partnership with the patient, careful attention to relational processes, and shared decision-making. Along these lines, the time spent is, in itself, not the most important element. What occurs during the visit to strengthen the patient–provider relationship is critical and may be just as important or more important than time spent.

Supporting this idea is a study by Parrish et al. (2016) who conducted surveys of patients

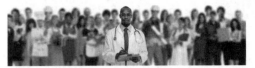

© Kurhan/Shutterstock

after a single new patient office visit with a hand surgeon. These investigators found that patient satisfaction was not associated with perceived visit duration but did correlate strongly with the surgeon's level of empathy. Addressing an issue long debated, the authors concluded that for these patients, patient-centeredness should be the focus and not necessarily making such visits longer.

When we shift to a consideration of what works best with poor, underserved communities and populations, the perspective needs to change based upon the assumption that many of these persons may not have access to or not use typical medical office visits.

Traditional methods of organization of health care services does not adequately reflect the perceived needs, realities of competing responsibilities, potential mistrust of traditional medical care services, and any barriers these communities face when physically accessing health care services. The following section of the chapter discusses the concept of bringing provider to patient versus patient to provider.

▶ Bringing Provider to Patient Meets Criteria for Quality Care and Health Promotion

As pointed out, the classic approach to the delivery of PC is an office visit. Not all persons have access to PC providers or services, and for some these services and the way they are organized do not meet the needs of various communities. Typically, these services would not be viewed as relevant or respectful of the life circumstances of underserved communities. The following discussion addresses home visitation as a key **health promotion programs** and an option to enhance quality care among hard to reach and underserved perinatal mothers and newborns.

The Patient Protection and Affordable Care Act established a Maternal, Infant, and Early Childhood Home Visiting Program initiative funded at the level of $1.5 billion over a 5-year period to states to establish home visiting programs for at-risk pregnant women and children from birth to age 5.

Furthermore, the Act requires that 75% of the funds distributed must be spent in home visiting programs with evidence of effectiveness based on sound research methods. Home Visiting Evidence of Effectiveness (HomVEE) was put into effect to conduct a thorough review of effectiveness literature.

According to Avellar and Supplee (2013), as of July 2012, 32 home visit program models were reviewed of which 12 met Department of Health and Human Services (DHHS) criteria, and most were shown to produce favorable effects on child development, health care usage, and reductions in child mistreatment. Less often found were favorable birth outcomes. In a later publication (2014), these

researchers reported on the effectiveness of 17 home visiting models that meet DHHS criteria for evidence-based early childhood home services delivery model. **EXHIBIT 26-1** contains a partial list of the 17 programs discussed.

The Scope and Focus of HV Programs

It should be noted that the scope and focus of HV programs is varied and dependent upon the mission of the private or public program funding and administering the program. HV programs are offered across all age groups (e.g., there are multiple programs aimed at improving the health and independency of older people). There are HV programs designed specifically for patients and families with dementia or Alzheimer's disease. However, in this chapter, we focus on maternal child HV programs, particularly those offering prenatal care and follow-up. There are a number of HV programs to decrease rates of preterm birth in young women, and specifically for at-risk vulnerable youth.

Considerable funds are awarded to HV programs to launch positive health outcomes in maternal and child health. The Federal Home Visiting Program is designed to give pregnant women and families, particularly those considered at risk, necessary resources and skills to raise children who are physically, socially, and emotionally healthy and ready to learn (mchb.hrsa.gov).

The goals of the program are (1) improve maternal and child health, (2) prevent child abuse and neglect, (3) encourage positive parenting, and (4) promote child development and school readiness. By participating in one of the local HV programs, families receive help from health, social service, and child developmental professionals. HV programs may include a number of different services including support for preventive health and prenatal services. Along these lines, evidence of program success is improvement in maternal and newborn health.

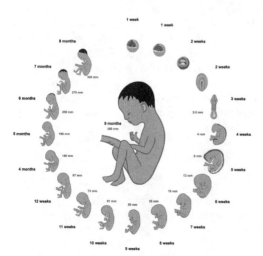

© Udaix/Shutterstock.

EXHIBIT 26-1 Selected HomVEE Identified Home Visiting Models Meeting DHHS Criteria

(1) Child FIRST, (2) Durham Connects/Family Connects, (3) Early Head Start-Home Visiting, (4) Early Intervention Program (EIP) for Adolescent Mothers, (5) Early Start (New Zealand), (6) Family Check-Up®, (7) Family Spirit®, (8) Healthy Families America® (HFA), (9) Healthy Steps, and (10) Home Instruction for Parents of Preschool Youngsters® (HIPPY).

These authors concluded that evidence indicated positive outcomes but gaps in the research were identified. These gaps were evidence of program effectiveness and needs of different types of families with a wide range of characteristics (e.g., immigrant families that have diverse cultural backgrounds or may not speak English as a first language or military families). More needs to be known about communities who are known not to access traditional medical services.

The following programs are in place, and more needs to be known about the outcomes of these projects. Those programs dealing with the needs of communities at risk (e.g., American Indian families) include Baby FACE (American Indian families with children from birth to age 3 and some sites to 5); Even Start-Tribal Program (families have other risk factors [e.g., chronic unemployment, low income, low adult literacy, and single or teen parent]), and Family Spirit focusing on pregnant Indian adolescents aged 12–19 at conception and at 28 weeks' or earlier gestation (Del Grosso, Kleinman, Esposito, Sama Martin, & Paulsell, 2011). Programs focusing on the needs of Hispanic families include Nurturing Parenting Programs (NPPs) and their offshoots (e.g., NPP for prenatal families; NPP for parents, infants, toddler, and preschoolers; and NPP for teen parents and their children).

Beyond the criteria set forth by HomVEE, additional direction for quality prenatal HV programs come from policies about the provision of quality care to at-risk populations. Important criteria directly impacting the topic of this chapter are: (1) access to health care must be available at all times, (2) care should be based on continuous healing relationships, (3) care should be customized to meet patient needs and values, and (4) the patient should be the source of control. A number of criteria are outlined in the original report entitled *Crossing the quality chasm: A new health system for the 21st century* (previously discussed in Chapters 2 and 3).

Furthermore, cooperation across health care professionals is a priority. Bringing health care communications to the patient, not the patient to the health provider, discussed in this chapter, demonstrates the importance of this approach to the goals of achieving quality health care.

While not designed to meet only the criteria listed, HV programs can significantly address these objectives. The organization and implementation is different from traditional health service delivery (e.g., the hospital, clinic, and medical office approach). HV programs are mechanisms to extend disease prevention and health promotion beyond the walls of the traditional health care service system.

According to the Council on Child and Adolescent Health, HV programs date back as far as the late 1800s in the United States when public health nurses and social workers provided in-home education and health care to women and their children, primarily in poor urban areas. While HV programs do not always provide medical care, they are often linked to private or public clinics and medical centers and provide some level of direct or indirect connection with these established public or private health care centers or clinics. HV programs are usually affiliated with community programs such as those associated with private or public schools and community service agencies.

HV programs address criteria set forth by Crossing the Quality Chasm report. *Access to health care must be available at all times* is bridged by the activities of HV programs. Furthermore, access to traditional health care services is eased by links to traditional treatment centers. *Care based on continuous healing relationships* is fostered by continuous relationships of patients and families with professional or paraprofessional health providers. Many of these programs serve clients for extended time periods. In the case of pregnant women, the entire pregnancy period including 3 months following a live birth serves to define the continuity of the relationship in HV programs. In selected instances, the program extends to future pregnancies.

Care customized to meet patient needs and values is achieved in unique ways by virtue of the fact that interaction occurs in the patient's home rather than a medical office which can be geographically distant. *The patient is the source of control* is an important criterion. Through HV programs based in the home, control over the time, duration, and even topics discussed become decidedly patient-centered versus institutional-focused.

It should be noted that any program's ability to address the quality care criterion is not only dependent upon the structure or delivery of the program, it is also contingent on the program elements and the skill and knowledge of the professionals and paraprofessionals and any supervising licensed health professionals guiding the delivery and outcomes of the program.

▶ Prenatal HV Programs and Improvement in Prenatal Care and Birth Outcomes

An important focus of HV programs is prenatal health care and corresponding improvements in birth outcomes in particular. The immediate and longer-term effects of negative birth outcomes of preterm birth and low birth weight are significant and were addressed in depth by the National Healthy Start Association (NHSA).

In the area of HV programs aimed at improving infant, child, and adolescent health, one can find an extensive list of prior or current HV programs. This list includes programs aimed at promoting birth health outcomes in at-risk first-time pregnant women: ChildFirst, Health Access Nurturing Development Services (HANDS), and Medicaid Obstetrical and Maternal Services (MOMS) programs. In most cases, mothers can go online to read about the program and find out if they are eligible.

Finello, Terteryan, and Riewerts (2015) summarize the dilemmas facing PC physicians who see a growing number of complexities in prenatal families. They explain that the majority of PC clinicians are practicing with limited training and a shortage of resources to support these families. Partnerships with evidence-based HV programs should be promoted to reduce the effect of early health inequities. Being nonresponsive to risks for poor birth outcomes is very serious.

Preterm births or low birth weight births, for example, are associated with increased risk for adverse developmental consequences including cognitive and neurologic impairments, behavioral and emotional problems, and attention-deficit/hyperactivity disorders. Many of these adverse problems can remain throughout the child's lifetime impacting their future development.

HV programs are offered throughout the United States and are typically voluntary which means that mothers are asked to participate; they are not required to participate. This participation, depending on the focus of the program, can extend up to 2–3 years. The programs offer education and support and are designed to be preventative in nature. They are found to be linked to various private or public community outreach centers, and evidence of their effectiveness in promoting positive outcomes can be found in the literature.

What makes these HV programs effective is best understood in the range of choices made available to mothers, particularly for mothers at risk for health disparities. Guo et al. (2017) explain that there are three different delivery approaches in the care of expectant mothers at risk for health disparities. First, there is the traditional approach which consists of the pregnant woman seeking care from a medical provider or medical provider group at the provider's office. Second, there are prenatal group education and support groups. In these groups, 8–12 women meet with an obstetric health provider to discuss their prenatal concerns and get support with their health and pregnancy assessments and education needs. These groups can meet for approximately up to 2 hours every 4 weeks and do so over the entire course of the pregnancy. These meetings are typically held in a clinic or hospital setting to accommodate the schedule of the professional health provider. The third option is the prenatal HV approach. This approach also offers health assessments, prenatal education, and support but most often from registered nurses or social workers. Additionally, **paraprofessionals health care providers** which are unlicensed, paid, or volunteer community health workers may be involved in conducting home visits. Guo et al. stressed that the HV approach is more beneficial because it provides timely intervention and continuous prenatal and in some cases postnatal care as well. The HV option can be particularly useful for isolated or disadvantaged families who lack accessibility to distant clinics and medical centers.

It is customary for HV programs to assess and respond to families with a predisposition for negative birth outcomes. Beyond this, there can be a great deal of variability in program format. Some HV programs meet the criteria established by the DHHS for an evidence-based early childhood home visiting service delivery model; however, others may not. Some target first-time parents, others do not. Generally, mothers join at the time of pregnancy, but some programs accept mothers and children as long as the child is under 3 months old (HANDS).

Most programs offer families education, support, and referrals as needed during pregnancy and early infancy. Some programs extend home visiting services before, during, and after pregnancy for up to 2 years (HANDS); others, to the infant's first birthday (MOMS). All programs aim to achieve healthy outcomes for both the mother and child though their focus may vary. For example, the HANDS and MOMS programs focus specifically on education and support to at-risk mothers with the aim to improve birth outcomes (infant birth weights and full-term deliveries). Preference is given to the enrollment of mothers who demonstrate multiple risk factors (e.g., single-parent status and low income).

Some programs recruit families coping with substance abuse and domestic violence (HANDS) and offer interventions addressing special issues. For example, HANDS offers a 15-session treatment called in-home cognitive behavioral therapy (IH-CBT). This program is conducted by a licensed therapist who travels to the mother's home to facilitate the sessions. A trained paraprofessional or professional home visitor, such as a social worker, conducts prenatal and postnatal home visits with parents; provides parenting information, problem-solving techniques, and parenting skill development; and addresses basic needs.

Some programs recruit women who are first-time mothers and extend well into the postpregnancy period (HANDS) while others terminate services at the child's first birthday (MOMS). Some programs employ paraprofessional home visitors supervised by licensed RNs (MOMS) while others use licensed registered nurses or social workers as home visitors or trained paraprofessional and professional home visitors. This work is supplemented with special program specialists (e.g., mental health professional conducting IH-CBT [HANDS]).

In a thoughtful landmark study of the usefulness of HV programs at the time, Sweet and Applebaum (2004) examined the efficacy of 60 programs described in their extensive review of the literature using a comprehensive meta-analytic approach to quantify the usefulness of HVs as a strategy for families across a range of child and parent outcomes. Only HV programs conducted and reported after 1965 were reviewed due to some significant shifts in focus of these programs from primarily health and safety to more multifaceted programs addressing a variety of growth and development and mental health support. The researchers reported that the two most frequently reported goals were parent education and child development.

Parent education goals included improvement of parenting skills and parent–child interaction. While programs were alike in their primary emphasis, there were some differences in such activities as in direct provision of health care; parent social support; and strategies to prevent child abuse and empowering interventions. In this chapter, we summarize what is known and what more needs to be known. Using reported study results, we provide a brief and cursory summary in the "Evidence for/More to Know Box."

🔎 26-1 CITED STUDY: More Visits, More Communication, and Better Care Outcomes

Home visitation (HV) approaches are employed to improve maternal-child health care delivery and management, particularly for families at high-risk for poor birth outcomes. Profound disparities in these outcomes have been reported and targeted in these populations. Negative health outcomes include high rates of preterm births and low birth weights.

Goyal, N. K., Hall, E. S., Meinzen-Derr, J. K., Kahn, R. S., Short, J. A., Van Ginkel, J. B., & Ammerman, R. T. (2013). Dosage effect of prenatal home visiting on pregnancy outcomes in at-risk, first-time mothers. *Pediatrics, 132*(Suppl 2), S118–S125. doi:10.1542/peds.2013-1021J

In this study by Goyal et al. (2013), the many factors that work together to result in high preterm birth rates are acknowledged but the investigators assert that HV programs providing education, training and support may make significant differences in the management of pregnancy outcomes in at-risk communities.

These researchers investigate the important component of what they refer to as "dosage." *Dosage* means the duration of patients' enrollment and intensity of participation. They stress that many of the modifiable lifestyle factors (e.g., nutrition, physical, and mental health can be amenable to change if exposure to the HV program is early and of sufficient intensity).

The aim of their study was to examine the impact of number of prenatal visits in the first and second trimesters on the likelihood of a preterm birth. They conducted a retrospective cohort study of first-time mothers in southwest Ohio enrolled in home visiting before 26 weeks of gestation.

These women (*n* = 441) had participated in a large community-based home visiting program managed by Cincinnati Children's Hospital Medical Center, Every Child Succeeds (ECS). Data was derived from state (Ohio) vital statistics available from the State Department of Health, and birth-related hospital discharge of both mothers and infants available from the Ohio Hospital Association for the period 2007–2010.

Findings from this study revealed that there was a statistically significant relationship between total number of home visits and birth outcomes where a high dose of home visits was associated with reduced odds of a preterm birth but not with birth weight. The limitations of the study are discussed as are the several ways the results contribute to understanding the impact of home visitation approaches. First, the findings provide additional data about an important aspect of HV programs, early intervention, and intensity of home visiting schedule. The authors clearly state that further conceptualization and measurement of prenatal delivery of home visiting is important to our understanding of the utility and relative costs of using this strategy.

🔍 *26-2 CITED STUDY: More Visits, More Communication, Better Care*

Using Paraprofessional/Licensed Nurses Coordinated Care Model

In a series of papers by Guo et al., the phenomena of HV and better outcomes were studied. Like Goyal et al. (2013), this study examined the relationship of *dose* of the prenatal HV program and birth outcomes as well. The MOMs program uses a coordinated model of HV services with trained paraprofessionals who serve as home visitors and licensed RNs who supervise these home visit assessments and interventions. In this collaborative model, paraprofessionals have ready access to the registered nurse (RN) if they discover or suspect problems

Guo, Y., Pimentel, P., & Olshansky, E. (2015, October). A community-based home visitation program's impact on birth outcomes. *The American Journal of Maternal Child Nursing, 41*(1). doi:10.1097 /NMC.0000000000000203

Guo et al. (2015) studied the impact of the MOMS Orange County coordinated HV program on birth outcomes in a largely at-risk community of Hispanic mothers. This program uses trained paraprofessional home visitors who are supervised closely by RNs. Their objective was to examine the impact of the program on birth outcomes measured by birth weight and age at gestation. They used a retrospective cohort design to study the relationship of home visits and these birth outcomes and found that *number of prenatal home visits* predicted higher birth weight and greater gestational age at birth.

According to Guo each mother is assigned a paraprofessional home visitor who assists the mother and prepares her for childbirth. The visitor meets the client in their home or, in some cases, another place most comfortable for the pregnant woman. Visitors meet with mothers once per month from the time they join the program through to the baby's first birthday. Education and support are foundational and assistance in seeking needed referrals is included. Topics can include how to have a healthy pregnancy, changes to be expected during the pregnancy and what childbirth is like, physical and mental health needs, and health education.

The health education portion of the program helps these expectant mothers (1) access prenatal care, (2) be aware of the signs of hypertensive disorders of pregnancy, (3) prepare for childbirth, (4) improve communication with their health care providers, (5) nutritional health and breastfeeding, and (6) enhance their parenting skills. Referrals are made to public health nurses or other health care providers and community services when needed. RN case managers provide supervision of the home visitors and review the accuracy of their assessments and client care plans and their appropriate use of referral resources and services.

Evaluations of this HV program supported the researchers' expectation that the program may be a promising approach to decrease negative birth outcomes and fewer premature births. They caution, however, that these findings were not statistically significant. They did find MOMS program participants had the lowest fetal and infant mortality rates.

In a follow-up analysis of the impact of the MOMs program, Guo et al. (2017) examined the relative costs of instituting MOMs by comparing the rates of preterm births using state (California) and county (Orange County) data. They found that pregnant women who received more prenatal home visits (*greater dose)* were more likely to have healthier birth outcomes (prematurity and low birth rates) relative to the countywide and statewide populations, controlling for maternal age and education and family income. Furthermore, in their analyses of the potential cost savings, they concluded that with better birth outcomes the relative cost savings seem to be anywhere from $1.1–2.1 million, countywide and statewide, respectively.

Guo, Y., Lee, J., Rousseau, J., Pimentel, P., Bojorquez, Y., Cabasaq, C., Silva, M., & Olshansky, E. (2017). The potential economic impact of a coordinated home visitation program: Preventing adverse birth outcomes. *California Journal of Health Promotion, 14*(2), 1–13.

🔎 26-3 EVIDENCE FOR/MORE TO KNOW BOX: Selected HV Programs Promote Positive Birth Outcomes in At-Risk Pregnant Women

Evidence for

- Impoverished underserved pregnant women have a higher risk for poor birth outcomes (preterm births and low birth weight babies).
- HV Programs alter patient–provider communications in the following ways:
  a. HV Programs provide face-to-face communication with the health care team.
  b. HVs increase the number of face-to-face contacts with pregnant women during the period before 26 weeks' gestation.
  c. There are two ways these HV contacts can be structured:
     1. A continuous relationship with a licensed provider (either RN or social worker).
     2. A continuous relationship with a paraprofessional who is indirectly supervised by a licensed RN.
- There is some evidence from research and evaluation studies that HV programs could be associated with better birth outcomes (lower rates of preterm births and lower rates of low birth weights).
- This evidence suggests that continuity (duration of enrollment) and high intensity (of participation) are instrumental in producing these outcomes.

More to Know

- Continuity of relationships between women participating in HV programs and professional or paraprofessional staff could provide opportunities for more frequent conversations and communication at a deeper level. This continuity and intensity might result in better assessment data and motivate mothers to use prenatal care and to improve lifestyle behaviors that impact risk factors for poor birth outcomes (e.g., nutritional status and drug and alcohol use).
- The level of relationship continuity in either approach (licensed provider or paraprofessional-licensed provider) is unknown.
- The level of intensity (beyond the number of completed home visits) is only one aspect of intensity; another dimension in the data derived in assessments and motivational goals met. These factors are intermediate. Altering the structure could impact the processes of care and these differences (in processes) might account for improved birth outcomes in high-risk pregnant women.

The potential benefits of HV approaches to positively impact child and family health and welfare outcomes is addressed in other studies as well. For example, Lowell, Carter, Paulicin and Briggs-Gowan (2011) studied the impact of the Child FIRST home-based intervention. In this program, a psychotherapeutic parent–child intervention is embedded in the system of care of multi-risk urban mothers and children (ages 6–36 months). They documented significant changes in program participant outcomes across a broad number of indicators: improved language skills, externalizing symptoms, less parenting stress, lower psychopathology symptoms, and less protective service involvement relative to usual care families at the same measurement points.

Overall, the evidence supporting the efficacy of HV programs is tentative but positive. Some studies reported associated positive outcomes: decrease in low birth rate; increase in birth weight (Guo, Pimentel, & Olshansky, 2015); or a decrease in preterm births, but not birth weight (Goyal et al., 2013). While there is much do be done to garner confidence in this approach across multiple communities and vulnerable populations, with different targets in mind (birth outcomes and/or child development and stress prevention), beginning evidence is positive.

It is important to keep in mind that not all at-risk expectant mothers may enroll in or stay the course through the entire program time period which in some cases may be 2–3 years. There are programs that report a reasonable completion rate of 80% or greater but as Ammerman (2016) points out, retention of mothers to the end of the service is a problem across the board. To support this conclusion, Ammerman pulls from the results of a study of 100 programs in 9 states having attrition rates of 50% at the first-year postenrollment. Further, Ammerman summarizes these findings and warns that more attention should be given to mothers' reasons for leaving HV programs.

There is more to be known about retention. For example, what factors contribute to failure to enroll, early dropout, and midprogram dropout. Several questions are worth exploration including patient satisfaction with the program, patient perceptions of the quality care received, differences in provider engagement with patients, and many other potential barriers to retention in HV programs.

Data about program outcomes and staff qualifications, cultural and linguistic differences between staff and patients, and competing needs of these mothers (including residential relocation) should be explored. What differences are there in mothers who are retained to the end of the program and those who leave the program early. McCurdy et al. (2006) summarized their findings of retention differences in a sample of mothers from nine HV programs across six states and concluded that the mothers who intended to use services look substantially different from those who do not. They found that lower infant birth weight and greater comfort with a provider in one's home were significant predictors of whether they expressed intention to use the program. They also draw attention to the lack of information regarding families who avoid services which may indicate higher need but avoidance or perceived competence and lower actual need for services.

▶ Summary

We introduced the idea that there is evidence to suggest that modifying communication approaches could yield different care outcomes. Namely, using HV programs as an adjunct to the prenatal care of vulnerable pregnant women at risk could strengthen communications with the health care provider team and subsequently, result in improved health outcomes.

HV programs have the potential to positively impact quality care to these women and families because (1) access to health care is provided at all times throughout the pregnancy and immediately thereafter, (2) they provide for a continuous healing relationship, (3) care can be customized to meet patient needs and values, and (4) because the care provider comes to the patient, the patient can be the source of control.

While there is evidence to support the idea that HV programs significantly alter the patients' and families' experience and enhance positive birth outcomes, findings are mixed. The heterogeneity of HV programs limits the generalizability of findings. In this discussion, we drew on and compared the results of two, what would seem to be, very similar evaluations of existing prenatal HV programs. But can these studies be compared in full or are there limitations in comparing the studies with one another and grouping findings together to conclude that prenatal HV programs can yield relatively better birth outcomes? The answer is that it may be too early to judge this potential positive effect of HV programs on birth outcomes.

A significant gap in the literature makes it difficult to judge either way. We know something about the patients, providers, and programs but need to know more. Missing from this complex puzzle is full disclosure of the processes of care that are a result of the structure (HV), and how these processes directly or indirectly positively or negatively impact outcomes. This chapter focused on health care services aimed at health promotion and disease prevention, particularly with at-risk vulnerable populations. In the next chapter, we address the elements of treatment of disease or illness with a focus on enhancing behavior change.

Discussion

1. Identify factors impacting effective communications with at-risk families and communities.
2. How might HV programs improve quality health care services to at-risk populations?
3. What are the different approaches to structuring HV programs?
4. Discuss the use of paraprofessionals in the provision of HVs versus licensed health professionals as the primary contact person for prenatal families.
5. Evidence of the impact of HV programs is promising. However, what key information is needed to judge, with confidence, the full adoption of these programs?

References

Ammerman, R. T. (2016). Commentary: Toward the next generation of home visiting programs—New developments and promising directions. *Current Problems in Pediatric and Adolescent Health Care, 46*(4), 126–129. doi:10.1016/j.cppeds.2015.12.010

Avellar, S. A., & Supplee, L. H. (2013). Effectiveness of home visiting in improving child health and reducing child maltreatment. *Pediatrics, 132*(Suppl 2: S90-9). doi: 10.1542/peds.2013-1021G

Del Grosso, P., Kleinman, R., Esposito, A. M., Sama Martin, E., & Paulsell, D. (2011). *Assessing the evidence of effectiveness of home visiting program models implemented in tribal communities.* Washington, DC: Office of Planning, Research and Evaluation, Administration for Children and Families, U.S. Department of Health and Human Services.

Goyal, N. K., Hall, E. S., Meinzen-Derr, J. K., Kahn, R. S., Short, J. A., Van Ginkel, J. B., & Ammerman, R. T. (2013). Dosage effect of prenatal home visiting on pregnancy outcomes in at-risk, first-time mothers. *Pediatrics, 132*(Suppl 2), S118–S125. doi:10.1542/peds.2013-1021J

Guo, Y., Lee, J, Rousseau, J., Pimentel, P., Bojorquez, Y., Cabasaq, C., … Olshansky, E. (2017). The potential economic impact of a coordinated home visitation program: Preventing adverse birth outcomes. *California Journal of Health Promotion, 14*(2), 1–13.

Guo, Y., Pimentel, P., & Olshansky, E. (2015, October). A community-based home visitation program's impact on birth outcomes. *The American Journal of Maternal Child Nursing, 41*(1), 16–23. doi:10.1097/NMC.0000000000000203

Finello, K. M., Terteryan, A., & Riewerts, R. J. (2015). Home visiting programs: What the primary care clinician should know. *Current Problems in Pediatric and Adolescent Health Care, 46*(4), 101–125. doi:10.1016/j.cppeds.2015.12.011

Institute of Medicine. (2001). *Crossing the quality chasm: A new health system for the 21st century. Crossing the quality chasm: A new health system for the 21st century.* Retrieved from: www.nap.edu. The full text of this report is available at http://www.nap.edu/books/0309072808/html/

McCurdy, K., Daro, D., Anisfeld, E., Katzev, A., Keim, A., LeCroy, C., … Winje, C. (2006). Understanding maternal intentions to engage in home visiting programs. *Children and Youth Services Review, 28*(10), 1195–1212. doi:10.1016/j.childyouth.2005.11.010

Parrish, R. C., Menendez, M. E., Mudgal, C. S., Jupiter, J. B., Chen, N. C., & Ring, D. (2016). Patient satisfaction and its relation to perceived visit duration with a hand surgeon. *Journal of Hand Surgery, 41* (2), 257–262, e4. doi:10.1016/j.jhsa.2015.11.015

Sweet, M. A., & Appelbaum, M. I. (2004). Is home visiting an effective strategy? A meta-analytic review of home visiting programs for families with young children. *Child Development, 75*(5), 1435–1456. doi:10.1111/j.1467-8624.2004.00750.x

Tai-Seale, M., McGuire, T. G., & Zhang, W. (2007). Time allocation in primary care office visits. *Health Services Research, 42*(5), 1871–1894. doi:10.1111/j.1475-6773.2006.00689.x

CHAPTER 27

Communications to Promote Behavior Change

CHAPTER OBJECTIVES

- Describe the motivational interviewing (MI) approach and identify the aims of this approach when used in a clinical setting.
- Identify the populations and clinical conditions for which health providers would consider the use of MI techniques.
- Describe the interviewing techniques most often used in MI.
- Discuss the literature reporting the potential benefits associated with MI techniques and approaches in diabetes self-management.
- Identify ways in which MI has been incorporated in the use of mobile devices or phone outreach with difficult to reach populations.

KEY TERMS

- Autonomy
- Client-centered counseling
- Develop discrepancy
- Empathy
- Motivational interviewing (MI)
- Primary and secondary outcomes
- Reflective listening
- Roll with resistance
- Self-efficacy
- Subjective reflections

▶ Introduction

Many of our behaviors are seen to reflect our motivation. For example, we attribute our success on an exam to be due, in part, to our motivation to do well and try hard. We perceive our unhealthy eating or lack of exercise as a lack of motivation. We are very familiar with the concept of motivation and often attempt to redirect our motivation to attain our goals. Sometimes it seems we are the unfortunate prisoner of lack of motivation with a discrepancy between what we want and how we behave.

To this end, any assistance in releasing us from lack of motivation is likely to make us feel better about ourselves and the world around us. An understanding of the role of motivation behind behavior gives us insight into problems patients and families have in making important lifestyle changes which could otherwise protect them from health problems and improve their recovery from current illnesses. This chapter focuses on **motivational interviewing (MI)**, a technique used to help patients explore and resolve any ambivalence they have about needed behavior change.

As simplistic as this phenomenon seems to be, it is a critical driving force in the counseling approach of MI in clinical settings. MI is a **client-centered** directive therapeutic approach to enhance individuals' potential for behavior change.

It is antithetical to what has been the traditional biomedical model practice to identify and define the patient's problem and give advice in the absence of the patient's perspective (Rubak, Sandboek, Lauritzaen, & Christensen, 2005).

MI has a substantial history. It was initially designed and used for the treatment of patients with drug and alcohol abuse disorders. Dr. William Miller introduced the principles and approach of MI in 1983 and later elaborated on the approach in the writings of Miller and Rollnick (1991). The goal of MI in clinical settings is to elicit behavior change in clients or patients struggling with ambivalence about an aspect of behavior that needs to be changed. MI typically aims to guide patients to approach and undertake behavior change through the use of several communication strategies. While MI is original in its approach, it has foundations in other theories of behavior change. For example, some describe MI as drawing from Carl Roger's client-centered approach (1972), which focuses on the counselor's role in unleashing the self-actualizing potential of individuals to make behavior changes and Albert Bandura's cultivating **self-efficacy** for behavior change (1977). In the mid-1980s through late 1990s, the Prochaska and DiClemente *transtheoretical model* expanded on the stages of change which is a key component of MI (1994).

According to Miller and Rollnick (2013), MI is a collaborative, goal-oriented style of communication designed to elicit motivation for and commitment to a specific goal. It achieves this objective by eliciting and exploring the patients' reasons for wanting to change in a patient-centered atmosphere characterized by acceptance and compassion (2013, p 29). It has been adapted for use in a variety of clinical settings where changes in patient behavior are critical to their good health. For example, clearly drug and alcohol abuse requires changes in lifestyle choices, as does weight management associated with certain medical diagnoses, particularly diabetes and heart disease. The underlying theory behind the MI approach is that ambivalence is at the core of

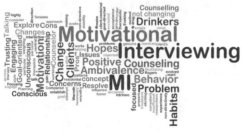

© Kheng Guan Toh/Shutterstock.

why patients cannot follow through to achieve and maintain behavior change which will lead to healthier behaviors and better quality of life.

Use of MI with Various Populations and Clinical Conditions

Early on, the MI counseling approach garnered interest and enthusiasm from mental health professionals and later a wide range of providers addressing the psychological and physiological aspects of illness. Beginning reports assessing the impact of MI occurred in the counseling of persons with alcohol-related disorders, marijuana- and tobacco-related problems, drug abuse, and gambling (Lundahl, Kun, Brownell, Tollefson, & Burke, 2010). Subsequently, there were reports of MI counseling with other lifestyle behaviors needing intervention (e.g., risky sexual practices, diet, exercise, and even poor dental health practices).

In each of these instances, patients may need support to resolve the ambivalence they have about making changes. Facing conflict between two or more courses of action (e.g., continuing to drink alcohol excessively and modifying or suspending drinking behavior) that represent opposite actions. With the use of MI, the patient is supported to uncover any resistance they have, and are encouraged to explore the costs and benefits of choosing one action over the other. MI approaches respect the patient's **autonomy** and freedom of choice about needed behavior change.

As previously indicated, the use of MI with addictive disorders is most notable. However, there is a collection of literature suggesting that it can also be effectively used with persons with other significant and chronic illnesses including depression and anxiety. Patients requiring adherence to treatment over extended periods of time, especially when this treatment includes a complex set of behaviors, are particularly helped with

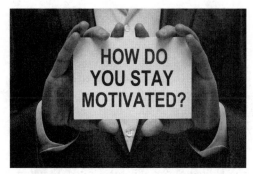

© SK Design/Shutterstock.

MI. Examples of these patients are those with obesity, asthma, diabetes, HIV/AIDS, and cardiovascular disease. In selected instances, medical outcomes (e.g., body mass index (BMI), blood glucose HbA1c levels, total blood cholesterol, and systolic blood pressure) were shown to improve in studies of patients receiving MI.

There are reports of the use of MI with adult populations of any age. An early pilot study to improve adherence to a behavioral weight-control program for older obese women with noninsulin-dependent diabetes mellitus (NIDDM), Smith, Heckemeyer, Kratt, and Mason (1997), reported improvements in the experimental group's attendance at group meetings, completion of food diaries, and recorded blood glucose levels. The researchers concluded that an MI component may significantly enhance adherence to the program and potentially, glycemic control indexed by A1c levels.

Other studies reported on the effectiveness of MI with adolescent populations. The potential use of MI, years later, with teenagers who have diabetes was reported by Channon et al. (2007). In this randomized controlled trial study of the use of MI with teenagers with diabetes, the 12-month mean A1c level was significantly lower in the group receiving MI than that in the control group. Furthermore, those in the MI group expressed more positive well-being and improved quality of life. Stewart, Siebert, Arit, Moise-Campbell, and

Lehinger (2016) examined the impact of a school-based MI intervention, Project READY, on reducing substance use in adolescents. They reported that their findings support the effectiveness of this school-based MI approach for adolescents using marijuana. MI was a critical component of these interventions.

It should be noted that while the bulk of the literature on the effectiveness of MI comes from developed countries, particularly the United States and the United Kingdom, beginning reports are surfacing from low- and mid-level income countries.

MI Principles and Techniques

As previously described, MI is a client-centered directive therapeutic approach to enhance individuals' potential for behavior change. The goal of MI in clinical settings is to elicit behavior change in clients or patients struggling with ambivalence about an aspect of behavior that needs to be changed. Typically, it aims to guide patients to approach and undertake behavior change through the use of several communication strategies and in the context of recovery. It should be stressed that addictions have physiological components that need to be accounted for in recovery while individuals are learning needed behavior change and participating in MI.

MI approaches, directly or indirectly, address the general principles laid out by the Institute of Medicine in the document *Crossing the Quality Chasm: A New Health System for the 21st Century* (2001). Specifically, the principles of (1) customizing care to meet patient needs and values and (2) respecting the patient as the source of control are supported in the MI principles of patient autonomy and patient self-efficacy. MI has both a unique philosophical approach and guiding principles directing the practice of MI in clinical settings.

Philosophical Underpinnings

Making the point that MI is more than just a technique, Rollnick, Miller, and Butler

(2008, p. 6) explain that MI is not a technique, it is a skillful clinical *style for eliciting from patients their own good motivations for making behavior changes in the interest of their health.* MI emphasizes the need to be patient-centered and respects patients' values and goals. Change if and when it occurs is a result of the individual's intrinsic need to change. A complete list of the characteristics of MI is outlined in the text by Miller and Rollnick (1991) and Miller and Rollnick (2013). Further, a summary of MI characteristics is also provided by Rubak, Sandboek, Lauritzwen, and Christensen (2005). **EXHIBIT 27-1** summarizes several principles and approaches foundational to the MI approach.

Practitioners using the MI approach view the provider's attempts to try to persuade the patient to change (by stressing the urgency or need to change or by confronting patient denial or giving advice only) results in patient resistance. It is by respecting patients' descriptions of the problem and formulating their own goals that change is possible. Otherwise, change comes from the patient and is not imposed or ordered by the provider.

The idea is that given support and guidance the patient is likely to choose a healthy option. Welch, Rose, and Ernst (2006) explain that **reflective listening** is the way that the provider can accurately understand a patient's story. Open questions, reflections, gentle probing for more detail, and the use of summaries is foundational to MI. Welch et al. state that this is "...*the means for understanding patient's unique connections to the targeted health behavior and develops rapport*" (p.6). (This was previously addressed in Part II—Chapters 4–6—and Chapter 13 of this text.)

Examples of Dialogue Using MI

As previously listed in Exhibit 27-1, MI includes both guiding principles and techniques and these shape providers' communications with patients. MI is sometimes described as a style that delivers a spirit of collaboration

EXHIBIT 27-1 Summary of MI Principles and Approaches

- MI is a client-centered approach which elicits behavior change.
- MI relies on identifying patient values and goals for behavior change.
- Change in behavior is not imposed on the patient; rather, it is a result of patient's intrinsic motivation to make behavior changes.
- The patient–provider relationship has a foundation in respect for the patient's autonomy.
- Traditional strategies relying on direct questioning, confrontation, and persuasion to mobilize a change in patient behaviors is antithetical to the MI approach.
- Resolving ambivalence to change is key to a MI approach and includes the patient's perspective on benefits and costs of the planned change.
- The patient's readiness to change may not be constant and is impacted by interpersonal interactions, including those between patient and provider.
- MI is a counseling style encompassing key techniques which include active listening, reflection, rolling with resistance, developing awareness of the discrepancy between current behavior and one's goals, supporting self-efficacy, or the patient's own beliefs that they can carry out and succeed in making behavior changes.

in patient–provider relationships. This spirit is described as collaborative, evocative, and honoring of patient autonomy (Rollnick, Miller, & Butler, 2008, p. 6). It is supported by four key guiding principles to shape provider communications with patients, what health professionals discuss with patients, and *how* they discuss it:

1. **Empathy**: To demonstrate empathy, health professionals must listen with empathy. They must communicate their interest in understanding and valuing the patient's perspective. It is through the practice of empathy that the provider–patient relationship is strengthened.

   Example: If the patient is talking about how stressful his or her overeating is, you might reply, "I think I hear you saying that you're eating is a stressful experience and that sometimes you have no control." This example illustrates how providers can show patients that they are listening and are getting a better understanding of what this situation means to them.

2. **Roll with resistance**: Rather than confront the patient with the undesired behavior, the provider addresses it with reflection. For example, when a patient admits to avoiding exercise rather than confront the patient with the resistance, the provider might reflect what the patient is saying.

   Example: If the patient said, "I haven't been exercising," rather than asking why or presenting the consequences of not exercising, an alternative response might be, "You say you haven't been exercising." This response is likely to open up a discussion about dealing with the patient's lack of motivation to exercise. Abruptly censoring the patient's resistance to exercise would likely lead to further avoidance of the topic and build a wedge between the patient and provider.

3. **Develop discrepancy**: In order for patients to commit to change they need to see the discrepancy or *mismatch* (incongruity) between what they are currently doing and what they want for themselves. In conducting MI, the provider assists the patient in understanding that the

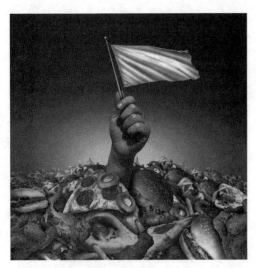

© Lightspring/Shutterstock

current behavior does not reflect the patient's stated values or goals.

Example: The patient might explain that his or her goal is to be able to lose enough weight to engage his or her child in play. The patient says, "I will never be able to run, chase, and play with my 5-year old; I can't even walk for very long." One response would be to link the patient's current overeating and lack of exercise to the patient's problems in meeting his or her goal to play with his or her child. *The provider* might follow up with an affirmation (e.g., "You are giving this a lot of thought and are understanding what it takes to meet your goal…this gives me the impression that you are motivated to exercise and are capable of moving forward from here.")

4. **Support self-efficacy:** Self-efficacy refers to patients' beliefs that they have the ability to make the desired change(s). If one believes they are capable of change, they are more likely to accomplish what it takes to make the change.

Example: The patient continues to express doubt that he or she can meet his or her goals. At this point it is helpful to support the patient's self-efficacy by recognizing his or her success in losing weight so far and starting a new exercise regimen. One response might be, "I am looking over your history during the last few months; I see you have made changes before. You have shown you can do it…and most likely will again."

In summary, the guiding principles and dialogue approaches of MI are designed to engage the patient in a collaborative relationship where talk of change is met with provider attentiveness and responsiveness. Rather than expecting the patient to make temporary changes, the focus is on change when the patient is ready, and this includes dealing effectively and with sensitivity to the conflicts and resistance the patient has about making behavior changes.

Structure of MI Programs

There is considerable detail in the structure of MI programs. These include method of delivery, duration of the program, number of MI encounters between patient and provider, and the profession of interventionists. It also includes the specific focus and targets of change. Method of delivery refers to whether the MI intervention is employed during direct one-to-one contacts with the provider, in a group with other patients with the same or similar condition, or indirectly through the use of phone or Internet transmission.

MI approaches have used all of these modes of delivery. However, the majority of studies reporting on the results of MI examined its use with individuals during one-to-one encounters ranging from one encounter to over five encounters. Rubak et al. (2005) reported that intervention periods can run anywhere from less than 3 months to over

2 years and the number of encounters can be only one up to 5 or greater. These authors also reported the professions of the MI interventionists to be either psychologist, physician, or other professional health care provider (e.g., nurse, midwife, and dietitian). However, in a more recent study by Do Valle Nascimento and colleagues (2017), MI interventions were conducted by trained community health agents in São Paulo, Brazil.

Group methods have also been employed. For example, MI to improve weight loss in women with type 2 diabetes was reported by West, DiLillo, Bursac, Gore, and Greene (2007). As previously stated, the duration of MI programs and number of encounters can vary significantly. In this study, all participants received a 42-session weight management group program (weekly encounters for the first 6 months, biweekly for 6 weeks, and then once a month for another 6 months). Weight loss was the focus of the first 6 months and weight loss maintenance in the remaining 12-month period.

The goal of this program is to elicit attainable and sustainable changes in diet and exercise with a specific focus on goal setting and problem-solving to achieve successful behavior change. Diaries were used and reviewed weekly. Topics in the groups included helpful behavior change perspectives including stimulus control, developing social support, cognitive restructuring, and relapse prevention. Education was provided about diabetes, obesity, and weight loss. Only the experimental group received the MI portion of the program. These group sessions focused on eliciting change talk and commitment language. The experimental group was also offered five individual-oriented MI interviewing sessions delivered by a licensed psychologist trained in MI.

The targets for change were behaviors and clinical indicators were used to measure change. The results of the study showed that women in the experimental condition (group meetings and MI) lost significantly more weight at 6 months and 18 months with significantly greater reductions in A1c at 6 months but not 18 months. An important finding was that there appeared to be ethnic differences in MI impact with African American women receiving diminished benefit from the addition of the MI component of the program.

The structure elements of MI also include which populations are receiving MI and what specific changes are targeted. As previously indicated, MI was originally used to treat patients with alcohol and drug abuse disorders. Still, we see documentation of its use in a variety of chronic illnesses where behavior change is needed. A study of MI for teens with diabetes type 1 adds to an understanding of MI use as does a study of low-income patients in a primary care setting in Brazil discussed later in this chapter. Finally, the structure of MI can be differentiated by the primary and secondary changes that are targeted.

Primary outcomes would include observations and self-reports of behavior change. In programs for patients with alcohol and drug abuse, primary outcomes include alterations in drinking and drug use (e.g., quantity and frequency of alcohol and drugs consumed). In studies of primary care patients who are facing problems of obesity, inadequate physical activity, or poor self-management of diabetes or asthma, the direct measures of changes are healthy diet, increased physical activity and/or exercise, diabetic dietary adherence, or medication adherence in the case of diabetes or asthma self-management.

Secondary outcomes are associated with the primary outcomes. As discussed here, secondary outcomes are a result of either short-term or long-term goal achievement. They are frequently biomarkers that are the results of changes in self-reported behavior change. Otherwise, with changes in diet and exercise behaviors one would expect concomitant weight loss and alterations in BMI values. Other secondary outcomes are dependent upon the behavior targeted and could include concomitant changes in other biomedical indicators: biomarkers for effective medication use in the case of improved medication adherence, positive changes in blood glucose levels HbA1c in patients with diabetes who have made needed dietary and exercise changes, and peak blood alcohol concentration in persons who have made significant changes in alcohol consumption.

Additional outcomes frequently measured in MI programs are **subjective reflections** of patients and/or interventionists. These outcomes include patient and/or interventionist satisfaction with the program and patient perceived well-being and quality of life, increased self-efficacy, or empowerment.

MI Principles and Techniques and Self-Management of Diabetes

Diabetes is a chronic health condition resulting from either the inability of the pancreas to make enough insulin (type 1 diabetes) or when the body cannot effectively use the insulin it produces (type 2 diabetes). When the body does not have enough insulin, or cannot use it effectively, the level of glucose (blood sugar) rises. Hyperglycemia (raised blood sugar) is a common result of uncontrolled diabetes. High blood sugar levels over time lead to serious damage to the body systems, particularly the neurological and cardiovascular systems. There are three major types of diabetes: type 1, type 2, and gestational diabetes (WHO, 2016).

Type 1 diabetes was previously referred to as insulin-dependent diabetes with juvenile or childhood onset. This type of diabetes is characterized by deficient insulin production. The cause is unknown and given what we know, there is currently no way to prevent this form of diabetes. Young people with type 1 diabetes show symptoms of excessive urination (polyuria), thirst (polydipsia), constant hunger, weight loss, vision changes, and fatigue which may occur suddenly.

In contrast, type 2 diabetes, formerly referred to as noninsulin-dependent diabetes, is the adult onset form of diabetes disease.

Type 2 diabetes is the result of the body's ineffective use of insulin. The majority of people with diabetes throughout the world have type 2 diabetes. Symptoms of type 2 diabetes disease are less pronounced and consequently can go undiagnosed for several years, even after diabetic complications have alerted the patient to a potential health problem.

Gestational diabetes occurs during pregnancy and places women at increased risk for complications during pregnancy and at delivery. These women and their children are also at greater risk for diabetes in the future (WHO, 2016). This form of diabetes is diagnosed through prenatal screening rather than through signs and symptoms of disease reported by patients.

According to the Centers for Disease Control and Prevention (CDC, 2015) as of 2014 29.1 million people in the United States (9.3% of the population) had diabetes, up from the previous estimate of 26 million in 2010. The number of undiagnosed cases of diabetes is estimated to be 8.1 million, and more than one in four (27.8%) people with diabetes do not know they have the disease. Furthermore, 86 million people are living with prediabetes, a condition that increases a person's risk of developing type 2 diabetes and other chronic conditions (e.g., heart disease and stroke) (CDC, 2016). About 95% of cases in adults are type 2 diabetes. There were 1.7 million people aged 20 years or older who were newly diagnosed in 2012.

If not reversed, CDC (2016) warns that one in three adults in the United States could have diabetes by 2050. Diabetes was the seventh leading cause of death in the United States in 2013 and the World Health Organization (WHO), citing projections of global mortality (Mathers & Loncar, 2006), states that diabetes will be the seventh leading cause of death in the world by 2030.

Of particular concern are the rising cases of diabetes, particularly type 2, growing at rates higher than expected which will have a significant impact on individuals' lives and early mortality. To this end, major medical and policy recommendations have put in place standards for diabetic management and prevention of diabetes in prediabetic conditions.

Complications from poor self-management of diabetes are increasing. These complications are serious potential health problems and include heart disease and stroke, diabetic retinopathy (resulting in vision loss or blindness), kidney disease which can lead to kidney failure, and hard to treat infections, particularly in the lower limbs (toes, feet, or legs) which may necessitate amputation to stop the spread of infection. Structured lifestyle change programs are important to the management of diabetes and can even cut the risk of developing type 2 diabetes disease by as much as 58% in people with prediabetes (CDC, 2016).

As early as 1998, literature on the potential positive effects of MI principles and approaches for patients with diabetes appeared. The implementation and mode of delivery of MI can differ when applied in medical settings. Early on, Miller and Rollick (2002, p. 254) explained that MI in public health and medical settings might be made a part of multicomponent interventions which include educational materials and nonmotivational interactions. They also explained that in medical settings, providers may not have the time or training to employ the full range of MI interventions, and their opportunity to develop the rapport needed to maximize the therapeutic effect of MI may be limited (Miller & Rollnick, 2002, p. 253). In the following review, examples of various means of integrating MI in clinical practice are presented and summarized. Some studies report on implementing select aspects of MI, and other studies report the results of employing MI in multicomponent programs.

In a prospective cohort study of patients with either type 1 or type 2 diabetes from a major diabetes treatment center at a university-affiliated community hospital, investigators examined the extent to which care provider support for autonomy was associated with increased perceived competence in self-managing diabetes. Furthermore, patient's perceived competence was reported to be related to significant reductions in their HbA1c (blood glucose) levels. Hemoglobin A1c tests are routine for people with diabetes. HbA1c levels are indicators of the risk of developing diabetes-related complications. Patients with diabetes are monitored for their A1c levels over time to avoid serious disease consequences.

A second study posted in *Diabetes Care* in 2007 sought to determine the impact of MI techniques in a behavioral weight control program. A randomized controlled clinical trial was conducted with 217 overweight women randomized to one of two approaches, MI or attention placebo. Furthermore, beyond studies of diabetes care and weight loss interventions, MI has been shown to be important in managing depression and anxiety experienced by many persons with diabetes.

Several examples of clinical research studies are highlighted in the following study boxes. These studies include the randomized controlled clinical trials integrating MI in a group-based behavioral obesity treatment program for women with type 2 diabetes (previously mentioned), a multicenter randomized controlled trial of MI with teens with type 1 diabetes, and a pilot study of a community health agent-led MI program with patients seen in primary care with type 2 diabetes in a low-income urban community in São Paulo, Brazil. Each of these studies is unique in their use of MI, including the delivery method (individual one-to-one and/or group), duration of encounter, population served (teens or adults with type 1 or type 2 diabetes), and MI primary interventionists (licensed clinical psychologists, nurses, or trained community health agents).

While there are significant differences in format and structure of these programs, all were intent on delivering *the spirit* of MI. Positive outcomes were identified in each reported research study including better weight loss and A1c reductions (weight loss women with type 2 diabetes), A1c reductions and more positive well-being and improved quality of life (teens with type 1 diabetes), and improvements in perceived quality of care, increases in physical activity, consumption of fruits and vegetables, and medication adherence (patients with type 2 diabetes seen in a public primary care center in São Paulo).

🔍 CITED STUDY: MI Improves Weight Loss in Women with Type 2 Diabetes

Group-Based Behavioral Weight Control Program with or Without MI

The authors conducted a randomized controlled clinical trial to determine whether adding a MI component to an existing behavioral weight loss program would improve weight loss outcomes and glycemic control in overweight women with type 2 diabetes. In a pilot study of a community-based type 2 diabetes self-management program, the investigators examine the likelihood of improving diabetes in at risk poorly self-managed clinical cases.

West, D.S., DiLillo, V., Bursac, Z., Gore, S.A., Greene, P.G. (2007). Motivational interviewing improves weight loss in women with type 2 diabetes. *Diabetes Care, 30*(5), 1081–1087.

The targets for change were both behaviors and clinical indicators to support the finding that change actually occurred. The results of the study showed that women in the experimental condition (group meetings and MI) lost significantly more weight at 6 months and 18 months with significantly greater reductions in A1c at 6 months but not 18 months. An important finding was that there appeared to be ethnic differences in MI. There was a diminished impact of adding the MI component for African American women. The researchers concluded that augmenting a standard behavioral weight loss program with an MI component may significantly enhance adherence to the weight loss program and glycemic control and that further investigation with larger samples and over a longer period of follow-up are needed.

🔍 CITED STUDY: A Pilot Study of a Community Health Agent-Led Type 2 Diabetes Self-Management Program Using MI-Based Approaches in a Public Primary Care Center in São Paulo, Brazil

Autonomy-Supportive Communications to Impact Poorly Controlled Diabetes Difference

In a pilot study of a community-based type 2 diabetes self-management program, the investigators examined the likelihood of improving diabetes in at risk poorly self-managed patients in São Paulo. The researchers stated that while there is evidence to support the effectiveness of MI-based brief counseling to improve health behaviors and outcomes among adults with type 2 diabetes, there is little evidence evaluating the feasibility, acceptability, and effectiveness of training community health agents (CHAs) in Brazil's Basic Health Units in these skills.

They conducted a pilot study to examine MI-based counseling delivered by CHAs and reported findings about the feasibility of offering the counseling as well as outcomes in a sample of 57 poorly controlled diabetes-treated patients at a primary care center. Nineteen CHAs participated in the training to offer MI and behavioral action planning to these patients during routine patient encounters.

Do Valle Nascimento, T. M. R., Resnicow, K., Nery, M., Brentani, A., Kaselitz, E., Agrawal, P., … Heisler, M. (2017). A pilot study of a community health agent-led type 2 diabetes self-management program using Motivational Interviewing-based approaches in a public primary care center in São Paulo, Brazil. *BMC Health Services Research, 17*, 32. Results of this pilot study showed evidence of the feasibility, acceptability, and potential effectiveness of this brief intervention to produce positive outcomes. Over a 6-month period, patients reported improvements in the quality of care received, an increase in physical activity, greater consumption of fresh fruits and vegetables, and increases in medication adherence. However, there was no decrease in the consumption of high-fat foods or sweets. Patient participants had significantly better blood glucose levels from baseline to 6 months. A1c levels were 0.34% points lower. Additionally, improvements occurred in mean LDL and triglyceride levels. Furthermore, CHAs expressed enthusiasm about learning these new skills, and according to the researchers, many described a shift from advice-giving to encouraging patients to define their own goals.

🔍 *CITED STUDY: A Multicenter Randomized Controlled Trial of MI in Teenagers with Diabetes*

MI includes awareness building, consideration of alternatives, problem-solving, making choices, realistic and achievable goal setting, and avoidance of confrontation. The authors of this study explain that type 1 diabetes is the third most common chronic disease in teenagers. While MI had demonstrated to be effective with adults and some data to support its efficacy with type 1 diabetes in teens, the researchers wanted to replicate these studies and extend the findings of the original pilot study by conducting a multicenter randomized controlled trial in the United Kingdom. This randomized controlled trial was conducted with 66 teenagers, aged 14–17, with type 1 diabetes; 38 were randomized to the intervention group and 28 to the control group. All participants received individual sessions over a 12-month period; the intervention group received MI and the control group received support visits.

Channon, S. J., Huws-Thomes, M. V., Rollnick, S., Hood, K., Cannings-John, R. L., Rogers, C. & Gregory, J. W. (2007). A multicenter randomized controlled trial of motivational interviewing in teenagers with diabetes. *Diabetes Care, 30*, 1390–1395.

At the end of the 12-month trial, the mean A1c level in the MI group was significantly lower than that for the control group. At 24 months the differences remained although the sample was reduced from 60 to 47. There were also differences in a number of psychosocial factors at 12 months: more positive well-being, improved quality of life, and differences in personal models of illness. The authors concluded that MI was an effective method of facilitating behavior changes in teens with type 1 diabetes, and these behavior changes could be evidenced in glycemic control.

$\wp$ *EVIDENCE FOR/MORE TO KNOW BOX: MI Approaches to Improve Diabetes Self-Management*

Evidence for

- There is evidence across research and evaluation studies that MI or programs incorporating MI principles and philosophy can lead to behavior change for increased physical activity, weight loss, treatment adherence, and cessation of drug and alcohol abuse.
- There is also evidence that MI approaches can facilitate self-management of diabetes in adults and adolescents with type 1 or type 2 diabetes. Reported outcomes have included a reduction in blood glucose levels, blood pressure, cholesterol, triglycerides, obesity, and improvements in a sense of well-being and perceived quality of life.

More to Know

- While reports of the positive results from using MI are extensive, particularly the use of MI in conjunction with other treatment programs, the effects are difficult to judge when there is no examination of how well the program met the standards for MI intervention approaches, differences in delivery mode and intervention intensity, and the qualifications of the interventionists.
- The extent to which behavior change is sustained over time and how this might vary across patient populations and behaviors targeted for change need further investigation.
- Whether and to what degree of variations in MI programs (e.g., ways MI is delivered [group setting, home, telephone, primary care setting or treatment center], duration of the program, number of intervention encounters, and provider [physician, mental health provider, or other health provider or lay educator]) influence program outcomes also needs to be evaluated.
- How MI approaches are currently combined with other behavioral approaches to effect behavior change in clinical populations needs further exploration.

▶ Summary

MI is a client-centered directive counseling approach to enhance individuals' potential for behavior change. It has promise for providing personalized care to a wide range of individuals whose health problems are, in part, a function of their decision-making and lifestyle behaviors. The use of MI, which is a psychological strategy, must always be centered in a psychosocial–physiological model of looking at disease and illness. This is important in judging the appropriate placement of strategies and evaluating potential outcomes. Diabetes, obesity, and drug and alcohol addictions, for example, have significant biopsychosocial interactions. Acquiring risky lifestyle behaviors as well as recovery and behavior changes should be seen from this perspective.

From the viewpoint of MI interventionists, individuals facing significant behavior change need help in setting relevant goals and gaining control over factors that limit their ability to achieve these goals. The result of this alliance is the potential for effective behavior change and subsequent improved health and quality of life. To the degree that these approaches favorably impact overuse of health care services, there is a possibility that there would be cost savings. Overuse of health care services is evidenced in preventable trips to urgent care and emergency services and the escalation of care from the uncontrolled self-management of disease.

MI approaches are antithetical to the long-held traditional biomedical model approach which is to identify and define the patient's problem and give advice in the absence of the patient's views and perspectives. Client-centered care that is personalized requires an effective patient–provider relationship where patients' perspectives are intimately linked to the therapeutic process. MI programs use a variety of therapeutic communication approaches including reflection, active listening, empathy, supporting self-efficacy, and rolling with resistance.

Because MI approaches run counter to the traditional biomedical model, health professionals need to be carefully guided and trained to reverse what might be a natural tendency to revert to the biomedical model. Using the MI approach requires specific knowledge and clinical competencies added to the vast medical knowledge health professionals already possess. Professionals need to know how to identify and highlight individuals' strengths and values which they bring to each patient–provider encounter.

Discussions of what matters to the patient and what they perceive to be the barriers to their needs and desires met is essential in the motivating process. Health professionals need to be aware that a number of factors will impact this process including the patient's level of education, health literacy, and cultural orientation. It may be that some patients are just as happy to be told what to do and how to do it in the context of the traditional model. The question remains to what extent will this approach be acceptable and successful with a range of patients and vulnerable populations with different cultural orientations.

In this chapter, the principles of MI were reviewed and the reported outcomes in behavior change were identified and discussed. Several examples of clinical research studies were presented, and specific studies examining the impact of MI with diabetes care were detailed and tabled. Studies of MI discussed in more depth were a randomized controlled clinical trial integrating MI in a group-based behavioral obesity treatment program for women with diabetes type 2, a multicenter randomized controlled trial of MI with teens with type 1 diabetes, and a pilot study of a CHA-led MI program with patients seen in primary care with type 2 diabetes in a low-income urban community in São Paulo, Brazil.

Each of these studies were unique in their use of MI including the delivery method (individual one-to-one and/or group), duration of encounter, population served (teens or adults with type 1 or type 2 diabetes), and MI primary interventionists (licensed clinical psychologists, nurses, or trained community health agents).

While there were significant differences in format and structure, all programs were intent on delivering *the spirit* of MI. Positive outcomes were identified in each reported research study including better weight loss and A1c reductions (weight loss women with type 2 diabetes), A1c reductions and more positive well-being and improved quality of life (teens with type 1 diabetes), and improvements in perceived quality of care, increases in physical activity, consumption of fruits and vegetables, and medication adherence (patients with type 2 diabetes seen in a public primary care center in São Paulo).

The reported results of employing MI appear promising. Still, there are important findings worth further investigation. Results showed that the program for women in the MI weight loss program was not as effective with a subsample of African American patients who lost less weight than their Caucasian women counterparts and appeared to have a diminished benefit from the addition of the MI component to the weight loss educational program. Additionally, patients in the primary care program in São Paulo showed significant positive changes but it was also noted there were no decreases in consumption of high-fat foods and sweets.

These studies as well as others emphasize the importance of a critical analysis of both the programs themselves and their reported outcomes in programs for diabetic patients. Along these lines, Rubak and colleagues (2005), in their meta-analysis of the results of 19 randomized controlled trials, indicated that MI diabetes programs show some consistent results but not all results are identical. They summarized the findings in the following way: MI studies have produced significant effects in BMI, total blood cholesterol, systolic blood pressure, blood alcohol concentration, and standard ethanol content, though there are limitations in study methodology.

In a systematic review of the literature on the effectiveness of MI for health behavior change in primary care settings with nonclinical populations to achieve behavior change for physical activity, diet, and/or alcohol intake, Morton et al. (2015) concluded the following. These authors examined reports in 33 published papers and found that 50% of the studies ($n = 18$) demonstrated positive effects. However, they warned that due to inconsistencies in how MI programs were described and what their intervention components might have been, it is difficult to judge the efficacy of MI in nonclinical populations.

Some researchers have gone to the extent to suggest that it would be premature to recommend wide dissemination of MI in diabetes care, and stressed the need for more studies with real-world settings with health care professionals of the field instead of intensively trained MI interventionists. This knowledge would further our understanding of adequate training and factors contributing to the implementation of MI in daily practice (Heinrich, Candel, Schaper, & de Vries, 2010).

Difficulties in judging efficacy because of lack of clarity of approaches are also addressed in other papers describing behavior change programs in primary care settings. For example, Rossen et al. (2015) discussed inconsistencies in the literature about the use of MI in diabetes care and in increasing physical activity.

They explained that it was difficult to judge effects due to failure to examine treatment fidelity (how well the program met the standards for MI intervention approaches), differences in delivery mode and intervention intensity, and the qualifications of the interventionists. They suggested that a flexible approach using various models is recommended along with tailoring the program to the individual patient. Their program included a framework incorporating the health belief model, the stages of change model, and the social cognitive theory. They included a person-centered individual counseling approach delivered by diabetes-specialist nurses. To address the need to ensure the fidelity of the MI approach they used notes about MI talk and at regular meetings examined the quality of the counseling sessions.

In summary, the purpose of this chapter is to heighten awareness of the possibility that altering communication approaches might improve our ability to assist patients to make needed behavior change which will impact both their health status and quality of life. While not conclusive, and unanswered questions remain, studies of MI programs show how programs can be designed to emphasize a personalized approach to diabetes care using a client-centeredness framework. The MI approach has received a considerable amount of attention in the clinical literature detailing both different philosophical underpinnings, skills, and techniques that may be produce better patient outcomes than other approaches, including usual care modalities.

Discussion

1. Identify key elements of the MI approach.

2. Discuss how a biopsychosocial framework is important when implementing MI interventions with patients.

3. Is it likely that MI approaches are most effective with major chronic illness (e.g., diabetes and asthma) when combined

with other behavior change and educational approaches.

4. Discuss the issues associated with training CHAs or other nonprofessional support persons to conduct MI with diabetic patients in primary care settings.

5. Evidence of the impact of MI approaches is promising; however, what key information is needed to judge, with confidence, the efficacy of these approaches in a wide range of patient populations?

References

Bandura, A. (1977). Self-efficacy: Toward a unifying theory of behavioral change. *Psychological Review, 84,* 191–215. PMID:847061

Do Valle Nascimento, T. M. R., Resnicow, K., Nery, M., Brentani, A., Kaselitz, E., Agrawal, P. … Heisler, M. (2017). A pilot study of a community health agent-led type 2 diabetes self-management program using Motivational Interviewing-based approaches in a public primary care center in São Paulo, Brazil. *BMC Health Services Research, 17,* 32. doi:10.1186/s12913-016-1968-3

Centers for Disease Control and Prevention. (2015). *National diabetes statistics report: Estimates of diabetes and its burden in the United States, 2014.* Atlanta, GA: US Department of Health and Human Services; 2014. Retrieved from www.cdc.gov/diabetes/data/statistics/2014StatisticsReport.html

Centers for Disease Control and Prevention. (2016). *Working to Reduce the US Epidemic at a Glance 2016.* Atlanta, GA: US Department of Health and Human Services; 2014. Retrieved from www.cdc.gov/Other/plugins/#pdf

Channon, S. J., Huws-Thomas, M. V., Rollnick, S., Hood, K., Cannings-John, R. L., Rogers, C., & Gregory, J. W. (2007). A multicenter randomized controlled trial of motivational interviewing in teenagers with diabetes. *Diabetes Care, 30,* 1390–1395. doi.org/10.2337/dc06-2260

Heinrich, E., Candel, M. J. J. M., Schaper, N. C., & de Vries, N. K. (2010). Effect evaluation of Motivational Interviewing based counseling strategy in diabetes care. *Diabetes Research and Clinical Practice, 90*(3), 270–278. doi: 10.1016/j.diabres.2010.09.012

Institute of Medicine. (2001). *Crossing the quality chasm: A new health system for the 21st century.* Washington, DC: The National Academies Press. doi.org/10.17226/10027

Lundahl, B. W., Kunz, C., Brownell, C., Tollefson, D., & Burke, B. L. (2010). A meta-analysis of motivational interviewing: Twenty-five years of empirical studies. *Research on Social Work Practice, 20*(2), 137–160. doi:10.1177/1049731509347850

Mathers, C. D., & Loncar, D. (2006). Projections of global mortality and burden of disease 2002 to 2030. *PloS Med, 3*(11), e442. doi:10.1371/journal.pmed.0030442

Miller, W. R., & Rollnick, S. (1991). *Motivational interviewing: Preparing people for change.* New York, NY: Guilford Press.

Miller, W. R. & Rollnick, S. (2002). *Motivational interviewing: Preparing people for change.* (2nd ed.). New York, NY: Guilford Press.

Miller, W. R., & Rollnick, S. (2013). *Motivational interviewing: Helping people change* (3rd ed.). New York. NY: Guilford Press.

Morton, K., Beauchamp, M., Prothero, A., Joyce, L., Saunders, L., Spencer-Bowdage, S., … Pedlar, C. (2015). The effectiveness of motivational interviewing for health behavior change in primary care settings: A systematic review. *Health Psychology Review, 9*(2), 205–223. doi:10.1080/17437199.2014.882006

Prochaska, J. O., Velicer, W. F., Rossi, J. S., Goldstein, M. G., Marcus, B. H., Rakowski, W., … Rossi, S. R. (1994). Stages of change and decisional balance for twelve problem behaviors. *Health Psychology, 13*(1), 39–46. PMID:8168470

Rogers, C. R. (1972). *On becoming a person.* Boston, MA: Houghton Mifflin.

Rollnick, S., Miller, W. R., & Butler, C. C. (2008). *Motivational interviewing in health care: Helping patients change behavior.* New York, NY: Guilford Press.

Rossen, J., Yngve, A., Hagströmer, M., Brismar, K., Ainsworth, B. E., Iskull, C., … Johansson, U.-B. (2015). Physical activity promotion in the primary care setting in pre- and type 2 diabetes—the Sophia step study, an RCT. *BMC Public Health, 15,* 647. doi:10.1186/s12889-015-1941-9

Rubak, S. Sandboek, A., Lauritzen, T., & Christensen, B. (2005). Motivational interviewing: A systematic review and meta-analysis. *British Journal of General Practice, 55*(513), 305–312. PMID:15826439

Smith, D. E., Heckemeyer, C. M., Kratt, P. P., & Mason, D. A. (1997). Motivational interviewing to improve adherence to a behavioral weight-control program for older obese women with NIDDM. A pilot study. *Diabetes Care, 20* (1), 52–54. PMID:9028693

Stewart, D. G., Siebert, E. C., Arit, V. K., Moise-Campbell, C., & Lehinger, E. (2016). READY or not: Findings from a school-based MI intervention for adolescent substance use. *Journal of Substance Abuse Treatment, 71,* 23–29. doi:10.1016/j.jsat.2016.08.007

Welch, G., Rose, G., & Ernst, D. (2006). Motivational interviewing and diabetes: What is it, how is it used, and does it work? *Diabetes Spectrum, 19*(1), 5–11. doi:10.2337/diaspect.19.1.5

West, D. S., DiLillo, V., Bursac, Z., Gore, S. A., & Greene, P. G. (2007). Motivational interviewing improves weight loss in women with type 2 diabetes. *Diabetes Care, 30*(5), 1081–1087. PMID:17337504

World Health Organization (WHO). (2016). *Global report: Diabetes Fact Sheet*. Geneva: World Health Organization. Retrieved from http://www.who.int /chp/chronic_disease_report/en/

CHAPTER 28

Collaborative Care to Promote Treatment Adherence and Effective Mental Health Care

CHAPTER OBJECTIVES

- Discuss the key elements of the collaborative care model which impact provider communications.
- Identify barriers to effective health care and treatment adherence for chronic diseases.
- Identify significant barriers to effective mental health care and medication adherence for persons with depressive disorders.
- Compare outcomes of collaborative care versus usual care for depression in primary care settings.
- Analyze the results of evidence-based evaluations of collaborative care programs, and the challenges ahead for providing underserved populations adequate collaborative care for depression.

KEY TERMS

- Adherence and nonadherence to treatment
- Adherence to medication
- Antidepressant medication
- Case manager
- Chronic disease
- Co-located mental health care

- Comorbidity
- Collaborative care model
- Evidence-based medical care
- Infectious disease
- Natural clusters of chronic illness
- Primary care settings

▶ Introduction

Communications in health care are significantly influenced by how care is organized and delivered. In Home visitation programs supplement traditional approaches, and have been shown, for example, to lead to better birth outcomes in high risk underserved populations (e.g., lower rates of preterm birth and higher birth weights). In Chapter 26, we explained how home visitation programs change communications for underserved pregnant women by essentially bringing the provider to the patient rather than relying solely on bringing the patient to the provider.

Home visitation (HV) approaches are different means of delivering needed health care services. They not only change the mode of communication but the exposure of the patient to health providers, essentially the amount of time spent or *dose* of provider time. This is important because more time spent can ultimately improve the relationship with the provider and yield substantially more information about the patient's needs. Furthermore, more information and a stronger patient–provider relationship can increase the patient's engagement in health care decision-making and **adherence** to treatment or lifestyle modifications.

Like HV programs, CC approaches are also different from the usual ways of delivering health care services. Like HV programs, CC approaches also significantly impact communication processes. Communications are different under CC compared to usual care. These differences occur at both the patient–family–provider and provider–provider level. Under CC, patients and families are exposed to a range of interventions varying in intensity and including several different health provider groups. The range of interventions can include scheduled telephone follow-up to encourage treatment adherence to complex arrangement of services to foster collaboration between health providers that are working on behalf of the patient's physical and psychological needs. Patients and their families are likely to be offered more opportunities to communicate with health providers and a wider range of provider specialists with whom to converse.

CC is unlike care as usual in **primary care settings** where one provider must respond to all presenting health conditions and medical management challenges. Historically, usual care is delivered by one provider specialty group (e.g., primary care specialists or specialists in internal medicine). These providers are not usually supported by ancillary service providers to meet the mental health needs of their primary care patients.

CC approaches work well with conditions in which there is a significant psychological component. This is particularly the case with **natural clusters of chronic illness**, e.g., depression and cardiovascular disease, cancer, or diabetes. Under **collaborative care models**, a *team* of providers interact to assess and provide necessary mental health care and follow-up to patients. CC facilitates communication between primary care providers and mental health specialists, either by virtue of physically locating them together as in **co-located systems** or by planned and executed exchange of information through multidisciplinary conferences, electronic message exchange, and telephone alert systems.

In this chapter, the focus is on CC models of health care as an option to care as usual for people with chronic illnesses. Specific attention is given to CC with depressed persons seen in primary care settings, and evidence of successful outcomes is enumerated. The evolution of

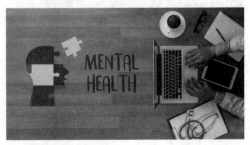

© One photo/Shutterstock.

the use of CC with depressed patient populations in primary care settings is best understood in the context of deficiencies that were documented during the previous two to three decades when primary care patient needs were addressed by primary care generalists, not mental health specialists. This approach was found to be inadequate in identifying and treating those patients with depression.

The CC model, designed to improve care outcomes, was a potential solution to improving the care of patients with depression who were only being seen in primary care settings and who would not encounter mental health services. In the section that follows, we explore elements of the care and treatment of chronic illnesses applicable to conditions requiring long-term assessment and monitoring for treatment adherence. The discussion focuses specifically on chronic illness, the need to assess and monitor treatment adherence in chronic illness, and how this is best achieved with CC.

▶ The Nature of Chronic Illness and Care Requirements

Chronic illness, the focus of this chapter on CC, is a major threat to health and well-being on both a national level and worldwide scale. According to the World Health Organization (WHO) **chronic disease** is the leading cause of mortality in the world (WHO, 2017).

Those diseases most often grouped in the category of chronic illness include cardiovascular disease, cancer, diabetes, and depression. The NIH explains that there are patterns in the distribution of chronic illness across groups, chronic conditions concern persons of all ages, from all incomes, and in every ethnic group. It is important to distinguish between groups that are likely to experience better outcomes as a result of better accessibility and more effective medical care. For example, although chronic conditions can be found in all populations, poor outcomes of care occur in some groups more than others. An example is the documented disparities in health and health care services among low-income populations, particularly those from underserved communities.

Chronic illnesses are distinguishable from communicable diseases. Chronic illnesses, regarded as non-communicable diseases, are frequently associated with certain lifestyle behaviors (e.g., smoking, diet, and exercise). Cardiovascular disease, obesity, and diabetes are examples. Unlike communicable diseases, chronic illnesses are not transmitted from one person to another. They also extend over longer periods, lasting 3 months or more. Adequate assessment and care of these conditions can prevent premature death and avoid unnecessary disability.

Infectious diseases or communicable diseases, on the other hand, are of shorter duration and can be prevented by vaccines or cured by medication. They include such diseases as tuberculosis, pneumonia, meningitis, Ebola virus, hepatitis, and sexually transmitted diseases and are particularly prevalent where access to vaccines, medication, clean water, and vector control is very limited. Certain communicable diseases occur in outbreaks or epidemics and are prevalent in underdeveloped countries but not in developed countries. There are exceptions; for example, upper respiratory disease is widespread in both underdeveloped and developed countries. In a recent report by WHO (2017), respiratory infections remained the most lethal communicable diseases, causing 3.2 million deaths worldwide in 2015.

Some upper respiratory conditions are quite prevalent in the United States and present a considerable public health problem; they include asthma and chronic obstructive pulmonary disease. Communicable diseases are both preventable and treatable. The prevalence of communicable disease is significantly reduced with immunization, public health awareness programs, outreach, and community engagement.

▶ The Importance of Treatment Adherence in the Management of Chronic Illness

Chronic illnesses require ongoing medical care and patient and family commitment to disease self-management if adequate control of symptoms and long-term disease management is to be achieved. The most important requirements in the effective management of chronic illness are the provision of **evidence-based medical care** and adequate self-management. Evidenced-based medical care meets professionally approved guidelines that are supported by clinical research evidence. These guidelines are generated from the scientific review and analysis of what works best. Health providers are responsible for evidenced-based care, but patients with chronic illness have an important role as well. Adequate self-management calls for patients and their families to follow prescribed treatments as instructed by health professionals. Adequate self-management includes continuous collaboration and communication with providers about effects of the treatment and any needs for change in the prescribed regimen.

Treatment adherence is recognized worldwide as essential to achieving treatment success. WHO (2003) defined adherence as "the extent to which a person's behavior—taking medication, following a diet, and/or executing lifestyle changes—corresponds with agreed recommendations from a health care provider." This definition was generated in a hallmark report on chronic disease and health promotion entitled *Adherence to Long-Term Therapies: Evidence for Action*. This call to action document stressed the point that treatment success relies on patient adherence.

Adherence to treatment is a significant predictor of adequate treatment and the reduction of disease-related morbidity. It is often discussed as either treatment or medication adherence, or both. Adherence to treatment guidelines (e.g., lifestyle changes, exercise and weight loss in the case of cardiovascular disease and diabetes) are ancillary requirements while **adherence to medication** regimens are primary. Medication adherence refers specifically to taking a medication or medications as directed in a prescription from an approved licensed health care professional.

Similar to the term *treatment adherence* is the term *medication adherence* which refers to patients taking their medications as prescribed with respect to timing, dosage, and frequency. The famous quote by Charles Everett Koop, M.D., former Surgeon General of the United States, "Drugs don't work in patients who don't take them" depicts the important principle underlying achieving effective medical care.

A term also seen in the literature to describe patient medication behavior patterns is *medication-taking persistence*. Medication-taking persistence refers to the extent to which patients continue to take a prescribed medication over time to achieve therapeutic outcomes. According to Cramer et al. (2008), it is the duration of time from initiation to discontinuation of therapy or drug treatment. Thus, adherence refers to the precision of drug use during treatment whereas *persistence* refers to the patient's dedication to medication therapy over time.

A critical and pervasive concern in health care worldwide is the extent to which proven treatment, if provided, is appropriately followed. The link between **nonadherence** and control over chronic illness is clear. Adequate treatment and medication adherence are complex phenomena influenced by many factors operating singularly or in combination. Medication and treatment adherence are not solely the responsibility of the patient and patient's family because the provider's lack of clear instructions, intolerable medication side effects, and demanding medication-taking schedules also contribute to whether patients do or do not follow their medication and treatment regimen.

Many factors have been examined for their association with treatment adherence

/nonadherence and are generally grouped into categories. WHO (2003) categorized these factors into five broad groupings: patient, condition, therapy, socioeconomic, and health system related. Understanding that there are many factors and their breadth and depth is important in designing strategies to improve medical care and enhance adherence behaviors. It also means that the search for only one solution is doomed from the outset. More realistically, a combination of patient-centered counseling along with system changes is needed. For example, the literature on improving medication adherence in patients with depression identifies the need for a system change as well as alterations in provider–patient relationships. Both changes are provided under CC and is the topic in the next section of this chapter.

▶ Depression: A Prominent Chronic Illness in Need of CC

Depression is a common condition worldwide. In fact, most people are surprised when they learn how common it is. WHO's recent fact sheet on depression (updated 2017) states that more than 300 million people of all ages suffer from depression. Furthermore, depression is the leading cause of disability and a major contributor to the overall global burden of disease worldwide. Pratt and Brody (2014), summarizing national survey data on the prevalence of depression in the United States. explained that for the period 2009–2012, 7.6% of Americans aged 12 and over had depression, defined as having moderate or severe depressive symptoms in the past 2 weeks.

Depression can either surface as a short-lived depressed mood or a long-term depressed condition. Based upon severity, it might present as either a mild depressive episode or major depression disorder. Most people will experience some level of depressed mood (feeling blue, down, empty, or sad) periodically but when these feelings persist for longer than two

consecutive weeks and are accompanied by feelings of hopelessness and failure to enjoy things previously eliciting pleasure, suspicion is raised that a more serious condition exists.

In its most severe versions, depression is a serious medical illness with a combination of mood, cognitive, and physical symptoms. Criteria used to distinguish a more serious condition include (1) depressed mood or loss of interest or pleasure present during at least two consecutive weeks; (2) feelings of hopelessness and pessimism, guilt, worthlessness, or helplessness; and (3) cognitive symptoms that include mild to moderate changes in concentration, memory, or ability to make decisions (American Psychiatric Association, 2013). Unlike other chronic conditions, there are no laboratory tests to provide a definitive diagnosis of depression. However, physical findings often include behaviors such as difficulty falling asleep or sleeping excessively (oversleeping) and appetite changes (e.g., overeating or lack of interest in eating which may be demonstrated in weight changes [e.g., weight gain or loss]).

There is evidence that depression is not declining significantly but rather, it may be escalating. The official document published by the U.S. Department of Health and Human Services (HHS), *Healthy People 2020*, has established definitive goals for reversing the escalating incidence of depression in every age group:

- Reduce the suicide rate.
- Reduce the proportion of persons who experience major depressive episodes among adolescents and among adults aged 18 years and older.
- Increase the proportion of adults aged 18 years and older with major depressive episodes who receive treatment.
- Increase depression screening by primary care providers.

Screening for depression is critical. Once screened and evaluated for the best possible treatment plan, patients are likely to be encouraged to take some category of **antidepressant medication** and/or participate in brief psychotherapy or counseling. In either case, treatment and medication adherence become significant concerns. As in the treatment of patients with chronic illnesses of many types, factors impacting treatment and medication adherence are multifaceted in patients experiencing depression.

Reviews of the literature on antidepressant medication adherence and programs that have been shown to improve antidepressant medication adherence illustrate this point. van Servellen, Heise, and Ellis (2011) found successful adherence enhancement programs to include similar targets of change as specified by WHO. These authors categorized factors as patient characteristics, patient health condition and **comorbidities**, therapy or treatment, patient–provider relationship, and health care system factors. Chong, Aslani, and Chen (2011) also summarized interventions that showed promise in promoting adherence to antidepressant medications. They identified and classified interventions as educational, behavioral, or multifaceted. Both articles described the value of multifaceted interventions over those that addressed only one factor known to improve adherence.

They also explained that multifaceted programs including patient education strategies, telephone follow-up to monitor patient response to treatment, and medication support and feedback to primary care providers were shown to significantly impact antidepressant medication adherence. Intervention programs showing significant improvement in outcomes were those that were more complex and multifaceted.

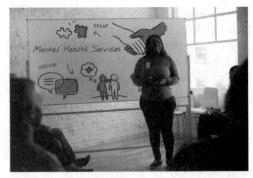

© Rawpixel.com/Shutterstock.

▶ CC Model: A Key to Improving Treatment Adherence and Quality of Depression Care

Multifaceted programs are believed to be critical in the delivery of quality depression care in primary care settings. In addition to adequate screening by primary care practitioners, proactive care management and involvement of mental health professionals are needed in promoting treatment adherence and improvements in depression symptoms in these patients.

In this chapter, CC approaches to improve depression care are explored. This approach in treating depression is particularly useful because it addresses the problem that mental health professionals are not involved in treating patients with depression who more likely go to primary care providers than mental health specialists. CC can make significant contributions by changing communications across provider groups. That is, primary care providers have better access to consultation from specialists trained in mental health.

A focus on CC does not mean that behavioral theories and approaches that have been shown to be efficacious counseling models to treat depression should be dismissed or set aside. As previously stated, depression is often treated with some form of counseling or psychotherapy using behavioral theories. These theories and psychotherapeutic approaches include: cognitive behavioral therapy (CBT), the interpersonal therapies, and problem-solving therapy. A focus on CC is in no way a suggestion that these therapies are no longer needed. Rather, they are frequently interventions used in conjunction with CC.

The CC model when applied to the treatment of persons with depression, illustrates how multifaceted programs can be effective in the organization of mental health services. From a communications perspective, CC emphasizes a team approach where care is designed and shared across an entire team of health providers including licensed mental health professionals and paraprofessionals. The major premise behind CC is that patients do better when care is organized to include a range of interventions varying in intensity from simple approaches (e.g., telephone intervention to encourage medication adherence) to a more complex arrangement of mental health services co-located with primary care.

The impetus for establishing CC as a model in the treatment of depression in primary care settings arose out of awareness that depression care was inaccessible to those who needed it and, when available, was very costly. The CC approach was viewed as a potential effective alternative. Early work by Wagner, Austin, Davis, Hindmarsh, Schaefer, and Bonomi (2001) outlined several important factors needed to improve the care of chronic illnesses, and this work laid a foundation for designing an effective CC approach for depression in primary care settings. They described obstacles patients faced in coping with their condition but also problems with current health care systems that do not adequately address patient and family needs for a wide range of services including psychological support and information.

This shared perspective was compatible with the observed needs to provide multifaceted programs in the organization of mental health care. CC was believed to enhance the systematic organization of primary care practice in the treatment of depression in primary care settings by providing closer follow-up, patient education, and monitoring of symptoms and treatment adherence by mental health specialists in primary care practice (Katon, Unützer, Wells, & Jones, 2010).

The CC model is an effective approach to organizing mental health services. It is particularly judicious because the largest proportion of people with depression is being treated in primary care settings, not mental health centers. With fewer if not any mental health services easily accessible to patients and their families something needed to change because primary care settings were not equipped to assess and meet the treatment needs of these patients.

Data showed that primary care physicians were likely to be the sole providers of care for many depressed patients, and early estimates suggested that 40% of those receiving mental health treatment were treated in the general medical health sector alone (Uebelacker, Wang, Berglund, & Kessler, 2006). More recent data on the treatment of depressed patients in primary care settings suggest that the bulk of mental health services for people with depression are still provided in primary care settings. In fact, Barkil-Oteo refers to primary care as the *de facto mental health system*. He further explains that primary care providers prescribe 79% of antidepressant medications and see nearly two-thirds of people in the United States being treated for depression (2013, p. 139).

While the majority of patients with depression could be receiving treatment from their primary care providers, this does not mean that this care meets professional treatment standards or that care is even minimally adequate. Psychiatrists are much more likely than primary care physicians and providers to provide adequate initial treatment and follow-up care after antidepressants are prescribed. The idea was then to pair these health professionals (primary care providers and psychiatrists) to maximize the possibility that primary care patients needing specialist care by a psychiatrist would receive this level of intervention. The change to organize care to suit a collaborative, integrated approach gained substantial professional support, and research funds from private and public sectors were distributed to implement and evaluate the outcomes of this multifaceted approach.

EXHIBIT 28-1 Summary of Elements of Depression Care in CC Programs

- Case management coordination of primary care and specialist care by social workers or nurses.
- Mental health specialist (usually a psychiatrist) serving as a consultant to primary care providers either proximally (co-located) or distally located to provide caseload supervision, and direct in-person follow-up with patients showing no improvement.
- Mental health specialist supervision of care including depression education, medication management, behavioral activation, and relapse prevention.
- Enhanced patient education with pamphlets, books, and video tapes.
- Allied health or mental health workers to provide closer patient follow-up to track care outcomes, adherence to medication regimens, and side effects of treatment frequently with the use of telephone contacts.
- Use of a formalized measurement tool: Patient Health Questionnaire-9 (PHQ-9). PHQ-9 systematically tracks treatment outcomes and patient progress.
- Development of an electronic depression register to enhance patient caseload supervision.
- Stepped-care approaches to provide incremental increases in intensity of care for those with persistent symptoms.
- In some cases, depression case manager provision of brief evidence-based psychotherapy to patients proactively identified through the screening process using the PHQ-9.

CC approaches harness a range of interventions to make a difference in depression care in primary care settings. As Gilbody, Bower, Fletcher, Richards, and Sutton explain (2006), CC approaches encompass interventions varying in intensity, ranging from something as basic as telephone follow-up to ensure medication adherence to more complex interventions that require extensive follow-up. These interventions may even incorporate psychosocial and psychotherapeutic interventions previously available in mental health centers and out of reach for many primary care patients.

A detailed list of CC interventions frequently implemented in these programs is provided in **EXHIBIT 28-1**. The list includes case management coordination of primary care and specialist care; mental health specialist intervention to provide patient assessment and treatment when needed but also primary care provider supervision of a caseload of depressed clients; education about depression and the importance of medication adherence which may include pamphlets, videotapes, or websites; close follow-up to track care outcomes;

adherence to and side effects of treatment; and the use of formalized measurement to assess levels of depression. The implementation of CC approaches created a significant reversal of lack of mental health specialist care in primary care settings.

▶ Evaluation of the Impact of CC on Depression Care in Primary Care Settings

CC approaches have been designed, implemented, and evaluated in a variety of settings in the United States and the United Kingdom. These approaches have included any number of the features outlined in Exhibit 28-1. In some studies, one or more interventions or elements might be missing. However, those features most often included are the provision of mental health specialists, team coordination between primary care and psychiatrist specialists, symptom recovery follow-up and treatment adherence monitoring, and enhanced patient education and self-care management skill training. Other, aspects (e.g., establishment of patient registries, brief psychotherapy [either group, individual, or both], and use of formalized measurement of depression symptoms) were also used but may not be incorporated in all CC models.

Most evaluations and research including summaries of literature reviews report significant positive effects of CC approaches over usual care in the short-term for adults with depression. There are also reports suggesting a number of positive secondary outcomes that occur including improved adherence to antidepressant medication regimens, mental health quality of life, and patient satisfaction. Examples of these studies are included in the Cited Study boxes. The following summaries provide details of two evidenced-based evaluations of CC approaches.

Bauer and colleagues (2006) evaluated the effectiveness of a CC approach compared to usual care in the treatment of bipolar patients discharged from 11 VA hospitals. The CC model included a specialty team consisting of a nurse care coordinator and psychiatrist, regular appointments supplemented by phone, and clinic contacts as needed. Elements of the program included enhancement of patients' skill in illness self-management through group psychoeducation and nurse **case manager** facilitation of information flow to the psychiatrist. The results showed that the length of mood episode (primarily mania) was reduced. Additionally, improvements were noted in social role function, mental quality of life, and treatment satisfaction.

Richards et al. (2016) examined the clinical effectiveness and cost-effectiveness of CC for depression in the United Kingdom; Collaborative Depression Trial care (CADET) compared usual care in the management of patients with moderate to severe depression in 51 primary care practices in three United Kingdom primary care districts. The intervention

included 14 weeks of 6–12 telephone contacts by care managers, mental health specialist supervision, depression education, medication management, behavioral activation, relapse prevention, and primary care liaison. Mean depression scores were lower for CC patients compared to usual care patients at 4 and 12 months. Quality of mental health but not physical health was better for CC patients, and CC patients were significantly more satisfied with their treatment. Cost estimates indicated that CC may be less costly and at the same time more clinically effective.

CC models have also been designed and studied for their effects on other mental health conditions (e.g., anxiety and panic disorders) (Roy-Byrne et al., 2009). In these instances, CC was also found to be more effective than care as usual. CC approaches with other chronic medical illnesses where depression and anxiety co-occur have been implemented and evaluated as well. These studies examined the impact of CC in patients with diabetes and depression (Kinder et al., 2006; Ell et al., 2010); cancer and depression (Dwight-Johnson, Ell, & Lee, 2005; Sharpe et al., 2014); and cardiovascular disease patients recently undergoing coronary artery bypass graft surgery who were experiencing depression (Rollman, Mazumdar, Belnap, Houck, Lenze, & Schulberg, 2010; Katon et al., 2010). The results of these studies and others supported the continued implementation of CC models in primary care settings and with a wide range of chronic illnesses.

There is substantial evidence to support the potential of CC approaches to remove the sizable gaps in care of patients with depression as both a primary and secondary condition in primary care settings. Archer and colleagues in their extensive review of the literature (2012) concluded that CC was more efficacious than routine care in treating patients with depression and anxiety. Mechanic (2012) explained that CC for mental health could reduce costs over time and across a range of both mental and physical health problems through the organization of collaborative services. Finally, Gilbody and colleagues (2006) warned that providing better clinical outcomes through changes in the way mental health services are provided means greater costs, not lower costs, but they also stressed that CC has been shown to be of "good economic value," and has demonstrated sufficient evidence to support wide-scale dissemination.

In summary, CC approaches have shown promise in addressing the gap of mental health services for people seen in primary care settings, and in providing better treatment of persons with a range of chronic medical illnesses where depression and/or anxiety occur. CC models have provided strong evidence of their effectiveness in improving depression symptoms, increasing treatment adherence, response to treatment, and remission and recovery from depressive disorders. In recognition of the effectiveness of CC approaches, the Community Preventive Services Task Force in 2012 supported the use and dissemination of CC in primary care settings.

Before concluding this review of CC approaches, it is important to provide cautionary remarks about generalizing these positive outcomes to all patient populations in all settings. First, caution is needed because in some cases short-term positive effects did not prevail over the long term, and recent documentation of problems in using CC approaches redirect our attention to the obvious and more subtle barriers to wide-scale dissemination of CC. In a thoughtful review of the state of the science, Sanchez (2017) enumerated various barriers to CC dissemination across systems of care and outside the parameters of funded and tightly controlled clinical trials. She listed three categories of barriers to wide-scale dissemination and sustainability of CC: (1) clinical barriers (e.g., lack of primary care provider knowledge of depression treatment guidelines) and patient-level barriers (e.g., fears of stigma associated with depression and its treatment); (2) organizational barriers (e.g.,

lack of provider time to conduct a comprehensive evaluation of mental health concerns and work force shortages); and (3) financial barriers (e.g., funding and reimbursement for mental health services provided). Attention to these barriers is important if there is to be progress in implementing CC.

▶ Summary

The efforts to transform mental health care in the United States have a substantial history dating back to studies describing the prevalence of depression in primary care patients that were without depression care or when this care was provided it was inadequate. CC is a multifaceted approach to quality care for persons with depression. It is distinguishable by its design which not only facilitates the possibility that patients with depression are identified, assessed, and appropriately treated but that primary care providers working with depressed persons communicate collaboratively with mental health specialists to deliver improved depression management of their primary care patients. This approach is also referred to as *integrated care* because it facilitates the provision of patient-centered care which is holistic and delivered by a multidisciplinary team of health care professionals.

The evolution of the use of CC with depressed patients and their families in primary care settings is best understood in the context of deficiencies that were documented during the previous two to three decades. The CC model, designed to improve care outcomes of people with chronic illness, was one potential answer to improving the care to patients with depression who were being seen in primary care settings and might not encounter professional mental health providers.

There is ample evidence of positive outcomes with CC programs in the literature spanning the last three or more decades. Much of the evidence reports significant positive outcomes that exceed those of usual care in primary care settings. Still, caution is important in generalizing positive findings across studies due to differences in how these programs are organized and implemented.

As previously explained, CC approaches can include a wide range of interventions (from simple telephone prompting to promote medication adherence to short-term psychiatric or psychosocial counseling). To date, identification of what interventions are vital to its success and which add less value needs to be addressed. Identifying what elements are most essential with which populations is necessary to ensure that the most effective aspects are retained, and this is done in the context of cost containment. Gilbody and colleagues (2006) stated that the effectiveness of CC approaches remain unclear as does knowledge of what elements determine effective outcomes, knowledge critical to those who want to establish CC in their communities, and primary care settings.

In conclusion, CC can potentially transform health care communications in the following ways. Both patient–family–provider and provider–provider communications are enhanced. Furthermore, CC adds to the number of patient–provider contacts, ensures the delivery of patient education and needed support services, and provides specialist supervision from mental health professionals trained and experienced in mental health assessments and antidepressant medication adherence.

🔎 CITED STUDY: Treatment of Depression in Low-Income Primary Care Patients with Co-located Care

One approach to facilitate the collaboration of care with depressed patients in primary care settings is co-located health care. In this study, the researchers describe CC in a large primary care practice in the United States with co-located mental health care. They also examined predictors of receiving any treatment and receiving adequate treatment. They approached patients with a minimum level of depression symptoms and asked them to assess their mental health service use, depression symptoms, and any related problems.

Uebelacker, L. A., Smith, M., Lewis, A. W., Sasaki, R., & Miller, I. W. (2009). Treatment of depression in a low-income primary care setting with co-located mental health care. *Families, Systems & Health: The Journal of Collaborative Family Healthcare, 27*(2), 161–171. doi:10.1037/a0015847

An important and positive finding was that most of the 91 patients (83%) with elevated depressive symptoms received some type of mental health care ($n = 91$). The investigators emphasized that these patients were appropriately identified as needing help.

The investigators speculated that reasons for improved care might include the feature that access to mental health services was effectively co-located in this primary care practice setting. Identifying patients' need for help is the first step in establishing a program of care. However, findings were not all positive in that only half of the patients in the sample were receiving "minimally adequate care."

Furthermore, minority patients were less likely to receive any care. The authors concluded that while co-located mental health care might be advantageous there is need for improvement. They stressed that an important step would be ensuring patients received at the minimum, adequate care. Furthermore, other more severely depressed patients may need more intensive mental health care.

🔎 *CITED STUDY: Clinical Effectiveness of a Collaborative Care Model for Depression Collaborative Depression Trial Care (CADET) in the United Kingdom*

These researchers indicated that while there was evidence of the effectiveness of CC in managing depression in the United States, there was little evidence that the same outcomes would occur in the United Kingdom where the delivery of care differs. Using a cluster randomized controlled trial they examined both the effectiveness and cost-effectiveness of a CADET in 51 primary care practices in three primary care districts. Researchers blinded to a treatment or control group collected data on depression, anxiety, and quality of life outcomes as well as patients' level of satisfaction with the quality of the care received in a sample of 581 adults ages 18 or older who had a current diagnosis of depressive episode.

Richards, D.A., Richards, D.A., Bower, P., Chew-Graham, C., Gask, L., Lovell, K., et al. (2016). Clinical effectiveness and cost-effectiveness of CC for depression in UK primary care (CADET): A cluster randomised controlled trial. *Health Technology Assessment, 20*(14), 1–192. doi:10.3310 /hta20140

The CC intervention included 14 weeks of 6–12 telephone contacts by case managers. Additionally, mental health specialists provided supervision which included depression education, medication management, behavioral activation, relapse prevention, and primary care liaison.

Results indicated that the CC group had significantly lower mean depression scores at 4 and 12 months. Also, patients reported quality of mental health but not physical health was significantly better in the CC group at 4 months but not 12 months. Patients in the CC group were also significantly more satisfied with their treatment compared to patients in the control (usual) care group. These investigators concluded that CADET had continuous positive effects up to 12 months on several of their outcome measures, and there was indication that the program would be preferred over usual care.

🔎 *EVIDENCE FOR/MORE TO KNOW BOX: CC and the Treatment of Depression in Primary Care Settings*

Evidence for

- CC approaches are organizational interventions that have a direct impact on the kind and amount of communication between health providers and patients, potentially enhancing care collaboration across the health team (e.g., between mental health specialists and primary care providers).
- There is evidence that CC approaches improve depression and can be significantly better in the care and management of depression in primary settings than care as usual.
- In some cases, improvements in depression with CC have been shown to persist up to 12 months, which is preferred by patients over usual care.

More to Know

- The similarities and differences between various CC models are not fully understood.
- The relative effectiveness of one model over the other is unknown. For example, are co-located CC models more effective than other CC models?
- The contributions of various components of CC to its overall effectiveness are unclear. For example, the relative contribution of telephone follow-up to assess and promote continued antidepressant medication adherence over all other aspects of the program is unclear.
- Recent discussions of the fate of depression CC approaches identify significant clinical, organizational, and financial barriers to its wide-scale implementation, the extent to which these barriers have or will interfere with implementation is unknown.

🔍 MUST READ BOX: Collaborative Depression Care: History and Evolution

Katon, W., Unützer, J., Wells, K., & Jones, L. (2010). Collaborative depression care: History, evolution and ways to enhance dissemination and sustainability. *General Hospital Psychiatry, 32*(5), 456–464. doi:10.1016/j.genhosppsych.2010.04.001

This informative summary of the evolution of CC approaches in the treatment of depression in primary care settings summarizes the implementation and evaluation of CC programs over a span of 30 years (1980s through 2010) in the United States. The article explains the impetus for major changes in how depression was assessed and treated due to serious gaps and ineffective access to depression care resources.

Data showed that the majority of persons needing depression care were being treated in primary care settings, not mental health centers. Specific CC practice examples are discussed such as the IMPACT (Improving Mood – Promoting Access to Collaborative Treatment) program, the DIAMOND (Depression Improvement Across Minnesota, Offering a New Direction) project, as well as comprehensive programs combining the treatment of diabetes and heart disease and comorbid depression. The importance of effective community engagement in populations of people of underserved impoverished patients when planning, designing, implementing, and evaluating CC approaches is emphasized.

Discussion

1. What factors impact health care and treatment adherence in persons with chronic illness?

2. What are the critical elements of CC approaches, and how do they impact communications between patient and provider and provider to provider?

3. Can CC models be routinely implemented in primary care settings? If not, why not?

4. Do CC approaches applied to the treatment of depression in primary care settings offer a sustained benefit over the long term? How would we study this question?

5. What is meant by the concept of implementing CC in "natural clusters of chronic illness"?

References

American Psychiatric Association. (2013). *Diagnostic and statistical manual of mental disorders (DSM–5)* (5th ed.). Arlington, VA: American Psychiatric Association.

Archer, J., Bower, P., Gilbody, S., Lovell, K., Richards, D., Gask, L., ... Coventry, P. (2012). Collaborative care for depression and anxiety problems. *Cochrane Database Systematic Review, 10*, CD006525. doi:10.1002/14651858.CD006525.pub2

Barkil-Oteo, A. (2013). Collaborative care for depression in primary care: How psychiatry could "troubleshoot" current treatments and practices. *The Yale Journal of Biology and Medicine, 86*(2), 139–146. PMID:23766735

Bauer, M. S., McBride, L., Williford, W. O., Glick, H., Kinosian, B., Altshuler, L., ... Sajatovic, M. (2006). Collaborative care for bipolar disorder: Part II. Impact on clinical outcome, function, and costs. *Psychiatric Services, 57*(7), 927–936. doi:10.1176/ps.2006.57.7.937

Chong, W. W., Aslani, P., & Chen, T. F. (2011). Effectiveness of interventions to improve antidepressant medication adherence: A systematic review. *International Journal of Clinical Practice, 65*(9), 954–975. doi:10.1111/j.1742-1241.2011.02746.x

Cramer, J. A., Roy, A., Burrell, A., Fairchild, C. J., Fuldeore, M. J., Ollendorf, D.A., ... Wong, P. K. (2008). Medication compliance and persistence: Terminology and definitions. *Value Health, 11*, 44–47. doi:10.1111/j.1524-4733.2007.00213.x

Dwight-Johnson, M., Ell, K., & Lee, P. J. (2005). Can collaborative care address the needs of low-income Latinas with comorbid depression and cancer? Results from a randomized pilot study. *Psychosomatics, 46*(3), 224–232.doi:10.1176/appi.psy.46.3.224

Ell, K., Katon, W., Xie, B., Lee, P. J., Kapetanovic, S., Guterman, J., & Chou, C. P. (2010). Collaborative care management of major depression among low- income, predominantly Hispanic subjects with diabetes: A randomized controlled trial. *Diabetes Care, 33*(4), 706–713. doi:10.2337/dc09-1711

Gilbody, S., Bower, P., Fletcher, J., Richards, D., & Sutton, A. J. (2006). Collaborative care for depression: A cumulative meta-analysis and review of longer-term outcomes. *Archives of Internal Medicine, 166*(21), 2314–2321. doi:10.1111/j.1742-1241.2011.02746.x

Healthy People 2020. Washington, DC: U.S. Department of Health and Human Services, Office of Disease Prevention and Health Promotion. Retrieved from Healthypeople.gov

Katon, W., Unützer, J., Wells, K., & Jones, L. (2010). Collaborative depression care: History, evolution and ways to enhance dissemination and sustainability. *General Hospital Psychiatry, 32*(5). doi:10.1016/j.genhosppsych.2010.04.001

Kinder, L. S., Katon, W. J., Ludman, E., Russo, J., Simon, G., Lin, E. H., ... Young, B. (2006). Improving depression care in patients with diabetes and multiple complications. *Journal of General Internal Medicine,21*(10), 1036–1041. doi:10.1111/j.1525-1497.2006.00552.x

Mechanic, D. (2012). Seizing opportunities under The Affordable Care Act for transforming the mental and behavioral health system. *Health Affairs, 31*(2), 376–382. doi:10.1377/hlthaff.2011.0623

Pratt, L. A., & Brody, D. J. (2014). *Depression in the U.S. household population, 2009–2012*. NCHS Data Brief No. 172. Hyattsville, MD: National Center for Health Statistics. 2014.

Richards, D. A., Richards, D. A., Bower, P., Chew-Graham, C., Gask, L., Lovell, K., & Russell, A. (2016). Clinical effectiveness and cost-effectiveness of collaborative care for depression in UK primary care (CADET): A cluster randomised controlled trial. *Health Technology Assessment, 20*(14), 1–192. doi:10.3310/hta20140

Rollman, B., Mazumdar, S., Belnap, B. H., Houck, P., Lenze, E., & Schulberg H. (2010). Main outcomes from the RELAX Trial of telephone-delivered collaborative care for panic and generalized anxiety disorder. *Journal of General Internal Medicine, 25*, S326. doi:10.1007/s11606-010-1355-4

Roy-Byrne, P., Veitengruber, J. P., Bystritsky, A., Edlund, M. J., Sullivan, G., Craske, M. G., ... Stein, M. B. (2009). Brief intervention for anxiety in primary care patients. *Journal of the American Board of Family Medicine : JABFM, 22*(2), 175–186. doi:10.3122/jabfm.2009.02.08007

Sanchez, K. (2017). Collaborative care in real-world settings: Barriers and opportunities for sustainability. *Patient Preference and Adherence, 11*, 71–74. doi:10.2147/PPA.S120070

Sharpe, M., Walker, J., Hansen, C. H., Martin, P., Symeonides, S., Gourley, C., ... Murray, G. (2014). Integrated collaborative care for comorbid major depression in patients with cancer (SMaRT Oncology-2): A multicentre randomised controlled effectiveness trial. *Lancet, 384*(99448), 1099–1108. doi:10.1016/S0140-6736(14)61231-9

Uebelacker, L. A., Smith, M., Lewis, A. W., Sasaki, R., & Miller, I. W. (2009). Treatment of depression in a low-income primary care setting with co-located mental health care. *Families, Systems & Health: The Journal of Collaborative Family Healthcare, 27*(2), 161–171. doi:10.1037/a0015847

Uebelacker, L. A., Wang, P. S., Berglund, P., Kessler, R. C. (2006). Clinical differences among patients treated for mental health problems in general medical and specialty mental health settings in the National Comorbidity Survey Replication. *General Hospital Psychiatry, 28*(5), 387–395. doi:10.1016/j.genhosppsych.2006.05.001

van Servellen, G., Heise, B. A., & Ellis, R. (2011). Factors associated with antidepressant medication adherence and adherence-enhancement programmes: A systematic literature review. *Mental Health in Family Medicine, 8*(4), 255–271. PMID:23205067

Wagner, E. H., Austin, B. T., Davis, C., Hindmarsh, M., Schaefer, J., & Bonomi, A. (2001). Improving chronic illness care: Translating evidence into action. *Health Affairs, 20*(6), 64–78. doi:10.1377/hlthaff.20.6.64

World Health Organization. (2003). *Adherence to Long-Term Therapies: Evidence for Action.* Retrieved from who.int World Health Organization (February 2017). Depression. Fact Sheet. Retrieved from www.who.int /topics/mental_health/factsheets/en/

CHAPTER 29

Communications for Advance Care Planning

CHAPTER OBJECTIVES

- Discuss the concept of shared decision-making in health care and advance care planning (ACP).
- Define the concept of patient-centered and family-centered care (PCFCC).
- Describe the impact of decisional conflict (DC) on health care decision-making and ACP.
- Discuss the role of decision aids (DAs) in facilitating communications about ACP.
- Analyze the results of evidence-based evaluations of the use of DAs in easing ACP.

KEY TERMS

- Advance care planning (ACP)
- Advance Directives (ADs)
- Bereavement counseling
- Comfort care
- Decision aids (DAs)
- Decisional conflict (DC)
- End-of-life care (EOLC)
- End-of-life (EOL) decision-making
- Hospice care
- Life-sustaining/life-prolonging treatment

- Palliative care
- Patient-centered and family-centered care (PCFCC)
- Patient Self-Determination Act (PSDA)
- Physician Orders for Life-Sustaining Treatment (POLST)
- Medical Orders for Life-Sustaining Treatment (MOLST)
- Shared decision-making (SDM)
- Transitional care

▶ Introduction

There are many instances in which compassionate communication is both appropriate and essential in assisting patients and their families facing serious illness. Clearly one instance is in the collaborative processes of **end-of-life (EOL) decision-making** and **advance care planning (ACP)**. These processes are not always clear to or accepted by patients and families. Patient and family cultural and religious beliefs play a role in their understanding and acceptance of EOL decision-making and ACP discussions with health providers. For example, some ethnic, cultural, and religious groups or individuals and families prefer not to be directly informed of a life-threatening diagnosis and prefer that the patient's condition and treatment decisions be discussed with family members only. Direct discussions of ACP and **advanced directives (ADs)** may be viewed as potentially harmful to the patient's well-being.

EOL and ACP refer to different processes. Typically, EOL decision-making involves discussions about the type of care desired at the EOL. ACP is the deliberate step to specify patients' preferences for care in the event that they are unable to articulate their wishes at a later time. EOL decision-making and ACP are often fraught with uncomfortable emotions which can include anticipatory grieving and regret on the part of the patient and patient's family (Djulbegovic, Tsalatsanis, Mhaskar, Hozo, Miladinovic, & Tuch, 2016). It is for these reasons and others that some families view these discussions as potentially harmful. For these reasons, health providers must be respectful of different cultural and religious beliefs and preferences while at the same time providing compassionate caring. Uncomfortable emotions, although natural and expected, are cushioned when health care providers can respect and engage patients and their families in compassionate ways.

ACP is an aspect of EOL decision-making which involves discussions about the type of care desired when faced with a wide range of options (e.g., choosing or refusing cardiopulmonary resuscitation, whether to go to the hospital or not, whether nutrition or hydration will be delivered with intravenous feeding, use of future interventions directed toward a cure, and discontinuing potentially other life-saving treatments).

In the current health care delivery system, there can be misalignment between what the care patients want during a serious illness and the medical care they actually receive from health care providers. Unfortunately, people do not know how or do not feel empowered to speak up about the kind of care they want. This

is due in part by their lack of understanding of this process. However, health care providers may not be adequately trained or have the opportunity to talk with patients about their treatment options and preferences and to discuss these issues with family members.

When it does happen, the process sometimes consists of discussions filled with medical jargon or hypotheticals because this is what providers understand and feel competent in discussing. What is absent is meaningful communications about patients' care preferences, cultural and religious beliefs and preferences, values, and goals over time. When communications are not clear and thorough, these conversations can short-circuit the process. Unfortunate outcomes include not only that these issues are not fully accounted for but that incomplete conversations can too easily lead to providers' use of aggressive care. Aggressive care provisions are not always compatible with patients' beliefs, interests, or values.

EOL and ACP discussions come to the forefront with the management of a chronic life-threatening illness (e.g., heart disease, kidney or liver failure, and cancers) at their advanced stage. These are times when failure to recover is clear but these processes are also relevant when considering that some unexpected accident might occur and render people incapable of verbalizing their preferences for care at that time.

In what can be a difficult time where communications might falter, beyond compassionate caring, **decision aids (DAs)** if appropriate can be used to guide patients, their families,

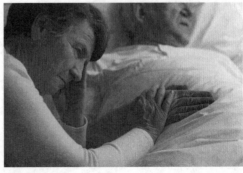

© Photographee.eu/Shutterstock.

and health care providers' discussions. In this chapter, issues and evidence related to providing ACP by minimizing **decisional conflict (DC)** and using DAs are addressed.

▶ Guided Health Care Decision-Making

Before discussing in depth the special circumstance of health care to patients facing EOL decisions, it is important to recognize that other medical situations call for similar approaches to ensure that patients' preferences are recognized and supported. Many patients, at some point, are presented with a wide range of decisions that may be very important but are not always EOL decisions. In these cases, decisions are also influenced by patients' specific cultural and religious beliefs.

Typically, these decisions focus on such treatment and health screening decisions to (1) enroll in a new treatment; (2) take or discontinue a medication; (3) have elective surgery; (4) choose invasive or noninvasive surgery; (5) undergo cancer screening and genetic testing; (6) prenatal screening; (7) terminate/not terminate a pregnancy; (8) decisions about contraception and immunization; and (9) choice of analgesic or anesthesia. These decisions are aided by discussions with various health professionals but never replace discussions with patients' physicians or board-certified specialists.

The general concept used to describe the process of decision-making is referred to as **shared decision-making (SDM)** and is appropriate for all health issues as well as **end-of-life care (EOLC)**. The goal of SDM is to better align patient preferences with treatment options. The following examples illustrate the issues inherent in achieving SDM. Consider what might be the appropriate provider-guided health care discussions in **EXHIBITS 29-1 to 29-3**.

EXHIBIT 29-1 Case Study: Facing Decisions About Initiating Kidney Dialysis

Making the decision to receive kidney dialysis treatment, like many other potentially life-extending treatments, requires SDM in the context of the patient's health status and treatment options. Kidney dialysis is a treatment or procedure to compensate for failing kidney function. It provides many patients a chance to live longer productive lives but the decision to go on kidney dialysis is not, in every instance, an easy one.

Typically, kidney dialysis requires three weekly visits to the dialysis center and results in fatigue as well as diet and travel restrictions. Increasing numbers of people over 75 years old with renal failure are having to decide whether to go on treatment or not. Mortality in the first year even on dialysis is high for this age group (approaching 40%).

Patients and their families are sometimes not adequately informed about the stringent treatment regimen and what this might mean for the patient's overall quality of life. They may only hear that if the patient does not go on dialysis they will die. For some patients, the possibility of living up to 1 or 2 years without discomfort, fatigue, and the imposition of frequent trips to the treatment center, the preferred option is to forego dialysis.

Still, other patients and/or families may choose a decision based upon what the health provider thinks is necessary to save a life even though this is not the primary concern of the patient. Also, providers may not always provide a clear picture of the treatment risks or burdens.

Provider-guided health care decision-making would include a complete review of the patient's health status including other chronic illness conditions impacting the quality of their life and life expectancy. Additionally, what kidney failure is and whether dialysis is a temporary treatment prior to kidney transplant surgery needs to be clarified either to the patient or in other cases to the family. The benefits of dialysis and the quality of life burden when receiving dialysis should be discussed. Patients and families need to know what happens if they choose to stop dialysis. Physicians have an obligation to recognize how cultural and religious beliefs might play a role and provide a clear and frank discussion with the patient and/or family.

EXHIBIT 29-2 Case Study: Genetic Testing Followed by Treatment for Prostate Cancer

Patients and their families interested in genetic testing in order to make the best decision about choices of preventive procedures for certain cancers will want and need to have open discussions with their health providers. Patients and families concerned about their risk for ovarian, breast, and prostate cancer need to be sufficiently educated and informed about genetic testing procedures. Each of these cancers has been shown to be linked to BRCA1 and 2 mutations. They will need to know how to interpret genetic findings and what next steps are advisable.

For example, men with BRCA1 or 2 mutations have a higher risk of prostate cancer. Genetic tests for these cancers are available, and in the case of prostate cancer, men at high-risk are advised to have discussions with their health care provider about plans for prostate cancer screening based upon all of risk factors that apply to them. Men, with or without a family history of prostate cancer, may seek genetic testing along with early monitoring of their prostate-specific antigen (PSA) level. However, there is evidence that prostate cancer, with the exception of more aggressive types, usually grows very slowing (men may not die from this form of cancer), so decisions about genetic testing might be seem irrelevant.

In fact, evidence about testing influenced decision-making. Reasons for initial concern about testing were that a high percentage of false positives could cause potentially harmful side effects from aggressive treatment. Hence, the decision to do PSA testing has been controversial. A federal panel recently changed its position and now recommends this decision be an individual one. An individual's decision is based upon their desire to avoid the chance of dying of prostate cancer. Still, no matter what the evidence says, they might choose aggressive prostate cancer treatment. Others may decide that the severe side effects from aggressive treatment are not worth it.

Provider-guided health care decision-making would include review of what is prostate cancer disease, explanations of what screening means, the chances of false positives, the treatment available, and its side effects. These are issues that must be discussed, and the discussion must be done in an open-minded, supportive manner. With men who have family members with prostate cancer or who may have died from the disease, compassionate understanding of how these events may have shaped the patient's and families' perspectives and decision is critical. Again, knowing the cultural and religious beliefs of these patients and their families will give providers additional insight in what these decisions might be.

EXHIBIT 29-3 Case Study: Choosing Between Noninvasive or Invasive Surgery with a Diagnosis of Breast Cancer

Too much concern about the likelihood of a life-threatening cancer is relevant to discussions about screening and treating for breast cancer as well as prostate cancer. Breast cancer is a common form of cancer, and while occurring mostly in women, may also be diagnosed in men. When a diagnosis of breast cancer is made, a sequence of steps is taken to ensure decision-making is consistent with clinical evidence but also respects the patient's unique beliefs, values, and fears. For example, some women prior to having a discussion of the clinical findings relevant to their specific case may choose a more aggressive but unnecessary surgical procedure.

Providers take into account all risk factors including the patient's history, size of tumor, how invasive the cancer is, genetic testing, and family history of ovarian and breast cancer. Their discussions with patients can significantly impact women's perceptions of their risk and what treatment they choose. In a publication by Esserman and colleagues (2014), the use of certain terminology might sway the patient in one direction or another.

Provider-guided health care decision-making would include a review of breast cancer and disease stages, explanations of what level of treatment matches the patient's clinical diagnosis, the likelihood that the cancer would return given each treatment option, and the side effects and consequences of choosing one treatment over another. These topics are covered with patients and/or their families.

As in the case of the decision about aggressive treatment to protect against prostate cancer these patients and families must also be spoken to in a supportive, nonjudgmental manner. Providers need to respect patients' underlying fears and beliefs. As with patients facing prostate cancer, women with breast cancer may have family members or close friends with aggressive breast cancer or who may have died from the disease. Compassionate understanding about how these events may have shaped the patient's and family's perspectives and decisions are also critical in these discussions.

The examples presented here are just a few of the several significant diagnostic and treatment decisions facing individuals and their families. The nature of the decision and recommended resolution highly depend upon the latest technology and advanced medical knowledge and research as well as the SDM process itself, whatever that might be. This shared decision-making process will need to consider all those unique and shared beliefs that influence the patient and family.

In summary, to encouráge patients and/or families to participate in the decision-making process, providers need to be fully aware of how these decisions interface with cultural and religious beliefs and family values. If patients and families are fully informed about decisions to be made they are more likely to feel confident in participating in these discussions. Feeling that one has no other choice than that recommended by the provider and no clear picture of the treatment benefits or risks are might defeat the intent of the SDM process but be appropriate if families prefer these decisions be made by their health providers. In the next section we focus on effective SDM under circumstances of ACP.

▶ SDM and ACP

SDM and ACP refer basically to the process of engaging patients and families in decisions and preferences about medical care. Patients and their families may express dissatisfaction with treatment when they feel excluded from this decision-making process. Other patients and families would not react in this way but welcome more extensive guidance by health professionals. In recognition of patients' lack of information about their medical care and in respect for their rights to be informed decision makers, the United States enacted the **Patient Self-Determination Act (PSDA)** in 1991. The PSDA requires patients be informed of their rights regarding decisions about their own medical care, and ensures that these rights are communicated by their health care provider.

The American Academy of Family Physicians strengthened these recommendations by maintaining that EOL and ACP decision-making reflect cultural values. To paraphrase this recommendation, care at the EOL should recognize, assess, and address the psychological, social, spiritual/religious issues, and cultural beliefs of patients and their families. This addition recognizes that different cultures may require significantly different approaches.

The concept of SDM is also detailed in the values for **patient-centered and family-centered care (PCFCC)**. PCFCC is an approach to patient care that requires that planning, delivery, and evaluation of health care is grounded in mutually beneficial partnerships between patients, families, and health care providers. This process speaks directly to the value of including family members, often the patient surrogates and/or caregivers at the EOL, in decisions about patient care. The inclusion of families is particularly helpful in understanding patients' decisions based upon personal values and cultural preferences.

Including families also address any uncertainty or stress they experience related to their family member's care.

Patient participation in informed SDM is vital in all health care and treatment decision, and particularly with ACP. As previously explained, ACP refers to patients' rights to express preferences for care in the event that they are unable to articulate their wishes at a later time. Aspects of ACP cover preferences for **life-sustaining treatments** and treatment for a life-limiting illness.

Decisions related to ACP also include the choice of **comfort care** over life-sustaining treatments. *Comfort care* is medical care given to persons near the end of their life while foregoing life-sustaining treatment to soothe the dying process. Note that comfort care is also provided to patients receiving **palliative care** who are suffering from symptoms such as pain but are not near the EOL. The goals are to prevent or relieve physical and emotional suffering as much as possible. It is done in the context of protecting the patients' quality of life and respecting their preferences.

Palliative care is a specific kind of medical intervention tailored to the seriously ill. Palliative care may be administered even when the patient is still receiving curative treatment. The intent of palliative care is to maintain or improve the quality of life of both patients and their families facing a serious illness. It includes relief from the symptoms, pain, and stress of a serious illness.

Palliative care is available even when patients are newly diagnosed with a serious illness and need comfort but also relief from the symptoms they are experiencing arising from the serious illness. Palliative care can include offering psychological and spiritual support to the patient and family to help them cope with the stresses of the diagnosis and implications of the diagnosis. **Bereavement counseling** is a specific type of support to families but is usually reserved for the stage when there is little hope for recovery and families are anticipating the loss of their loved one.

As the health of patients worsen, care may be transferred to different settings. The process of transitioning from one care setting to another is addressed specifically in the guidelines for **transitional care**. Transitional care refers to the coordination and continuity of medical and health care when the patient leaves one care setting and moves to another. For example, patients may be transferred from the hospital to home or hospital to nursing home or assisted living facility, home to assisted living, or hospital to rehabilitation center. Patients may move multiple times from one care setting to another.

In the case that the patient's health is declining without the possibility of improvement, patients may be transferred to **hospice care**. Hospice care may include comfort care as well. It can be given in the home, a separate free-standing hospice care center, the hospital, nursing home, or other long-term care facility.

In most cases it is given in the home. Hospice care focuses on caring, not curing and is available to patients of all ages and with all illnesses. In skilled nursing facilities, trained hospice staff members are dedicated to providing compassionate care. There is no attempt to treat the illness. Comfort care is at the core of hospice care or EOLC. The primary purpose is to provide supportive, compassion care to the patient and family caregivers, and bereavement counseling may be continued or begun depending upon the family's needs and preferences.

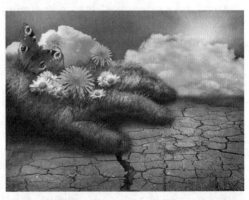

© SidlikS/Shutterstock.

▶ Compassion and Its Role in Advance Care Planning

Compassionate caring is a value and ethical principle underlying all health care delivery. Health care professionals need skill and knowledge in communicating with patients facing controversial treatment decisions and **end of life (EOL) decision-making**. The term compassionate care stems from the concept of compassion as a feeling, sometimes described as empathy or sympathy, and the action that stems from this feeling. Sinclair and colleagues (2016b) explain that compassion is defined as the "suffering with" or a deep awareness of the suffering of another person together with a desire to relieve this suffering.

ACP provides an opportunity for providers to engage the patient and/or patient's family in SDM. This action uses cognitive skills to present evidence and explain the probability of treatment effect but most importantly it calls for providers' abilities to communicate with empathy and understanding. It must include openness and appreciation of patients' and families' unique experience, fears and concerns, and their religious and cultural beliefs that shape their perceptions.

There is a clear role for compassionate caring in the process of facilitating ACP which occurs in the context of the human experience of life and death. For patients and families whose religious and cultural beliefs are central to their experience, these beliefs may or may not be mixed with powerful emotions. These emotions may impact their very ability to focus on the tasks of decision-making. Denying the presence of these feelings and their potential role in the ACP process is not only detrimental to the patient and family but unethical. Showing compassion is vital to this process and when needed is rarely forgotten by the patient and family.

Compassionate care is a professional prerequisite and is necessary to achieving quality patient care. It is expected and needed by patients and their families. While these skills are very important, there is evidence that providers neither fully understand compassion nor are they competent in delivering compassionate care. These concerns stem from observations that patients are ill-informed, feel they have little choice in their treatment, and observations of providers' lack of compassion in discussions with patients and their families.

These observations raise questions about whether health professionals are actually equipped to adequately communicate and prepared to address the increasing challenges they will face in the future. Concerns have also been directed at gaps in health care professional education and training with the suspicion that preparation in delivering compassionate care is lacking. In recognition of the potential inadequate preparation of health professionals, the skills and ethics of communicating effectively with their patients have received greater attention both in university prelicensure training programs as well as postgraduate education and quality improvement hospital- or professional organization-sponsored programs. An understanding of patients' perceptions and expressed needs for compassion is important and can inform students, practicing clinicians, health care institutions, and health care policy about the integral role of compassion.

In their in-depth study of the literature addressing the state of the research on compassion in clinical caregiving, Sinclair and colleagues (2016b) outlined what is known about the nature of compassionate health care and the limited understanding of the concept. They raised doubt about what constitutes compassionate care and how patients would describe its essential elements. They indicated that a major deficit in the literature is the lack of patient and family voices. That is, what would they say about compassion, what health provider behaviors to them would constitute compassion, and what advice would they give providers on being compassionate. In fact, patients' views were relatively underrepresented as few studies looked at patient perspectives or included patients' definitions of compassionate care.

In a follow-up study conducted by Sinclair and colleagues (2016a), patients' views of compassionate care were examined. These researchers asked patients a series of 10 open-ended questions about what compassion and compassionate care meant to them (e.g., "In terms of your own illness experience what does compassion mean to you?" "How do you know when a health care professional is being compassionate?" "What advice would you give health care providers on being compassionate?") (Sinclair et al., p. 196).

These researchers identified the core variable of compassion that emerged from their study and defined compassion as "a virtuous response that seeks to address the suffering and needs of a person through relational understanding and action" (Ibid, p. 195). Patient responses included statements such as "I would have to say I know it intuitively. You feel it coming off them," and "They stop and listen, they establish a relationship and get to know who you are, they get to know me as a person and vice versa" (Sinclair et al., 2016a, p. 196).

Attention has been given to effectively teaching compassionate care, and these efforts have measured the impact of different skill-learning approaches on health providers' communications. The use of clinical mentors to demonstrate compassionate approaches, personal reflection about clinical care experiences, and experiential learning using real-life scenarios have been used and tested.

Sinclair et al. (2016b) explained that compassion is optimal when developed through experiential and reflective learning and includes the student's personal life experiences with the human condition, life circumstances, and threats to health and well-being. EOL discussions create a special circumstance in which students' personal and clinical experience can serve to provide the needed compassion for both patient and provider. Sanso, Galiana, Oliver, Pascual, Sinclair, and Benito (2015) describe the value and impact that palliative

care clinicians' inner life experience can have on their professional practice and manner of delivering compassionate care as well as on their own quality of life. These authors suggest that a "reflective practice" can both benefit patients and serve a protective function for clinicians who are frequently exposed to EOL distress.

▶ Skills to Assist Patients in Discussions of EOL Decision-Making

Over the last 30 years, recognition of the need for EOLC and EOL decision-making have increased significantly. Once felt important in selected instances such as with patients in the final stages of cancer, these needs have expanded to include people dying from other chronic illnesses.

Changes in the approach to EOLC planning is a function of advanced technology prolonging the lives of persons with a wide range of chronic illnesses but is also due to the population aging. In addition to patients dying of cancer, the number of people dying from other chronic illnesses has increased significantly. Even illnesses not previously seen to be relevant to EOL decision-making such as dementia and other slow progressing debilitating diseases, have drawn attention to the need of earlier EOL decision-making. While the issue of planning for EOLC seems initially irrelevant. Due to patient incapacity at later stages rendering them incapable of entering into informed decision-making, early planning for EOLC preferences is essential for these patients as well.

Formal course work to prepare health professionals, including nurses and nurse practitioners, for EOLC discussions have been implemented and tested. Some of these programs have focused upon decisions to be made throughout a long course of treatment.

For example, in a study by Cohen and colleagues (2016), fellows in nephrology received a communication skill course to improve communication skills with patients facing advanced kidney disease. This course was offered as part of an educational quality improvement project with first year nephrology fellows enrolled in Harvard University-affiliated training programs.

Annual workshops were conducted and focused on didactic information, discussion, and practice with simulated patients providing a real-life context for the training. The content included skills in delivering bad news, acknowledging emotion, discussing care goals in dialysis decision-making when prognosis is uncertain, and addressing dialysis therapy withdrawal and EOLC. Feedback from the nephrology fellows indicated that there was improvement in all areas with sustained improvement at 3 months.

Participants reported integrating specific ACP skills in their discussions with patients, including the *Ask–Tell–Ask* technique and the use of open-ended questions. These results suggested that the program could enhance physician communication skills over the entire course of treatment for advanced kidney disease.

▸ Addressing Barriers to Communications About EOL: Decisional Conflict

Decisional Conflict (DC) is one of the most important barriers to effective EOL decision-making discussions. DC, by definition, is a state of uncertainty about a course of action (O'Connor, 1993 and updated, 2010), and this uncertainty is more likely when a person and/or family is confronted with decisions that are risky or have uncertain outcomes. It occurs more often than not and can lead to a breakdown in communications and even decisional delay. All parties, patients, providers, and families are affected by DC, yet it is the role of the provider to take the lead in identifying the conflict and acting to resolve or minimize this conflict.

EOLC presents a number of what could be regarded as high-risk options where significant potential benefits or losses can result. EOLC planning requires answers to what will be done under the following circumstances where options for medical care exist and desires for life-sustaining treatments must be known. Specially, decisions about such interventions as cardiopulmonary resuscitation (CPR) or ventilation must be made. O'Connor further explains that when there is a need to make value-tradeoffs in selecting a course of action or when there is regret over the positive aspects of any option not chosen, DC is likely.

DC can lead to ineffective decision-making about EOLC and is highly likely in the following situations:

- Deficits in information where patients may be unclear about benefits and risks and treatment options.
- Unclear about personal values.
- Feeling unsupported in the decision chosen or forced to make a decision when not ready (LeBlanc, Kenny, O'Connor, & Legare, 2009).

While uncertainty associated with DC may not cause significant anxiety, behavioral manifestations of DC can include a range of uncomfortable responses. Patients may verbalize uncertainty about their choices, vacillate between courses of action, or delay decision-making (O'Connor, 1995). Negative emotional responses may include anxiety if patients perceive that their conflict or uncertainty will in some way threaten or endanger their care. Although rare, this conflict can escalate to a sense of panic. Because of the potential detrimental effects of DC, health providers have a key role in managing patients' and families' responses to it.

▶ Minimizing Decisional Conflict Through Decision-Supporting Interventions

In this section we turn our attention to how DC in ACP can be minimized. DC can be successfully addressed through decision-supporting approaches. Interventions to minimize DC include assessment tools to identify the level of patient conflict experienced by patients and DAs that educate and prepare patients to make decisions. DAs are useful to people facing a wide range of health treatment or screening decisions, and there is documentation about their usefulness in the literature (Stacey et al., 2017). The focus of this discussion is on their use in supporting persons facing ACP.

▶ Use of the Decisional Conflict Scale

Various versions of DC scales have been designed and studied for their effectiveness in measuring patients' DC. *The DC scale* (O'Connor, 1995) was among the first scales. This scale was designed to describe health care consumers' uncertainty in making health-related decisions. It also identified factors contributing to patients' experience of uncertainty and perceptions of effective decision-making.

The scale was pilot tested with 909 individuals contemplating various low-risk procedures: patients deciding on either influenza immunization or breast cancer screening. This scale captures five key phenomena: (1) how informed patients perceive themselves to be (e.g., "I know which options are available to me"), (2) their clarity about what matters to them most (e.g., "I am clear about which benefits matter most to me"), (3) their perception of the level of support they have in making

decisions (e.g., "I have enough support from others to make a choice"), (4) how clear they are about the best choice for them (e.g., "I am clear about the best choice for me"), and (5) the extent to which they feel they made an informed choice and plan to stick to their choice (e.g., "I feel I have made an informed choice").

▶ DAs Help Inform Patients and Families About EOLC Decisions

DAs help patients and families consider different health care options available to them. Butler, Ratner, McCreedy, Shippee, and Kane (2014) explained that DAs do this by supporting the following steps in the decision process. Patients' and families' need to (1) learn more about anticipated conditions, (2) consider these options, and (3) communicate their decisions about available options. Several DAs can help minimize DC while supporting effective EOL decision-making. These communication tools exist in different formats. A summary of DA formats is provided in **EXHIBIT 29-4**. DAs have been designed to structure communications about EOLC and guide patients and surrogate decision makers' discussions with health professionals.

They come in a variety of formats or mixed formats, and when evaluated in clinical trial studies are compared with what has been *usual care.* These aids may be in the form of (1) videotapes depicting true-to-life decision situations with video scenes addressing issues of life-prolonging care, basic care or comfort care (Volandes et al., 2012); self-directed computer programs (Green & Levi, 2011; Levi, Heverley, & Green, 2011; Hossler, Levi, Simmons, & Green, 2011; Vogel et al., 2013); take-home booklets with audio recordings, reviewed by an oncologist (Leighl et al., 2011); DVDs and booklets about facing advanced or terminal illness such as *Looking ahead: Choices for medical care when you're seriously ill* (Matlock, Keech, McKenzie,

EXHIBIT 29-4 Summary of Elements of DAs to Support Advanced Care Planning

- Videotapes depicting true-to-life decision situations with video scenes portraying basic medical care addressing issues of life-prolonging care, basic care, or comfort care (Volandes et al., 2012).
- Self-directed computer programs (Green & Levi, 2011; Levi et al., 2011; Hossler, Levi, Simmons, & Green, 2011; Vogel et al., 2013).
- Take-home booklet with audio recording reviewed by an oncologist (Leighl et al., 2011).
- DVD and booklet for patients facing advanced or terminal illness entitled *Looking ahead: Choices for medical care when you're seriously ill* (Matlock et al., 2014).
- Video for patient decision-making about future care in dementia entitled *It helps me see with my heart* (Deep et al., 2010).

Bronsert, Nowels, & Kutner, 2014); and videos for decision-making about future dementia care such as *It helps me see with my heart* (Deep, Hunter, Murphy, & Volandes, 2010).

While these formats have been evaluated, it is unclear how useful they might be with a wide range of patient populations. This is because they need to be tested further with other populations. For example, in the Leighl and colleagues study (2011) of DAs for patients

with advanced colorectal cancer considering chemotherapy, patients were primarily Christian, White, aged 60, and had some level of education beyond high school.

On the whole, DAs have been seen to be effective in eliciting patients' preferences, enhancing patients' understanding of treatment options, and minimizing DC associated with selecting care options in some patient populations. Three cited studies describe different and sometimes overlapping approaches to easing EOL decision-making.

In summary, DAs can provide a number of important benefits to some patients and their families when used in ACP discussions: (1) they inform patients and families about situations they will or are currently facing including available treatment options, the benefits and potential burden of any one treatment path, and what will or could happen if one or another treatment is not chosen; (2) the patients and their families are encouraged to express their personal values and preferences for treatment which may be influenced by religious or cultural values; and (3) they enable patients and families to feel more supported in their decisions through the process of shared decision-making. Furthermore, DAs have the potential of decreasing potential DCs. The following case study examples present evidence about several different DA scenarios detailing the nature of the DAs and potential impact of their use in advanced care planning.

🔎 *CITED STUDY: DA Designed for People Facing Advanced or Terminal Illness*

The purpose of this study was to evaluate the feasibility and acceptability of a DA for patients facing advanced or terminal illness. Patients and families are confronted with a range of complicated decisions with advanced or terminal illness. These include whether to use life-prolonging therapies which include chemotherapy, artificial nutrition, and hydration.

The researchers explained that these decisions occur at a difficult time when patients experience significant symptoms and diminished decisional capacity even though they desire information and

(continues)

🔍 *CITED STUDY: DA Designed for People Facing Advanced or Terminal Illness* *(continued)*

control near the end of their lives. These investigators conducted a pilot randomized clinical trial to evaluate the DA entitled *Looking Ahead: Choices for Medical Care When You're Seriously Ill*.

Matlock, D. D., Keech, T. A. E., McKenzie, M. B., Bronsert, M. R., Nowels, C. T., Kutner, J. S. (2014). Feasibility and acceptability of a decision aid designed for people facing advanced or terminal illness: A pilot randomized trial. *Health Expectations, 17*, 49–59.

From a group of 239 patients or decision-makers, 51 (21%) participants on an inpatient palliative care service in a major university hospital enrolled in this study and were either randomized to the control group receiving standard patient consultation or the intervention group receiving standard consultation and the DA. The DA was a DVD and booklet encouraging conversations, ACP, and patient-centered decision-making. Exit interviews were conducted and found the DA acceptable but feasibility was limited by late-life illness challenges. There were no significant differences in knowledge or DC. Participants described an increased sense of empowerment and control and explained that receiving the DA at an earlier point in time would have been more useful.

🔍 *CITED STUDY: Augmenting Advanced Care Planning with Video DA*

These researchers described the inevitable situation of having to plan with patients the needs for future medical care in situations that neither the time nor circumstance can be predicted. They evaluated the impact of an educational video addressing goals for ACP among patients with advanced cancer.

A sample of 80 patients recruited from the ambulatory oncology practices affiliated with a major comprehensive cancer center were recruited and were surveyed before and after viewing the educational video. The video included video scenes which portrayed basic medical care and addressed issues of life-prolonging care, basic care, or comfort care. The pre- and post-video changes in patients' preferences and knowledge of goals of care and resuscitation were reported.

Volandes, A. E., Levin, T. T., Slovin, S., Carvajal, R. D., O'Reilly, E. M., Keohan, M. L., ... Noy, A. (2012), Augmenting advance care planning in poor prognosis cancer with a video decision aid. *Cancer, 118* (17), 4331–4338.

Results showed that patients did not change their preferences for their level of care but after the video, more patients did not want CPR or ventilation. Knowledge about the goals of care choices and individual choices for resuscitation did increase. Patients rated the video as acceptable, commented that they would recommend it to other cancer patients, and found it helpful. The researchers concluded that the video may be feasible and effective but that preferred goals needed to be translated to medical orders for "do not resuscitate." They indicated that the visual medium offered a powerful aid to providers to ground ACP discussions with patients.

🔍 *CITED STUDY: Supporting Treatment Decision-Making in Advanced Cancer*

The purpose of this study was to examine the impact of a DA for patients with advanced colorectal cancer who were considering treatment options. Specifically, the authors wanted to know how this DA impacted patients' understanding, treatment decisions, DC, decision-making, and other outcomes. The 207 persons who were deciding on chemotherapy for metastatic disease were randomized to receive the DA or care as usual. The DA consisted of a take-home booklet with an audio recording that was reviewed by an oncologist.

Leighl, N. B., Shepherd, H. L., Butow, P. N., Clarke, S. J., McJannett, M., Beale, P. J., ... Tattersall, M. H. (2011). Supporting treatment decision making in advanced cancer: A randomized trial of a decision aid for patients with advanced colorectal cancer considering chemotherapy. *Journal of Clinical Oncology*, *29*(15), 2077–2084.

Patients receiving the DA were reported to show a greater increase in their understanding of prognosis, treatment options, risks, benefits, and higher overall understanding. The DA did not increase patient anxiety. There were no differences in DC, treatment decisions, and achievement of involvement preferences.

In addition to the DA approaches listed in Exhibit 29-4, other commonly used clinical and legal forms exist to guide physicians and patients in advance care decision-making. The most widely used form is the AD. In some contexts, ADs are also referred to as living wills. As previously explained, they are made during ACP, regardless of the current health status of the patient, and are legal documents giving written instructions detailing the type of care desired when one is seriously ill or dying, and are no longer able to make decisions for themselves because of illness or incapacity.

Patients and families can complete ADs without the assistance from their health care provider and no discussion with their health care provider is required. However, patients are responsible for giving a copy of their AD to their health care provider to put into the medical record at the hospital or facility where they are being treated. ADs are shared with family who are expected to respect the patient's preferences. An example of a statement that may be found in a living will is, "If I suffer an incurable, irreversible illness, disease, or condition and my attending physician determines

that my condition is terminal, I direct that life-sustaining measures that would serve only to prolong my dying be withheld or discontinued."

In addition to ADs, there are two additional forms that may be used. These forms are available in some states, but not all. Some states use a form known as **Physician Orders for Life-Sustaining Treatment (POLST)** or Practitioner Orders for Life-Sustaining Treatment in states where POLST can be ordered by not only physicians, but nurse practitioners.

In other states, the **Medical Orders for Life-Sustaining Treatment (MOLST)** are used. These forms provide detailed guidance to patients and providers in making patients' medical preferences known. Unlike ADs which are legal documents, these forms are medical orders. These medical orders are filled out by the patient's physician or sometimes a nurse practitioner or physician's assistant but always after discussing the patients' wishes with them.

Once signed by the patient's physician, this form has the same authority as any other established medical order. These forms, depending upon the state, are signed by the patient as well. A difference between POLST or MOLST forms and an AD is that the POLST or MOLST forms are designed to apply outside the medical facility. They can be used by first responders (paramedics, firemen, and police), as well as by emergency rooms, hospitals, and nursing homes as the patient's expressed desires for **life-prolonging treatment**. In using these forms, patients and providers systematically follow a three-step procedure.

First, the completion of the form starts with a conversation between the health care professionals and patients or the patients' authorized surrogate about the patient's current condition and health status. Second, patients are encouraged to provide their preferences for treatments, and these preferences are recorded on a standardized form and kept in an official medical record and/or with the patient if living at home. Third, the form goes with patients as they are transferred from one treatment setting to another to promote continuity of care and response throughout the process on the part of all medical personnel and first responders. It has been shown that these forms are honored appropriately and when used, can even reduce unwanted hospitalizations.

In summary, DAs along with other supporting documents are available to all patients, and when used to support patients' health care decisions are both useful and beneficial. They can provide structure to potentially uncomfortable dialog. They inform patients and their families about the care decisions which can be made in advance of a time when patients may be unable to instruct others about their preferences for treatment.

DAs seem to be useful to a wide range of patient situations from choosing treatment options when there is controversy over the best option but the patient's condition is not terminal to advanced care planning for patients needing EOLC. There is much more to be learned about the impact of various DAs and select-ACP forms. Their use in different patient populations and for a wide range of patient situations and conditions is still unclear. Likewise, patients' preferences for one DA over another should be explored. The factors influencing patients' decisions to choose one over another need to be explored extensively.

Oczkowski, Chung, Hanvey, Mbuagbaw, and You (2016) explained that further information is needed to determine whether structured communication tools such as DAs are better than *ad hoc* discussions in providing patient, family, and system-level high-quality outcomes in critical care settings. Finally, in a recent review of the range of DAs available to facilitate EOLC decisions in older patients, Cardona-Morrell, Benfatti-Olivato, Jansen, Turner, Fajardo-Pulido, and Hillman (2017) warned of a number of important issues. The sensitivities of these decisions may make self-administered DAs inappropriate for older patients, and continued evaluation of existing DAs is needed to ensure they meet their intended purpose.

🔍 *EVIDENCE FOR/MORE TO KNOW BOX: The Impact of DAs in Supporting Patient Advance Care Planning*

Evidence for

- DAs can provide structure to an uncomfortable topic for both providers and patients and their families.
- Several DA formats have been shown to increase patient and family knowledge and comfort. Most have been reported to be acceptable, and would be recommended by patients to others facing similar circumstances.
- DAs may not necessarily alter DC or change patient preferences for life-sustaining treatment.

More to know

- Less is known about the impact of DAs on patients' families.
- Few studies report health professionals' opinions and perceived ease in using these DAs in clinical settings.
- The exact timing of the use of DAs is unclear. A conceptual framework describing the timing of EOL decision-making discussions may be helpful.
- DAs seem to be useful in a wide range of patient situations from choosing health care screening and treatment options to ACP. More needs to be known about with which patient groups DAs are appropriate, and whether DAs surpass usual care in supporting effective advance care decision-making by patients and their families.

🔍 MUST READ BOX: EOLC: From Patients' Rights to Systemic Reform

Wolf, S. M., Berlinger, N., & Jennings, B. (2015). Forty years of work on end-of-life care—From patients' rights to systemic reform. *New England Journal of Medicine, 372*, 678–682.

This informative summary of the evolution of work to improve EOLC and protect the rights and preferences of patients examines key phases in the process: (1) securing rights (1976–1994), (2) facing clinical realities (1995–2009), and (3) reforming EOLC systems (2010–present) over a 40-year period in the United States. The article describes how securing patient rights was insufficient to ensure these rights were protected in the clinical arena. It became increasingly evident that system changes were needed and should include structures to support high quality of care near the EOL and fully trained clinicians to inform, support, and facilitate patient and family members' decision-making. Skill training and the use of DAs to assist health professionals structure processes of decision-making, goal setting, document preferences, and care planning were required. It was recognized that all providers across shifts of care, during patient transfers, and with family care providers during discharge planning should receive training and be able to actively engage patients and caregivers in EOLC decisions.

▶ Summary

Effective communication in ACP entails understanding the tasks involved, assessing patients' and families' capacity to engage in shared decision-making processes, and the various DAs available. It also includes knowledge and appreciation of the unique concerns and cultural and religious beliefs that influence patient and family experiences.

Advance care decision-making involves discussions about the type of care desired at the EOL and includes a wide range of issues (e.g., choosing or refusing cardiopulmonary resuscitation, whether to go to the hospitalize or not, whether nutrition or hydration be delivered with intravenous feeding, use of future interventions directed towards a cure, and discontinuing potentially other life-saving treatments). These discussions become applicable potentially early on as well as later in the management of chronic illnesses (e.g., diabetes, heart disease, and cancers), at their advanced stage.

Patient, family, and health providers' recognition of the impending failure to medically recover from a life-threatening illness comes at a time when both instrumental tasks, completing necessary paperwork, and emotional coping are at their highest. It can be a difficult time, and communications might falter, resulting in incomplete recognition and respect for patients' rights.

DAs are tools that can be used to prepare and guide patient, family, and health care provider discussions. While DAs address the cognitive aspects of decision-making, they may be inadequate in dealing with the emotional aspects of this decision-making process. In this chapter, the context of shared decision-making is outlined, and issues and evidence related to promoting ACP by minimizing DC and using DAs are addressed. An important feature of this discussion and the intent of the chapter is the emphasis on *how* shared decision-making occurs. Very simply, carefully positioned compassionate caring is critical to the process and the well-being of patients, their families, and health care providers themselves.

Discussion

1. What is meant by patient- and family-centered care and why is it important in shared decision-making in general and with EOLC?
2. What is the role of DC in making ACP more difficult?
3. How do DAs help providers, patients, and families complete ACP?
4. What key outcomes have been reported in studies evaluating the effects of DAs?
5. Discuss ways in which compassionate caring can be helpful in palliative care and ease advance care decision-making.

References

Butler, M., Ratner, E., McCreedy, E., Shippee, N., & Kane, R. L. (2014). Decision aids for advance care planning. Technical Brief No. 16. (Prepared by the Minnesota Evidence-based Practice Center under Contract No. 290–2012–00016-I.) AHRQ Publication No. 14-EHC039-EF. Rockville, MD: Agency for Healthcare Research and Quality. July 2014. www.effectivehealthcare.ahrq.gov/reports/final.cfm

Cardona-Morrell, M., Benfatti-Olivato, G., Jansen, J., Turner, R. M., Fajardo-Pulido, D., & Hillman, K. (2017). A systematic review of effectiveness of decision aids to assist older patients at the end of life. *Patient Education and Counseling, 100*(3), 425–435. doi:10.1016/j.pec.2016.10.007

Cohen, R. A., Jackson, V. A., Norwich, D., Schell, J. O., Schaefer, K., Ship, A. N., & Sullivan, A. M. (2016). A nephrology fellows' communication skills course: An educational quality improvement report. *American Journal of Kidney Disease, 68*(2), 203–211. doi:10.1053/j.ajkd.2016.01.025

Deep, K. S., Hunter, A., Murphy, K., & Volandes, A. (2010). "It helps me see with my heart": How video informs patients' rationale for decisions about future care in advanced dementia. *Patient Education and Counseling, 81*, 229–234. doi:10.1016/j.pec.2010.02.004

Djulbegovic, B., Tsalatsanis, A., Mhaskar, R., Hozo, I., Miladinovic, B., & Tuch, H. (2016). Eliciting regret improves decision-making at end of life. *European Journal of Cancer, 68*, 27–37. doi:10.1016/j.ejca.2016.08.027

Esserman, L. J., Thompson, I. M., Reid, B., Nelson, P., Ransohoff, D. F., Welch, H. G., ... Srivastava, S. (2014). Addressing overdiagnosis and overtreatment in cancer: A prescription for change. *The Lancet. Oncology, 15*(6), e234–e242. doi:10.1016/S1470-2045(13)70598-9

Green, M. J., & Levi, B. H. (2011). Teaching advance care planning to medical students with a computer-based decision aid. *Journal of Cancer Education, 26*, 82–91. doi:10.1007/s13187-010-0146-2

Hossler, C., Levi, B. H., Simmons, Z., & Green, M. J. (2011). Advance care planning for patients with ALS: Feasibility of an interactive computer program. *Amyotrophic Lateral Sclerosis, 12*, 172–177. doi:10.3109/17482968.2010.509865

LeBlanc, A., Kenny, D. A., O'Connor, A. M., & Legare, F. (2009). Decisional conflict in patients and their physicians: A dyadic approach to shared decision-making. *Medical Decision-Making, 29*, 61–68. doi:10.1177/0272989x08327067

Leighl, N. B., Shepherd, H. L., Butow, P. N., Clarke, S. J., McJannett, M., Beale, P. J., ... Tattersall, M. H. (2011). Supporting treatment decision-making in advanced cancer: A randomized trial of a decision aid for patients with advanced colorectal cancer considering chemotherapy. *Journal of Clinical Oncology, 29*(15), 2077–2084. doi:10.1200/JCO.2010.32.0754

Levi, B. H., Heverley, S. R., & Green, M. J. (2011). Accuracy of a decision aid for advance care planning: Simulated end-of-life decision-making. *Journal of Clinical Ethics, 22*, 223–238. PMID:22167985

Matlock, D. D., Keech, T. A. E., McKenzie, M. B., Bronsert, M. R., Nowels, C. T., & Kutner, J. S. (2014). Feasibility and acceptability of a decision aid designed for people facing advanced or terminal illness: A pilot randomized trial. *Health Expectations, 17*, 49–59. doi:10.1111/j.1369-7625.2011.00732.x

O'Connor, A. M. (1993 updated 2010). *User manual-decisional conflict scale.* Retrieved from www.ohri.ca/decisionaid

O'Connor A. M. (1995). Validation of a decisional conflict scale. *Medical Decision-making, 15*(1), 25–30. doi:10.1177/0272989x9501500105

Oczkowski, S. J. W., Chung, H., Hanvey, L., Mbuagbaw, L., & You, J. J. (2016). Communication tools for end-of-life decision-making in the intensive care unit: A systematic review and meta-analysis. *Critical Care, 20*(97), 1–19. doi:10.1186/s13054-016-1264-y

Sanso, N., Galiana, L., Oliver, A., Pascual, A., Sinclair, S., & Benito, E. (2015). Palliative care professionals' inner life: Exploring the relationships among awareness, self-care and compassion satisfaction and fatigue, burn out, and coping with death. *Journal of Pain and Symptom Management, 50*(2), 200–207. doi:10.1016/j.jpainsymman.2015.02.013

Sinclair, S., McClement, S., Raffin-Bouchal, S. M., Hack, T. F., Hagen, N. A., McConnell, S., & Chochinov, H. M. (2016a). Compassion in health care: An empirical model. *Journal of Pain and Symptom Management, 51*(2), 193–203. doi:10.1016/j.jpainsymman.2015.10.009

Sinclair, S., Norris, J. M., McConnell, S. J., Chochinov, H. M., Hack, T. F., Hagen, N. A., ... Bouchal, S. R. (2016b). Compassion: A scoping review of the healthcare literature. *BMC Palliative Care, 15*, 6. doi:10.1186/s12904-016-0080-0

Stacey, D., Légaré, F., Lewis, K., Barry, M. J., Bennett, C. L., Eden, K. B., ... Trevena, L. (2017). Decision aids for people facing health treatment or screening decisions. *Cochrane Database of Systematic Reviews, 2017*(4), CD001431. doi:10.1002/14651858.CD001431.pub5

Vogel, R. I., Petzel, S. V., Cragg, J., McClellan, M., Chan, D., Dickson, E., ... Geller, M. A. (2013). Development and pilot of an advance care planning website for women with ovarian cancer: A randomized controlled trial. *Gynecologic Oncology, 131*, 430–436. doi:10.1016/j.ygyno.2013.08.017

Volandes, A. E., Levin, T. T., Slovin, S., Carvajal, R. D., O'Reilly, E. M., Keohan, M. L., ... Noy, A. (2012), Augmenting advance care planning in poor prognosis cancer with a video decision aid. *Cancer, 118* (17), 4331–4338. doi:10.1002/cncr.27423

Glossary

Access and utilization of health care systems
Access to health care is more than just how easily patients can physically reach the location of health care centers and health providers. Access refers more generally to the timely use of health care services to achieve quality care. According to *Healthy People 2020*, it includes the ability to gain entry into the health care system (usually thought of as having insurance coverage), accessing the location where needed health care services can be found (geographic availability), and finding a health care provider who the patient trusts and can communicate (personal relationship).

Accessibility of health care or **Access to health care** Access to health care is sometimes a term used to refer to how easily the patient and family can physically reach the health provider's location. In actuality, access is more general and not just the notion of geographic accessibility. It refers to the timely use of health care services to achieve quality care.

Accountability in health care Accountability in health care delivery systems includes measuring and reporting health care outcomes but also controlling the many factors that result in negative health outcomes related to system-based factors (e.g., hospital and health care service system approaches to measure and curb avoidable medical errors).

Acculturation Acculturation is a process of social, psychological, and cultural adaptation that stems from a blending of cultures. The original culture is modified to some degree to adopt new beliefs of the host culture.

Active listening Active listening is the process of fully understanding what another is communicating. It enables providers to be fully attuned not only to what the patient is saying but also to what the patient feels. Active listening is also referred to as *empathic listening* or *reflective listening*.

Adaptation to illness The process of adapting to the diagnosis of a chronic-debilitating or life-threatening illness is called psychological adaptation to illness. It involves appraisal of threat. There are a number of stages, commonly referred to in different terminology but including denial, anger, bargaining, depression, and resolution and acceptance.

Adaptive coping Patients and families coping with serious illness or injury face the need to cope not only with new physical and emotional conditions but with the impact of treatment as a result of illness or injury. Coping is a deliberate effort to reduce stressful situations. Adaptive coping responses are those that reduce stress; they include strategies such as: seeking appropriate help and adapting self-care strategies to reduce stress.

Adherence and nonadherence to treatment
The World Health Organization (WHO) defines adherence to treatment as "the extent to which a person's behavior – taking medication, following a diet, and/or executing lifestyle changes, corresponds with agreed recommendations from a health care provider." When patients are nonadherent to treatment, or only partially adherent, they run the risk for suboptimal recovery, relapse, and increase the odds of disease-related morbidity. A concept frequently used in conjunction with adherence is *persistence*. Persistence, more precisely, refers to continuation of treatment for the prescribed period of time while adherence refers to following the designated treatment plan as prescribed (e.g., dose and timing of medication taking).

Adherence to medication Adherence to treatment when it includes medications is termed medication adherence. A person is adherent to their medication regimen when they take their medication as prescribed. Nonadherence refers to patients who are only partially following their medication regimen or discontinue their medication without the explicit guidance of a professional health care provider.

Advance care planning (ACP) Advance care planning refers to the process of planning one's preferences for care in the event that they are unable to articulate their wishes at a later time. ACP covers preferences for life-sustaining treatments and treatment for a life-limiting illness. These decisions are based upon the patient's personal values and care preferences and are transmitted to family members and health care providers.

Advance directives (ADs) Everyone should be encouraged to have an AD early on and not wait for a time when they are terminally ill. ADs are legal documents giving written instructions detailing the type of care desired when one is seriously ill or dying and are no longer able to make decisions for themselves because of illness or incapacity. They are shared with family and health providers who are to respect the patient's preferences. An example of a statement that may be found in an AD or living will is, "If I suffer an incurable, irreversible illness, disease, or condition and my attending physician determines that my condition is terminal, I direct that life-sustaining measures that would serve only to prolong my dying be withheld or discontinued."

Advice or directive Advice can frequently appear as a directive. The first basic principle in using advisement is the less direct the advice, the less likely it is patients will resist taking the advice. To hold to this principle, providers must have an open style—a willingness to have their advice rejected. Advice that *must* be followed is not advice but rather a command or directive, and when the advice must be adhered to, providers must clearly say so.

Advisement Advisement is the act of communicating what one thinks or feels about another's experience, namely, what they should or should not feel, think, or do. In the patient–provider relationship it is most often unilateral in that most of the data and facts come from the provider to the patient in a statement of advice.

Advisement purpose (of questions) Questions used not to gather patient information but to communicate a judgment or advise are questions with the purpose of advisement. They can be confusing to patients who may not understand whether there is a real question behind the words of the provider.

Affordability Affordability of health care refers to individual, family, or community capacity to purchase needed health care in a timely manner. A primary aim of national health care reform has been to make health care affordable to everyone. Affordability of health care services from a broader context refers to the relative costs of delivering care as a portion of the nation's gross national product (GNP).

Affordability of health care Affordability of health care refers to individual, family, or community capacity to purchase needed health care in a timely manner. A primary aim of national health care reform has been to make health care affordable to everyone.

Analogic communication When one refers to objects as representations or likenesses and observes and responds nonverbally and contextually, they are using analogic communication capacities.

Anonymity Anonymity refers to the specific privacy rights of patients wherein their exact identity is not made known to others.

Antidepressant medication Antidepressants are medications used to treat the symptoms of depression. They may be used in cases of major depression but also other less debilitating depressions (e.g., dysthymia, or even anxiety disorders, eating disorders, or other chronic medical conditions). In instances where depression is associated with other chronic illness (e.g., diabetes, cardiovascular disease, and arthritis), depressive symptoms are considered secondary to the primary illness. There are a variety of classes of antidepressants available to successfully alleviate symptoms of depression.

Anxiety Anxiety is characterized as a distressed state accompanied by diffuse feelings of uncertainty, apprehension, and sometimes fear of imminent danger.

Autonomic nervous system (ANS) The nervous system that is responsible for regulating the functioning of internal organs is the ANS. The intensity of behavior is largely governed by the functions of the ANS. The ANS has two systems: (1) the sympathetic and (2) parasympathetic processes.

Autonomy In motivational interviewing (MI), it is not the role of the provider to tell the patient what to do; rather, it is the patient's right and responsibility to decide for themselves whether to change or not and how to go about it. In this way, the patient's sense of autonomy is honored and protected.

Availability of health care Availability of health care services refers to the existence of health care resources to meet the needs of individuals and communities, and can be described as both the availability of appropriately trained health providers and health care facilities to meet the current and changing needs of the population.

Avoidable suffering Avoidable suffering refers to harm to the patient from an imperfect health care system. This suffering can be prevented by organizing care around meeting the needs of patients.

Bargaining Bargaining can be either *positional* or *interest* based. When faced with a conflict, parties may negotiate in favor of their position which involves holding onto a fixed idea or position of what one wants and arguing for it and it alone. In contrast, with interest-based bargaining, all parties give their ideas about the problem but attempt to come to a solution which deals with the interests of all parties.

Behavior control Behavioral control is the perception of the ease or difficulty of particular behaviors. High levels of perceived behavioral control are likely to mobilize patients to adapt and cope effectively.

Bereavement counseling Bereavement counseling, sometimes referred to as grief counseling, is a form of support and counseling to help people who have experienced a death of a loved one cope with the associated emotional and psychological stress (including grief and bereavement) due to their loss. It should be distinguished from bereavement or grief therapy which is designed to help individuals who are experiencing more complicated grief reactions including prolonged grief or is manifested in other psychological or bodily symptoms.

Bilateral symmetry of the brain Bilateral symmetry of the brain refers to the fact that the two lobes or hemispheres of the brain are similar anatomical parts arranged on opposite sides of the brain.

Caregiver burden Caregiver burden is the stress felt by giving physical and emotional care to those who are unable to care for themselves. It is usually given in a home care situation. Caregiver burden has been associated with emotional distress (depression) and poor health in the caregiver and poor care outcomes. Caregiver syndrome is a condition of exhaustion, anger, and guilt resulting from giving care under difficult circumstances and for extended periods of time. It has also been referred to as caregiver burnout.

Caring confrontations Caring confrontation is a term used in clinical psychology, social work, and other health professions to indicate the act of presenting to patients something they are not aware of, and is done in a gentle caring manner.

Case management Case management is a broad term used to describe a wide range of health care services including case management, treatment planning, referral, and follow-up to ensure comprehensive and continuous services and coordinated payment for these services.

Case manager Care management, or case management, refers to the designation of an experienced care manager to a caseload of primary care patients. Depression case managers may screen patients, assess severity of symptoms, and/or in some cases, provide grief counseling or therapy interventions. Care or case managers connect patients, primary care providers, and mental health specialists to ensure quality patient care for depressed patients.

Chronic disease Chronic illnesses, frequently regarded as noncommunicable diseases, are sometimes considered a consequence of lifestyle behaviors and require ongoing medical and self-care management. They include medical conditions such as cardiovascular disease, diabetes, and chronic respiratory diseases.

Client-centered counseling Client-centered counseling is also known as person-centered counseling or client-centered therapy. It refers to the approach of focusing on the client's perspective.

Close-ended questions Questions that are phrased to evoke a narrow range of possible responses and that frequently elicit one word or "yes"/"no" responses are closed-ended.

Coding Coding is a term in neurophysiology that is used to describe the correspondence of some part of a stimulus and some aspect of action in the nervous system.

Cognitive appraisal Cognitive appraisal is the person's interpretation or understanding of a situation. High levels of positive appraisal are likely to increase patients' experience of cognitive control.

Cognitive control These aspects are linked to one another. A persons' perceptions that they are capable of cognitive functioning (e.g., understanding and problem-solving) are more likely to experience decisional control in matters of managing their illness.

Collaborative care model The collaborative care model is a multifaceted program to meet the needs of patients, particularly those persons with chronic illness. CC has been found to be more efficacious than care as usual in a primary care setting. The major premise behind CC is that patients do better when care is organized to include a range of interventions. These interventions can vary in intensity from such simple approaches as telephone interventions to encourage medication adherence to a more complex arrangement of services to foster better communication and collaboration between health providers. The term *stepped collaborative care* refers more specially to the process of escalating the intensity of treatment when it is shown that the patient does not meet certain expected outcomes by a certain period of time. For example, in the treatment of persons with depression in primary care settings, if the patient does not achieve remission (a significant reduction in depression symptoms) by taking selected medications after 18 weeks, the patient is referred to mental health specialist intervention.

Co-located mental health care Co-located care refers to services located at the same physical space or complex (e.g., health center or multidisciplinary clinic). Although not fully integrated with one another, they increase the possibility of fluid communication between all health care providers who are providing care. Co-located care is particularly important for persons with chronic illness or complex care requirements. Co-located mental health care refers to the organization of behavioral health services within primary care practices so as to create a seamless transition between mental health services and primary care.

Comfort care Comfort care is a part of medical care and is given to persons when experiencing severe symptoms of illness. It is also a part of end-of-life (EOL) care to soothe the dying process. The goals are to prevent or relieve physical and emotional suffering as much as possible. It is done in the context of protecting the patients' quality of life and respecting their preferences for care.

Commands Like orders, commands are directives that must be followed. They are different from orders in that they demand immediate action.

Community-based programs Community-based programs are those designed, facilitated, and evaluated, at least in part, by community leaders who have earned a respected voice from community residents and partner with existing community or health care centers. These programs are often successful in achieving health care outcomes for at-risk communities.

Comorbidity Comorbidity refers to the simultaneous occurrence of two conditions or illnesses, such as one or more diseases that occur in addition to the primary condition which is the first to be diagnosed. Comorbidity also refers to the interactions of two or more conditions that will impact the course or outcome of the primary diagnosis. Comorbidity is usually associated with worse outcomes. For example, the occurrence of obesity with heart disease will impact the course and outcomes of heart disease.

Compassion Compassion is the concern shown for the suffering of patients and includes sensitivity, warmth, tolerance, and empathy.

Competitive or attention-getting disclosures Patients generally want to focus attention on themselves and learn that the way to do this is to disclose important information about themselves. However, during patient–provider encounters, providers can self-disclose, averting the attention away from the patient. Providers may not always realize they may be competing with patients for attention. Some provider self-disclosures are problematic.

Complaining and demanding patient behaviors This is a common negative stance. Patients can frequently exhibit unrealistic expectations, and fear and anxiety are often the inner feelings of complaining and demanding patients.

Comprehensive care Comprehensive care is a critical element of quality patient care. It refers to the extent to which care includes attention to multiple factors that influence quality of life such as psychological, physical, spiritual, and social domains.

Compromise A compromise is a solution that produces relatively the same losses and gains for both parties.

Confidentiality Confidentiality in health care communication implies that the patient may either assume or be explicitly assured that his private communications with the provider will not be transmitted to others except in specific instances. Providers have a moral, ethical, and legal responsibility to protect the confidentiality of these communications.

Confirmation Confirmation is a way of communicating acknowledgment and acceptance of others. Confirming communicative responses acknowledge and validate the other person.

Conflict Conflict or interpersonal conflict exists when two or more interdependent parties have opposing interests or positions on an issue. Conflicts can be latent, emerging, or manifest.

Conflict resolution Conflict resolution is the process taken to reach a mutual acceptable solution. Settlements are agreements that come with conflict resolution and can be either *binding* or *nonbinding* decisions.

Confrontations Confrontations are acts of presenting differing observations of discrepancies. These discrepancies can be differences between (1) what patients say they do and what they actually do, (2) patients' statements or behaviors observed over time, and (3) differences between what patients should do and what they are actually doing. Telling patients that their behaviors are discrepant is an act of confrontation. They are either low, moderate, or high intensity. Unlike high-intensity confrontations, low-level confrontations are less intense and consequently arouse lower intensity of emotional response.

Consensus Consensus refers to reaching an agreement on issues through the process of blending each party's views.

Continuity of care Continuity of care, like coordinated care and comprehensive care, is concerned with the quality of care. It is achieved when patients and providers or provider teams work cooperatively to ensure uninterrupted care over time. Continuity is possible when coordination is also in place. Continuity of care is sometimes referred to as "continuance of care," "continuum of care," or "continuing care."

Coordinated care To achieve coordinated care, all providers must practice as a coherent, harmonizing team with shared responsibility for patient care outcomes. Coordinated care refers to the durability and effective interaction of many, including patient and family.

Corpus callosum The two hemispheres of the brain are connected by a large network of axons called the corpus callosum.

Crisis Crisis occurs when a person is presented with a critical incident or stressful event that is perceived as overwhelming and outside the individual's abilities to cope and function. Crisis can occur for patients and their families at any point in time: at diagnosis but also when illness takes a turn for the worse.

Crisis-prone Crisis prone is a term used to describe individuals who seek out crisis or find themselves in ongoing crisis situations.

Cues to action Cues to action is a concept of the *health belief model (HBM)*. Perceived cues to action are important in eliciting behavior change and maintaining this change as well. Cues to action can include something as simple as posting a note on a refrigerator to remind oneself to eat more vegetables and fruit.

Culture Culture is a term used to describe identifiable integrated patterns of human behavior that include customs, beliefs, values, behaviors, and communications.

Cultural competence Cultural competency defines a developmental sequence detailing levels of novice, intermediate, and advanced cultural competency.

Cultural competence continuum The cultural competence continuum refers specifically to a negative–positive sequence: on the one hand cultural destructiveness and at the other end of the continuum, cultural proficiency.

Cultural identity Cultural identity refers to the extent to which individuals subscribe to a given culture. Everyone is said to have a cultural identity. More often than not, individuals have several cultural identities due, in part, to the fact that one's cultural heritage is rich.

Deadlocks, stalemates, or impasses These terms are used to refer to the state of inertia that is experienced by disputants. They are unable to move forward in resolving their issues and/or disagreements.

Decision aids (DAs) DAs are sometimes used in the process of making screening or treatment decisions and particularly EOL decision-making. They include structured tools (e.g., videotapes and booklets) designed to guide patients and health professionals in discussions about EOL decision-making.

Decisional conflict (DC) Decisions before and at EOL can be stressful and fraught with many emotions including uncertainty, fear, and confusion. When patients have insufficient information, feel forced to make a certain choice, or their values are counter to the decision to be made, decisional conflict is more likely. Health professionals can ease decisional conflict and help patients to reach a renewed sense of certainty about their care decisions.

Decoding The process of deciphering the meaning of a message is known as decoding. The receiver decodes messages.

Defensive silence Defensive silence is silence that occurs when the patient or provider feels threaten by the topic or manner in which they are addressed.

Denial (first, second, and third order) First-order denial refers to denying facts (e.g., lab test results). Second-order denial is denial of the implications of the facts or data (that they must be treated for a serious condition). Third-order denial is denial of the ultimate outcome (e.g., the prognosis of their illness regardless of treatment).

Develop discrepancy In conducting MI, the provider may assist patients in understanding that the current behavior does not reflect the patient's values or goals. Otherwise, there is a difference between how patients are behaving and what they verbalize as their desired state or outcome. When patients are enabled to recognize this discrepant, they are more likely to shift their behaviors to ones that reflect their desired values or goals.

Difficult patient behaviors Patients can display one or more difficult responses which could include: rage and anger, manipulation, demanding, aggression.

Digital communication Humans utilize both digital communication and analogic communication. Digital communication refers to perceiving and expressing oneself in concrete terms (e.g., referring to things by their names).

Directives Directives are absolute statements made to patients about the preferred course of action. Providers expect directives to be followed. Directives are simply statements that tell patients what is expected of them. Directives are different from advice. Advice is offered without explicit expectations while directives describe what providers expect patients to do.

Direct/indirect questions Direct questions leave little doubt about what information the provider is looking for. Indirect questions may not be worded in ways to inform patients what information the provider is seeking.

Disagreements, tensions, and disputes *Disagreements* and *tensions* are different from conflict. Although many conflicts might have started as disagreements, they may not always escalate to the level of a conflict. *Disputes* are conflicts in which the parties have dealt directly with their differences but are unwilling or unable to resolve the issues.

Disclosures in service of aggression or manipulation These types of disclosures are frequently used to communicate negative judgments. In the context of patient–provider discussions, they tend to be confusing to the patient and disruptive to any level of empathy that was previously established.

Disparities in access health care Disparities in access refers to differences across individuals, communities, and countries in the opportunity to access health care resulting in inequities with the understanding that without opportunity and access the health and well-being for the less privileged will suffer.

Disturbed communication Disturbances in patients' communications can occur in any or all sensory functions (i.e., perception, processing, or expression). A disturbance in one sensory modality will affect the functioning of other senses functions by changing sensory strengths and preferences.

Effective health care communications Effective communications between patients and health professionals are the foundation for quality patient care. Effective communications refer not only to the exchange of information but also the process connecting a patient with a provider on a deeper level and include the capacity to listen and understand messages and the metacommunication behind the transmitted message.

Electronic health records (EHRs) EHR systems are centralized databases containing a collective and comprehensive medical history and related information that can be shared across different health care systems as well as with the patient. Because data can be shared and electronically submitted, EHRs have the potential to improve coordination of patient care and therefore, quality care and patient safety.

Electronic medical records (EMRs) EMRs were the precursor to EHRs. They also played a significant role in coordinating patient care. However, EMRs are more limited in that the record typically stores data from one provider or provider group and is collected, monitored, and stored in the provider's office. Unlike EHRs, the data collected, maintained, and stored are specific to what patient care was delivered at the office or clinic in question. Additionally, the details of other conditions including data on prevention and support services are rarely contained in these records unless this data was deliberately provided by the patient or a referring provider.

Emotional knowing Emotional knowing or emotional intelligence is the capability of recognizing one's own and other person's emotions being able to identify and label them appropriately and is often used to describe empathy.

Emotion-focused coping Emotion-focused coping is that which centers on the emotions related to the stressor rather than the stressor itself. While it is expected in initial phases of adaptation to a serious illness if not changing to problem-focused coping, it may result in maladaptive behaviors.

Empathy Empathy is both a cognitive and emotional state of understanding of the experiences of others. Empathic understanding refers to the condition of knowing the other person through insight achieved in the process of empathic listening to identify what it must be like to be that person. To demonstrate empathy, health professionals communicate their interest in understanding and valuing the patient's perspective.

Encoding This is the process of forming a message that transmits a specific meaning. The sender encodes messages.

End-of-life care (EOLC) EOLC refers to health care not only in the final hours of patients' lives, but care to those with terminal illness whose illness has become more advanced, progressive, and incurable. All physicians, nurses, and other allied health professions are assigned to provide this form of care when it is deemed appropriate.

End-of-life care (EOL) decision-making EOL decision-making involves discussions about the type of care desired at the EOL. It includes a range of issues (e.g., choosing or refusing cardiopulmonary resuscitation, do or do not hospitalize, whether to provide nutrition or hydration by intravenous feeding, whether to use future interventions directed towards a cure, and discontinuing potentially life-saving treatments). EOL decision-making includes conversations about ADs.

Evidence-based medical care Evidenced-based medical care refers to professionally approved guidelines for the diagnosis and treatment of conditions that are supported by evidence from clinical research.

Experiential confrontation Confrontations can also be described as either experiential or factual. When providers speak from their first-hand experience of patients' behavior they are using experiential confrontation or data of a factual nature about something the provider has experienced.

Extrospective and introspective tendencies Extrospectively skilled persons can easily recognize stimuli outside oneself. In contrast, introspectively skilled persons may be more aware of their own needs (introspective). However, the result may be dysfunctional perceptivity in either case.

Factual confrontation Providers use factual confrontation when they present data of a factual nature derived from experience- and evidence-based practice.

Families in crisis Families experiencing crisis are those whose lives have been disrupted by a mental health or an acute, or chronic physical illness. They are experiencing a shift in equilibrium that potentially renders them unable to fulfill their roles and make informed decisions, at least temporarily.

Family and kinship Family and kinship ties are defined through genetic lines, adoption, or through marriage and household partnerships. They range in size from a singular family unit to multiple family ties in a community or a single residence.

Family engagement in health care Family engagement in health care refers to the participation of families along with patients and providers in the planning and delivery of health care to the patient. Engaging both patients of all ages and their families in health care has been shown to result in higher quality and safer patient care.

Formal groups and informal groups Formal groups are composed of members working to achieve a known and approved goal. In health care institutions, they are often listed in organizational charts and policy and procedure manuals and are organized around institutional aims. In contrast, informal groups function in more oblique ways and serve to meet members' needs for affiliation. They are also found in institutional settings along with formal task groups.

Fragmentation of health care delivery Fragmented health care refers to the lack of coordination of health care services (largely due to misalignment of incentives) having serious implications for unnecessary and unsafe care emphasizing the needs to improve quality care and reducing health care costs.

Functional and dysfunctional aspects of families Functional families appear "healthy." They communicate effectively, make decisions, and follow-through. In the broadest context, dysfunctional families are those that fail to be effective along various dimensions. Their communication and decision-making capacities within the family structure are limited. Function and dysfunction can occur at different levels and vary over time.

Functional communication or dysfunctional communication Functional communication is characterized by an absence of disturbances in perception, processing, and expression of thoughts and feelings. When communication is functional a basic level of health is presumed. However, when dysfunctional, poor health is suspected.

Functional health literacy Rather than reflecting simply the reading level of the individual, health literacy refers to how one will be able to understand health care communications and will be able to successfully navigate the health care delivery system. When functional health literacy is low, further consideration of how to impart information is needed.

Functional or dysfunctional group communications Group members can display a number of behaviors that promote communication as well as disrupt communication. Sometimes they reach the level of dysfunctional role behavior not just temporary or momentary behaviors. Thus, positive or negative group behaviors can be seen as transitory as in destructive work behaviors or more permanent as consistent role behaviors.

General literacy Literacy generally refers to the ability to read and write. Persons at risk for low literacy come from populations living in poverty, older age groups, non-English speaking, minorities, and those who have not completed high school.

Generalized self-efficacy (GSE) scale Self-efficacy is the confidence in oneself to master a change or new behavior. There are modifications of this scale that are appropriate for different conditions (e.g., alcohol cessation, physical exercise, and condom use).

Genuineness Genuineness in the patient–provider relationship is key in demonstrating providers' capacity to be trustworthy.

Global trust Global trust is the inherent human capacity to trust others. This kind of trust is consistent much like a trait characteristic.

Group conflict Group conflict can arise in either formal or informal groups. If not resolved it can interfere with achieving group agreed-upon goals. Destructive group behaviors or dysfunctional role behavior can result in group conflict.

Group content Group content refers to the explicit goals and tasks of the group and make up the majority of communication exchanges within the group.

Group maintenance Behavior in a group may be directed toward maintaining and encouraging the group. These behaviors include gate-keeping and harmonizing. Both behaviors encourage members to sustain their participation.

Group process Group process refers to the dynamic unfolding of interaction within a group. It is the interpersonal aspect of the group and is frequently observed as group dynamics with stages of development over time.

Health belief model (HBM) The HBM originates from the work of Rosenstock and others and offers an expanded view of the change process by identifying motivations to change and barriers to making changes.

Health care delivery system Health care delivery system is a term which describes the major way health care is provided. Aspects of a delivery system would include inpatient, outpatient, and home care programs. It is the organization of people, institutions, and resources that deliver health care services to meet the health needs of selected populations and communities.

Health care quality The Institute of Medicine defines quality health care as the degree to which health services for individuals and populations increase the desired health outcomes and are consistent with current professional knowledge and research. Quality care is dependent upon effective patient–provider and provider communications.

Health care reform Health care reform in the United States has a long history with many attempts to design a system to support the goal of health care for everyone. While in transition, the evolution to promote access to care by limiting costs is complex. Previous attempts have shown weaknesses in providing access to care without increasing deductibles and copayments for health care.

Health information technology (HIT) Health information technology is a generic term used to describe health information storage and management and the secure exchange of this information between patient and health professional and across health care systems. An example is electronic health records (EHRs) which are believed to improve care quality, patient safety, and effectiveness.

Health Insurance Portability and Accountability Act (HIPAA) The Health Insurance Portability and Accountability Act of 1996 is legislation that provides for privacy and security of patients' medical information.

Health literacy Health literacy is the degree to which an individual has the capacity to obtain, communicate, process, and understand basic health information and services to make appropriate health decisions.

Health maintenance organizations (HMOs) HMOs are comprehensively designed structures for financing and delivering health care. These services are provided to enrollees within a specific geographical area.

Health promotion Health promotion is a term used frequently in the context of disease prevention. It is generally agreed that the U.S. health care system should be reflected in the number of years people can remain healthy. This goal includes an investment in community based health promotion programs to serve at-risk communities and populations.

Health promotion programs Health promotion programs are those strategies which enable people to increase control over their health and level of wellness. Such programs are frequently found in small- or large-scale public health initiatives and involve public health policy as it applies to issues of income, housing, and nutrition. Many programs provide education and support aimed at empowering patients and improving health literacy.

Home visitation (HV) programs HV can be a promising approach to removing disparities in health care access. The emphasis however is on education, support, and when appropriate, linking individuals to either traditional public community services or traditional health care facilities.

Hospice care Hospice care is provided when the patient's doctor makes the judgment that the patient is likely to die within 6 months. Hospice care provides comfort care to the patient as well as support to the family. This includes direct care delivery and help with daily living activities and often respite care to family members caring for the patient. Respite care provides a short-term, temporary break for family caregivers and has been shown to help sustain the family member's ongoing involvement and well-being. Unlike palliative care, during hospice care, attempts to cure the patient are stopped. Hospice care can be delivered at the patient's home or a nursing home, hospital, or separate hospice facility.

Identification Identification is the first condition or step in establishing empathy and is stated as the need for the provider to first comprehend the situation and feelings of the other.

Implementation phase The implementation phase is the second phase of a therapeutic relationship and follows from the first phase, initiation. Implementation activities include beginning a course of action (e.g., assessing health, treating disease, or referral). Ideally it is grounded in a relationship of mutual trust. During this phase, assuming that trust is in place, the provider and patient are mutually engaged in confronting and working on health problems.

Incorporation The second step in establishing empathy is incorporation. The process of incorporation means that the experience of the patient that is now known to the provider is taken into the self of the provider.

Increasing connectedness The impact of empathy is achieved through the patients' feelings of connectedness with the provider. Feelings of connectedness are reinforced by confirmation.

Infectious disease Infectious diseases or communicable diseases, compared to chronic health conditions, are of shorter duration and can be prevented by vaccines or cured by medication. They include such diseases as tuberculosis, pneumonia, meningitis, Ebola virus, hepatitis, and sexually transmitted diseases and are particularly prevalent in underdeveloped countries where access to vaccines, medication, clean water, and vector control is very limited.

Informational continuity Informational continuity refers to the use of information about a patient on past events and personal circumstances to make the current patient care appropriate.

Informed choice It is generally understood that patients who have the capacity to make decisions about their care must be permitted to do so. Patient choice is not absolute.

Informed consent Informed consent is the permission from the patient to conduct a test, treatment, or procedure after the provider has fully informed the patient, in ways that the patient can understand, about the actions that will be taken. Informed consent can be obtained in writing or orally. Some situations require written consent (e.g., in the case of research studies).

Inherent suffering Inherent suffering is the consequences of patients' diagnosis (e.g., pain and treatment [e.g., painful and frightening surgery]). While it can be modified, it cannot be eliminated altogether.

Initiation phase The initiation phase is the first phase in developing a therapeutic relationship with patients. Trust in the relationship is key to successful care management in the implementation phase to follow.

Integrated delivery system (IDS) The aim of an IDS is to address aspects of fragmented health care. An IDS is a network of health care organizations within a larger service system. Managed care was an early example of integrated care but drew disapproval. Integrated care seeks to improve continuity, coordination, and comprehensive care. IDSs are seen to result in high-quality care.

Intensity of advisement Advisement can be characterized by level of intensity. Low-intensity advisement is the process of giving information, opinions, and recommendations but the patient has maximum control over the ultimate course of action. This form of advisement is usually very nondirective. Providers get more directive in their advice-giving with patients who have already developed a health problem and they want their professional advice to be followed.

Interpersonal continuity Interpersonal continuity of care, sometimes referred to as relational continuity of care, refers to an ongoing therapeutic relationship between patient and one or more providers. It provides the patient with a sense of predictability and coherence.

Interpersonal space Silence can provide interpersonal space. This refers to a hypothetical, changing degree of psychosocial distance that occurs whenever individuals communicating turn to silence or remain silent.

Interpretations Interpretations convey an understanding of the individual that is not within his or her immediate awareness. In therapeutic encounters, interpretations are offered less frequently than reflections and when substantial data has been gathered.

Interprofessional collaboration Interprofessional collaboration refers to the collaboration and cooperation of a wide range of health professionals to plan, deliver, and evaluate health outcomes and health care delivery.

Interresponse time Interresponse time is the period of time that elapses after a speaker makes a statement and before another speaker replies or the same speaker talks again. Interresponse times can vary. They include pauses as short as 1–2 seconds or therapeutic silences lasting up to 10 seconds.

Interruptive response Interruptive responses are disruptions of another individual's speech that generally have the impact of cutting short the expression of the senders' thoughts and feelings.

Irresponsible or accidental disclosures Irresponsible disclosures on the part of providers are made without real regard for the patient receiver. They are sometimes accidental. In the patient–provider relationship, they can be considered boundary transgressions because too much personal information is shared by the provider when there is no therapeutic intention.

Leadership styles (transformational and inter-actional) Transformational leadership is a style of leadership recognizing members' perceptions of the need for change and the ways to go about it. It inspires rather than prescribes goals and goal behavior. Transactional leaders micromanage a team to ensure the fulfillment of preset goals.

Leading or loaded questions Leading or loaded questions restrict or influence patient responses. The wording of these questions suggests what answers are sought or desired.

Life-sustaining/life-prolonging treatment Life-sustaining care refers to that care or treatment given to patients to sustain their life and bodily functions. When people are experiencing treatable or curable illness, any life-sustaining treatment is only temporary. Life-sustaining treatment for those whose illness is terminal and untreatable is prolonged until it is withheld. Withholding or forgoing life-sustaining treatment occurs when death is unavoidable and predicted. Advanced directives and living wills document those treatments the patient prefers not be rendered. They may include cardiopulmonary resuscitation, mechanical ventilation, surgery, dialysis, and even antibiotics. Decisions to forego life-sustaining treatment are frequently very challenging for all involved: patients, providers, and family members.

Limbic system The limbic system is responsible for emotional experience and expression. It consists of a set of subcortical structures in the forebrain that includes the hypothalamus, hippocampus, amygdala, olfactory bulb, septum, part of the thalamus, and the cerebral cortex.

Maladaptive coping Maladaptive coping strategies tend to create further problems without addressing the problems causing the stressful life event. For example, illicit drug use or binge eating in order to dull the emotions associated with the stressor can worsen the illness and inhibits effective coping.

Maladaptive coping responses Patients and families coping with serious illness or injury may cope in ways that increase stress and/or even deter their use of appropriate health care services. One such response is prolonged denial which can interfere with patients' accessing needed health care services.

Managed care Managed care is a term describing a health care delivery system aimed at reducing costs of providing health care benefits while providing quality care. Over the last two decades, managed care has been the predominate form of health care delivery in the United States.

Management continuity There are three types of continuity: interpersonal, informational, and management continuity. Management continuity refers to a consistent and coherent approach to the management of care that is responsive to the patient's changing needs and that can transcend health care settings.

Manipulative-dependent patient behaviors Manipulative patients generally have self-centered attitudes. They frequently attempt to control providers' actions, sometimes in passive-aggressive ways. They may anticipate loss of control and are usually fearful. Their concerns of losing control may cause or escalate their manipulative-dependent behaviors.

Mathematical literacy Health numeracy is the degree to which individuals have the capacity to access, process, interpret, communicate, and act on numerical, quantitative, graphical, biostatistical, and probabilistic health information needed to make effective health care decisions. Health numeracy is sometimes referred to as mathematical literacy.

Meditation Mediation refers to the process by which an impartial third person with authority assists disputants to reach mutually acceptable solutions.

Meta-disclosures Metadisclosures are disclosures about a disclosure. For example, "I lied to you because I wanted you to think I was better than I am" is a metadisclosure. It reveals something about a previous self-disclosing statement.

m-Health m-Health or mobile health is a generic term that applies to the use of devices to collect and transmit health information, frequently with the use of health-related apps. m-Health is supported by mobile communication devices including mobile phones, tablet computers, and wearable devices. It is characteristically a different way in which patients and providers communicate. One usually thinks about patients and providers communicating face-to-face (in person) where the collection of health information occurs in the context of health care visits.

Mistrust Mistrust in the patient–provider relationship occurs when trust in providers' clinical competence or providers' commitment to the best interests of patients, or both, is lacking.

Motivational interviewing MI is an intervention to elicit behavior change in clients or patients. It is typically patient-centered and aims to guide patients to approach and undertake behavior change through the use of several communication strategies.

Multicultural environment Multicultural environments refer to the multiple cultural orientations in a single group, community, or population. The United States is currently referred to as a *salad bowl*. This term describes the multicultural environment in the United States.

Multidimensional communication The assumption that communication occurs on multiple levels (e.g., the verbal and nonverbal levels) exemplify that interpersonal communication is indeed complex.

Multiple-choice questions These questions are phrased in ways to require patients to consider several possibilities, usually between two or more options, simultaneously. For example, "Are you feeling better, the same as yesterday, or the worse you have felt since your surgery?"

Natural clusters of chronic illness Chronic diseases often co-occur; otherwise they can appear in groups. When they do, they can make treatment more complex, as well as costly. People seeking care at primary care settings may be treated for diabetes or cardiovascular disease but must also be assessed for clinical depression because both diabetes and cardiovascular disease can cluster with each other and with depression. This cluster can result in worse diabetic care outcomes because untreated depression can lead to poor adherence to diabetes treatment.

Navigating the health care system Getting the best health care possible requires patients and families to effectively navigate the health care system. Finding one's way through the system is essential and difficult in the current complex and often-fragmented system of care. This includes knowing how the system works, what you will be asked and why, and who is available to assist the patient at each juncture of the care-giving process.

Nonadherent patient behaviors Adherence to treatment refers to the degree to which the patient follows the treatment as prescribed. Nonadherence is the action of not following treatment or medication regimens as prescribed. Nonadherent patient behaviors are difficult because they

sabotage any chance of treatment working the way it is intended to.

Open-ended questions Open-ended questions are phrased to evoke a wide range of possible responses, and encourage patients to elaborate upon their concerns or needs. An example is, "What can I do for you?" Patients are encouraged with this free-form question to describe their experiences and needs in depth.

Optical Illusions An optical illusion is a visual account of something seen but what is visually perceived is different from the object observed.

Orders Orders are directives that the patient must follow. Giving orders is a critical aspect of providers' roles.

Overtalk Overtalk is one person's conversation competing with that of another. It is intended to overrule or cut short the sender in order to provide time for the next person to speak either on the same topic (an aspect of the topic) or on an entirely different topic. While overtalk occurs in social exchanges it is counter-productive in therapeutic encounters.

Palliative care The intent of palliative care is to maintain or improve the quality of life of both patients and their families facing a serious illness. It includes relief from the symptoms, pain, and stress of a serious illness. It may include offering psychological and spiritual aspects of patient care, a support system to help the family cope with the impending loss of the patient, and bereavement support through counseling. Palliative care can be administered even when the patient is still receiving curative treatment.

Paraphrasing Paraphrasing consists of selecting among several statements that the patient has made, summarizing these statements, and giving them meaning in another form.

Paraprofessional health care providers Paraprofessionals are unlicensed members of a health care team. An aspect of health care may be delegated to a paraprofessional. They are not fully qualified to practice without supervision. Health promotion programs in community or school settings frequently hire or enlist volunteer paraprofessionals to support their goals.

Parasympathetic nervous system This neuro-network to the internal organs tends to work to conserve energy and produce relaxation.

Patient's Bill of Rights There are several conceptual models of patients' rights that depict ethical and legal parameters for health care providers. Among the most well known is the American Hospital Association's "Patient's Bill of Rights," later renamed The Patient Care Partnership: Understanding Expectations, Rights and Responsibilities.

Patient-centered and family-centered care (PCFCC) PCFCC is a concept and approach to patient care that requires planning, delivery, and evaluation of health care to be grounded in mutually beneficial partnerships between patients, families, and health care providers.

Patient portals Patient portals are systems of electronically entering and storing medical and health-related information. Through these portals, providers are able to communicate to patients the results of lab test results, an outline of identified patient health conditions, and the treatment that is planned. Patients can introduce their own entries. These systems also provide patients the opportunity to message their provider, refill a current medication, request an appointment or referral, and find information about a previous visit and upcoming appointments.

Patient Self-Determination Act (PSDA) The PSDA was legislated in 1991 to require patients be informed of their rights regarding decisions about their own medical care, and ensure that these rights are communicated by the health care provider.

Pauses Pauses are temporary disruptions in the flow of communication that are short-lived. They frequently allow for gathering thoughts and reflection.

Perinatal health care outcomes This concept refers to health care outcomes associated with care of relating to being the period around childbirth, especially the 5 months prior to delivery and 1 month following a live birth. Prenatal care refers to the care prior to birth. Postnatal or postpartum care refers to the care given immediately after birth.

Personal health records (PHRs) Unlike either EMRs or EHRs, PHRs are created by the patient using either their own format or one that is available through an official organization (e.g., Medicare).

Generally, a PHR is a record with information about the patient's health that is entered by the patient or someone helping the patient (e.g., a close friend or family member). This health record format is described in detail on the website Medicare.gov.

Person-centered approach Rogers's person-centered approach establishes the concept that individual change comes from individuals' overriding belief that humans have an underlying *actualizing tendency* and will approach change as a natural result of this tendency.

Physician orders for life-sustaining treatment (POLST) or Medical orders for life-sustaining treatment (MOLST) In attempts to improve care reflecting patients' preferred EOLC options, physicians are encouraged to speak with patients and create specific medical orders to be honored by health care workers should a medical crisis arise. The POLST or MOLST are medical orders, not legal documents as is the AD.

Plain language Providers may use very complicated sentences to explain disease and treatment. Using plain language increases the likelihood that the information will be understood by both patients and their families. Plain language expresses ideas simply and avoids jargon.

Preferred provider organizations (PPOs) PPOs are managed care approaches that contract with independent providers (health professionals and ancillary services) for negotiated fees for services.

Primary and secondary outcomes Primary outcomes are the first and usually the most important set of outcomes. They are generally the most important targets in clinical trials. Secondary outcomes are those that are related to primary outcomes or are a result of primary outcomes. For example, primary outcomes associated with adherence to a weight reduction program would be weight lost, but subsequent to weight reduction, secondary outcomes may include improvements in mobility and quality of life. Additionally, biomarkers may reveal alterations in BMI levels. In programs for patients with alcohol and drug abuse, primary outcomes include alterations in drinking and drug use (e.g., quantity and frequency of alcohol and drugs consumed). Secondary outcomes would be the result of either short-term or long-term goal achievement. In this case they may include improved social and occupational functioning and positive changes in medical biomarkers for liver functioning. Primary and secondary health outcomes should not be confused with primary and secondary health care.

Primary care settings Primary care settings refer to the patient's first point of contact when seeking medical care and also their principal point of continuing care. Health screening, health promotion, disease prevention, health maintenance, counseling, patient education, initial diagnosis, and referral to specialty care is provided at primary care settings. Primary care providers (primary care physicians and nurse practitioners) often coordinate care with any specialty care the patient is receiving.

Principle of multidimensionality Multidimensionality in communication refers to three levels for each message: (1) the content level, (2) the feeling or emotional level, and (3) a level that describes the perceived relationship of one communicant to another.

Privileged communication in health care The doctrine of privileged communication refers to the legal right by statute that is provided to patients from having confidences revealed publicly (e.g., from the witness stand without their expressed permission).

Problem-focused coping Problem-focused coping strategies target the causes of the stress and solve the problem creating the stress. It aims to remove the stressor or problem by effective problem-solving solutions.

Protection of patient privacy The concept of privacy refers to the right of the patients to limit others having access to their personal and medical knowledge.

Question response burden Question response burden is the level of demand placed on the patient to answer the provider's question. For example, the question, "How are you?" may be more demanding for a patient in severe pain than the question, "Are you feeling relief from the pain medication I gave you?" The reason is the first question requires the patient to sort through and label feelings and experiences while the second question might be easier to answer because it is focused and requires a "yes" or "no" reply.

Questions used as self-disclosure statements Self-disclosure questions are telling questions. They disclose something personal about the provider while asking the patient to respond to a question. "Did you know that when you change your position in bed that makes it harder on me?" is an example of a question that appears to ask for information but also tells the patient something about the provider.

Reception Reception refers to the absorption of physical energy (e.g., light and sound). Receptor cells receive sensory information from stimuli. Coding occurs to get messages from receptors to the brain.

Reducing alienation Empathic responses reduce patients' feelings of alienation. Feelings of alienation can arise in patients for many reasons including isolation from others due to illness.

Reflections Reflections are responses that direct back to the patient the patient's ideas and feelings about the verbal content (as well as the verbal content itself).

Reflective listening Reflective listening is a communication strategy consisting of seeking the patient's perspective and then offering the idea or what the provider thinks is the perspective back to the patient so the patient can confirm or alter what was said. The purpose is to ensure that the provider actually understands the patient's perspective. It can also serve the function of reassuring the patient that the provider is interested and fully committed to the therapeutic relationship.

Reframing The strategy of reframing is used to alter disputants' views on an issue. It is used to move parties out of a stalemate and toward new solutions.

Respect Respect is the positive regard of another. In the patient–provider relationship, respect of patients is critical to trust building.

Response matching Response matching refers to the tendency of the receiver to imitate the sender's level of disclosure.

Restatement Restating or stating again what the patient has said or using a slightly different wording to reiterate what the patient has said, is making restatements. Restatements are limited to the expressed content. They do not require reference to the feelings that the patient is either expressing or may have expressed.

Reverberation Reverberation is the third step in showing empathy. The provider's past experience interacts with that which is known to the provider from the patient. The provider's history with similar patient situations contributes further insight to understanding the patient's experience.

Role reversal Role reversal is the reversal of the helper–helpee relationship where the provider is seeking assistance from the patient by disclosing some personal issue or problem. It is nontherapeutic and can lead to the patient's mistrust of the provider.

Roll with resistance Roll with resistance is a key principle of MI. Rather than confront the patient with the undesired behavior, the provider addresses it with reflection. When a patient admits to avoiding exercise rather than confront the patient with the resistance, the provider might reflect what the patient is saying. For example, if the patient said, "I haven't been exercising," the provider would not ask why or present the consequences of not exercising. An alternative response might be, "You say you haven't been exercising?"

Ruling out/ruling in questions Ruling out or ruling in questions are used to clarify and specify patients' needs and concerns. The question beginning with, "Is it this…or is it that?" enables providers to better understand patients' experiences by ruling out irrelevant data.

Sacrosanctity of provider–patient communications This term refers to the sacred nature given patient and provider communications emphasizing that it should not be infringed upon.

Selective attention/selective inattention Selective attention refers to the idea that persons have a capacity to focus on parts of an experience or only some stimuli. When this occurs as a result of reaction to stimuli, it is referred to as selective inattention. It means that certain stimuli are ignored or not registered in order to avoid any mental distress associated with the stimuli.

Self-care Self-care refers to the actions performed by patients themselves (or their significant others) directed at alleviating the effects of illness and its treatment.

Self-disclosure Provider self-disclosures refer to instances of openly sharing personal information including personal preferences, experiences, attitudes, and feelings. They can have therapeutic

or problematic outcomes and should be used judiciously by the provider and be purposeful.

Self-efficacy Self-efficacy refers to patients' beliefs that they have the ability to make the desired change(s). If one believes they are capable of change, they are more likely to accomplish what it takes to make the change.

Self-reflection Self-reflection is the process of pausing to carefully consider what you are feeling or thinking or about what the patient is experiencing. Silence can provide time for self-reflection. Formal approaches believed to promote self-reflection are meditation, yoga, hypnosis, and mindfulness awareness.

Self-service kiosks Patient-managed self-monitoring tools are accessible in kiosks which offer up information which may or may not be previously known by the patient. A classic example of a simple kiosk is the public's access and use of monitors found in drugstores to measure weight, blood pressure, heart rate, and body mass index (BMI). The options and features available with kiosks can be extensive and are tailored to the needs of the average person frequenting these sites. Information is provided on multimedia touch screens that can be saved and transported on a USB port.

Sensor technology Sensory technology devices, sometimes accompanied with an app for recording and tracking changes, allow patients to view health data on the spot. This advantage is particularly important when it comes to managing certain chronic conditions (e.g., asthma, high blood pressure, and diabetes). They may come in the form of wearable watches or a more formal assessment apparatus. Sensory devices can monitor homebound patient falls or problems in a diabetic's blood sugar levels which could activate a call to the provider for further assessment.

Sensory modalities There are five sensory modalities that transmit information for data processing in the brain. They include sight, smell, taste, touch, and hearing.

Sensory modality strength Among all senses there are some modalities stronger than others and this may be different across individuals and over time. For example, hearing is a preferred sensory modality in young children. Adults are more likely to use multiple modalities simultaneously such as vision and hearing. Multimodal strength refers to exhibiting strength in more than one modality at a time (e.g., having strength in visual and auditory channels simultaneously).

Sensory transduction Sensory transduction refers to the conversion of a sensory stimulus from one form to another. For example, our capacities to change the energy from a physical stimulus to an electrochemical pattern in the brain's neurons is the process of transduction. Transduction in the next process after reception. Messages must be translated during transduction through the process of coding.

Shared decision-making (SDM) SDM refers to the process of engaging the patient in decisions about their care. It is encouraged in every situation where decisions about care are to be made. When SDM is absent, patients can experience low treatment satisfaction and perceive that their treatment decisions belong only to their physicians.

Significant others (SOs) Significant other refers to individuals who may or may not be related by blood or marriage but who act as family members.

Silence Silence is the absence of audible speech experienced as quiet, stillness, and sometimes peacefulness and tranquility.

Social cognitive theory The *social learning* and *social cognitive* theory maintains that change occurs in the context of a cost–benefit analysis where perceived positive consequences of changing offset any negative consequences that the change may produce. Environmental factors, personal factors, and attributes of the behavior itself all affect the process of behavior change. Concepts relevant to this theory are social support, self-efficacy, outcome expectancies, and perceived self-regulation.

Social ecological model (SEM) The *SEM* is a theoretical model that considers multiple and interactive effects of the many personal and environmental factors that influence health behaviors at several levels such as individual, family, and population.

Specific trust Specific trust is trust an individual has of another person in a specific relationship. People who mistrust a provider would be categorized as possessing low specific trust. Trust of this kind depends on the state of current affairs and the specific interaction in the here-and-now.

Split-brain This term is used to refer to conditions where a portion of the corpus callosum has been damaged or destroyed.

Stages of group development Groups develop in stages. These stages depict the maturity of the group's development and reflect a group at any one point in its history.

Subjective norm A subjective norm is a concept from the theory of reasoned action (TRA) model. Attitudes, intentions, and subjective norms influence behavior. Salient attitudes are those relevant to the change target. *Attitudes* are influenced by the opinions of others and *intentions* shape behavior. *Intention* is the probability that the individual will perform a behavior which is influenced by both *attitudes* and *subjective norms*. Subjective norms are what individuals perceive others will think of previous behaviors or new behavioral change.

Subjective reflections Subjective norm refers to the perceived social pressure to behave or not behave in a certain way. It may not be the social norm which is the widely held belief.

Symmetrical or complementary communications People take either symmetrical or complementary roles in relationships and communicate accordingly. When people mirror each other's communication or behavior they are displaying symmetry. When they are behaving in a complementary manner, one person's behavior complements the other.

Sympathetic nervous system The sympathetic nervous system includes the neuronetwork to the internal organs. This system prepares the body for vigorous activity (e.g., running, lifting, or exercising).

Sympathy This is a term used to refer to the act of feeling the feelings or needs of another. It is usually accompanied by responses of sadness or pity.

Telemedicine and telehealth Telemedicine or telehealth generally refers to health care that is given remotely. It is delivered by means of telecommunication technology and can include a clinical diagnosis and/or treatment. Telemedicine or telehealth is associated with improving access to medical services particularly when access is limited due to distance, such as for persons living in rural communities. In some cases, patient data derived through telehealth technology is regarded sufficient to assess the patient. However, health data derived from m-Health devices alone is not considered accurate enough to be used in making a medical diagnosis or to monitor patients' health.

Termination phase The termination phase is the last phase in the patient–provider relationship when providers are referring a patient to another provider and discharging them from treatment. It is important that providers clearly explain the process of discharge, and patients understand that they are no longer under the care of the provider.

Theory of reasoned action (TRA) The basic tenet underlying TRA is that individuals' beliefs that a behavior leads to certain outcomes and positive attitudes about these outcomes influence attitudes toward the behavior which in turn influences their behavior.

Therapeutic communication Therapeutic communication in the patient–provider relationship is interpersonal exchange, using verbal and nonverbal messages, that culminates in the patient being helped.

Therapeutic interviewing skills Therapeutic interviewing differs from therapeutic communication. Therapeutic communication refers to an extensive and foundational set of skills used in therapeutic relationships. Therapeutic interviewing skills refer more specifically to strategies in conducting clinical interviews for the purpose of patient assessment.

Transitional care Transitional care refers to the coordination and continuity of medical and health care when the patient leaves one care setting and moves to another. For example, patients may be transferred from the hospital to home or hospital to nursing home or assisted living facility, home to assisted living, or hospital to rehabilitation center. Patients may, in fact, move frequently from one care setting to another and receive care from multiple health professionals. Because of this, high levels of continuity of care and coordination of care are needed to provide or sustain care quality and patient safety.

Transtheoretical model (TTM) of change TTM establishes a temporal dimension for behavioral change. Otherwise, individuals progress through a series of stages to arrive at change. These stages include precontemplation, contemplation, preparation, action, maintenance, and termination.

Trust Trust is the reliance on the veracity and integrity of another individual. In patient–provider relationships, it includes both confidence in providers' competence and perceptions that providers have the patients' best interests in mind.

Trust in patient scale The trust in patient scale is a measure of the level of trust providers have of patients. It includes providers' judgments that patients will or will not fully inform them about changes in their condition, will follow the treatment plan as directed, and will be honest about the information they give providers.

Trust–mistrust continuum Trust and mistrust can be viewed on a continuum. Otherwise, levels of trust can be measured as very high (complete trust) to very low (mistrust).

Types of groups Groups are commonly categorized as either reference groups or work/task groups. Reference groups are those that typically represent an aspect of one's personal life and include religious, ethnic, gender, and age groups. Work/task groups provide identity through their unique purpose and role in an organization.

Usability (utilization) of health care While related to the concept of access to care, utilization is not the question of whether health care services are physically accessible but rather whether these accessible services are actually used. There are numerous reasons why health care which is accessible, within reach, is not used. They include characteristics of the consumer and health care system that either facilitate or deter service utilization.

Index